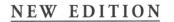

NEW EDITION

COMPLETELY REVISED AND EXPANDED

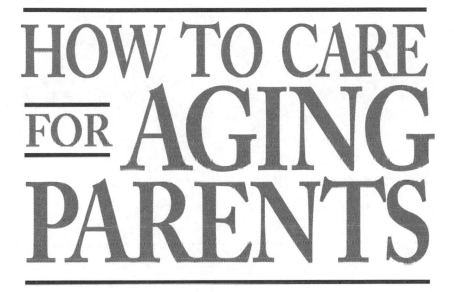

HOW TO CARE
FOR AGING
PARENTS

Praise for HOW TO CARE FOR AGING PARENTS

"A health-care journalist who cared for her own father through a terminal illness offers this smart, compassionate, and timely book for every child who must care for an aging parent."

—THE SEATTLE TIMES

"An excellent resource . . ." —THE FAMILY CAREGIVER ALLIANCE

"Morris' book, How to Care for Aging Parents, *may contain the most valuable advice anyone in that situation can get."*

—HARRY ROSENTHAL, ASSOCIATED PRESS

"How to Care for Aging Parents *is well-researched and comprehensive. . . . an excellent guide that will continue to be of enormous assistance to contemporary older persons as well as their adult children and the generations that follow."*

—ROBERT N. BUTLER, M.D., FOUNDER,
NATIONAL INSTITUTE ON AGING

". . . the most complete, yet easy-to-read, publication on the subject that I have yet to see." —BUSINESS FIRST

"Combining personal experience with expertise in healthcare and social and political issues, Morris has produced a thoroughly researched, well-organized, and comprehensive manual."

—LIBRARY JOURNAL

"Thoroughly researched and packed with practical and from-the-heart ideas and information, How to Care for Aging Parents *helps pave a difficult road by forthright discussion of issues such as death, new roles, emotional minefields, doctors, hospitals, social services, etc."* —GOOD TIMES

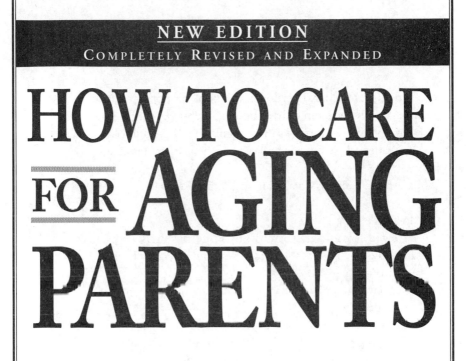

NEW EDITION
COMPLETELY REVISED AND EXPANDED

HOW TO CARE FOR AGING PARENTS

VIRGINIA MORRIS

FOREWORD BY
ROBERT N. BUTLER, M.D.

Workman Publishing • New York

Library of Congress Cataloging-in-Publication Data

Morris, Virginia.
   How to care for aging parents / by Virginia Morris; with a new
introduction by Robert Butler.—New 2nd ed., completely rev. and
updated.
      p. cm.
   Includes index.
   ISBN 0-7611-3426-3 (alk. paper)
      1. Aging parents—Family relationships—Handbooks, manuals, etc.
   2. Aging parents—Care—Handbooks, manuals, etc. I. Title.

HQ1063.6.M66 2004
362.6—dc22   2004049653

Workman books are available at special discounts when purchased in
bulk for premiums and sales promotions as well as for fundraising or
educational use. Special editions or book excerpts can also be created to
specification. For details, contact the Special Sales Director at the address
below.

Cover photograph © Mara Lavitt.

Workman Publishing Company, Inc.
708 Broadway
New York, NY 10003-9555
www.workman.com

Printed in the United States
First printing October 2004
10 9 8 7 6 5 4 3 2 1

To Dr. John McLean Morris (1914–1993)

In your living, you taught me about courage,
determination, philanthropy, and truth. In your dying,
you taught me about love. I will miss you, always

Many Thanks

At the end of one of his comedy shows, Steve Martin faced his audience to say good-bye. "You've been a wonderful audience and I'd like to thank each and every one of you," he said. He then proceeded to point at each individual in the audience saying, "Thank you. Thank you. Thank you. Thank you. Thank you. Thank you. Thank you. . . ."

I, too, would like to thank each and every person who helped create this book—the dozens of doctors, lawyers, researchers, advocates, and social workers who shared their wisdom and time; the public relations people at groups like the Alzheimer's Association, the National Institute on Aging, and AARP, who fielded my endless stream of questions with patience and thoroughness; and, in particular, the dozens of caregivers who opened their hearts and homes and shared their pain, joy, and sorrow with me. These people have all created this book. To each and every one of them, I am grateful. But because it is impossible to offer so many individual thank-you's here, I have limited my acknowledgments to a few essential players.

In getting out this new edition, I am enormously grateful to Dr. Leo M. Cooney Jr., Humana Foundation Professor of Geriatric Medicine and Chief of Geriatrics at Yale University School of Medicine; Daniel Fish, past president of the National Academy of Elder Law Attorneys and partner in Freedman and Fish, in New York; and Elinor Ginzler, manager of AARP's independent living and long-term care program.

I also want to thank those who not only provided insight, but also pored over chapters of my manuscript, checking the facts and adding new ideas: Dr. Margaret Drickamer, a remarkable geriatrician who spent so much time answering my questions that she should be listed as a coauthor; Dr. Ronald Miller, who generously opened the doors of his geriatric assessment center and library at Yale to me; Dr. Sherwin B. Nuland, surgeon, friend, and author of several outstanding books, including *How We Die*, who provided not only information, but also enormous moral support; Lea Nordlicht Shedd, an elder law attorney whose thoroughness and patience with this project reflects her dedication to her work; Tim Casserly, elder law attorney and financial planner, who tirelessly guided me through the complexities of finance and law; Sara Stadler, estate planner, who selflessly helped with this project even when she was behind in her own work; Mary Pat Tracy, a social worker who provided tremendous insight into the needs and dilemmas of caregivers; and Sarah Berger of the National Citizens' Coalition for Nursing Home Reform, whose entire organization helped me to understand the ins and outs of how nursing homes operate.

I am also indebted to Calvin Cobb, partner in Craighill, Mayfield, Fenwick, Cromelin & Cobb, in Washington, D.C.; and Lenise Dolen, president of the National Association of Professional Geriatric Care Managers and director of Dolen Consulting Systems in Tarrytown, New York.

I am grateful to all sorts of people at Workman Publishing. Robbin Reynolds came up with the idea for this book; Peter Workman not only trusted me to write it, but wanted me to write it a second time for this new edition; and Ruth Sullivan, my editor, pored meticulously through untold pages of manuscript and truly helped make this book what it is. Sara Blackburn added her own professional and personal touches to the editing process. Diane Botnick provided much-needed laughter and coolly handled my steady stream of phone calls. Micah Hales has been at my side, electronically, throughout this second writing, looking up information and patiently handling my fits of neurosis and anxiety. Publicists Kim Hicks and Sarah O'Leary somehow remain calm and enthusiastic despite all the demands on their time. And Jenny Mandel, both Special Markets Director and dear friend, is an endless source of optimism, energy, and insight. Many thanks also to the art designer of the second edition, Janet Parker, for her keen eye and patience, and to all the Workman typesetters who have devoted tremendous hours and skill to this book.

Other readers who deserve great thanks are Mary Miner, a geriatric social worker; Anna Kavolius, nurse and attorney with Choice in Dying (now Last Acts Partnership); Colleen Pierre, dietitian; and Beth Burrell, my friend and colleague.

Finally, I want to thank my wonderful husband, Bob Plumb, who saw me through—and put up with me through—every step of this project. Enormous, suffocating hugs to Jack and Emma, who are absolutely the best children in the world and heroically handle a mom on a deadline (which is a pretty scary thing). And I am always grateful for my dear, wonderful mother and my siblings, who are not only my family, but better yet, my friends. They have advised me, encouraged me, and believed in me, even when I didn't believe in myself.

To each and every one of you, thank you.

Contents

Foreword

Whon the clock strikes midnight on January 1, 2011, the oldest of the baby boomers will turn sixty-five. This remarkable generation, the largest in American history, will continue to have an enormous impact on the nation socially, economically, and politically as it ages, transforming old age as no other generation has before in history.

At the same time, as these men and women born between 1946 and 1964 grow older, their parents are also aging, and those who have not already experienced the impact of aging on their parents will do so in the next decade. Some of their experiences will be positive, as more people remain active and productively involved in their later years. In a recent study, nearly half of Americans age sixty-five and older described their lives as "the best years of my life," and 84 percent said they would be happy if they lived to be ninety. Statistics show that disability rates are decreasing, and, for the first time in history, four-generation families are becoming common.

Still, as their parents grow very old and become vulnerable to disease and frailty, the caregiver burden on the baby boom generation will rise rapidly. There are few role models to follow, since aging itself is a relatively new development. It is only very recently that people could be assured of reaching their mid-seventies, due to advances in health care and technology. Being among the first to deal with this phenomenon, the baby boomers will confront issues for which they are poorly prepared. Yet, all along, the baby boom generation has altered or redefined social issues, and, in the new task of parentcare, they are likely to continue their role as a transformative generation and alter the very face of old age.

When it was first published in 1996, *How to Care for Aging Parents* offered practical advice and wisdom to adult children who were turning fifty and just beginning to come up against issues with which they had little experience. Now, totally revised, updated, and expanded, this book continues to be an excellent guide for dealing with the financial, legal, medical, and psychological issues facing women and men as they care for their aging parents.

Well-researched and comprehensive, this invaluable resource also offers an up-to-date guide to hard-to-find services and subsidies.

As the baby boom generation grows older, Virginia Morris's book will undoubtedly continue to be of enormous assistance to contemporary older persons as well as to their adult children and the generations that follow.

—Robert N. Butler

Robert N. Butler, M.D. is the founder of the National Institute on Aging and is President and CEO of the International Longevity Center and Co-Chair of the Alliance for Health & the Future.

Introduction

While I was writing the first edition of this book, my father died at the age of seventy-eight. It was strange writing those last chapters on death and grief when my own loss was so consuming. Nearly ten years later, as I wrap up this revised edition, I am haunted once again by my personal life.

As I pore over the new information about osteoporosis, Medicare, and memory loss, my own mother is seventy-eight and has acute lung disease. Her doctor says that at some point soon she will need an oxygen tank and help with all the tasks of daily life. She is looking at apartments in a full-spectrum "retirement community." I am looking for a larger house so that she can move in with me. I keep telling myself she shouldn't be in an institution. I can take care of her. It is time for her to sit back and let her children do this for her.

Well, all I can say is, woe to the author who doesn't take her own advice, who doesn't dodge the very pitfalls that she describes. For as I step back from my immersion in each page and paragraph of this book, I see that we, as individual caregivers and as a society, make two mistakes. We make them because we are caught between old, firmly held beliefs and a new and rapidly changing reality.

The first mistake we make is the belief that caring for an aging parent is simply a matter of being a family, of caring for one's own, of fulfilling one's filial duty. *She's my mother, for Pete's sake. She took care of me; I can take care of her. I don't need help. This is what families do.* We may know better, but some voice in us—and in me, as it turns out—holds tight to this belief.

This attitude made sense throughout most of history. We could care for our aging parents ourselves, thank you very much. But in a short period of time, really in a generation or two, everything has changed.

Not long ago (and still, today, in some developing countries), family members lived near one another, their days were fairly flexible, and, most important, aged parents were never very aged. People didn't grow old; they grew up and they died. Caring for a parent meant sharing meals, helping out with some chores, and then, for a few weeks, seeing him through sickness and death.

Today, people are living much longer than ever before. They don't get sick and die; they grow old, grow frail, and need almost constant care and assistance, not for weeks but for years. They don't simply need a loving touch and some hot food; they need catheters, oxygen tanks, and eight different medications. They need someone to put the spoon in their mouth, get them on the toilet, pull their socks on, and remind them what day it is. The average caregiver (if there is such a thing) devotes more than twenty hours a week to this task, for nearly five years. Many, of course, do even more than that.

That's not the only thing that's changed. Our society has become increasingly mobile. Adult children no longer live down the street from their parents; they live two hours away, often by plane. And women, the traditional caregivers, are working and they are having children later, making them less available to help aging parents.

As a result of all this, caregivers jump in and help, and then can't figure out why they have so much trouble with the task, why they feel so frustrated, anxious, depressed, and overwhelmed. They jeopardize their careers, incomes, marriages, savings, and their own health. Studies show that caregivers have a higher rate of depression, insomnia, illness, and, yes, mortality. This task is literally killing them.

We take it all on without realizing that today this enormous undertaking goes well beyond the realm of filial bonds. Surely we should care for our parents as they age. But this is not something anyone should do on his or her own. As I must remind myself, a working mom with two young children, we need lots of help, support, and services. We need an entirely new approach because the demands of caregiving, the amount of time involved, and the structure of our lives have all changed. Drastically.

Before delving into the second mistake, let me note that things are only going to change more. This massive transformation of society, and of caregiving, is not over. In fact, it's accelerating.

In 1900, the average life span in the United States was forty-seven. Today it is seventy-seven. That's a gain of more than thirty years, or more than 60 percent, in only one century—and much of it in the latter half of the century. This change in life expectancy is greater than the gain seen during the previous five thousand years.

And now, perhaps within our lifetime, and certainly within our children's lifetime, the average life span is expected to extend another ten or twenty years. People will routinely make it to eighty-five, and thousands will surpass one hundred.

Why? People are leading healthier lives (although obesity may erase some of those gains). Doctors have better diagnostic tools. A host of new sciences—the map of the human genome, stem cell research, gene therapy, cloning, regenerative medicine, nano-technology—will help eradicate disease and keep people living longer. Scientists also expect that within the next ten or twenty years, they will develop a drug that will actually slow the aging process itself.

On top of all this, on January 1, 2011, the first of some 76 million baby boomers will turn sixty-five, graying America to all-new shades of whiteness.

Clearly, this means change, on many levels, for all of us.

Society, as a whole, must adapt. In the past ten years, since the first edition of this book came out, there's been a marked increase in assisted-living facilities, technological gadgets to help people remain independent, agencies catering to the needs of caregivers, and information available to families. (The Internet has been a great boon to both the elderly and their caregivers.) But so much more is needed—financial relief for family caregivers, more respite programs, better housing options, job support, etc.

As individuals, of course, we need to prepare for our own extended lives and prolonged retirement. We also need to prepare for years of eldercare. Before long, people who are sixty-five will be caring for parents who are eighty-five and grandparents who are 105. People will be choosing nursing homes for themselves and their parents at the same time. Caring for an aging parent, for years, will be a normal part of life's stages, as expected as marriage, kids, and retirement. But we can't do it all ourselves; we'll need help from both traditional sources as well as new and creative programs.

We also need to rethink our definition of *old* and our attitudes about aging, for herein lies the second mistake we make simply because ingrained attitudes die hard.

While researching for this new edition, I was surprised to find numerous books and studies of "the elderly" and "seniors" that turned out to be based on people in their sixties. (Some were about people over fifty!) With the average life expectancy inching its way over eighty and people often surpassing one hundred, sixty is hardly senior. In fact, these days seventy isn't all that old, and lots of people are still working, playing sports, and yes, having sex, at eighty and ninety.

We make a grave mistake in assuming that old age is some waiting station between life and death, that just because a person is eighty and has diabetes, heart disease, and a touch of arthritis, his mind and body are shot; he can't be an active and productive member of society; exercise and green, leafy vegetables won't make a difference; and he should really just sit in his Barcalounger because, Lord knows, he might break. Of course, this is a self-fulfilling prophecy. When people are made to feel useless, they become useless (and frailer and sicker and more dependent). In fact, this sedentary, isolated, unproductive lifestyle is more detrimental than aging itself.

Perhaps the most important change in the past ten years is the realization that older people can be productive, remain active, and benefit enormously from lifestyle changes. A number of recent books (*Successful Aging* by Dr. John Rowe and Dr. Robert Kahn, *The Virtues of Aging* by Jimmy Carter, and *Age Power* by Ken Dychtwald) argue that people have the power to age "successfully," to remain independent and active into their sixties, seventies, and beyond.

But we shouldn't stop there, for all sorts of research now shows that even the old-old—people who are eighty and ninety years old and suffering from various ailments—can benefit enormously from doing simple exercise, eating healthful foods, getting outdoors, staying active, having a sense of purpose, and expressing their creativity. They need, desperately, to be "a part of" rather than "apart from."

This is the challenge we face as caregivers, as members of this changing society, and as people who will be wearing orthopedic shoes ourselves one day. We mustn't prematurely age our parents, creating helplessness and further decline, by assuming that life is, for all intents and purposes, over at eighty.

As I said at the beginning of all this, I too am guilty. Without thinking, I make assumptions about old age and infirmity when it comes to my own mother. Three years ago, when she lay in a hospital bed, small and weak, her doctor told me that things didn't look good, and she had about three years left to live. Today, he tells me that her lungs are in very bad shape, and she could be on a ventilator at any moment.

I want to say, *Stay home, Mom, don't push yourself, what can I get for you, did you take your pills, I don't think you should be doing that, let me do that for you, and really, who cares what you eat because you're almost eighty.* But she still works occasionally, plays tennis, snorkels, goes to the ballet, reads the paper cover to cover, spends weekends with her eighty-three-year-old boyfriend, wants to take a painting class, sticks with skim milk, eats a lot of green, leafy vegetables, and is, as I write, planning a trip to South America.

It feels all wrong, but of course it's all perfectly, exactly right. My mother is probably alive today and will live another ten years because she doesn't listen to me or her doctor, with our ageist attitudes. She's alive, really alive, because she simply refuses to grow old in any traditional sense. She's happy not to dye her hair or wear makeup or get a face-lift (or even use the antiwrinkle cream that I pile on with great hope every night). She doesn't mind aging; she simply refuses to be old. She refuses to let lung disease, a hard cough that sounds like it might be her last, and nearly eight decades of wear and tear slow her down one whit.

If I had had my way, she would have been sedentary three years ago, and then perhaps the doctor's prediction would have been right on track.

So, Mom, go on. Have fun. I'll be here when you get back from Venezuela or Brazil or wherever it is you're headed, still trying to figure out how to move you into my house and make a bathroom wheelchair accessible. I'll be worrying about fevers and coughs and pneumonia and whether or not you're still okay. And I will, somewhat reluctantly, go look at a life-care center with you. But you go do your thing, because I am starting to realize, to really accept, that you're not old until you stop living.

✳   ✳   ✳   ✳

Author's Note: While reading the information and recommendations offered in these pages, keep in mind that they are addressed to a widely diverse population. Some caregivers live under the same roof with a parent and do this job without break, while others manage home-care services from afar. Some people are just heading into this job with a relatively healthy parent, while others are already well-versed in matters of geriatric care. Most of the advice is aimed at people caring for a lone parent, but some is directed at people who are helping one parent take care of another. The demands of the job, the strengths and strains of your relationship with your parent, and the support you receive from others all make your job unique. Which advice you follow, how much you give, and how you give it is something only you can decide. Do only what feels right for you—no more, no different—and you will be doing it right.

Chapter One

GET READY, GET SET

Talking with Your Parent
• Gathering Paperwork • Researching the Options
• Organizing Your Life • When You Can't Be There

....

NO ONE PLANS TO TAKE CARE OF A PARENT. WE DON'T SET aside money or time for the task, or begin reading books such as this one as soon as a parent turns seventy-five. For the most part, a parent's old age, and the needs and dilemmas that typically accompany it, come as a surprise. In fact, even when events begin to unfold, and the reality of the situation becomes apparent, most of us still look the other way, hoping that perhaps things will take care of themselves, that Dad will be all right and our services will not be needed. As a result, most people find themselves reacting to each crisis only as it arises.

No matter where you are in the process, whether you're just starting out or already deeply enmeshed, the most important thing you can do for your aging parent, and for yourself, is this: Be prepared for what might come. If your father's arthritis is getting worse, talk with him about what he might do when he can no longer manage alone, and start exploring community programs and services that he might need. If your mother has Alzheimer's, talk about her wishes concerning her future care and where she will live once the disease is advanced, and start making plans. When you use this book, don't read only the section that applies to your current situation; read about issues that you are not yet dealing with—but may very well have to tackle one day.

Delaying and denying are natural, but very risky, approaches to take. Your parent will grow older, his health will decline, and his needs will intensify. Staying one day ahead, one question ahead, one chapter ahead will give you and your parent time to consider the options carefully. It will ensure that your parent receives the best care possible. And, while it may not seem so, it will mean less stress and anxiety for you in the future. At a time like this, a little peace of mind is a priceless commodity.

Critical Conversations

Although it can become too late quite suddenly, it is never too soon to talk to your parent about the future—her medical care, housing, finances, and personal concerns. Obviously, if your mother is extremely sick and frail, these talks are urgent. But even if she is still relatively healthy and independent, discussing her current situation and her future is vital.

First of all, many preparations, such as buying long-term care insurance, getting on a waiting list for certain services or a particular nursing home, and setting up your parent's house to prevent falls, must be done in advance. Second, an accident or illness can come on suddenly. You need to be ready to respond, and you need to know how your parent wants things handled.

These conversations are much, much easier to have when there is no dire issue at hand. The subject is still relatively safe, and you can approach it with some detachment. *Mom, what if one day you needed full-time care, or had to move, or couldn't make decisions for yourself?* "What if" is not threatening. You are not talking about some immediate situation, but some distant possibility. Not only is the door easier to open at this point, but by talking early you establish a communication channel. Then, when a serious situation does arise, you are on familiar turf. The issue has been discussed. *Mom, remember when we talked about this? At that time you said such and such. Do you still feel that way?*

Discussing the future early also helps prepare your parent emotionally for what may come. If your father is encouraged to think about the possibility of moving out of his house before such a move is even an issue, it will be easier for him to make the move if it does, one day, become necessary. You can start the wheels turning, start the process of adjustment and acceptance, before any great change has to take place.

And finally, these talks give your parent and family members a chance to air their worries, to reassure one another, and to learn the truth about any haunting questions.

YOUR RELUCTANCE

ADMITTEDLY, ASKING YOUR FATHER about his finances, or anticipating a time when he can no longer take care of himself, is not easy. You may have a relationship in which personal issues, particularly *his* personal issues, are not discussed. Raising them may upset a fragile but relatively comfortable balance. If he is a domineering or protective force in your life, you risk losing—at least for a moment—the role of the child and you may find yourself taking on a strange new role. But more difficult than anything else, such conversations force you and your parent to acknowledge that he will decline, that he will need help, and that he is, indeed, mortal.

Certain issues may make you particularly uncomfortable. For example, you may be reluctant to ask about assets and wills out of respect for your parent's privacy or out of fear of sounding like a gold digger. Or you may not want to bring up the subject of death for fear of upsetting your parent. But the truth is that your parent and other family members probably share your concerns as well as your reluctance to discuss them. In fact, your mother may be keeping silent because she is worried about upsetting you. Your breaking the silence and initiating discussions may be awkward and painful but, at the same time, a welcome relief for all concerned.

Think about your reluctance and the reasons for it. Contemplate your role and the risks of both talking and failing to talk. Remember, as uncomfortable as it may be, talking about the worst-case scenarios won't make them come true, and refusing to talk about them won't make them go away. Ignoring the inevitable will only leave you unprepared for a crisis that is sure to come.

FINDING THE WORDS

IF YOU ARE CARING FOR A PARENT who is already quite frail or has a serious diagnosis, and questions and problems are already obvious or hovering, you might be able to tackle this head-on. *Mom, given your health and what the doctor's told us, I think we need to talk about some things.* If siblings or other family are involved, get everyone together to discuss the issues. (See page 174 for more on holding a family meeting.)

If you can't come right out and say what you need to, use an indirect approach. For example, you might express your concern about a friend or family member who is elderly and frail or ill. Talk about his situation and

BREAKING THE SILENCE

◆ Pick a time to discuss your parent's health, finances, or other matters when you won't be interrupted, and when you and your parent (and siblings) are calm and rested.

◆ Listen carefully, even when you have firm convictions about what should be done. You may have ideas about where your mother should live or how she should handle her finances, but it's important to listen now. Be open-minded and make a point of really hearing what she says, then let her know that you hear her.

◆ Keep the discussion focused on your parent's concerns, at least at the start. You may worry about who is going to take care of him once his Parkinson's disease gets worse, but he may be frightened about becoming helpless, losing people's respect, or becoming a burden. Give him ample room to express his thoughts, for these are crucial issues that need your undivided attention.

◆ Whenever possible, phrase your concerns as questions, letting your parent draw conclusions and make choices. Ask what she thinks should be done rather than telling her what should be done.

◆ Be open and clear with the facts—a poor medical prognosis, a major financial hurdle, a less-than-optimal selection of housing options. Be gentle, but don't lie or hide information to protect your parent. Misinformation, lack of information, and half-truths will only hurt him in the long run.

◆ End each discussion before you or your parent becomes tired or overwhelmed.

◆ Leave the conversation open. One discussion breaks the ice, but these topics need to be revisited again and again.

◆ If your parent changes the subject or makes it clear that she doesn't want to talk about something, let her know you are concerned and then back off and try again another time.

what is good or bad about it, as well as what problems might have been avoided had his family planned ahead and talked about them earlier. *Mom, what would you want if something like that happened to you?* You might also describe your own situation, your plans to buy additional insurance or draft a will, or your concerns about your own retirement. *Dad, I'm worried about how I will ever retire. How did you set up your finances? Do you have enough to cover all your expenses?* Or, use a magazine article or television show as a springboard. *I was reading an interesting article on hospice care. Have you heard much about that, Mom?* If your parent had elderly parents, ask how he handled certain matters for them, what was frustrating about it, and what was rewarding about it.

If talking face-to-face is too difficult, write a list of questions for your mother. Tell her that these are some issues you've been concerned about and ask her to think about each of them. Then plan a time to sit down with her and discuss them.

YOUR PARENT'S DENIAL

WHEN YOUR PARENT IS HIDING behind denial—*Oh, honey, why do you have to bring up such dreadful things? Let's talk about something more pleasant*—grant her some of that protection. Be patient and try to understand her fears and the reasons why she might not want to face these issues. Old age and the disability and dependence that often come with it are, obviously, painful and difficult to accept. Denial is a natural response.

If the subject isn't pressing, simply remind her that you care and you want to be helpful, then ask her to please think about the matter. You have planted a seed. She will surely give the subject some thought (if she hasn't already). Give her a couple of weeks and then bring it up again. *Mom, I know this is difficult for you. But if we talk about these things, I'll know what you want, and we can plan together for the future.*

If you still are not successful, ask another family member to talk with her. For whatever reasons, she may be more receptive to someone else. Or perhaps a close family friend can launch this conversation. You might also suggest that she talk with a member of the clergy, a social worker, a lawyer, or a doctor about certain matters. Or, you can call these people yourself and ask them to raise the subject with her. It's often easier for people to talk to and accept the advice of someone outside the family circle, especially if that person is a trusted professional.

When denial stands in the way of specific actions that absolutely have to be taken—your father refuses to stop driving even though he's practically blind—then you have to step in and take action, regardless of your parent's wishes. Push, tenderly and compassionately, but very firmly. *Dad, we cannot ignore this any longer. We have got to deal with it.* At some point, you might have to take away the car keys, or the car. (See page 28 for more on when to intervene.)

If, no matter what you do, your parent continues to deny the facts and the issue isn't life-threatening, find a new approach. There's no sense banging your head against the wall. You cannot force her to see things that she simply is not willing to face. So prepare on your own. Think about what will happen if your mother becomes seriously ill or dependent. What help might she need? How much will you and others be able to help her? And where will the rest of the help (community services, hired professionals, volunteers, etc.) come from? Who will pay for it?

WHAT TO TALK ABOUT

YOU MAY KNOW YOU NEED TO HAVE some discussions with Dad, but where do you begin and what do you ask? Here are a few major topics to get you started. (All of these topics are discussed in detail in individual chapters, including thoughts on how to talk about them.) Depending upon your parent's situation, you might want to do a little research into some of these issues first, so that you can explain some of the options.

◆ **Your parent's needs and concerns.** Before you do anything else, listen, listen, listen. This is a whole new stage of life (one you haven't experienced and are hard-pressed to even imagine). Your parent is likely

> " *After my father died I was very worried about my mom's finances. My dad always took care of everything that had to do with money. Mom never knew about his accounts; I don't think she ever balanced the checkbook.*
>
> *I said to Mom over and over, 'Let's review your financial situation,' and I offered repeatedly to take care of her bills for her. She would say, 'Brenda, don't worry about it. I'm fine.' And then she would change the subject.*
>
> *Then my brother came to visit, and within a day he had Mom pulling out folders and showing him bank statements. By the time he left, she had handed over almost all of her financial stuff to him.*
>
> *I was stunned. I mean, I was glad to have it settled, but I was also a little annoyed. I'm an accountant. He's a teacher. I guess she feels that money is men's work. I probably should have thought to get him involved right from the start."*
>
> —BRENDA S.

to have fears and hopes that are new, ones that she has never voiced before, ones that you are completely unaware of. You want to talk about her finances, but she's so focused on feelings of vulnerability, afraid of falling or becoming confused, or mired in grief over the losses in her life that she can't even think about financial issues right now. Listen to your parent—really listen—and then address her concerns before you move on to whatever is on your mind. Be careful not to dismiss her concerns by suggesting that they are silly or by offering quick and easy "solutions."

She might also open the door to the issues you want to discuss, which makes it easier. But more important, her concerns are vital and need addressing. Finally, listening to her will make her more willing to, in turn, listen to what you have to say.

What are your mother's biggest worries about the present and the future? What goals in her life does she feel are unmet, what tasks unfinished or conflicts unresolved? What aspects of your father's life are most important to him at this stage of life—being near family, hearing the opera, seeing certain friends, practicing his religion? What is hardest about growing older for him? What might be positive about it? You might be surprised at what your parent is worrying about, what his needs are, and what both of you can do to address them.

◆ **Daily activities.** Can your parent get through his day okay? Can he bathe and groom himself, or is the help that is provided right now enough? Can he get to the grocery store and prepare reasonably healthful meals? Or are the meals that others are preparing appetizing and nutritious? Is he still

driving? If so, it's best (and easier) to begin conversations now about how he might retain his driving skills and what he will do if, at some point, he can no longer drive. Does he fall now and then or feel unstable? How might he improve his balance and cut the risk of falls? Can he get into and out of a chair or bed? How about paying his bills—can he keep track of bills and write checks? There are solutions to many of these problems (discussed throughout the book), but you can't help him if you don't know what his problems are. Your parent might be embarrassed and not know that these are common problems with various solutions, so probe gently. Assure him that many of these kinds of problems are fixable, and admitting them doesn't mean you'll cart him off to a "home."

Your parent might not admit to some problems or may not be fully aware of them, so you need to observe what's happening, in addition to talking to him.

◆ **Housing.** How important is it to your parent to remain in his own home? What could be done to make his home more manageable for him and to keep him as independent as possible? Where would he want to live if he could no longer live at home? What if it isn't possible for him to live with other family members? What is most important to him in regards to housing (staying in his hometown; proximity to a certain friend, relative, or doctor; ability to keep a pet with him; climate; etc.)?

Even if you think you will never, ever put your parent into a nursing home, assisted-living facility, or other "senior" housing, consider the options with your parent. Visit a few facilities. See what's around. You don't know what is to come, and you can't make decisions if you don't know what choices exist. Be prepared, because you don't want to have to find alternative housing in the midst of a crisis. Talk now, examine the choices, and be ready.

◆ **Finances.** What are your parent's current financial needs and potential future needs? Is she in a financial position to meet these needs? Should she revise her investments, try to get cash out of her house, or simplify her finances? Should your parent buy long-term care insurance? Is she nearing Medicaid eligibility? Is her insurance—including life, health, home, and auto insurance—adequate and current?

One of the most pressing financial issues is long-term care. Most people drastically underestimate what this costs, and they overestimate what Medicare and other insurance programs cover. Medicare covers most doctor bills, hospital bills, laboratory tests, etc., but it does not cover the kind of long-term care most elderly people eventually need—nurses, aides, companions, and homemakers, or care in a nursing home or other facility. These bills can be astronomical. It is easy to spend $40,000 to $120,000 a year, devouring what might have seemed like a fairly comfortable savings account. Most people pay out-of-pocket until they are broke and then go on Medicaid, the government's insurance for the poor. Consider how your parent and family might handle such expenses.

Also, has your parent executed all necessary legal papers, including a will, durable power of attorney, and advance directives? Is there anything she might do to protect her estate from excessive taxes or, if she has little savings, to prepare herself to get on Medicaid and other government programs for low-income people?

◆ **Health care.** Does your parent have a good doctor who oversees all her medical care and whom she trusts? Do her other doctors all communicate with this primary physician? If she is currently disabled or sick, what is her prognosis, and how will that affect her independence, housing, finances, and future care?

If she couldn't make medical decisions for herself at some point, whom does she trust to do that for her? Has she legally named a health-care proxy to make these decisions for her? Has she talked to that person in depth about her wishes? If it's you, what would she want you to know? Does she dread the prospect of a particular disability or treatment? Is she more apprehensive about being in pain or about being groggy from painkillers? How far should you go in continuing to fight an illness?

◆ **Death.** This is a tough subject to discuss, but it is a crucial one. Many people in this country die alone, in

CRUCIAL DOCUMENTS

Whatever else you do, be sure your parent has the following:

◆ **An updated and valid will,** which ensures that his belongings (no matter how extensive or meager) will be allocated according to his wishes. A current will reduces the likelihood of family conflict and an extended and complicated probate process. In the case of a larger estate, a properly drafted will can also help avoid some taxes.	◆ **A durable power of attorney,** which authorizes someone to act on your parent's behalf, from signing checks to making housing choices, should he become incapacitated. Having power of attorney means the family can avoid the harrowing process of going to court to have a guardian named to oversee his care and finances.	◆ **Advance directives,** which include a **living will** and **a durable power of attorney for health care.** The first outlines your parent's wishes concerning end-of-life medical care, and the second gives some trusted relative or friend the authority to make health-care decisions for your parent, should he not be able to make them for himself at some point.

(See Chapter Seventeen for a full explanation of these documents.)

pain, afraid, and hooked to tubes. Living wills and other legal documents won't, by themselves, protect your parent from such a death. But he can dramatically improve his odds of having a peaceful and even meaningful death if this issue is discussed now.

Bring it up, however obliquely, and encourage your parent to talk. You may be surprised to find that he's thought about this quite a bit. Most people have. But even if he's given it considerable thought, he might still be resistant to open conversation, or he might not have given particular and very important issues much thought. In other words, you will probably have to make several attempts before you get any useful information about your parent's wishes regarding death. Still, keep at it. Do not stop at vague comments like, "Just don't drag it out," or, "When I'm at that point, pull the plug." Push the conversation further and get some helpful insight.

Be sure that your parent has signed advance directives (a living will and a power of attorney for health care) outlining his general wishes and authorizing someone to make decisions in his stead. Then, get into some specifics. What, if anything, frightens him or concerns him about dying? Why do these things worry him? Is there some way that you might be able to alleviate his fears? Is he more concerned about death or what the end of his life will be like? Is there a certain point after which he would no longer want life-sustaining medical care, such as a ventilator, artificial nutrition and hydration, surgery, transfusions, or antibiotics?

Gathering Information

As your parent grows increasingly frail, your family will need certain financial records and other information. (See the checklist on pages 12–13.) Find out whether your parent has all the relevant papers and make sure that you or another family member knows where they are.

If both of your parents are alive, you might simply remind them that these papers are important and suggest that they get them in order and ensure that each has easy access to them. If only one of your parents is alive, offer to find these documents. If your parent doesn't want help, impress upon her the importance of gathering these materials, then follow

FALLING ON DEAF EARS

Talking about these issues may not be a problem; getting your parent to heed any advice, however, may be extremely frustrating. Your parent might not be denying what is happening; she just has different views on how to deal with it. You know your mother should sign a will. You are certain that your father should buy additional insurance. But they refuse to budge. What could be more maddening than a parent who simply won't do what she's told?

You may need to act if the situation is truly dire or if your parent is mentally incompetent, but in many situations you will have to do something far more difficult: Accept your parent's autonomy and acknowledge the limits of your control over his life. Do what you can. Cajole, beg, push, bribe, and threaten. And then, depending upon the situation, you might have to drop it. You may be convinced that he's making a mistake, but unless he is in real danger, your parent has a right to make decisions, even ones that you consider to be foolish.

up later to make sure that she has done it. (This might require repeated attempts and a bit of aggravation, but stay with it.) Again, be sure that you can put your hands on these documents when you need them.

If your parent is infirm, and you have to look for these papers without his help, you might become upset as you hunt through his personal papers. If so, get a sibling or friend to help, and do it on whatever sort of schedule is manageable for you—all at once, like swallowing a pill, or in a series of small doses.

If you have trouble locating certain documents, call your parent's lawyer, accountant, or anyone else who has or has had a hand in his financial or legal affairs. Then look in the obvious places—a safe-deposit box, desk and bureau drawers, office files, and papers stacked on tables and in corners. If you don't find everything you need, look for leads such as bills, canceled checks, receipts, address books, and letters.

You might be able to track down some documents on the Internet. The federal government's Web site, www. firstgov.gov, has a state-by-state list of addresses to write to for vital records. The Veterans Administration and Social Security Administration also have information. ElderWeb, www. elderweb.com, has some helpful links.

Insurance companies will often provide information about a policy even when the request comes from a family member of the insured. The Social Security office, former employers, and the local office of veterans' affairs may be willing to send you information about pensions and other benefits. Unfortunately, banks are not very helpful in these situations unless you are dealing with a local bank where the manager knows your family. By law, banks can give out account information only to the owner of the account or the owner's legal guardian.

During my mother's illness, I accumulated so much stuff—brochures from nursing homes, documents from lawyers, forms from Medicare, pamphlets from social service agencies. Every time I got something, I just tossed it into this giant box in my bedroom. Then whenever something came up, like when I wanted to get meals delivered to her while I was away, I would think, 'Oh yeah, I have something on that,' but I could never find it.

A friend came over one day and dumped out my box and started sorting through it. She spent the entire day organizing the whole mess. That was the best thing anyone did for me during those two years. Not only could I find things quickly, but it made me feel better. I'd been feeling so out of control, and that gave me a little edge. It made an enormous difference."

—TERRY B.

CHECKLIST

Documents and information that your parent should gather (or you should gather for him) and file where family members can find them:

☐ Names, addresses, and phone numbers of
—doctors, dentists, and other medical providers, such as optometrists, hearing aid suppliers, and pharmacists
—lawyers, financial advisors and accountants, insurance agents, real estate agents
—banks, investment firms, and any other financial institutions your parent has dealings with
—the religious organization your parent is affiliated with, along with names of particularly important clergy
—clubs, associations, boards, community groups in which your parent might be involved
—your parent's close friends and relatives

☐ Medical history, including allergies, immunizations, illnesses, surgeries, and past doctors (who might have old medical information on your parent)

☐ Certificates of birth, marriage, divorce/separation, and citizenship

☐ Military/veterans papers

☐ Driver's license

☐ Passport

☐ Your parent's will and any codicils (amendments) to the will and letter of instruction that goes with the will

☐ Durable power of attorney, living will, and power of attorney for health care

☐ The keys to his house (or houses), office, safe-deposit boxes, and post office boxes, and combinations to safes

☐ Insurance policies, including life, health, disability, mortgage or loan, homeowner's, accident, and auto

☐ Social Security, Medicare, and Medicaid numbers and identification cards

☐ A list of employers, dates of employment, and terms of employment

☐ Contracts with any current and past employees

☐ Any business contracts

☐ Any rental agreements

☐ Deeds to real estate

☐ Titles to automobiles, boats, and other vehicles

☐ The location of any hidden valuables

☐ A list of all charge, debit, and banking cards

☐ Internet passwords, online banking access codes, PIN numbers

☐ Any automatic bill-paying arrangements or electronic transfer accounts

☐ Any appraisals of personal property

☐ Copies of federal and state tax returns from the past three to five years

☐ Receipts from property taxes and other large recent payments

☐ Instructions on how to care for a pet, plants, house, and dependents

☐ Burial and funeral instructions, if any, and any arrangements made for prepayment of a funeral

You should also have

☐ A list of all monthly bills, such as utilities, property taxes, mortgage payments, and insurance premiums

☐ A complete list of your parent's assets, including
—savings, checking, and money market balances
—stocks, bonds, and other securities
—estimated value of all real estate
—value of automobiles, boats, and other vehicles
—business ownership and partnership agreements
—profit-sharing and pension plans
—trust agreements
—retirement accounts (pensions, IRA, Keogh, SEP, 401(k), etc.)
—records of any loans (financial or property) your parent may have made to family members, business associates, or others

☐ A list of debts, including mortgages and other loans, credit card debts, outstanding bills, and other liabilities (credit card and charge account numbers)

Scoping Out the Scene

Wherever you are in this process, learn about services in your parent's community and housing options *NOW*. Most people assume they don't need outside help (*This is my father; I can take care of him myself*), or don't know that such help is available. Then, when they finally go to sign up, it's so late in the game that they are frazzled and burned out, perhaps in debt and sick themselves.

Don't wait until there is a crisis—say, your parent is lying in a hospital bed about to be discharged, and you don't know the first thing about what options exist for her care at home, or your parent needs help and you live more than three hours away and haven't a clue where to turn. Don't wait until your parent is so frail or confused that changing schedules or moving is like shifting the Rock of Gibraltar. Don't wait until the options are dismal, or there are no options. (Some programs and residences have waiting lists, some with waits of several years.)

Learning about the options early means that when your parent needs help (or you do), you have some idea of what exists. You might be surprised at what sorts of help is available—from free delivery of books on tape, to rides to the grocery store, to all-day care and home companions.

STARTING POINTS

YOUR PARENT'S DOCTOR MAY KNOW about some of the services in the community, or should at least be able to direct you to someone who does. Friends who have been in a similar situation may also be helpful. Beyond that:

◆ **The area agency on aging** is the best place to start. These agencies, which are overseen by state units on aging, go by a medley of names—bureau on aging, council of senior services, commission on the elderly, etc. They can be found by calling the Eldercare Locator (800-677-1116) or visiting www.eldercare.gov online, or by calling the state unit on aging, listed on page 628. These agencies have information about many of the services, programs, and senior housing options available in your parent's community. Staff should be able to answer specific questions about your parent's care. Be prepared to provide detailed information about your parent's needs and resources; the more information they have, the better they can help you. Many of these agencies have their own Web sites.

◆ **Local senior centers, community groups, and religious organizations,** such as Jewish Family Services and the United Way, usually know quite a bit about local services, programs, volunteers, courses, and organizations. Senior centers, which can be found through the phone book or area agency on aging, often provide services directly.

◆ **The local hospital's discharge planner** or social services department is responsible for making sure that patients have the services they need and move into proper housing when they leave the hospital. They know a great deal about services in your parent's community. Some hospital social workers will guide you whether or not your parent is in the hospital. Case managers at geriatric assessment centers do similar work. Beware, however, that some hospitals have agreements with certain agencies and facilities, and the planners might be biased. Get information from them, but then do your own research, if possible. Your parent's doctor should be able to direct you to a case manager.

◆ **Many larger companies** offer information on eldercare through their employee assistance plans. Some also have referral programs for information about services in other areas, and some will actually put you in touch with a trained care manager who can guide you. Don't be afraid to tap into this. It's there for you.

◆ **The state long-term care ombudsman's office,** which represents residents of nursing homes and their families, can give you information about local nursing homes and other types of housing for the elderly. (The state offices are listed in Appendix B, page 628.)

◆ **Medicare's Web site and hotline** (877-267-2323 or www.medicare. gov) are very helpful in explaining coverage and benefits and providing information about home care and housing options.

◆ **Foundations and organizations for a particular disease** often have local chapters that offer information about services and programs. Many of these organizations are listed in Appendix A, page 600. You can also get referrals to national organizations from the National Health Information Center (800-336-4797 or www.health.gov/nhic) or the National Rehabilitation Information Center (800-346-2742 or www.naric.com). AARP (which is no longer called the American Association of Retired Persons) has a wealth of information on its Web site, www.aarp.org.

◆ **A geriatric care manager** can assess your parent's needs and identify services she needs or take over your parent's care almost entirely. You may be able to find one in the local Yellow Pages, or through the National Association of Professional Geriatric Care Managers (520-881-8008 or www.caremanager.org). You can also search on the Internet for "geriatric care manager" and the name of your parent's hometown. Care managers' services are not inexpensive, but they are often well worth the price.

◆ **211.** Many states are establishing, and some have already established, human service information lines, which are contacted by dialing 211. Operators are trained to link people to social services and local programs.

The Key Is Organization

If you diligently write lists of "Things to Do" on scraps of paper and then misplace them, or you're constantly remembering things that you shouldn't have forgotten, know that life is only going to get crazier now. When a parent needs care, the reminders, names and numbers, appointments, bits of information, and to-do lists start pouring into your life like confetti. Organization is the only way you will survive this. Here are a few tips:

◆ Keep a small spiral notebook in your purse or back pocket at all times. When you think of an essential errand while driving to the grocery store, jot it down at the next traffic light. As a reward for your efforts, you get to cross things off as you accomplish them. Remember, if this book is left at home on your desk, it will be of little use to you.

◆ Have a small calendar on your desk or by your kitchen phone (preferably one that travels in your purse or briefcase with the aforementioned spiral notebook). Record not just the obvious dates and appointments, but every task that must be done on a certain day. If bottles and cans get picked up every other Thursday morning for recycling, make a note to yourself to put them out on Wednesday night. With so much on your mind now, sometimes remembering your own name can be an effort.

◆ Each time you call a home-care agency, lawyer, or social worker, make a note about the call on your calendar or on a legal pad, including the name of the person you spoke with and what you talked about, so you can refer to it later if necessary. (*But I spoke to Anne Preston on March 18, and she confirmed that the home health aide would start tomorrow.*)

◆ Whenever you make calls to agencies, doctors, etc., have all the necessary information in front of you, and have all of your questions written out. Otherwise, you may forget an important question and have to go through all the secretaries and recorded announcements to make contact again. Then write down the information so you can remember it and relay it reliably to others. Get into the habit of asking for people's direct lines or extensions, and keep note of them.

◆ Confirm, confirm, confirm. It's better to confirm an appointment the day before than to find out that your father's hearing aid specialist has taken an unscheduled vacation and his temporary assistant forgot to cancel his appointments.

◆ Buy some folders and a sturdy file box or an accordion file and use it to store all information regarding your parent's care. Label each folder or section in a way that makes sense to you—Medical Information, Nursing Home Brochures, Legal Papers, Community Resources, Letters to Siblings, etc. If you hate to throw things out (you never know when you might need it), keep a file called Information No Longer Needed, or Trash File, just so your other files are current and not overstuffed. (Once you have your files set up, use them. They may look efficient, but they aren't much good if they are empty. And keep them up-to-date rather than just stacking papers in a "to be filed" pile. That pile can become rather large and nasty-looking very quickly.)

◆ Make a master list of all essential names and phone numbers and store one copy at the beginning of the file box and one copy beside the telephone. (If you're calling certain people or agencies regularly, and if your telephone has a memory feature, you might want to store their numbers into your automatic dialing system.)

◆ If you work better on a computer and pocket organizer, set up a computer file that includes all the information and accounts concerning your parent. Be sure to make a backup disk copy and keep it in a safe place.

◆ Make copies of important papers —receipts, insurance claims, nursing-home applications—before sending them off.

◆ Write a daily schedule. Before scoffing at this idea, try it for a couple of weeks. You may not adhere to it precisely, but it will help structure your day so you are not constantly thinking, "I've got to get to the grocery store. I can't believe I forgot to call the Social Security office. Wasn't someone supposed to pick up Mom's dentures?"

The task—or the breather you so desperately need—will already be assigned to a time slot. Even if you don't use it, writing a schedule for a few weeks will help you see where your day is going and why you don't have time for all the things you need to do. And it may give you ideas for how you can be more efficient. For example:

7:00 A.M.	up and at 'em
7:15-8:00	breakfast, kids off to school, clean up
8:00-8:45	shower, check e-mail, make phone calls
8:45	take Mom to the eye doctor for 9 a.m. appointment, read mail in waiting room
10:00	drop Mom at day care, stop at pharmacy
10:30-11:15	grocery store, other errands
11:30	meeting with Ed Walker
1:30-5:00 P.M.	work on Copeland report—no interruptions!
5:00	pick up Mom at day care, kids at after-school program
5:30	laundry, clean up, deal with kids and Mom
6:30	fix dinner, still dealing with kids and Mom
7:00	dinner is served
8:00	help everyone get ready for bed
8:30	pay bills
9:00	call Wendy for a chat
10:00	watch TV
11:00	bed

Be reasonable when making your schedule. Give yourself more than the minimum time required to do a chore or to get someplace. If you have an appointment, expect to wait. And finally, if you're a morning scrambler,

HAVE A PLAN B

If your parent depends upon you for her care, be sure to have a contingency plan ready in case you are suddenly laid up, go out of town, or face some other emergency. Make plans for someone else to step in on short notice, for your parent to go to a senior center or adult day-care center, or for her to go to someone else's house or into a senior residence for a temporary stay.

Likewise, if you are going away on business or on a vacation, and you've made plans for another relative or caregiver to step into your spot, have some other option available as well in case your original plan for your parent's care falls through.

If your parent depends upon someone else for her care—an aide or companion—be sure to have the name of a backup person who can fill in, or someplace where your parent can go if her companion can't or doesn't show up for work for some reason. Too many caregivers don't have a Plan B and are caught in dire straights when life takes an unexpected turn.

get up fifteen minutes earlier than usual to give yourself time to organize the day and start it off calmly.

When You Can't Be There

If you live far away from your parent or if you work—in other words, if you are like most caregivers—you have to be extra organized. You absolutely must plan ahead, because you won't have the luxury of responding instantly to a crisis. What are you going to do when you're sitting at work, three hundred miles away and you get a call that your father has taken a turn for the worse and needs help?

At least a third of all family caregivers care from afar—at least an hour away and usually four or more hours away. And about half of caregivers work either full time or part time. Not being with an elderly parent day in and day out can make life easier in some ways (ask anyone who lives with an aged parent), but it increases the burden in other ways. The cost of travel, phone calls, and hired help are compounded, of course, but it's the additional load of worrying and guilt that can be unbearable. (*Is she all right? How will I know if she isn't? Should I be visiting more often? Should I take time off from work? Am I not giving enough?*)

Forget the guilt trip, but do make the most of your visits and the time you can give. Now more than ever, organization and preparation are the keys to your success—and your survival.

Take a good look at what's been discussed so far in this chapter. Here are a few additional tips for organizing from a distance:

◆ Have a list of all important phone numbers with you at all times—doctor, lawyer, accountant, insurance companies, emergency hotlines, the area agency on aging, etc.

Be sure that your parent, her doctor, and anyone involved in her care know how to reach you. Invest in a cell phone or pager and have it with you at all times so people can reach you in case of an emergency.

◆ Establish a local support network as soon as possible. Make a list of friends, family, or neighbors who live near your parent. Let these people know of your concern. They can be extra cars and eyes, as well as caring friends. They can alert you when they notice signs of trouble and be available if there is an emergency.

◆ Phone calls don't always tell you what you need to know. Visit your parent so you can see for yourself what's really going on, and so you can make adjustments to your parent's home or get additional help when necessary.

◆ If you live far away, organize your visits in advance so you can accomplish as much as possible. If you

need to meet with a doctor, lawyer, social worker, or other professional, set up appointments at least a month in advance, as their schedules get filled quickly. Be sure to confirm these appointments closer to the date.

◆ In advance of visiting, plan what you want to accomplish and anything you might need to discuss with your parent.

◆ When you are with your parent, take a mental inventory of her health and living situation. Try to foresee trouble before it happens. Does your mother seem wobbly or dizzy? Is she well groomed, or has her personal hygiene deteriorated? Is there ample food in the refrigerator? Is the food spoiled and moldy? Are there piles of unopened mail or unpaid bills? Does she still do the things she used to, like read, knit, and do the crossword puzzle? Does it appear that she's getting out, seeing friends? If things seem askew or different than they used to be, it may be a sign of underlying trouble—depression, confusion, illness, diminishing eyesight— or simply a signal to you that she needs more help at home and opportunities to get out.

◆ Include some time during your visit to talk with nearby relatives, friends, or others who see your parent regularly, both to hear their thoughts and concerns and to thank them for helping in any way that they do.

◆ Check out local services and facilities. See what hospital is best, what nursing homes are acceptable, and what community services are offered.

◆ Even though your life is busy, be sure to spend some time simply being with your parent, chatting, listening, watching a movie, or just sitting quietly. A trip that's all business misses a critical element. Find time to relax, to listen, to offer support.

◆ Enlist the help of at least two people who live nearby and might be counted on when your parent suddenly needs help, or when you suspect trouble and need someone to check in on her.

◆ Learn to distinguish real emergencies from unfounded complaints or cries of loneliness or other guilt-inducing calls. It's okay to say that you can't come right now, that you were just there last week, that you know your parent is okay, that you will be there next week or next month. Learn how to reassure her without feeling guilty. (Beware, however, that unending complaints and requests for reassurance may be an early sign of dementia. See page 460.)

◆ If your parent lives alone, see if a relative, friend, or neighbor will stop by occasionally to see how your parent is doing, or perhaps drop off a meal or offer a ride into town. A local church, community organization, senior center, or religious organization might know of volunteers who can check on your parent. You also might hire a companion to spend time with your parent.

◆ Learn about any local elder-watch programs. Some post offices and gas and electric companies train employees to watch for trouble at homes where they know an elderly person lives alone. People who deliver meals to homebound elderly people are also often trained to spot problems. A bank manager might be willing to keep an eye out if you are concerned about your parent's finances—is the account suddenly being used up, or has it lain dormant for some time (meaning that bills are not being paid)?

◆ If your parent has in-home care or lives in a nursing home or other institutional residence, it is no less important that someone check in on her regularly. Staff from home-care agencies or nursing homes can be neglectful and even abusive. Someone should check in regularly and at unexpected times to see how things are going.

◆ Buy your parent an emergency response system (see page 105) so if she is in trouble when she is alone, she will be able to get help immediately.

◆ If your parent has trouble dialing the phone, either because of dexterity, memory, or vision problems, buy a phone with an extra-large dial pad or one that has automatic dial buttons. You can tape photos of people and emergency service symbols onto automatic-dial buttons so she doesn't have to remember or read phone numbers.

◆ Leave a duplicate of your parent's house key (or code number to a lock or security system) with a trusted neighbor or friend, and/or hide one outside of her house or apartment in case there is an emergency and someone needs to get in. (Hide it very discreetly; forget the fake rock.)

◆ Have on hand a copy of the phone book—both White and Yellow Pages—from your parent's hometown. This is helpful in case you suddenly need to find a home-care agency or track down a particular doctor. You can also gain access to White and Yellow Pages on the Internet, although this often isn't as useful (www.yellowpages.com, www.superpages.com, www.switchboard.com).

◆ If you don't have an inclusive, one-price telephone plan (and you might want to switch to one if you are calling your parent and various caregivers often) or if you travel out of the country frequently, you'll want to keep long-distance calls brief. Be ready with information and questions when you call doctors or lawyers.

◆ If your parent can handle it, get her connected to the Internet. This is an easy (and relatively stress-free) way for the two of you to communicate, and it enables your parent to communicate with others and do some of her own research into health or financial questions. You might buy an inexpensive computer that provides only Internet access. (Or if she can get to the library, encourage her to use public Internet access.) Despite the adage "you can't teach an old dog new tricks," the elderly are the fastest growing group of Internet users. It helps keep them in touch with friends and family, which is vital in old age. If your parent balks, find out why. It might be that she has trouble reading the small print or managing the keypad. You can buy a variety of gadgets to make it all easier. You can also buy Web cameras, or webcams, that attach to her computer and yours so you can communicate and see each other at the same time, which is fun, and allows you to actually see how she is.

◆ When things begin to get unwieldy, look into hiring a geriatric care manager, or find out if a local government agency or charitable group offers subsidized care management. A manager can assess her needs, organize local services, handle emergencies, and keep you up to date.

◆ Above all, take care of yourself. Recognize and accept the limits of what you can do and give yourself credit for all you are doing. Don't hesitate to ask for help or use community services. And finally, get support from friends or a professional counselor to help you alleviate stress and guilt.

Chapter Two

YOUR PARENT AND YOU

*Adapting to New Roles • Knowing When to Intervene
• Defusing Old Struggles • Managing Day-to-Day
• The Difficult Parent*

....

P ARENT-CHILD RELATIONSHIPS ARE, BY THEIR VERY NATURE, stressful. Your father doesn't understand you, expects too much from you, or refuses to accept help. Your mother makes you feel guilty, embarrasses you, or perhaps reminds you too much of yourself. Whatever the issue, it stays with you. Long after you think you have outgrown the parent-child power dance, and after you think you've resolved it or let go of it, a casual comment or a certain look can trigger a familiar surge of adrenaline.

Now that your parent is growing frail and needs you, the bond may be stronger, but the aggravation may be greater as well. This is the paradox of parentcare. On one hand, the prospect of losing your parent intensifies your love, and this time together is precious. On the other hand, the issues are painful and sometimes contentious. Both of you may be feeling exhausted, unsure, and crabby. And your roles—who is in charge, who is the "parent"—are unclear and sometimes uncomfortable.

You can't change your parent, especially not at her age, but you may be able to change some of your reactions to her, which should greatly ease daily tensions. You can also define the scope of your duties so that you protect your own needs while also helping her. All of this might help you form, not an entirely different relationship with your parent, but perhaps a more peaceful one.

Adapting to New Roles

When a parent grows frail, roles shift uncomfortably, and both parent and child can become disoriented and unsure about how to behave. Who is in charge? When should you intervene? Are you the parent now?

ARE YOU PARENTING YOUR PARENT?

IT IS A COMMON REMARK AND A thought that is hard to avoid, especially if you are changing diapers, tying shoelaces, or dealing with incompetence or irrational outbursts. But regardless of the circumstances, the answer is a flat-out and very definite NO. You are not parenting your parent.

If your parent is no longer able to care for herself, you may have new responsibilities, ones that may at times resemble those of parenting. But your parent is and always will be your parent, and you will always be her child. Go ahead and use some of the same

tricks that help in parenting—diversions to get her onto a new subject, a baby monitor so you can hear trouble, or crib sheets for incontinence. But allowing yourself to think that the roles have reversed, that you are now the parent and your parent is a child, is a potentially disastrous way to look at this situation—for both of you.

For your parent, it is dehumanizing to be treated or spoken to as a child, to be nagged, scolded, or bossed around, even if it's done in subtle ways. No matter how disease and age may have altered your parent's body or mind, no matter how much or how little she can do or think for herself, and no matter how much you are doing for her, she is an adult and deserves to be treated as one. She has a lifetime of experience and a wealth of time-tested opinions. She has earned her autonomy and pride. She may have reverted to childish ways, but that does not make her a child.

For you, reversing the roles will only lead to dead ends and frustration. After all, children grow and learn and (usually) do what their parents tell them to do. If you try to parent

REMEMBER THE GOOD OLD DAYS

If your parent is quite ill, if he has gotten crotchety in his old age, or if dementia has distorted his personality, find a photo from when he was younger—a photo of him at his best, a photo of him holding you when you were a child, a photo of him strong and well. Or put together a collage of photos. Then put it on your refrigerator or on your desk, someplace where you will see it often. It will help you remember better times, when he was stronger. It will help you recall the father who laughed with you and cared for you and taught you things. It will help you remember why you are doing so much for him now.

your parent as you would a child, without perceiving the vast differences in the two situations, you will make things much harder for yourself. You will beat yourself up wondering why you are having such trouble with the task, and you will be angry with your parent for not behaving as you want her to. *Why doesn't she listen to me and do what I say?*

If you behave as an adult and treat your parent as an adult—an aged adult who needs your respect, as well as your care—both of you will fare better.

FOSTER INDEPENDENCE

NOT ONLY SHOULD YOU AVOID parenting your parent, but you should go a step further and make a point of reinforcing any independence that remains. Rather than cleaning his room, making his lunch, or getting him dressed, find a way for your parent to do some things for himself. (See Chapter Six for ways to make daily tasks more manageable.) Rather than completely taking over his finances and legal affairs, keep him at the helm as much as possible.

Whatever your parent's situation, your job is not to control his life, but to help him maintain as much control over it as possible.

Activity and independence are good for your parent's body, mind, and spirit. Physically, it is good for him to move, lift, bend, walk, and carry things in any way that he still can. He may not want to take his plate to the kitchen or walk to the mailbox because his arthritis makes it difficult, and you may want to help by doing these things for him. But the truth is that inactivity is deadly. Movement, any movement at all and as much of it as possible, is valuable medicine.

This applies to the mind as well as the body. Mental exercise, such as keeping track of one's checkbook, composing letters, or listening to the newspaper read aloud (if she can't read it for herself anymore) can keep the mind well oiled and running more smoothly, ward off depression, and possibly slow the onset of dementia.

More than anything else, independence boosts the soul. Your parent may welcome your help, but when people are constantly catered to, when they no longer make their own decisions, when they are treated as needy and helpless, they grow only more needy and helpless. As they give up increasing amounts of control, they also give up their self-esteem, spirit, and drive. They wither.

Your parent is shouldering so much. Aging is difficult work. Help him hang on to whatever abilities and autonomy he still has. Help him to help himself, whenever possible.

Of course, this may mean more work for you, not less, as you might have to wait while he struggles to put on his pants or clean up after he spills the juice, but it is a great gift to him, and should, in other ways, make everyone's life better.

OFFER RESPECT

WHATEVER YOUR PARENT'S SITUATION, whatever your relationship, try to treat him with respect and make him feel that he still wields some control. He is losing so much else; he cannot afford to lose your respect. If he can't handle his finances alone or make decisions regarding his own health care, keep him involved. Ask what he thinks. Listen to his thoughts. Always keep his needs and preferences at the forefront of any decision.

> *"The only time I wasn't the daughter was when I turned into the mother, and that was the best feeling ever. It was October. My mother was very sick, so I brought her to the hospital, and the doctor ordered some X-rays. They had taken Mother's clothes off, and she was so weak that I had to hold her up. Her body, which used to be so strong and lean, was thin, her skin was loose, and I could feel her bones. I was holding her little body in my arms, and there was a great poignancy, a closeness, which I was so happy about. She was finally trusting me to care for her. She wasn't fighting me. On that day, I felt what I had always wanted to feel with her. It was like a pouring out of tenderness."*
>
> —BETTY H.

If he can't communicate, assume that he can understand you, explain simply what is going on, and reassure him that you are moving forward, guided by his wishes as he has told you about them in the past.

Be careful not to boss your parent around as if he were a child, nag him about bad habits, or instruct him on how to behave. And never talk about him as if he were not in the room.

Ask that others treat your parent with respect as well. If you witness behaviors on the part of a caregiver that you think might trouble your parent,

> ❝ *Now that my mother's dementia is worse, she's given up and wants me to take over. I have to help her dress and get her to day care and feed her. It's to the point now that if someone asks her a question, she'll answer but look to me to make sure it's right.*
>
> *Sometimes I get so frustrated and tired that I yell at her. I tell her what to do and then get mad when she doesn't do it right. And then I feel awful and I think, 'What in the world is happening here?'*
>
> *I have to keep reminding myself over and over that she's my mother and I love her dearly and I respect her. But it's hard."*
>
> —Linda K.

talk with the caregiver. Give him or her some specific suggestions for protecting your parent's dignity. Caregivers might call your parent by a formal name if that is what he or she is used to—Mr. Hughes, Dr. Johnston, Mrs. Weber. They should place towels strategically when helping with a bath or caring for a wound. They should explain things at all times, telling your parent what is happening and what they are doing even if your parent doesn't seem to hear or understand. And they should avoid calling your parent "honey" or "doll" or other expressions that might seem condescending or inappropriate to your parent.

PUT YOURSELF IN HIS SHOES

Perhaps this book should be called, *Be Nice; You're Next.* Think about it. We treat children with a certain kindness because we have been there. The memories may be faint, but we understand what it is like to be a child. Most of us don't, however, have any idea what it is like to be truly old and frail. But, most likely, we will one day.

Put yourself in your parent's shoes—literally (or use your imagination). First of all, imagine you've lost most or all of your friends, your spouse, your job, and any sports or hobbies you once enjoyed. Now put on some very scratched-up glasses, perhaps with toilet paper tubes glued to each lens so you can only see what's directly in front of you. Plug your ears with cotton. Wrap your knees so tightly with bandages that walking is difficult and stairs are impossible. Breathe through a straw so only a bit of air is getting in. Plug your nose and try tasting your favorite foods. Now get—or imagine—yourself in a situation where you are uncomfortable or in pain much of the time. With all this, you're still not even halfway there.

Your parent has lived a long life, has struggled and suffered, and, recently, has lost so very much. He stands to lose only more—his health, his home, more friends, more abilities. He is, ultimately, facing death.

As you try on his shoes, remember, too, that your parent comes from a different time and place. He has different habits and beliefs and ways of

SOME REWARDS

C aring for an aging parent is trying, without a doubt. It is exhausting, stressful, frustrating, and, at times, completely overwhelming. Beyond the day-to-day pressures and practical questions that arise, there are complex emotional issues to deal with—guilt, resentment, and grief, the strains of family relationships, the echoes of one's childhood, and the stark, painful visions of one's own old age and death.

However, there are often unexpected rewards. This is, after all, your parent, and no matter how he might infuriate you at times, no matter how he might have erred in his role as parent, and no matter how much you must do for him now, no one will ever love you in quite the same way, and, in truth, you will never love anyone else in this way. Helping him now is an opportunity to reciprocate some of that love and attention. It is a chance to say, during quiet moments, things that you might not have said otherwise, and to care for him in tender ways that you never have before. Caring for your parent allows you to reaffirm family bonds and, in some cases, to strengthen those bonds.

Of course, these rewards may be hard to see or even imagine when you are in the thick of this. But when they come, cherish them. If you get a word of thanks, remember it. When there is some closeness, make a note of it. These are the moments that will get you through all this.

While it may be hard to conceive of now, when you look back on your parent's life and this time you had together, you may be glad that you had the chance to give in such an intimate way.

dealing with things. He might not understand your frustration that he won't emote openly or discuss certain issues because he was brought up to believe that people didn't do that; it was in bad taste or weak to talk about such things. Your parent might fret about money constantly not because he's irrational, but because he struggled through the Depression and because he is not getting a paycheck anymore.

In other words, have empathy and try to be understanding as you deal with your parent. View things from his perspective. Think how he might feel, and why he might behave as he does. And then think how you might feel. How you would want your children and others to treat you if you were at this point in life.

Be nice because, in fact, you will one day be in his shoes.

When to Intervene

The need to protect your parent's independence and respect his autonomy can collide with the need to look out for his safety and welfare. What do you do if your father insists on staying in an unsafe home, or refuses to call the doctor after a fall? What if your mother is losing her vision but refuses to stop driving? When do you intervene and when do you bow out? And how do you step in without taking over?

If your parent has a mentally competent spouse, remember that it is largely the spouse's job to decide when and how to intervene. Don't usurp her role. She will make decisions, as well as she can, about her husband's care. It is your role to support her, nurture her, and help her to do what she thinks is best. Offer information and advice, prod when necessary, but remember that you're in the backseat.

If you are caring for a lone parent or handling the care of two disabled parents, you must step in when your parent is deemed incompetent and can no longer understand options, make a rational decision, or communicate her views. (See page 396 for information on competency and obtaining guardianship.) If you question the sanity of her actions, consider having her evaluated for depression and dementia. Often, these ailments affect people's judgment.

If she is deemed incompetent, you may have to make important decisions about her health care, housing, and finances.

You also have to step in when your parent's (or someone else's) safety or health is seriously threatened. You should be sure your parent's bills are paid to protect him from utility cut-offs and eviction. You have to disconnect the gas to the stove if your mother, in her distracted state, is at risk of burning the house down. You must stop her from driving if she is a hazard to herself and others. You may need to find some way to get her to take her medications if she is forgetting them.

But beyond these issues of dire risk and mental incompetence, your duty to protect your parent is superceded by his right to make his own decisions. All of us make decisions about personal health, finances, and safety every day—when we get into a car, or have a cigarette, or decide to go bungee jumping, or invest in something new— and some of these choices are unwise. Your parent, even at her advanced age, retains the right to take risks—even ones you may consider foolhardy. One day you will have the same rights, and you will be allowed to make your own decisions, despite the better judgment of your children.

So what do you do? First, assess your concerns. Why do you think she shouldn't do whatever it is that she is doing? (Or do what she isn't doing?) Why shouldn't she, for example, take fewer baths or save her money under her mattress? What are the risks? How serious are they? Can they be reduced? Why do you think some other option is preferable?

When you think about the problem, focus on your parent's needs, not yours. Do you want your parent to move for her sake, or because it will be easier for you if she moves? When it comes to her spending money, are you concerned about her financial security or worried about your own inheritance? Refocus your thoughts on what is best for your parent and what she needs and wants.

Then, talk with your parent. How does she feel about this? Listen to her thoughts and reasoning. Try to understand how *she* sees it.

Discuss the risks and benefits involved. Perhaps she doesn't know that breaking a hip can be fatal. Perhaps she hasn't thought about how a move might provide her with companionship and activity. Talk about the options. If she can't manage the stairs, perhaps her bedroom can be moved to the first floor. If she can't shop and cook for herself, maybe she can have meals delivered.

If you hit a wall, get others in the family involved, as well as her doctor, lawyer, or anyone else whom your parent respects. Sometimes people will listen only to certain people. And sometimes they will only listen to professionals.

After all of this, if your parent is competent and the risks are not dire, the final decision is hers. Keep in mind that your parent is basing her decisions on different criteria than you

are. Your main concern is her health and safety (or it should be), but at this point in her life she may place greater value on familiar routines, old habits, control, and independence.

You might worry because your mother insists on taking her regular morning walk and refuses to use a cane, even though she's tripped a

---

❝ My mother had a stroke about a year ago that left her very unsteady. She needed a cane to get around, and climbing stairs was almost impossible for her. What was difficult for me was that she started going back to her old routines almost immediately. She lives in the city and loves the theater, the opera, going out with her friends. About two weeks after her stroke, I realized that she had resumed her old social life. I was worried sick. It was winter and the sidewalks were slippery, and I was afraid she was going to fall or have another stroke.

But she got around pretty well, with the help of friends. And I began to realize that for her to stay in her apartment, to sit alone and watch television, would be a fate worse than death. My mother is going to get out and do things as long as she is alive. That's her nature. I worry, but I respect her immensely for it. I hope I have her gusto when I'm her age.❞

—FRAN M.

WHOSE LIFE IS THIS, ANYWAY?

E arly on, when a parent is newly ill or suddenly widowed, adult children often jump in with both feet to help. With all the best intentions, they discuss Dad's living situation, his social life, his health, his finances, and his future—often among themselves, with little or no input from Dad. After a number of conversations and a little research, they call Dad with their consensus: "Now that Mom's gone, we've been thinking that you should move. Andy knows of a wonderful place with golf and a swimming pool on the west coast of Florida. It would be just perfect for you. And, if your arthritis gets worse, there is an assisted-living section. It will be much better for you than living in that old house."

The problem is that Dad loves his old house, and he has no intention of moving. The conversation immediately becomes touchy. He feels betrayed and justifiably angry over the fact that discussions are being held about him, as if he were a problem that needed a solution. His children are hurt that he is not happy about this plan they have worked so hard to develop, and annoyed that he refuses to do what is clearly best.

Unless your parent is mentally incompetent, he is still an adult and still in control of his own life. He doesn't need anyone making decisions for him—and certainly not without him. If you are concerned about an aspect of your parent's life, express your concerns, but don't instruct him. Include him in discussions about his future. It is his life, after all.

couple of times. But if she's relatively stable and doesn't have osteoporosis, the benefits of such a routine probably outweigh any risk. Indeed, you might celebrate the fact that she still has such spirit.

Your father might not be willing to sign a durable power of attorney because he is not comfortable relinquishing any power at this point. Perhaps he doesn't truly understand the value of such a document. But his feeling of control, however irrational, may be more important than the legal protection.

Likewise, your parent may be willing to take certain risks in order to stay in her own home. Or she may be unwilling to give up cigarettes. Or she may not want a certain surgery. She may be more interested in living fully than in living longer. Understanding her point of view will help you let go of futile battles.

You are wasting your energy and perhaps not helping your parent by pushing and pushing. It's annoying and, at times, terrifying, but once you've tried all you can try, there is little you can do about it. For your own sake, as much as your parent's, let it go. For a while, at least.

For now, make other arrangements whenever possible. Do what you can to reduce any risk. Find other options. And learn to live with her decision.

In time, raise the issue again. See if her thoughts have changed.

The question of when to intervene can get tricky when a person lingers in the gray area between competency and incompetence. Or when a behavior is not life-threatening but still very serious (say, your mother is handing out chunks of cash to "that nice mail carrier," or buying into minor financial scams).

If you face a troubling situation and don't know how much to intervene, ask a geriatric care manager who is well versed in these matters. These professionals can help you determine the true level of risk and your parent's competency, as well as help come up with solutions. You can hire a geriatric care manager, or find a case manager who may offer free guidance, through a local hospital's social work or geriatric department or through your area's agency on aging. (For more on geriatric care managers, see page 149.)

If you can't find a solution and your parent's life is in danger, call Adult Protective Services, which is part of the Department of Social Services.

> *Very late one night as I was returning to the city, I saw an elderly man I knew getting off the train. He was very frail, and I was astonished to see that he was not only traveling alone, but that no one was there to meet him at the station. I took him home in a taxi, and he seemed very grateful.*
>
> *I was furious at his kids, affluent people whom I also knew slightly, for letting him travel on his own at that hour. I hated to think what might have happened to him, out alone in the city so late at night.*
>
> *A few years later, when my own father became old and frail, he insisted on traveling on his own. He wouldn't put up with our telling him that it wasn't safe, and we finally realized that we couldn't cover his activities in a way that made us feel secure. I understood the man's kids for the first time and felt foolish that I'd been so self-righteous and critical. What can you do? You have to contain your anxiety. You have no choice."*
>
> —SARA B.

To find the office near your parent, call the area agency on aging (see page 628). Adult Protective Services will generally send a nurse or social worker to your parent's home to determine the risks and find ways to protect your parent from harm.

Defusing Old Struggles

This may not be the time to enter into therapy with your parent. He's sick. You're a wreck. And time is running out. It's all you can do to just get from one day to the next.

Of course, if you have the time and energy and think it might help resolve some conflicts, go for it. Find a therapist and talk it out, on your own or, if possible, with your parent. Sorting through some of the struggles in this relationship may help you survive and perhaps even grow during this stressful time. After all, this is a primal bond; it is the basis of all the other bonds in your life. Understanding it may help

> *No matter how difficult she is or how much we disagree, I can't shut her out. Never. It would be like shutting something in myself out. She needs me now tremendously. The most I'll miss is about three days, and then I have to see her or call her.*
>
> *There must be something so deep in this relationship between mothers and daughters, more than we can ever realize. We're so connected, even when we're so different."*
>
> —BETTY H.

strengthen other intimate relationships in your life.

If therapy isn't an option, just take a look at some of the tensions involved. Parent-child relationships are, obviously, complex, even when the parent is well into her nineties and the "child" is in her seventies. The issues, for some reason, don't fade away and, at times like this, can grow only larger. Even strong relationships come with little buttons and nagging questions. *Why does she irritate me so much? Why does he set me off like this? Why does he say things like that?*

Even a quick review and some insight may help you find a little peace, patience, and forgiveness.

◆ **Pinpoint the problem.** What is it that troubles you about your parent and the way you relate to him? What is it that you want and are not getting? What exasperates you, and why does it affect you so much? Think very carefully about this. Try to be precise. Does your parent's personality bother you because it is grating, because it has stood in the way of your being close, or because you see the same trait in yourself? Do you withdraw from your mother's helplessness because it places too much of a burden on you or because it has caused you to become painfully self-sufficient? Do you cringe because of the way your father behaves now or because you still feel wounded by something he did in the past?

Or is the root of your anguish simply your parent's power over you?

WHAT HAVE YOU GOT TO LOSE?

I f there is an issue that you've wanted to raise with your parent but you haven't done it, think about what may be stopping you. What's the worst thing that could happen? What do you fear? Are you afraid of breaking some unwritten family rule? *We don't talk about Dad's drinking. We don't discuss their divorce.* Are you afraid that your parent will be hurt, get angry, or be disappointed in you? Are you worried about getting into the kind of painful argument that always ends in tears? Are you afraid of hearing what your parent has to say, or of losing your role as the child?

Weigh the potential cost and gain of raising the subject or leaving it alone. Then decide which way you want to go. If you leave it alone, do so because you have considered the matter and made a conscious decision, not because you put it off or avoided it. Then, try to accept the consequences of your decision and move on.

Few of us adequately break away from our parents; instead, we continue to fight for autonomy well into our own old age. Perhaps the real trouble lies not in your parent's actions, but in your own need to sever childhood ties.

◆ **Tackle some issues.** If your parent is able to take part in this, and there is a specific issue you want to deal with—a recurring argument or an unresolved conflict—go ahead and try. You may get somewhere, but even if you don't, you will find some peace of mind in knowing that you tried, that you broke the Code of Silence and did what you could to settle the matter.

Keep your expectations low. If the subject is taboo or deeply painful, you may want to do this with a ther-apist who specializes in family relationships. However you choose to handle it, here are a few thoughts that might help:

◆ Bring up the topic at a time when you are calm. Instead of jumping into a heated discussion just when your mother has said the one thing that really exasperates or hurts you, wait until the emotional climate is more temperate.

◆ Stay composed. If you are confrontational or accusatory, or simply hysterical, you will only put your parent on the defensive, and blaming her will prevent you from moving forward.

As a general rule, use statements that begin with "I" rather than those that begin with "You." Instead of telling your mother that she is never

For years I thought I would finally have a really wonderful relationship with my mother. I envied people who had such relationships, and I was sure that I could have one too. But I've gotten a little more perspective on that. I'm doing the best I can by my mother, but I realize that we can never be close. We are just too different from one another.

Now I don't expect her to understand me. I used to open up to her, tell her something that I felt deeply or was upset by, and she would say, 'But you're doing fine, aren't you?' And that would be the end of it. She would end the conversation. She doesn't want to hear about any of the darker sides of my life. It makes her anxious, and she needs me to be happy and effervescent. But I don't expect intimate conversations anymore. And things are much better between us. The less need I bring to this, the better it is for the relationship."

—KAREN L.

satisfied and that she manipulates you, tell her that you often feel guilty and how bad that feels. Ask her if she ever felt that way around her mother, and if so, how she handled it.

◆ Avoid old arguments. Steer the conversation away from familiar eddies with a history of going nowhere. As soon as you sense things slipping into old patterns, change the topic.

◆ Let go of unreasonable hopes. There will be issues, especially those having to do with your parent's personality or past events, that you can't change. You can make an effort, but do so with minimal expectations. And then, try to let go of whatever it is.

Personality traits are hard to change at any age, but they tend to become only more fixed later in life, and for some reason this seems to be particularly true of less desirable traits. Someone who is gentle, giving, and selfless may become more saintly as the years pass, but more often someone who is a little trying will become very difficult indeed.

A parent who has never asked you about your life or your feelings is not apt to get to know you now. A parent who has been frugal with compliments is not likely to shower, or even sprinkle, you with praise. A parent who has been needy may be only more needy now. And a parent who has avoided a specific topic for a lifetime will be hard-pressed to venture into painful territory at this stage of life.

Of course, somewhere in your logical mind, you know all this, but accepting it in your heart can be wrenching. Recognizing that your parent won't change means accepting that this will never be the kind of relationship that you wanted. All of us want, deeply and profoundly, to have a loving, intimate bond with a parent,

WHAT DOES HE WANT FROM ME?

You have just spent the day racing around your parent's house, doing her laundry, changing the bed, and fixing her dinner. Two days later, she says that you never visit her. What's a daughter to do?

It may be that your parent doesn't want more of your time, just more of you. That is, your company and affection may be more important to her than clean socks and hot meals. So while you are busy as a bee, she is feeling ignored. Later, she wonders why she never sees you because, the truth is, she hasn't seen you.

The dilemma is that these tasks have to be done and, truth be told, it may be easier to be in the kitchen cooking than in the living room sitting with your parent. Find a compromise—a little time in the laundry room, a few minutes by her side. Or talk with her while you fold the laundry. Also, ask your parent what household chores she most wants done, and then cut out some of the others. By addressing her most fundamental needs for companionship and affection, you will be giving her far more help, and you may head off some of the I-never-see-you laments.

If she still complains that you don't visit enough, avoid arguing—*I was here just two days ago! What do you want from me?* Simply reassure her that you love her and that you will come to see her again as soon as you can. Her comments are more a reflection of her loneliness and insecurity than a criticism of you.

one that is based on mutual respect and trust. Accepting that such a tie will never exist, at least not in the way you believe it should, is almost like accepting the death of your parent—the parent you had hoped for and the parent you can never have.

Recognizing all this may leave you feeling intensely alone, and perhaps betrayed. But accepting, and then mourning, this loss allows you to move on. Once you let go of your hopes, you can stop struggling to make this relationship into something it isn't. And once you stop looking to your parent for approval and validation, you are free to get these things from yourself.

Ironically, when you no longer have any expectations, you may find that your relationship with your parent develops new strengths. You may notice qualities in your parent that you never saw before. Without that old tension,

> *After my father died, I found his old letters and journals, and as I read them I realized that there was this whole other side of him that I never knew, a sensitive and caring and emotional side that he never, even once, revealed to me. It makes me sad because I keep thinking, if only I had known this part of him, we might have had a very different relationship."*
>
> —ALICIA B.

your parent may be able to appreciate certain qualities in you for the first time. You may find that you actually enjoy what is, rather than constantly feeling cheated by what isn't.

◆ **Learn about him**. Sometimes we expect our parents to understand and respect us for who we are, but we fail to give them the same courtesy. While there is still time—if there is still time—get to know your parent, really know him, as an individual. Ask your father about his life—his upbringing, his parents, his childhood home, his schooling, his friends, and his loves. Ask him about his dreams, travels, successes, failures, challenges, hardships, and role models.

Get him to tell you stories he's never told you or to add new details to the old stories. Next time he begins a story that you've heard many times before, rather than rolling your eyes in exasperation and walking out of the room, nudge him to tell a different angle of the story, or ask why that moment in time was so important to him. Find out about his life and his history, because it will tell you so much about him, about your relationship, and about yourself.

While you are at it, get him to talk about his current situation. Perhaps he is grieving losses or afraid of what he believes his future now holds. Is growing old what he thought it would be? What makes him happy now?

Hearing about your parent's past, getting to know what makes him who he is, understanding something about how he feels now, all of this should help you to see your parent as an individual. You will begin to see him as both strong and vulnerable, a person who did the best he could by you and who is still doing the best he can.

It won't change what has happened, but it might help you to let go of some anger and be more forgiving. It might give you a little more patience and tolerance. And it might just help him to see you as an individual.

Sometimes learning about a person like this, really for the first time, will also take conversations into directions and topics that you never expected.

If your parent is able and willing to open up as a result of your gentle probing, these talks will be enjoyable for him. Not only does he get to talk about himself, which is glorious, he gets to pass his stories, and his life, on to future generations. Finally, he will feel heard, and he will know that you care, really care.

◆ **Stop blaming.** Whatever your mother did in the past is done. She probably intended to be a good parent, just as you want to be a good parent to your own children. If you need an apology, or if you think it would make you feel better if you told her what you are feeling, then discuss the subject with her, but do it carefully.

Not only is the past over, but your parent has a lot on her plate right now. Yes, whatever is troubling you might be painful for her, too. But beyond that, she may be at a point in her life where she is letting go of the past. She may be spending her emotional energy preparing for what lies ahead. Try to let it be.

◆ **Improve thyself.** Even though your parent may not be able or willing to change, you still can. It's a major step to accept who he is—even accept that you may not ever understand exactly why he is the way he is—and let it be. Work on your own personality and relationships. Learn from his mistakes and be more open, honest, loving, or tolerant yourself.

In other words, you are not your parent. You are your own person, and you make your own choices.

Managing Day-to-Day

Moving from the big picture to the small picture, if your parent has a trait or habit that makes your chest tighten and your shoulders tense,

> ❝ *My mother is very dependent, always has been, but she never says thank-you or shows any appreciation or cares that she is putting you out. I said to her, 'Mom, don't you realize what you are putting us through? Don't you realize the anxiety and worry that you cause?' And she said, 'That's your problem.'*
>
> *I had to laugh at that. I mean, she's your mother. What are you going to do?"*
>
> —RHODA B.

there are steps you can take, day-to-day, to ease the stress and lower your blood pressure.

◆ **Pass by the hooks.** Find ways to ignore those little comments or looks that make you so hopping mad. Pretend you are a fish swimming along a mountain stream on a beautiful day and that you spot a fat, scrumptious worm. It lures you, but you are no dummy. You know that there's a big, sharp hook behind it. You have two choices: Bite at the hook and get hurt, or swim on by and enjoy your day.

Next time your parent says something that makes your blood pressure rise, say to yourself, "Aha, that is a hook, and as much as I am drawn to it, I have no intention of biting." Swim on by. Count how many hooks you pass by (one is awfully good) and then try to do better the next time. It will be your own inner victory. With each hook you pass, unfazed and unaffected, you win.

◆ **Pause before responding.** When your parent does or says something that's abrasive, count to ten before responding. Take a deep breath, and then exhale slowly as you count. That brief pause will help you to stay calm and give you a moment to consider your response (and decide whether you will pass by that hook).

◆ **Recognize your habits.** How do you typically react to problems in this relationship? Do you become angry and combative? Do you withdraw? Or do you tense up? Do you throw yourself into your work? Do you take it out on other people? Or do you head straight for the nearest quart of ice cream?

Once you're aware of your reaction, you will be better prepared to alter it. If you start yelling at the children or shutting out your friends, ask yourself, "What is this about?" Perhaps you'll notice that it's not about the kids being demanding, but about your visit with your mother that afternoon.

◆ **Forget victory.** Instead of trying to win a fight with your parent, make it your goal simply to end the discussion peacefully. That will be a true victory. Rather than saying, once again, "Why do you always bring up that same story? Why can't you just let it go?" say, in your calmest voice: "You know, whenever you tell that story, we end up in an argument. I really don't want to fight with you. I want to have a nice time with you. I wonder if there's some way we can either resolve or avoid this discussion. What do you think?"

◆ **Head for new ground.** If you find yourself falling into the same uncomfortable or annoying ruts with your parent, change the pattern. Play cards, go for a walk, talk about something new, or plan your visits for a different place and time. If you always visit in the evening when your parent is tired or has had a drink, stop by in the morning instead. If you always visit in her bedroom, bring her down to the living room or go out for lunch. The change may do you both good.

◆ **Reward yourself.** Ignoring the hooks, staying calm, avoiding old fights, and generally being more tolerant are no small feats. They require enormous patience and personal strength. Reward yourself for a job well done. Buy yourself a little present, treat yourself to a bubble bath, take a drive in the country, immerse yourself in some activity that has nothing to do with your parent and her illness.

◆ **Introduce your parent to you, the adult.** If you constantly fall into the childhood role you played in the family, pull your parent into your adulthood. If she is mobile, take her with you to your office or bring her to a local meeting in which you are involved. It's easier to be you on your own turf. If she is less mobile, introduce her to your friends, show her your latest business report, or bring her some of your artwork. Let her see you as an adult, be firm in your resolve to act as an adult, and she may start to think of you as one and treat you accordingly.

◆ **Adjust your expectations.** Not just your grand expectations about this relationship, but your hopes about each visit, about holiday gatherings, about family togetherness. Lower your expectations to as close to zero as possible.

If you envision your family as a Norman Rockwell painting, you are doomed to disappointment. Likewise, if you approach your parent's door poised for a fight, it will probably happen. Family arguments can be ignited simply because you are primed for them. When it happens, you explode. *I knew that's what you would say. You always. . . .*

When you visit, keep your mind open and let things go as they will. Enjoy what's good and try not to make too much of the bad.

◆ **Resort to humor.** Humor is the great defuser. When things are getting hot, a little lightness, as long as it is not mean, can temper the heat instantly. When your father makes the same critical remark or complains, yet again, about your lack of devotion, be prepared with a light response. When things head into a familiar impasse, tell him a joke or a funny story. Find hysterical movies to watch together. Read humorous books aloud. Laughing together will break many barriers.

◆ **Make note of the good times.** When you have a wonderful visit or a moment of closeness, share a warm hug, or receive a rare word of praise or thanks, don't sell it short. Make a note on your calendar or write a brief description of it, and keep it close at hand. It will help get you through the tougher times.

While you are at it, write a little note to your parent about that special moment or warm feeling you shared. Mail it or leave it by her bed. When a relationship is tense, this is an opportunity to connect in a positive way.

Exceptionally Difficult Parents

There is no scale for rating difficulty when it comes to eldercare. Who has the most challenging parent? What situation is most taxing? There's no way to judge. Indeed, caring for a saint can be tough when she's your parent. She doesn't want to be a bother, she doesn't tell you what she needs, and you're busy with a million other things. And let's remember that even the nicest parents can become irascible when they are debilitated, confused, sick, afraid, depressed, and in pain. Then those thorny parent-child issues come into play. Basically, it's all a challenge.

Nevertheless, some parents are doozies. They refuse to accept help or need constant attention. They cannot be left alone or don't want anyone around. The aides stink. The food stinks. Life stinks. And they want you to know it, over and over again.

Many of the tips already offered in this chapter should help, but here

MEDICAL ALERT

Bad moods and annoying behaviors may signal depression or other mental health problems. Unremitting orneriness, social withdrawal, refusal to eat or see friends, frequent complaints and criticisms, can all signal depression, which is common among the elderly. Have your parent tested and appropriately treated. (See page 281 for more on depression.)

Sometimes these behaviors are also signs of early dementia. Discuss the symptoms with her doctor and, if necessary, have her tested or take her to a geriatric assessment center.

are some additional thoughts for truly extreme cases.

As we've noted, complaining or criticizing is often misdirected, so it's important that you find out what is underlying your parent's grumpiness. Your mother says she hates your clothes, but it may be because they remind her that you used to go shopping together, and now she can't do that, or because she can no longer wear clothes that have those small buttons. Your father says you don't visit enough, but it may be because he is afraid of being abandoned. Your mother says she hates the dinner you made, but perhaps it's because she misses cooking for herself. Your parent claims that you stole her money, but maybe it's because she is becoming forgetful and explains away these lapses by blaming you.

See if you can't get to the root of the anger or bitterness or neediness. Ask your mother why she hated the dinner. What would be her perfect dinner, and where would she have it? Ask her what she used to like to cook and who she liked to cook for.

It's vital that you remain calm. Remember the hooks. Know them. Watch for them. Do not go there. You do not want to become a bickering, battling, angry person. Rise above it. Your calm response may catch your parent off guard; she was looking for a fight, and you've taken the wind out of her disgruntled sails.

Silence in this case, in particular, truly is golden. You don't need to respond to anything immediately. When your parent gripes, be quiet for a moment. It gives you time to calm yourself and gives your parent an opening to delve into some fears or concerns that may be behind her comments. When she goes at you, demanding that you say something, simply answer that you are thinking about what she's said. Eventually, she may actually tell you why she's really complaining.

Rather than disagreeing with your parent or pushing him to change, let him know that you hear what he is saying and that you understand, or are trying to understand, what he is feeling and all he is going through.

For example, next time your father accuses you of neglecting him and says that you don't love him, just listen quietly, let him know that you hear him, and even encourage him to explain his comments—*It must be very hard living here alone. I imagine it would be nice to have someone else around and more visitors. I'm sorry things are this way right now.*

If particular activities or situations tend to trigger battles between the two of you, avoid those activities. Find new things to do together. Rather than sitting in his living room, bickering with each other, go to a movie or a friend's house. Rather than talking about his health, pull out a photo album and get him to tell you about some better time in his life.

Sometimes complaining, calling constantly, or becoming sick at just the wrong moment (for example, when you are about to leave on vacation) is a way to control other people. Your parent complains, and you come running, or cancel your vacation, or tell him he doesn't have to move after all. He got what he wanted. And so he complains more, or needs you more, or ruins your next vacation as well. He controls so little in his life these days, and this behavior works to his advantage. He may not be doing it consciously or maliciously. It just happens.

However, don't fall victim to it. Set firm, clear limits as to what you will do for your parent, and stick to them. Don't cancel your vacation or leave work for the eighth time this week.

> " *The difficult thing for me is the nonstop talking. I've heard the same conversation over and over, the same exact stories. My mother is a compulsive talker, and those are long hours.*
>
> *What I do now when I'm visiting is to ration myself. After I've been with her for a while, listening to her talk, I'll either go out and take a long, long walk by myself, which is great, or I'll try to get her out of the house. This is a new thing, and it works quite well. I now get her out every day.*
>
> *It was so important to break that pattern of sitting in the living room, with her in her chair and me on the couch, opposite each other. It opened things up a little.*"
>
> —ANNE C.

Next time your mother gripes that you are a lousy daughter and don't do enough for her, stay calm (always calm). Do not get into a shouting match. And do not rearrange your life to do more for her. Rather, let her know that you heard her, and then acknowledge her feelings. Give her a hug. Tell her that you will see her next week. And then depart as planned.

Between 2 and 5 percent of elderly people living in the community (that is, not in nursing homes and other facilities, where the rate is higher) are excessively suspicious or paranoid, or have delusions about people trying to harm them. They may believe that their children are cheating them or planning to desert them. They may believe people are stealing things or giving them dangerous medicines.

Once again, stay calm. Listen. Be empathetic. But at some point, you need to seek professional help for your parent. Do not try to reason with her or argue with her no matter how irrational she is. Let her talk about her concerns and why she feels the way she does. Let her know that you hear her. *It must be very frightening to feel that way. What else worries you?*

Then get her to a good doctor, preferably a psychiatrist who has a lot of experience with elderly people. Drugs are often effective in treating excessive anxiety, paranoia, delusions, or suspiciousness. But drugs for the elderly must be prescribed with great care, keeping doses low and balancing any unwanted side effects.

At least 5 percent of people over sixty-five suffer from hypochondria or a related problem called "undifferentiated somatoform disorder." In the first, called hypochondriasis, a person is obsessed with the idea that he has a serious illness. In the latter, a person complains about symptoms (fatigue, abdominal pain, loss of appetite, etc.) that have no medical basis.

Obviously, you must be sure that your parent isn't actually sick. Then find an experienced doctor who is both sympathetic and firm. Psychotherapy is generally not all that helpful in these situations, so a good doctor is your best bet. He or she must steer your parent away from unnecessary tests and treatments, but treat certain symptoms, such as insomnia or pain. Appointments should be regular, but brief and to the point.

Keep in mind that even though symptoms may not have a biological basis, they are still real. Just because your parent gets upset whenever you are away, and her anxiety leads to nausea, that doesn't mean that she isn't really nauseated. Be sympathetic, but don't reinforce the behavior (i.e., canceling your business trip because she has abdominal pain).

Your parent is not being mean; she is afraid and sad, and she is trying to regain control of her life in any way she can. Let her know that you are sorry she feels so horrible and make arrangements for someone to check on her while you're gone.

Whatever your situation, every caregiver needs to pay utmost attention to the next chapter. When dealing with a particularly difficult parent, caring for yourself is the only way to retain some sanity for yourself.

CARING FOR THE CAREGIVER

Setting Limits • The Male Caregiver
• Emotional Minefields • When One Parent Is Well
• 12 Steps to a Healthy Mind-Set

THOUGH IT MAY SEEM TO BE A CONTRADICTION, CARING for yourself during this time is the most important thing you can do—both for you and for your parent. And yet, it is the one thing most caregivers fail to do.

Don't flip past this chapter too quickly, thinking that you simply don't have time for such things. *My mother needs me. I can't worry about myself right now. I'll be fine.* Your parent's care can easily consume an ever-expanding part of your life. It may begin with a few calls here, some visits there, and questions for doctors and lawyers. Then, more visits. More worrying. More phone calls. Before you know it—and sometimes without your even realizing it—you are too busy for friends, distant from your spouse, distracted at work, and constantly trying to shake a cold.

You cannot take good care of your parent if you are not taking care of yourself. The stress and strain of caregiving makes people exhausted, irritable, isolated, depressed, resentful, and, more often than you imagine, physically sick. (More than sick; it actually increases mortality rates.) In such a state, you will be of little use to your parent. Numerous studies show that the caregivers who offer the best care to their parents are the ones who take care of themselves and take advantage of available help and support.

Setting Limits

If there were such a thing as Caregivers Anonymous, the first step in the program would be getting rid of that little voice inside you that says, "I can do it all. I am responsible for everything, and, whatever I do, it's never enough."

Of course you want to make your parent well, make her happy, make her safe. In fact, if it were possible for you to be with her every minute of the day, perhaps you would be. This is your parent, after all. But the truth is that you can't personally do everything that needs to be done for her, and trying to do so will only exhaust and frustrate you without really helping your parent over the long haul.

So how do you use your energies most effectively? If your mother has a sudden and severe illness, of course you'll want to be there. But when her needs are more chronic, when you find yourself taking on more and more responsibility over a matter of months or even years, you must step back, take a realistic look at the situation, and establish some boundaries for yourself.

Determine what you can reasonably do for your parent and, more important, what you have to stop trying to do. As hard as this is, you may be surprised to discover that setting some limits will relieve your guilt and ease some tension. And you will have more patience and energy for those things that only you can give.

◆ **Examine your motivation.** Why are you helping your parent? It sounds like an odd question, but it's a healthy one to mull over. Do you view your parent's care as a burden that was dumped upon you? Do you feel that you have a duty to care for her? *She's my mother, after all.* Or are you helping because, given your parent's situation and your feelings for her, this is what you choose to do?

If you are running in circles caring for your parent because you are hoping to get the praise, respect, or love you never had before, you're headed for disappointment. This relationship isn't likely to change at this point, especially not in that direction. In fact, you may find that you are criticized more than ever now.

If you are trying to repay your parent for all she did during your

> *For a long time, I visited my mother twice a week, but I was always running and always tired. I started to dread each visit, and I was angry with her because I felt it was all her fault. She was ruining my life.*
>
> *Then a friend said to me, 'This isn't her fault. It's your fault.' And, you know, she was right."*
>
> —FRAN M.

childhood, think about the reality of that. While you may have a duty to be sure your parent is safe, fed, clothed, and sheltered, there is no *quid pro quo* between your childhood and her senior years. Raising a child, and all the labor and constant attention it entails, is not a debt anyone ever intended for you to repay.

Some people work around the clock caring for a parent because they are trying to make up for lost time, or because they believe they are fending off illness and death.

Perhaps you feel, on some unconscious level, that this is what "good people" do, "good girls" in particular. If you don't do it, others will think badly of you.

Your motivation may be complicated, but take a moment to think about it, consider your options, and make a conscious choice about your involvement in your parent's care. Then, accept this as your choice, something you decided to do, not as something your parent or an unfair world has dumped on you. The work you do for your parent will still be difficult, and it may still seem a bit unfair, but it will feel more like an interruption and less like an imposition. It will be a conscious decision that is more about love and family and less about old debts and unmet needs.

◆ **Identify your parent's needs.** You know what needs to be done, but what on that list is essential? What does your parent really need, and what is a luxury or perceived need? Does she need you at her house every afternoon? Does she need help with bathing and dressing? Make a checklist of her real needs—the musts—and then a second list of what would be nice—the extras.

This is not as simple as it sounds. Your parent might need someone to make or deliver meals because she can't cook for herself. She may need someone to clean her house because she can't do it herself, but this doesn't have to happen weekly. In fact, how often it needs cleaning is a matter of judgment. It might be more important that she sees her grandchildren or gets out for some fresh air occasionally.

Writing it all down, and perhaps getting her input, will help you to see what is crucial and what is not. You can then determine what is necessary, what is valuable, and what can be skipped.

◆ **Accept and enlist help, early.** Love and devotion can only come from you. Other care can come from others. Don't hesitate to ask others to help, use community services, and hire workers.

Siblings, in particular, should be called on right away. They might have different ideas about your father's care or different ways of doing things, but they have a right to care for him. Besides, he needs them now. You need them, too. If you begin this as a family effort when the tasks are smaller, you will have each other further down the road when the needs and responsibilities tend to be more monumental. (See page 170 for more on dealing with siblings.)

" I used to spend hours trying to convince my parents to move out of their big house and to organize their finances. But they didn't do anything. They would ask me questions and listen and act like they were going to do something about it. But they never did.

And then I realized, they are not going to change. They are not going to move until something forces them to. And there is nothing I can do about it. It was terribly difficult to back off. You want so much to help, and you know things are only going to get worse. It took me three years to give up and let go, and I still struggle with it sometimes. I just have to go along and see what happens next."

—DIANE P.

If you don't have siblings, or your siblings can't or won't help for some reason, draw on neighbors, aunts, uncles, cousins, local volunteers, and friends. When more help is needed, sign your parent up for meal delivery, housekeeping, adult day care, and other local services. It's important that you get your parent hooked up with such supports early because it gives him time to get used to them before his health declines further, and it makes him less dependent upon a sole caregiver—you.

Caregivers are often reluctant to use outside help. They feel they should do it themselves. They wait until they are at their wits' end to ask, and by then, they and their parents have already suffered needlessly. Worse, they sometimes can't get the services they need because of paperwork and waiting lists. So seek help early.

Let other people give *you* a hand as well—someone might pick up your dog at the vet, bring over a casserole, water your plants, or stay with your parent on occasion so you can get some rest.

◆ **Rein yourself in.** Once you've established a network of helpful family members and community services, be candid with yourself in determining what it is that you actually need to do yourself. Day-to-day, your parent's care may seem more pressing than other matters in your life—everything you do for your parent at this point may seem essential—but think about it. Visiting your mother every day may be ideal, but wouldn't she be okay with fewer visits? (Don't base this on what she says; determine it for yourself.) Try to distinguish between your anxiety about your parent's welfare and the real demands of the situation.

As you decide what's truly necessary, consider what you may be ignoring or giving up because of your parent's care. Are you willing to jeopardize your own health? Neglect your children? Damage your career? You may decide to skip a trip to Florida because your father is in the hospital, but when he is in the midst of a prolonged illness, should you cancel a special dinner out with your husband or miss a deadline at work?

Create a pared-down schedule for yourself that meets your parent's most pressing needs—the things that only you can do for her—while still respecting your own needs. Even if you live with your parent, set some parameters—what hours you will be with her each day, which tasks you will do for her. Schedule time away from her just for yourself.

Be conservative in your plan; it always feels better to increase your commitment than to decrease it. Don't promise to make three visits a week or a month if that puts you over the edge; keep it at two.

◆ **Let go of futile efforts.** Don't waste precious energy trying to get your parent to change her ways if it's clear that she won't. Talk with your parent about your concerns, get others to help in the effort, and show

> ❝ *When I retired, I didn't tell my mother. I didn't want her to think I was more available, that I had more time for her. I had been taking care of her for several years, and when I retired, I realized there was a lot that I wanted to do for myself, a lot that I had neglected because of her.*
>
> *I told her that I was working from home more, in case she called and found me there, but I didn't tell her that I had retired. And I have never regretted it.*"
>
> —BARBARA F.

her other options. If she still won't budge, and she is mentally competent, you may have to give up. There is no point in banging your head against a wall.

For example, if you are spending a lot of time researching group homes for the elderly, and your mother has absolutely no intention of moving, at some point you need to stop the hunt and get on with more productive tasks, like safeguarding her house and finding community and in-home assistance.

You may feel that you have failed. But you haven't. Your mother may be in a somewhat risky situation. She may fall or run out of money. But you have done all you can, and you cannot do anything more. You can't blame yourself if your parent's decisions are, in your mind, poor ones. (See page 28 for more on when to intervene.)

THE MALE CAREGIVER

Men are more involved in eldercare than they used to be, although the shift is occurring slowly. While husbands care for elderly wives, most of the grown children who provide regular, hands-on care for an aging parent are still, unfortunately, daughters. Women not only care for their own parents, but they care for their aging in-laws as well.

Sons help, to be sure, and, as a population, they are helping far more than they used to. Some are even providing the full scope of care. But men generally help with "hands-off" care, like finances, legal matters, transportation, and hiring outside help. They might do some shopping and home maintenance for their parents. But daughters are usually the primary caregivers and handle most of the hands-on care, like dressing, bathing, feeding, toileting, and just plain being present.

As men join the caregiving workforce and take on more and more tasks, it is becoming clear that they have very different approaches and issues than women do. Some things they do better; some things, worse.

Because most men grew up in an environment where women played the role of primary caregiver, they tend to be a little slow in getting involved and, once there, question their competency as caregivers. They feel helpless and uncertain. They don't know what to do or how to begin. It's a new and unfamiliar role.

Most sons are also reluctant to provide personal care—such as helping a parent to bathe or dress—or even to talk about such issues. They will, however, go grocery shopping or figure out how to get Mom to her doctor's appointment, and they might even make some meals.

The research available suggests that men are often reluctant or unwilling to let others know that they are caring for a parent. They are particularly silent at work, fearful perhaps that revealing the situation will hurt their careers.

They are also less willing to get emotional support when they feel overwhelmed. They don't talk with their male friends about the stresses of parentcare or join support groups as readily as women do. Likewise, they are less likely to talk with a doctor or other professional about depression or anxiety, or to take medication for it. Instead, they turn to alcohol (bad), work longer hours (bad), or release their stress on a playing field (good).

There are aspects of parentcare that men do better than their female counterparts. Men are more apt to deal with issues matter-of-factly. They see a problem, take it head-on, find solutions, and plan ahead. *What is the issue? What do I need to do to solve it? Who do I need to call? What services do I need?*

Sons are generally better at getting outside help, using community services, hiring outsiders, and delegating responsibilities. While a son is more apt to hire home-care workers right away, a daughter might feel that she should do it all herself and that she doesn't need help or doesn't want to bother people.

The sexes need to take lessons from each other. While women should try to foresee problems, delegate, and get help with daily tasks earlier (and they might even benefit from a good game of hoops now and then), men need to learn to talk and find support when the going gets tough.

Some support groups are tailored just for men, and these can be very useful. If a support group is too touchy-feely, online support groups provide anonymity and don't require that you leave the house or office. (See page 54 for more on support groups.)

Letting go of hopeless crusades is an enormous accomplishment. You and your parent can accept life as it is and work within existing parameters.

◆ **Learn to say no.** Caregivers are often as bad at saying no to requests for help as they are at saying yes to offers of help. Learn to say no to your parent, certainly, but also learn to say no to yourself. It may be your own psyche and your own needs that drive you to do more than you can handle, while your parent may be okay with less help, with assistance from a community service, and with fewer visits.

Women, in particular, often have trouble saying no; they feel they must be the "good girl" or "strong daughter." This martyr syndrome is neither helpful nor good.

Convince yourself that saying no to certain things is not only okay, but necessary. Practice. Try it out on the dog. Say no to the mirror. Just get the word out.

Confronted with a parent's escalating needs, you may learn, perhaps for the first time in your life, how to act on your own behalf.

◆ **Stick to your guns.** Sure, you can decide to cut back on some visits, even put a plan in writing, but how do you stick to it, especially if you have a parent who questions your plan or criticizes you for not doing enough?

Say you decide that your marriage needs more attention, but just as you

> *The last time I went to my support group, this woman was talking about her father, who has dementia. She was taking care of him twenty-four hours a day, and she was so warm and had such a nice sense of humor about it all that I thought, 'This woman is a saint.' It made me feel terrible."*
>
> —LINDA K.

and your spouse settle in for a quiet evening together, the first in weeks, you find yourself wondering if your father is all right and feeling guilty for not being with him. You're short with your husband when he asks what's troubling you, and end up calling your father, just to check in.

Be firm in your resolve. If you decide that you are not going to concern yourself with your father's financial affairs anymore because you have handed that job over to another family member, don't spend an evening researching home equity loans. If you've told your mother you cannot be interrupted during work, and she continues to call hourly, remind her quickly and gently that this is not the time to talk and that you'll call her when you get home. Then hang up. (Be aware, however, that this constant need for reassurance may be an early sign of dementia.)

Important: Don't be unduly influenced by how someone else is handling a comparable situation. Just because a friend sees her mother every weekend and once during the week doesn't mean that you should change your schedule. Just because your cousin cared for her mother at home for twelve years and is critical that you aren't doing the same, don't be apologetic. Every situation is different; every relationship is different. Only you can create the right balance for yourself. Find it and keep to it.

Emotional Minefields

Taking care of yourself, simply surviving parentcare, requires that you deal with some potent emotions. Believe it or not, reactions you are experiencing now, even the ones that seem disturbingly out of character for you, illogical or childish, are normal and quite common. And most of them can be tempered once you recognize what it is you are feeling and why.

GUILT AND HELPLESSNESS

THESE ARE THE CONSTANT COMPANIONS of caregivers, with women more often plagued by guilt and men more often frustrated by feelings of helplessness. Women seem to have inherited a burden of guilt from their mothers, and their grandmothers before them. *I'm not doing enough, I'm not doing it right, I should have done something else.* Men, on the other

THOSE UNTHINKABLE THOUGHTS

M any people caring for an aged parent wish, at some point along the way, that their parent would die. It may be a fleeting thought or a constant presence. Either way, it can be very disturbing.

If you are hoping that your father will die soon because he is terminally ill and his existence is pretty miserable, then you shouldn't have any guilt about such thoughts. They are normal and, in most cases, merciful.

The trouble comes when you are wishing that your parent would die because he is overbearing, because he is a burden, because you want an inheritance, or because you are simply tired of waiting and wondering. In other words, you want him to die not for his sake, but for yours. This is a common and natural reaction, but it is jolting when the thought first comes into your mind, and it can produce a great deal of guilt and shame.

Caring for a frail parent, even if you are not providing hands-on care, is draining on many levels. Since there is really no other possible outcome, it is natural to want the struggle to end, for everybody's sake. You are not a bad person for feeling this way. You are only human.

hand, tend to want to fix problems, and they become exasperated when problems can't be fixed. In general, they also aren't as experienced as women in the hands-on care and empathy that is required when a parent is frail or sick, so they feel all the more helpless. Whatever your gender, distance can compound feelings of guilt and helplessness.

Getting a grip on these emotions is essential, and you'll have to do so again and again, for they have a habit of resurfacing. Consider for a moment whatever it is that you think you should be doing for your parent and are not. How reasonable are your expectations? Can you real-istically do these tasks? Would performing them help your parent significantly?

Now look at the situation from the opposite perspective. Instead of berating yourself for not doing something, focus on what you *are* doing for your parent. Make a list of these things and be sure to include absolutely everything that you provide—emotional support, regular phone calls, visits, letters, talks with doctors, help with financial matters, assurance that your parent will be cared for in the future and that his wishes will be respected. Recognize and be proud of what you are giving and give it generously. But dump the guilt.

> ❝ *I wish I was there with my father. Absolutely. I saw him a lot over the summer, and that really made me happy. I loved being there for him. But I guess that's easy for me to say from a distance. While I feel a bit at a loss, the grind of being there on a daily basis is very hard on my brother. Because I'm far away, I appreciate each visit, each minute. I am always afraid when I leave that it might be the last time."*
>
> —JANE C.

ANGER AND RESENTMENT

TRY TO DEFUSE ANGER OR RESENTMENT as soon as you recognize it. (Your spouse or kids or siblings might spot it before you do; listen to them.)

Reframe your resentment. That is, rather than wishing that the person or the situation that you resent would change, think about what you can do to change things. If you resent your parent because you are doing too much and missing out on your own life, then back off. Do less. If you resent your spouse for not sympathizing or doing more, talk with him about specific ways in which he can help and exactly what it is you need from him. And then lower your expectations significantly. (Listen, too, to his issues and views.)

Anger is more difficult to deal with because it is so hot and blinding. Be careful. Anger can lead to rash acts and regrettable words, even abuse. When you are angry, try not to take any action right away. Walk away from the situation and wait until you simmer down. Once you're calmer, address the reason for your feelings. You don't want to explode, but you also don't want your anger to implode.

Ask yourself what makes you so stomping mad. What would ease the fury? Can the situation be changed? If not, how can you respond to it differently so you don't become quite so angry the next time?

If you have trouble thinking clearly about this, write about it. Just vent all over the page about how unfair life is and how angry you feel. Writing can help blow off a little steam without burning anyone in the process. It can also, with time, help to clarify some issues—and sometimes, as a result, lead to solutions.

Keep a diary for several months, or just let loose on any handy piece of paper whenever you find yourself on emotional overload. If you are uncomfortable addressing a diary, write a letter to the person who caused the anger and then don't send it. Or direct it at a friend, some made-up therapist or, if you are religious, your particular god. While you write, don't think about sentence structure or grammar or legibility, just scribble down the thoughts as they come to you—and they will come fast once you let it happen. If it's easier, talk into a tape recorder that you keep by the bed or take along in the car.

AROUND AND AROUND WE GO

Don't fall into the anger-guilt-anger cycle. *My mother annoys me. I get angry with her. I feel guilty for getting angry. I resent her for making me feel bad, so I find her even more annoying. Then I get angry. . . .*

Recognize the cycle, determine what gets you on this merry-go-round, and then next time, try to stop it before it starts. If you do get angry, forgive yourself immediately. Don't feel guilty. Snapping at your parent and other emotional outbursts are typical reactions to this kind of stress.

If anger, or the situation that is precipitating it, gets beyond your control, talk to a therapist. Therapy can be enormously helpful in sorting out overwhelming feelings of anger.

SORROW AND GRIEF

PARENTCARE IS, IN THE END, ABOUT loss and grief. You are losing your parent, a little bit at a time. And no matter what that relationship may be, you are likely to be mourning it in some way, on some level. You may be grieving the impending loss of a parent you love, or grieving the relationship you never had with this parent and the loss of any chance of having such a relationship. You may be grieving the loss of your own childhood, even though you're a grown adult.

This grief, called "anticipatory grief," is important to recognize and allow. All of us grieve in our own way, at our own pace. The sadness can be constant, or it may crash over you in waves at odd times. Allow yourself time to grieve. There is nothing weak or selfish about this. And holding in the feelings may make you tense or withdrawn from your parent, when it's the opposite you want.

Take some time away from work. Spend time alone if you feel the need,

---

My mother has always been my best friend, and after my father died, we only became closer. The idea of losing her is too painful for me to bear. She has always been there for me, always understood me. When she is gone, no one will do that for me. I can't imagine my world without her.

Sometimes after I hang up the phone when she sounds down or weak, I feel helpless and sad. I cry so hard that I can't breathe. I guess I'm lucky to have a mother that I love this deeply, but sometimes I think that if I didn't, it wouldn't hurt so much."

—CAROL P.

or share your thoughts with others (friends, support groups, therapists, spouse). Then, while you still have time, let your mother know that you are sad, that you love her, that you will miss her. Don't miss this opportunity to tell her how you feel. (See Chapter Twenty-Six for more on grief.)

SUPPORT GROUPS

MORE THAN ANYTHING ELSE, CARE-giver support or self-help groups help you to see that your situation is not unique, that others face many of the same difficult issues and turbulent feelings. This in itself can be an enormous relief. Because group members are usually strangers, it's a safe arena in which to air intimate problems, vent anger, or talk about feelings you might be ashamed of. And because you all face similar situations, you

> *Sometimes in the evening I reach a point when I think, 'I'd just rather not go out tonight.' But I always come home from the support group feeling better. Because everyone in the group is dealing with someone with dementia, it helps me see that what my mom is doing is perfectly normal for this disease. I also see that what I'm feeling isn't cruel or selfish or crazy. Even if I never see these people again when this is over, I'll never forget them."*
>
> —BARBARA F.

understand each other in a way that others, even best friends, cannot.

Support groups are particularly wonderful for people who feel isolated either because they have no other friends in the same situation or because they aren't interested in opening up to friends, mates, or siblings about the subject. They are also a godsend for people who simply feel overwhelmed by the situation at hand and want to see how others handle it (or fail to handle it). People garner all sorts of helpful caregiving tips at these meetings as well.

The nature of support groups varies widely in terms of purpose and membership, and you may need to try two or three before finding one that meets your needs. Some groups are designed for anyone caring for a sick parent, while others zero in on specific issues—family relationships, Alzheimer's, cancer, grief. Some are set up so people can share practical information and resources, while others function purely as emotional outlets. Some have leaders, others are group led. Although support groups are usually for the caregiver, some encourage the parent to attend as well.

To find a support group, contact your area agency on aging (see page 628), Children of Aging Parents (800-227-7294 or www.caps4caregivers.org), or the National Self-Help Clearinghouse (212-817-1822 or www.selfhelpweb.org). Most nursing homes, adult day-care centers, senior centers, and mental health clinics should also be able to refer you to nearby support groups. If you are

DEEP IN DEPRESSION

 Depression is a physical illness that needs immediate medical attention. The rate of depression among family caregivers is at least twice as high as for the general population. The problem is, studies fail to capture the extent of the problem because caregivers are so caught up in their duties that they fail to report depression to their doctors or get help. There is no question, however, that if you are caring for your parent, you have greatly increased your risk of depression.

If you have symptoms of depression—feelings of extreme sadness, relentless waves of self-criticism, apathy and hopelessness, changes in eating or sleeping habits, trouble concentrating, irritability, teary bouts, thoughts about death—consult a doctor immediately. Depression can be treated effectively with counseling and/or medication. (See page 281 for more on depression.) It may also be avoided or alleviated by many of the tips in this chapter. Take care of yourself. Get some exercise, see friends, talk about your feelings, set realistic goals, do things you enjoy.

For immediate help, call the local crisis intervention, suicide, or depression hotline, or call 911. For information about depression and a referral to a local specialist, contact:

**The National Foundation for Depressive Illness
800-248-4381
www.depression.org**

**The National Mental Health Association
800-969-6642
www.nmha.org**

interested in a specific topic, look in the phone book for the appropriate association, many of which either run support groups themselves or can refer you to one (for example, the Alzheimer's Association, the American Cancer Society, Alcoholics Anonymous).

You can also find a variety of support groups online, which are anonymous and more convenient, albeit a bit less personal.

12 Steps to a Healthy Mind-Set

Setting limits and coping with guilt take a lot of discipline and practice. These emotions can also quickly wear you down, not only mentally,

MAINTAINING A SOCIAL LIFE

If you and your parent live together, you can still have a social life. You just have to be a little flexible.

Leave your parent at home and get a sitter or companion to stay with her, rather than skipping a night out or dragging her into a social situation that will be tiring for her. Even though it may seem like an extravagance (*I don't really have to go out tonight*), make yourself do it. It's a worthwhile investment in your mental health.

If you want your parent to be involved in a social event, have the guests come to your house rather than going out. Home is a more familiar and comfortable setting for your parent. It also means she can leave the room when she needs to rest, without breaking up the party.

Have a potluck supper, with each guest bringing a course, so you're not cooking everything yourself. (If these are good friends, they can help prepare and clean up, too.)

If you decide to cook dinner for guests yourself, make something that's easy to prepare in advance, like lasagna or stew, or put something on the grill. Better yet, buy prepared food or order out. Paper and plastic tableware make for much easier cleanup. (No, they are not great for the environment, but this is a war zone.)

See page 491 for tips on socializing when your parent has dementia.

---

but physically. Here are some other ways to take care of yourself. Think of it as your own 12-Step Caregiver's Anonymous Program.

I *TAKE FIVE*

IF YOU ARE CARING FOR YOUR PARENT on a regular basis, especially if you are living with her, remove yourself completely from the situation once in a while. You need to refuel, and you can't do it without some distance. Do get away before you are too distraught to plan or enjoy such a break.

You might take a vacation—a week or even a couple of days—or you might simply take off an afternoon to sit in the park, see a friend, or have a pedicure. A break can also mean setting aside an hour a few times a week that is all yours, to do as you please. Make arrangements for any necessary fill-in help (a schedule of family, friends, volunteers, home-care workers), or get your parent into a respite program (see page 167).

Then, while you are away, be completely away. Do something just for yourself. Think about something else. Talk about anything else. Clear your head.

2 *A FRIEND INDEED*

WHEN YOU ARE CARING FOR AN AGING parent, quite often the first thing that goes is your social life. Invitations are turned down and friendships are put on hold because you simply do not have the time or the energy for them. If you are living with your parent, social isolation can become a serious problem.

But friends are more important now than ever. They can provide a sympathetic ear, make you laugh, get you thinking about other things, and remind you that you are not alone. Studies show that caregivers who have social supports, and use them, experience less depression and illness and generally are less overwhelmed by their responsibilities than those who don't. So rather than cutting yourself off, reach out to your friends. Find a way. Make it a priority. Go out for lunch with them, go for a walk, or at least call them on the phone. Just as you would be there for them, your friends want to be there for you.

3 *SHIFT GEARS*

WHENEVER YOU ARE FEELING TYPE A, think Type B. Researchers have actually timed people who run through red lights and blast their horns at pedestrians, and they have found that these racers don't save themselves any time at all. In fact, hurrying often slows things down because, in the rush, you are more apt to spill food on your shirt or misplace your car keys.

It seems contradictory, but sometimes when life is hectic, it helps to slow down. Stay calm. Breathe. Learn to meditate. (Meditation is especially helpful at times of stress.)

If you are driving somewhere, and it takes twenty minutes to get there, don't try to make it in nineteen. Leave extra time and then relax. Use that time to listen to your favorite music or a book on tape, or to think about an issue that needs some solitary thought. Or simply relish the silence. Stay in the slow lane, wait until the light turns green, and leave the honking to the geese.

4 *THE WORRY HOUR*

CARING FOR A PARENT MEANS worrying—lots and lots of worrying. Most of it is useless, but nonetheless unavoidable. Rather than stewing during a meeting at work or lying awake at three o'clock in the morning, set aside a specific time, fifteen minutes or half an hour each day, just for worrying. It sounds ridiculous, but it works. When you can't stop fretting, jot down whatever it is you are thinking about and know that you will contemplate it during your "worry hour." Then, go back to sleep. You'll probably discover that it wasn't all that critical after all.

HEALTHY BODY, HEALTHY MIND

The mind-body connection works in two directions. You can boost your physical health with a positive outlook, but you can also improve your outlook by tending to your physical health. Now, when your energy and optimism are taking a beating, it is more important than ever that you eat well, exercise, and get plenty of rest. Yes, you've heard it all before, but now give it a real try. Make a concerted effort to take care of your body, and see if you don't notice a dramatic difference in your mood.

GOOD EATING

Good eating habits take very little time, so you have no excuses.

◆ Don't eat on the run, wolfing down a sandwich in the car or eating stew out of a pot while you talk on the phone. Slow down. Savor the moment.

◆ Keep your shelves and freezer packed with good, healthful food (pasta, canned tomatoes, tuna, frozen vegetables, etc.) so there is always something healthful for dinner.

◆ When buying prepared foods, look for ones with the least amount of fat and sodium.

◆ Make better choices, even when you're in a hurry. Rather than racing out the door in the morning with a cup of coffee and a muffin (most muffins are full of fat), have a slice of toast and a glass of orange juice. Rather than getting a burger at the lunch wagon, bring your own healthful meal to work.

◆ A carton of ice cream fills a void, especially late at night, but not for long. Before throwing yourself face first into the sugar bag, consider your options. Do a few stretches and see if you can't beat the demons.

◆ To save time, plan the week's meals in advance, and when you cook, make plenty. Freeze extra portions for another day, or turn leftovers into new meals.

A LITTLE SWEAT

There is nothing like a workout to shed pent-up emotions, clear a muddled head, and revive a tired body. Exercise protects people from the harmful effects of stress, elevates mood, lowers anxiety, and promotes self-esteem.

◆ Make it challenging. Every now and then, push yourself. Challenging yourself physically seems to have a beneficial effect on stress and resiliency.

◆ Make it doable. Weight training and rigorous workouts are great, but if you hate that sort of thing, find something else. It's better to walk two miles a few times a week and stick to it than to run four miles daily and give up after a week. An exercise regime should last at least twenty minutes and be varied.

◆ Make it social. Find an exercise partner. You will be less apt to excuse yourself from the routine, and you get to socialize while you sweat.

◆ Make it useful. If you simply don't have time for the gym, rake the yard, walk to work, read the newspaper on a stationary bike, or talk to a co-worker while you walk.

◆ Make it fun. Exercise doesn't have to be boring. Play tennis, swim, skate or dance.

REGULAR CHECKUPS

Are you urging your parent to see a doctor but neglecting your own health? Stop postponing that physical checkup, mammogram or your eye exam any longer. Your parent may provide a handy excuse for you to cancel (or fail to make) medical appointments, but don't.

ZZZZZS

In studies of laboratory rats, scientists have found that severe sleep deprivation is always fatal. It is more harmful than starvation. For humans, life without sleep certainly feels deadly, causing irritability, poor concentration, lack of coordination, and forgetfulness. Make sleep a priority.

If you are having trouble sleeping, exercise will help, and see the tips on pages 240 and 241.

AVOIDING PITFALLS

For people under stress, a cup of coffee each morning can gradually turn into three. A glass of wine with dinner can become a scotch before dinner and half a bottle of wine during the meal. Be aware of how much caffeine and alcohol you are consuming, because without realizing it, you can start imbibing more and more.

Avoid using drugs, including sedatives, antidepressants, and antianxiety pills, unless you are taking them under the supervision of a doctor.

And be careful that you don't use food to calm your frazzled nerves. When you reach the bottom of the Pepperidge Farm bag, you won't feel any better; in fact, you'll probably feel a little sick.

5 LOVE TO LAUGH

LAUGHTER IS A FORGOTTEN HEALER. It makes the world sane (or at least it makes the insanity more fun), and it makes the body healthier. A good dose of humor bolsters the spirit, and hysterical laughter strengthens the immune system, improves circulation, and relieves stress.

Of course, howling with laughter when someone you love is ill or dying can feel like a sacrilege. You may think that you have to be solemn to reflect the seriousness of the situation and to show respect for your parent. But you don't. You really don't. It's okay to laugh, no matter how sick or incompetent your parent may be. In fact, the worse things get, the more aggressively you should seek out things to laugh about.

Find something funny about the situation, and your parent probably will, too. (Dentures are funny, especially when your parent isn't wearing them. Certain sourpuss nurses are funny. The Jell-O served in hospitals is funny. Sagging, loose skin under the arm is mildly amusing when it's not your own.) See a slapstick movie, visit a goofy friend, scan the comics, play a joke on someone, read a Dave Barry or Molly Ivins book, clown around with your sisters. Whenever you are feeling that you just can't take it anymore (and long before that point) find some way to laugh—a long, side-splitting, teary, wet-your-pants kind of laugh. It's good medicine.

6 GET SOME PERSPECTIVE

TAKE TIME TO READ THE MORNING paper or listen to the news. Stay abreast of what's happening in the world, in your community, and with your friends. It will help put your problems into perspective and get your mind off your situation.

Likewise, if your parent's illness and needs are a major topic of conversation in your house, or the only topic, plan a meal during which you agree they will not be discussed. Talk about the school play, world events, or just gossip. Do whatever it takes to get away from the subject from time to time.

7 TAKE ACTION

ANYONE CARING FOR A PARENT IS bound to have disagreements with professionals, disputes with institutions, and arguments with relatives. Don't just complain to your friends about a chronically late home-care worker, a rude orderly, or a poorly run meal service. Talk to the person involved, and if he's not responsive, speak to a supervisor. Take action. Without being belligerent, move up the ranks until you get an acceptable response. Be pleasant, but persistent.

Don't hesitate to ask questions when dealing with professionals. Learn about your parent's ailments, ways to appeal Medicare decisions, and patients' rights within a nursing home. Be an educated advocate for yourself and your parent, and don't be afraid to speak up when necessary.

Getting answers and taking action is far better than letting problems fester. It will give you some sense of control (and thus, less frustration and anger). Most important, it often leads to solutions.

8 AVOID THE COULDA-SHOULDA-WOULDAS

ALSO KNOWN AS THE IF-ONLYS OR the More-better-different syndrome, it's a dangerous mind-set. *I should have . . . If only . . . I might have . . .* ad infinitum.

Wishing for things that can't be, regretting what is, or daydreaming about what might have been is futile and potentially destructive if it keeps you from more productive tasks. It's human nature to think this way, but try not to focus on what isn't, and look instead at what is and what can be.

9 PURSUE OTHER INTERESTS

HOBBIES, SPORTS, CRAFTS, AND OTHER such pursuits are not frivolous pastimes. They help clear your mind of your worries—even for brief interludes—which allows you to regain some balance and energy. So don't forgo your pottery, gardening, painting, tennis, or javelin throwing. And don't feel guilty about enjoying them. Make it a point to find time for them. Take pleasure in them.

> " *My mother had a mastectomy, and sometimes she forgets to put her prosthesis in. She'll come downstairs with her shirt all askew and sagging and, after standing there for a minute or two, she'll say, 'Something is not right.'*
>
> *And I look at her and I have to laugh. 'Mom,' I say, 'you forgot your boob.' And we'll both laugh. She thinks it's funny, too. It could happen to anyone. If we didn't laugh, we would cry. It's that sort of thing"*
>
> —CAROL G.

10 SPIRITUAL SUPPORT

WHETHER YOU ARE RELIGIOUS OR not, spiritual issues often arise when a parent is sick, for the situation provokes troubling questions: *Why would a loving God do this? How do I ease my anguish or grief? How do I face my own mortality?* Caring for an aging parent can also try one's patience and kindness. A little guidance may help strengthen your will and focus your life. Nearly 75 percent of caregivers say they use prayer as a way of coping. And it is, for most people, a very effective way of coping.

If going to religious services doesn't interest you, or if you simply want a more personal discussion, most clergy are happy to meet with people individually. Just call. (You can send a little donation if you want to repay the

WHEN ONE PARENT IS WELL

When one parent is ill or just very frail and the other is still competent and relatively healthy, everyone's attention naturally turns to the patient, but your primary focus should be on the healthier parent. If your father is sick, your mother will be his primary caregiver. Your job is to help her so that she can do her job well.

The person who is healthier is often ignored in these situations, but her life has taken a dramatic turn. She stands to lose her mate and may already have lost many vital aspects of their relationship together. She has also taken on enormous work and responsibilities as the primary caregiver and decision maker at a time when she may have her own health problems. She may be working around the clock tending to her spouse, and she may be shouldering duties that she never had before, such as paying bills, handling home maintenance, dealing with lawyers, and planning for the future. (Or, if your father is the caregiver, he might not be used to cleaning, shopping, cooking, and providing personal care.)

Sit down and talk about the situation. Make a list of what jobs need to be done, which ones your parent feels that only she can do, and which jobs others in the family or outsiders can do.

Your parent might be unwilling to hand over any tasks at first. She might insist that she's fine and that she can handle this. Talk to her about why she feels that she must do it all. It may be that she doesn't want to burden you. Or she may feel that only she can do it right, and giving anything up would jeopardize her spouse's care. She may, on some level, believe that the harder

favor.) Sometimes it helps to simply sit quietly in a place that you feel is spiritual, a place where you can listen to your soul and remember your priorities.

II MEDITATION, MASSAGE, AND RELAXANTS

YOU DON'T KNOW HOW MUCH STRESS you are carrying around until you sit in a relaxation or meditation class and let go of it. The techniques you learn there can be used anywhere, anytime, to ease the pressure. Classes in tai chi, meditation, and yoga, as well as in general relaxation, all relieve stress.

In fact, you can actually permanently change your responses to stress and become a more calm and relaxed person. Scientists have found that

she works, the longer her spouse will live. Or she might simply be running from the truth; by working day and night, she doesn't have to face the reality of the situation and all that lies ahead. Ask her what she thinks will happen if you help. What does she fear?

You may need to inch your way into this, taking over one small task and then another very slowly, or nudging her gradually toward community services and in-home help—one helper, one hour, one day at a time.

Give her whatever support you can. Listen to her tears and needs. And pry her away from the job occasionally so that she can get some sleep, see friends, do something else. Offer to take care of your father for certain shifts or for several days at a time. You might also take over peripheral duties, like home maintenance and bill paying, so that she can focus her energies on your father's needs.

Monitor her health, as she may be neglecting it now. Get her to eat well, sleep, exercise, and see the doctor when necessary.

Helping your parent now will not only allow her to give her best to her spouse, it may also head off disaster. What often happens is that the well parent works so hard that her health declines. You may find yourself with two ailing parents instead of one.

The Well Spouse Foundation (800-838-0879 or www.wellspouse.org) can offer help. It hooks members up with support groups and pen pals and issues a newsletter. If you are having trouble getting your parent to take care of herself and take breaks, you might want to talk with a geriatric care manager about easing your mother's workload.

meditation, for example, causes long-term changes in the brain that are enormously beneficial. So this is not only an opportunity to help yourself during this stressful time, but an opportunity for personal growth.

To find out about such classes, call local gyms, spas, and recreation centers, or check the Yellow Pages or the bulletin board at a local health food store.

If you can afford it, give yourself a real treat by having a massage. You can get the name of a good masseuse or masseur from a doctor or physical therapist or sports medicine center, or by getting trusted references from friends, or by calling or contacting the American Massage Therapy Association in Illinois (847-864-0123 or www.amtamassage.org).

12 *INDULGENT NECESSITIES*

IT MAY SOUND LIKE AN OXYMORON, but some indulgence is a necessity. Everyone needs some pampering occasionally, for both physical and mental health, especially at times like these. So treat yourself to a long, hot bath, a shopping spree, an exquisite dinner, room service in a hotel, a facial, an afternoon in the sun, a morning lounging in bed, a new hairstyle—whatever brings you that special, mischievous pleasure that comes only from indulging yourself. Go ahead. You deserve it.

> *During my father's illness I got very depressed and closed in. I realized that I needed some outlet, some way of dealing with the constant anxiety. So I started drawing.*
>
> *I hadn't done any sketches for years, but I bought a pad and pencils and dug in. I find I can express my rage and fear in drawings better than I can with words. I sketch each night. It's my sanity. I've actually gotten pretty good at it."*
>
> —ELEANOR R.

HEALTHY AGING

Pumping Iron • The ABCs of Diet • The Liquor Cabinet • Up in Smoke

YOUR PARENT IS OLD, FRAIL, AND HAS A MEDICAL FILE AS thick as a New York phone book. She has real problems, and you have serious concerns. She can't hear well, she can barely walk, money's a problem, she's confused, and she's got a life-threatening illness, not to mention several seriously annoying habits. You are sleepless from worry and more than a bit overwhelmed. *Healthy aging* is really not a concern right now; your parent is well beyond needing a few vitamins and is certainly not about to go to the gym.

Well, hold on just a minute.

Eating well, exercising, dealing with stress, and otherwise taking care of oneself are no less important at eighty-five than they are at age fifty. The old adage is right: Use it or lose it. And if your parent has already lost most of it, she might get some of it back, or at least enjoy what remains a little more. The truth is that much of the decline that we attribute to aging—frailty, imbalance, immobility, confusion, anxiety, depression, forgetfulness, and illness—is the result of poor lifestyle and isolation as much as passing years.

Most people wrongly assume that people over seventy-five or eighty can no longer enjoy life or benefit from healthful habits. Their mission is simply to keep Mom from falling out of her chair. But by tending to her body, and particularly to her heart, mind, and soul (see Chapter Five), your parent may be able to improve her mobility, independence, optimism, and energy. You won't cure her Alzheimer's or cancer, but you will make the most of what she still has and make these final years as good as they can be.

Do not assume that she can't do it, or that she won't do it, or that she's too old to do it. New leaves get turned over every day, even by people like your parent. She doesn't have to turn over the entire leaf; she can improve her life by simply eating a little better, stretching a tiny bit, getting some fresh air, seeing a friend from time to time, and doing something she enjoys. Small lifestyle changes can reap big rewards.

Pumping Iron

Even if your parent can't hobble across the hallway or push herself out of a wheelchair, she can still benefit from some gentle exercises. It's one of the most important things she can do for her physical health and general well-being. Don't be overprotective here—*But my parent is really too feeble for this.* And don't let her fear stand in the way, either. If she can't or won't go to a gym or pool, maybe she can walk to the mailbox, sway to her favorite music, sweep her own front step, or do some easy stretches at home.

Even if your parent is confined to a wheelchair or bed, she might be able to do neck rotations, arm stretches, and foot flexes each day. Pretty much everyone can do something, and every little bit helps.

But remember, with all of this, you are not your parent's parent. Make suggestions, explain the benefits, show her the path, make it possible, and join in whenever you can, but don't be an unrelenting nag. Positive reinforcement, support, and encouragement are best. Being bossy is not helpful.

Also, keep your expectations reasonable—in other words, low. None of this will cure your parent of disease or revive her failing mind. It will not make her young again. However, it is an option, if she is interested, that should give her more energy and make these days a little more pleasant.

WHY BOTHER?

THE BENEFITS OF EXERCISE FOR VERY elderly people (or anyone for that matter—so get out of that chair) are enormous. Your parent might groan at the thought, but exercise is more effective than many of the medications he takes. Here are just a few benefits of exercise for even extremely frail people:

◆ Increased mobility, stamina, and energy
◆ More independence and a higher level of functioning
◆ Less depression and anxiety
◆ Enhanced self-esteem and optimism
◆ Reduced risk of heart disease, diabetes, osteoporosis, and some types of cancer
◆ Improvement of existing vascular or heart disease, osteoarthritis, and diabetes
◆ Better balance and coordination, which reduces the risk of falls
◆ Stronger bones, muscles, and joints
◆ Loss of extra weight
◆ Relief of pain
◆ Deeper, more restful sleep
◆ Improved bowel function (less constipation)
◆ Boosted immunity
◆ In some cases, improved memory and less confusion
◆ A bonus: kinder interactions with caregivers

Numerous studies have demonstrated the vast benefits of flexing, lifting, and stretching very late in life.

In one study, a group of frail nursing-home residents in their eighties and nineties worked out for ten weeks in a highly supervised program of weight lifting. These patients, many of whom had been written off as barely mobile, dramatically improved their strength, muscle mass, walking speed, and stair-climbing ability. Some gave up their canes and walkers. Others found they could climb stairs or get out of a chair without help for the first time in years.

Another large study of elderly people found that exercise reduced the risk of falls considerably. Tai chi, which is very easy on the body (see the box on page 69), was found to be the most helpful. Those practicing tai chi lowered their risk of falls by 25 percent.

Other studies have shown exercise to work as well as antidepressants in some people, to lower cholesterol levels, and to work better than drugs in treating diabetes, among other things.

A couple of smaller studies have found that when people with Alzheimer's disease started a light exercise program, it reduced depression, withdrawal, aggression, and anxiety; increased optimism and independence; and improved their relationships with caregivers.

If your parent is reluctant or downright refuses to move a muscle, find out his reasons. Some elderly people are afraid they will get hurt; some worry that they will have to join a gym or buy special equipment, and they don't want to spend the money; still others are embarrassed because they think exercising is only for young

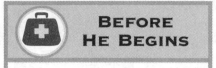

BEFORE HE BEGINS

Before your parent embarks on any exercise regime, he should first talk with his doctor, a physical therapist, or a sports medicine specialist.

people; and some are just used to their sedentary way of life. All of these issues and concerns can be addressed. Your parent can stick to slow and simple exercises, and do them at home if he prefers. With time, he should overcome his reluctance and fears. If he still won't budge, let him be. You can only influence him to a certain extent, and you can always go hiking by yourself.

FINDING THE RIGHT EXERCISE PROGRAM

A GOOD EXERCISE REGIME SUITS THE specific needs of your parent and is something she will stay with. She should talk with a physical therapist or doctor first to come up with a plan.

Some people will enjoy a short walk, while others will be drawn to the gentle, meditative quality of tai chi. Your parent might spend ten minutes in the morning stretching and doing resistance exercises in bed. Anything at all is better than nothing.

If your parent is bedridden or in a wheelchair, she obviously needs something very simple. A physical

therapist can help (ask her doctor to recommend one). She might try an exercise video. Some are made especially for people who are older or have physical disabilities (see page 73). You'll find further suggestions throughout this chapter.

Sometimes exercising is simply a matter of doing more for oneself—getting up and about, taking care of the house or garden, walking to the grocery store. Your instincts might tell you that your parent should sit down, but don't listen to them. Let him sweep the walkway or rake the leaves or hobble to the kitchen. It's good for him.

If your parent is willing and able to be serious about exercising (remember that those nursing-home residents were lifting weights, so don't sell him short), a good regime has four components: *aerobic, strength, flexibility,* and *balance* exercises. If possible, he should alternate, doing aerobic exercise one day and strength exercises the next.

◆ **Aerobic.** Aerobic exercises give the heart and lungs a workout and improve endurance. Walking, riding a stationary bicycle, swimming or other water exercises (which are especially good for people with arthritis, osteoporosis, or back, knee, or hip problems) are all good choices, but so are raking, dancing, and mopping the floor.

◆ **Strength.** Lifting weights is not simply for those seeking rippling abs and bulging biceps. In fact, after lifting weights, your parent might not notice any visible increase in muscle, but the effect will still be there—more strength, better metabolism, less risk of osteoporosis.

Strength exercises can be done with small weights, a large band of rubber for resistance (these can be found at sports stores), or jugs, bottles, or socks filled with sand, beans, or water (but don't put water in the socks!). Your parent can also stand in a doorway and push against the doorjambs, squeeze his palms together, let someone else act as an immovable barrier, or work against the weight of his own body by doing push-ups or sit-ups.

If your parent is particularly frail, he can keep repetitions simple—he can lift his shoulders slowly and lower them, make a fist and release it, and so on.

◆ **Flexibility.** Bending and stretching improve range of motion, alleviate arthritis, and relieve tension. With the lack of use that comes with age, muscles and bones shrink, and tendons and ligaments fail to extend. As a result, older people often stoop over, have trouble with their balance, and experience back pain.

TAI CHI

Tai chi, a Chinese martial art, involves slow, synchronized, almost dancelike movements that help both the body and mind. According to ancient Chinese thinking, focusing one's concentration and breathing, and moving deliberately through the various postures, improves the flow of *qi* (pronounced "chee"), which is the vital life force.

Whatever the reasons, tai chi helps coordination and balance, significantly reducing the risk of falls among the elderly. It has also been shown to be helpful in reducing stress, alleviating depression, lowering blood pressure, easing arthritis pain, improving immune function, and increasing independence.

The moves are easy to learn and easy to do. Tai chi can be done anywhere at any time in any clothing, and by anyone who can stand up. The moves are gentle, graceful, and soothing, with names like "white crane spreads its wings" and "waving hand in the cloud." (Very frail people might want to avoid the Chen style of tai chi, which is a faster version.)

It is best learned with an instructor. Classes are available through local Arthritis Foundation chapters, YMCAs, recreation centers, senior centers, some churches and synagogues, community centers, and gyms. You can also purchase tai chi videos so your parent can do this at home or with friends at a nursing home.

RULES OF THE GAME

NO MATTER WHAT EXERCISE PROGRAM
is followed, an easy beginning, safe surroundings, and a slow ending are especially important when the exerciser is
aged. Your parent should be sure to
observe the following guidelines:

◆ Start slowly and work up gradually, doing a little more each week.
It might take only a few minutes of
walking, for example, for your parent
to become winded. That's okay. It's
important to go slowly. It might take
several weeks for her to build up more
stamina.

◆ Rest whenever necessary. Your
parent should stop exercising immediately if he has palpitations, chest
pains or cramps, or if he becomes
nauseous, dizzy, faint, light-headed,
breathless, or exhausted.

◆ Drink ample fluids, especially
if it's a warm day (but avoid ice-cold
fluids, which can cause cramping).
Elderly people tend to lose their sense
of thirst, so drinking water might not
come naturally to your parent. She
might need a reminder from you.

◆ Stay balanced. Stand with legs
planted slightly apart, back straight, body
aligned, and eyes focused ahead. Your
parent should have something nearby
that he can grab if he feels off balance.

◆ Begin and end with simple, easy
stretches, warming up beforehand and
then cooling down slowly toward the
end.

*My mom is almost eighty
and has a list of medical
problems, and somehow she just
keeps on going. She's amazing. She
swims in the pool at the senior home
she's at and rides a stationary bike.
She's always seeing friends, going out
to dinner, going to lectures. I call her
and she's like, 'Oh, I can't talk right
now. So-and-so's coming for lunch.'
It's as though she decided that she
is not going to get old, and so she
doesn't. I think, Please, please let
me be like her!"*

—ANNE C.

Your parent should take it easy,
stretching gently until he feels a slight
pull, then hold it for anywhere from
eight to thirty counts, depending on
how it feels, and then release it. He
can stretch his fingers, rotate his head,
arch his back, reach for his toes, raise
his arms upward, pull his elbows back,
lift his toes off the floor, and so on.
Yoga classes are also a great way to
improve flexibility, and some are
geared for seniors.

◆ **Balance.** This is critical for the
elderly, as it helps prevent falls (which
in the elderly are extremely serious
and often fatal). Balance exercises are
often part of strength exercises, but
they also include things like holding
the back of a chair and going slowly
onto tiptoe, or bending one leg up
and back. Again, tai chi is a great exercise for improving balance.

WALKING FOR LIFE

Walking is a great form of exercise for an elderly person. It's easy on joints, it's entertaining, it's cheap, and it can be social. It requires no special skills and can be done virtually anywhere. Your parent might just walk to the end of the driveway and back. For more serious walkers, schools often have outdoor tracks, and some malls are open during certain hours just for walkers. (Scenic routes are more enjoyable, but your parent should avoid wooded paths where rocks, roots, and stumps can trip him up.)

Get your parent to start with a short walk—which may be a few paces or a few blocks, depending upon his abilities—three times a week, and then add a little more each week. If possible, he should pick up the pace from a leisurely stroll to a more determined stride. As he walks, he should stand straight, with his head erect and arms swinging loosely at his sides. Tell him to lift his feet rather than shuffle, so he docsn't trip on cracks and bumps.

Make sure your parent has comfortable sneakers with arch supports and thick rubber soles. Find sneakers made of nylon, mesh, canvas, or other material that lets the air circulate. He should wear layers of clothing that he can shed as he warms up. If he needs to carry things with him, get him a fanny pack.

Someone should always know where he is headed, and he should keep to well-populated, well-lit, safe areas. And remember, your parent should drink plenty of liquids so he doesn't dehydrate. Remind him to drink before he's thirsty, because once he's thirsty, his body is already seriously low on fluids.

◆ Vary exercises. If your parent is doing strength exercises, he should work on different muscle groups each time. Don't work on the same muscles two days in a row.

◆ Avoid getting dizzy. Your parent shouldn't get up too fast or change directions too rapidly.

◆ Keep breathing! People tend to hold their breath when exercising. Your parent should breathe regularly with each repetition. Inhale just before exertion and exhale at the maximum point of exertion.

◆ Exercises should not be painful.

◆ Watch the temperature. Choose a comfortable time of day, when it's not too hot or cold, and the sun isn't too strong. If your parent is exercising outdoors, he should remember to apply sunscreen.

◆ Wear loose, comfortable clothing that doesn't impede movement,

"When I was pregnant, I did stretching exercises from a video. My mother, who is in a wheelchair, would watch me. She enjoyed the music and energy of it. And it was something for her to do. I encouraged her to join in and, with some reluctance, she finally did. She did simple versions of what I was doing, or she would swing her arm out to the side when I was swinging my leg, that sort of thing. But she had fun with it.

After the baby was born and I wasn't using the tape anymore, I gave it to her. She says she still uses it most days. I know it helps her keep moving, and it's entertaining."

—JANE D.

and wear layers that can be shed as the body warms up.

◆ Use the right equipment—good walking shoes, a helmet for bike riding, etc.

◆ If your parent is exercising in his house, he should clear plenty of space to allow for safety and freedom of movement.

STICKING WITH IT

YES, YOUR MOTHER STARTED EXERcising, but after a week it was no longer novel, and there were so many reasons not to do it. How can you help get her back on track?

◆ Remind your parent, repeatedly, of all the benefits.

◆ Make sure her exercises are not too burdensome or painful.

◆ Make exercising part of each day's routine. It might be helpful to keep a daily record—how many minutes, what movements, how many repetitions, etc.

◆ Suggest that she exercise to music, if she enjoys that. Turn on some music, or get your parent a pair of headphones if she's walking or doing exercises outside. If not music, perhaps a book on tape.

◆ Encourage her to exercise with friends or to join a class or gym. Exercising with others is more fun and is more likely to remain part of a routine. (She might even do it with you.)

◆ Find an exercise that your parent enjoys. If not walking or doing stretches, then perhaps a class in yoga or pilates.

◆ She might set a goal and then get some reward (her favorite dinner, perhaps?) when she reaches it.

◆ Have options for bad weather (exercise tapes, the gym, climbing the stairs, walking in a mall).

◆ If your parent refuses to exercise, encourage her to do more around the house and yard, like walking to the corner store, weeding the garden, climbing the stairs, and vacuuming. You don't actually have to *call* it exercise, but that's what it is.

WHERE DO WE SIGN UP?

IF YOUR PARENT IS INTERESTED IN A group activity, find a community exercise program for elders that is oriented toward his particular needs and abilities. It should be a safe and structured workout. Doing it in a group will add a nice social aspect to the sport.

Call a local senior center, community center, department of recreation, Jewish center, or YMCA, to find out about such classes. Ask at local gyms and health clubs about exercise classes that might be appropriate, or ask about a fitness trainer who specializes in working with elderly people.

For more information and free booklets on exercises for seniors, contact AARP (888-687-2277 or www.aarp.org) or The National Institute on Aging (800-222-2225 or www.nia.nih.gov).

If your parent is living in a senior facility, many have workout rooms or access to a gym. Ask the activities director.

VIDEO EXERCISE

There are dozens of exercise videos especially for older people and those with disabilities. Look for them at your local library or video store, or search online. If possible, be sure the video is aimed at any disability your parent might have. For example, the Arthritis Foundation has several videos for people with arthritis (800-283-7800 or www.arthritis.org). The National Institute on Aging (800-222-2225 or www.nia.nih.gov) has a general exercise video for seniors for only $7 (others can cost up to $40).

There are also many videos on tai chi for seniors, wheelchair exercises, and exercises for seniors with osteoporosis, breast cancer, and other ailments.

The ABCs of Diet

Does your parent skip breakfast, dine on a half of yesterday's saved sandwich, or return meal trays that have barely been touched? Is your mother living on tea and toast? Is she growing thinner by the day? Or is your father obese and piling up his Oreos despite diabetes, arthritis, and repeated warnings from his doctor? Perhaps your parent complains of problems like constipation or fatigue, or his doctor has mentioned something about vitamin deficiencies. If any of this sounds familiar, it is time to act.

While most of the country is talking about obesity and buying diet books by the boatload, the elderly have very different weight and nutrition issues. Perhaps the most important difference is that when it comes to the

DIETARY ADVICE

 If you are worried about your parent's eating habits and the doctor isn't much help, your parent, or you, may want to consult a nutritionist. Since anyone can hang up a shingle, be sure to look for a "registered dietitian," a certification that means the person has, at the very least, received a bachelor's degree in nutrition or a related field and has passed a special exam.

To find a registered dietitian, call the state dietetic association, look through the Yellow Pages, ask at the doctor's office, or contact the American Dietetic Association (800-366-1655 or www.eatright.org), which can refer you to a registered dietitian in your parent's hometown.

elderly, extra weight is not the biggest concern; malnutrition and weight loss are.

Studies suggest that nearly a quarter of the elderly in this country are malnourished. That doesn't mean they are bone-thin and starving. Malnourished simply means that your parent, for various reasons, is failing to get the vitamins, minerals, and other nutrients that his body needs.

The problem is often overlooked by doctors, who examine heart func-

tion and brain waves, not lunch plates. It is even overlooked in hospitals, where, according to at least two studies, nearly half of elderly patients do not get proper nutrition. So, it's up to you to be aware of your parent's eating habits and any weight changes, and to ask the doctor about any concerns you have.

NOT TOO FAT FOR ME

MOM'S APRON STRINGS DON'T REACH around the back? Dad has a protruding midriff? One good thing about old age is that, finally, a little pudge is not a bad thing. The body stores calories in fat, and that extra reserve can be useful in times of illness or surgery. It also makes a nice padding, possibly protecting frail bones and vital organs from falls. And fat helps a person maintain body temperature, which is a plus in one's older years.

Whatever the reasons, the evidence suggests that elderly people who are a little overweight fare better than those who are underweight. So unless there are compelling reasons for your parent to lose weight (see below), don't bug her, and tell her not to worry about it. Just buy her longer apron strings.

WHEN THE WEIGHT SHOULD GO

IF, HOWEVER, YOUR PARENT HAS arthritis, osteoporosis, heart disease, diabetes, or another condition that requires weight control, and he is more than a little plump—20 to 30 percent over one's desirable weight is considered obese—or if he is dangerously overweight, then it is time for a change.

Forget the fad diets, which tend to fail and usually aren't healthful. Have a doctor or registered dietitian work out a meal plan for your parent, or use your common sense. Basically, he needs to skim some fat and calories from his daily diet, while being sure he gets the nutrients he needs. He should also add some exercise to his day, if possible.

Your parent shouldn't aim for major weight loss. Losing 5 to 10 percent of his weight, a more attainable goal, is plenty. That alone should lower his blood pressure, reduce his cholesterol level, improve his diabetes, and relieve the pressure on his joints.

If your parent has put weight on suddenly, he should see his doctor. There are various conditions and medications that might be behind sudden weight gain.

WHEN THE WEIGHT SHOULD NOT GO

AMONG THE ELDERLY, SUDDEN AND unintentional weight loss is the most serious nutritional concern. Weight loss is a warning sign of a number of serious illnesses, including depression, cancer, heart failure, or dementia. If you notice weight loss, urge your parent to talk with his doctor about it or speak to the doctor yourself. Even if his weight seems okay, ask the doctor about possible nutritional deficiencies.

WHEN EATING SLOWS

If your parent is not eating well, be sure you know why.

You can make shopping, cooking, and eating more manageable for your parent, or you can have meals delivered. If he has trouble eating, find foods that are easier for him to handle and special utensils that might help, or see if someone could sit with him at mealtime and help him eat.

When your parent can't or won't eat much at all, nutritional drinks, like Ensure or Boost, may be helpful. But use them sparingly as they do not replace real food and proper nutrition.

Finally, talk with his doctor. Poor eating, especially if this is a new habit, may be a sign of illness or disability.

(For more tips on making shopping, cooking, and eating more manageable for your parent, see page 119.)

HEALTHY EATING

IN GENERAL, IF YOUR PARENT HAS A reasonably good diet, and the doctor says he's fine, let him be. As we've noted, a few extra pounds are not a worry. Some Fritos in the afternoon or

NUTRITIONAL SUPPLEMENTS

The experts are still hemming, hawing, and disagreeing about the virtues and dangers of dietary supplements. Meanwhile, the business of dietary supplements is exploding. It's not just vitamins and minerals anymore, but amino acids, hormones, herbs, antioxidants, and a whole assortment of unpronounceable and unrecognizable items. And they are not just found in pills, injections, and patches sold at the pharmacy, but in "energy bars" and drinks sold at convenience stores and markets across the country.

The best way to get nutrients is still through healthful food. However, many elderly people have health and other problems that make it almost impossible for them to get all the nutrients they need through diet alone.

A daily multivitamin—and some are specifically designed for the elderly—may help. But before taking any kind of supplement, your parent should talk to her doctor or a registered dietician.

As for the vast number of other supplements claiming to boost memory, energy, happiness, and well-being, and the thousands that promise to cure illness and reverse aging, be highly skeptical. Very few dietary supplements have been scientifically shown to do anything beneficial. Most are a waste of money, some are dangerous, and, as with megadoses of vitamins, many can interfere with the work of medications. Just because something says "herbal" or is sold in a health-food store does not mean it is safe. According to the National Institute on Aging, some supplements can cause high blood pressure, nausea, diarrhea, constipation, fainting, headaches, seizures, heart attacks, or strokes.

a slice of cake after dinner may be nothing to worry about. Someone who's never had heart problems probably doesn't need to start worrying about cholesterol and forgoing egg yolks at eighty. And with everything else that's going on, your parent doesn't need you nagging him about this.

Having said this, the fact is that most elderly people do not eat well, or their bodies do not absorb the vitamins and other nutrients they need, or they have health problems that would be alleviated by better nutrition.

As people age, they don't get the nutrition they need for a variety of reasons. For starters, they often aren't hungry. Chemical changes in the body are largely to blame, although certain medications and illness can certainly dampen one's appetite. A more sedentary lifestyle also leaves one less hungry—you burn fewer calories, and so you need fewer calories. And let's remember, institutional food—such as that served in a nursing home—is generally pretty dreadful. The prepared foods that your father might be heating up in the microwave aren't very exciting either, and probably not very nutritious.

With age, the sense of smell diminishes, and with it goes taste, making food less appetizing. Loneliness and depression can also make eating less enjoyable and interesting.

Your dad might say he's not hungry, but in truth he might have trouble getting to the grocery store, affording food (for real or perceived reasons), preparing food, and using utensils. If he is acutely ill or has trouble with his dentures or other oral problems, he may have difficulty chewing and swallowing. If your parent has dementia, he might simply forget to eat.

And finally, old age, disease, and medications can hinder the body's ability to absorb certain vitamins and minerals.

If your parent is eating very little, every bite counts. He cannot afford to indulge in too many "empty calories"—those foods that fill without providing nourishment, such as chips, candy, soda, cookies, cake, etc. The foods he eats should be packed with as much nutrition as possible.

Eating well reduces the risk of disease, improves recovery from illness or surgery, and generally makes peo-

FOR MORE INFORMATION ON DIET AND NUTRITION

American Dietetic Association
800-366-1655
www.eatright.org

USDA Food and Nutrition Information Center
www.nal.usda.gov/fnic

Federal Government's Nutrition Website
www.nutrition.gov

Nutrition Hotline of the American Institute for Cancer Research
800-843-8114
www.aicr.org

ple feel more energetic. But what is a good diet for an elderly person?

Your parent should stick with a few basic principles (and any special medical orders). Stated most simply, he should have plenty of fruits and vegetables, fiber, fluids and whole grains, while limiting fat and salt. Beyond that, there are two key words: *variation* and *moderation*. That is, don't let your parent fall into a rut, even if it's a healthful rut. A good diet includes lots of different vegetables, fruits, rice, grains, nuts, etc. And as for moderation, don't go to extremes. An occasional doughnut is fine; a pound of broccoli a day is not necessary.

For information about specific vitamins, minerals, proteins, and other dietary details, as well as a list of food groups and daily servings specifically for the elderly, see Appendix I, page 658.

The Liquor Cabinet

While it might seem that sipping a couple of scotches every evening is one of your father's last little pleasures in life, beware. Alcohol, even seemingly reasonable amounts of it, can cause serious health problems in the elderly and exacerbate some of the more routine aggravations that come with old age. In other words, those highballs might be making your dad's day-to-day life more miserable than you—or he—imagine.

Alcohol is a drug, and as with other drugs, it has a more pronounced effect in older bodies, which absorb, use, and dispose of alcohol differently than do younger bodies. Even if your father has always had an evening cocktail without any trouble, it might simply be too much for him now. Studies show that when a sixty-year-old and a twenty-year-old drink the same amount of alcohol, the older person's blood-alcohol level is 20 percent higher than the younger person's. A ninety-year-old is apt to have a blood-alcohol level that is 50 percent higher.

Although one drink with dinner may not be cause for alarm (and, yes, a small amount may even reduce car-

MEDICAL ALERT

If your parent routinely drinks alcohol and is placed in a situation in which alcohol is not available, such as a nursing home or hospital, he may go through withdrawal. The symptoms include shakiness, sweating, rapid breathing, agitation, and sometimes delirium, hallucinations, and seizures. Alert the personnel about his previous drinking habits, because they may not understand the cause of his problems. Be sure the information is entered in his record so you're not depending on the person you've told to pass it along to other staff. Withdrawal is a medical emergency that requires immediate treatment.

diovascular risk), even small amounts of alcohol can intensify problems that your parent might already be struggling with (confusion, incontinence, insomnia, poor appetite, and depression). It also hinders coordination and slows a person's reactions, increasing the chances of a serious fall. In addition, alcohol can also make a person more susceptible to infections, colds, and other illness.

Perhaps most disconcerting, alcohol and medications, including over-the-counter (nonprescription) medications, can be a dangerous mix—and most elderly people take between two and seven medications a day.

Because of all of this, the National Institute on Alcohol Abuse and Alcoholism recommends that people over sixty-five have no more than one drink per day. One drink, by the way, is defined as one 12-ounce beer, 5 ounces of wine, or 1.5 ounces of distilled spirits—gin, vodka, scotch, etc. Go measure 5 ounces; it's not as much as you think.

Unfortunately, boredom, pain, and insomnia can make alcohol a welcome analgesic. Those who have routinely had one drink every evening begin to have two or three; former teetotalers decide that a little nip each evening might help them sleep.

If your parent is a casual drinker, be aware of the extra dangers and talk to him about it, or have his doctor mention it to him.

As for heavy drinking, there is no question that this is very serious. In addition to all the risks mentioned above—confusion, falling, malnutrition, problems with medications, etc.—your parent now faces a higher risk of liver disease, stroke, immune disorders, hypertension, vitamin deficiency, certain types of cancer, and permanent brain damage.

While alcoholism seems to be less prevalent among those over sixty-five than in younger age groups, it is hard to know for sure. There is little solid data, in part because alcoholism and what is called "heavy drinking" often go undetected in the elderly. Older people are often alone, and so are not seen by friends and colleagues. They are less apt to be driving, and so are not discovered by police. Furthermore, people either excuse the behavior (*Hey, it helps her sleep at night.*) or they mistake drunkenness for other problems that come with aging. So when Dad forgets what he said last night, stumbles across the living room, or falls asleep at the dinner table, others think it's all just part of old age.

Some signs of trouble: Your parent gulps his drinks, he seems to have a heightened reaction to alcohol (he appears flushed, confused, or unstable

---

❝ My mother used to love to have a couple of old-fashioneds every night. Then we decided that her drinking might be contributing to the dizziness and the falls, so Elizabeth, Mom's companion, got her down to one small glass of sherry. I was amazed, but Elizabeth can get Mom to do almost anything—things that I could never convince her to do.

One evening when I was visiting, Mom said, 'Oh, I think I'll have a real drink tonight.' And I said, 'No, Mom, please don't do that.' I was a little nervous about what her reaction would be, but she didn't say a word, and she didn't have the drink. I was truly shocked. And very relieved."

—GRETA N.

FOR MORE HELP

For information about alcoholism or referrals to treatment centers and self-help groups, contact:

Alcoholics Anonymous
212-870-3400
www.aa.org

Al-Anon Family Groups
800-356-9996
www.al-anon.org

National Institute on Alcohol Abuse and Alcoholism (NIAAA)
301-443-3860
www.niaaa.nih.gov

National Council on Alcoholism and Drug Dependence Hope Line
800-622-2255
www.ncadd.org

National Clearinghouse for Alcohol and Drug Information
800-729-6686
www.health.org

after only one cocktail), he tries to hide or lies about his drinking, he loses interest in food, he is irritable or unreasonable, he begins to withdraw socially, or he starts to neglect his personal hygiene and care.

If you are worried about your parent's drinking, talk with him about your concerns or ask his doctor to talk with him. If the problem is dire, have a family meeting where you all confront the issue and talk about the effect his drinking is having on the family. Point out the medical risks he is taking and what he is doing to his body. Talk about the benefits of quitting, how it will affect his life and his relationships. Let your parent know that if he decides to quit, you will all support and encourage him. You can also seek help from one of the groups listed on this page.

Your parent might be able to cut back or abstain on his own (although it's unlikely). Counseling from a doctor is often helpful. (Sometimes seeing the results of a liver function test or some other clear indication of the consequences of his drinking is useful.)

Structured programs or more intensive counseling is just as effective among the elderly as it is among younger people; however, those who started drinking recently will be helped more easily than those who have an entrenched drinking problem. Some research suggests that treatment is more effective when it is done in a setting with other elderly people, where they can talk about pertinent issues (life in retirement, physical ailments, family life, etc.).

There are prescription drugs that help alcoholics abstain, in particular benzodiazepines, which are calming and ease the shaking and rapid heart rate that often come with withdrawal. Naltrexone helps to ease the craving for alcohol. These should be used in combination with counseling or support groups.

Because withdrawal can lead to medical complications in the elderly, such as delirium, hospitalization is sometimes recommended.

Up in Smoke

Everyone knows the perils of cigarette smoking, but what's the point of stopping late in life? After all, your mother has smoked for nearly forty years. Isn't the damage done? Is there any real benefit to stopping at her age? Surely you know the answer: Absolutely. The rewards are enormous at any age.

Sure, if your father is lying in a bed, weeks or months away from death, perhaps you should just let him be. It's agonizing to see people with acute emphysema or late-stage lung cancer lighting up a cigarette, but this might not be the time to make a fuss about it.

But for others, who maybe aren't so far gone, the benefits of quitting— even at an advanced age, even after years of smoking—start immediately. As soon as that last cigarette is put out, the body begins to repair and restore itself. Within minutes, blood flow improves and blood pressure drops, reducing the risk of heart attack, stroke, and other circulatory disease. Within hours, carbon monoxide levels in the blood return to normal. Within a few weeks, a person's sense of taste and smell return, and breathing becomes easier. Within months, coughing and shortness of breath improve. According to one study, someone who quits at age sixty-five adds about four years onto his life.

(There are no similar studies for those who are eighty-five or ninety-five.)

If he can quit smoking, your parent will not only be much healthier, but he will be more energetic, have a better appetite, sleep better, and, goodness knows, smell a whole lot better (and not only will he smell better to others, but he'll have a better sense of smell himself). He will be less prone to infectious diseases like flu and pneumonia, which are very dangerous for older people. And just think of the money that he'll save. (It's not a bad idea to do the math with him so he'll see how much he'll be saving each year.) By quitting, he will also safeguard other family members, particularly grandchildren, from diseases caused by his smoking.

While kicking the habit will, with time, dramatically reduce his risk of getting lung cancer and other serious lung disease, it won't reverse the damage that's been done. However, by quitting, he won't be making his condition worse and he lowers his risk of developing some new, primary cancer.

While some people can quit on their own, most people need help. Nicotine replacement therapy (patches, inhalers, lozenges, nasal sprays, and gums) is effective. These substitutes allow a person to get the nicotine he craves without the toxic effects of smoking (although they do cause some side effects of their own). He can quit with fewer withdrawal symptoms and then slowly taper off the amount of nicotine. But given your parent's age and other health concerns, it is vital that he talk to his doctor before starting such treatment.

FOR MORE HELP

For more information about quitting, supporting someone who's quitting, local classes, counselors, and telephone "quitlines," contact the American Cancer Society (800-227-2345 or www.cancer.org). Numerous other groups offer guidance and information, including the American Lung Association (800-586-4872 or www.lungusa.org) and the National Cancer Institute's Cancer Information Service (800-422-6237 or www.cancer.gov).

Bupropion, an antidepressant, also helps reduce the symptoms of withdrawal. It can be used alone or in combination with nicotine substitutes. But again, a doctor needs to be consulted.

Nicotine substitutes alone, however, are not usually enough, for they fail to address the emotional and social aspects of smoking. To be successful, most people also need some sort of cessation class, counseling, and/or support group. At the very least, it helps to have a smoking buddy who is quitting at the same time or who knows what your parent is going through. Some people also find techniques like acupuncture and hypnosis to be helpful. If it works, go for it.

If your parent decides to quit, he will need enormous support and encouragement from loved ones. Nicotine is very addictive. Until his body adjusts, the craving will be powerful. The first few weeks will be the hardest, for everyone. Your parent is likely to be cranky, angry, and tired. He might swear and yell or just retreat into his smoke-free hell. Some people have headaches. Some have trouble breathing in the beginning, although this will vastly improve with time. He may have trouble sleeping and concentrating, and may feel anxious and depressed. He might gain some weight, but not enough to worry about; the pounds are a whole lot healthier than the tar and nicotine.

Put up with his moods. Tell him you're proud of him. Keep him busy and distracted. Support him. Set goals or milestones (one week without cigarettes, etc.) and then celebrate when he reaches them. Remind him of all the good things he is doing for his body (and yours) and for his wallet. Avoid situations that he associates with smoking. Find some substitutes for that hand-to-mouth habit, like popcorn, carrot sticks, and sunflower seeds. If he's willing, exercise will help distract him and relieve some of the stress he's now under.

And finally, cigars, snuff, chewing tobacco, and pipes are *not* safe alternatives to cigarettes. These habits are also addictive and can cause cancer and heart disease.

HEART, MIND, AND SOUL

Staying Involved • Family and Friends • Spirituality • Creativity • Volunteering • Expanding the Mind • Dating, Sex, and Marriage

I T'S TERRIFIC IF YOUR PARENT LIFTS WEIGHTS, EATS SPINACH and tofu stew, and throws out his cigarettes. Scientific research shows that this will all contribute to a healthier and more independent life. But the anecdotal evidence, the stuff the doctors see in their offices every day, suggests that tickling a devoted grandchild, going to church, seeing an old friend, or volunteering might be the strongest medicine of all.

Quite simply, those who have close family ties, social contacts, a hobby or intellectual pursuit, optimism and humor, and a spiritual base—or at least one or two of these ingredients—get sick less often, recover faster, live longer, and generally enjoy life more. People who read, play cards, do crossword puzzles, plant flowers, or keep their minds active in other ways are also less apt to suffer from memory loss.

People need family and friends, and they need opportunities to learn, teach, do, create, or reminisce. In other words, they need to feel that their lives have meaning. Frederick Nietzsche once said, "He who has a *why* to live can bear almost any *how*."

The Quest

We're not talking about anything major. You don't need to arrange for your parent to visit the Galapagos Islands (although if he likes that kind of thing, there are trips for the disabled, as well as terrific videos). Even minor activities or events can have a major impact.

Talk with your parent about what she enjoys now and what she used to enjoy in her younger days. (Or, try to remember this yourself.) What made life interesting? What gave it meaning? What made her happy?

If it was raising her children, maybe she can become a foster grandparent, or she can dictate her memoirs for her grandchildren or sort through family photos. If she loves her church, arrange for her to get there, have tapes of services recorded for her, or see if a member of the clergy will visit her. If she was always involved in politics, call local political offices to see if she can volunteer in some small way, perhaps by stuffing envelopes. If she loves nature, get her out to a park or preserve, rent nature videos, or buy her an ant farm.

If your parent is in a nursing home, she might receive visits from a grandchild, listen to her favorite music, arrange flowers, or, if she can get around at all, she might volunteer by delivering books or visiting other residents.

Look through the newspaper, read bulletin boards, and scan community calendars. Ask her friends or other elderly people in her community what they do with their days. Don't give up. You may have to try a couple of ideas before something strikes your parent's fancy. But eventually you will find something, or someone, to warm her heart.

STAYING IN THE FAMILY LOOP

This is the most critical element. At the end of the day, what humans need more than anything else are social bonds. They need friends and family. They need to love and be loved. This need is written deeply into our genetic codes, and it is basic to our survival. It is with us throughout life, but it seems to be most acute at both the beginning of life and toward the end, when the body is weak, life is uncluttered, and one's needs are primal.

Sit with your parent. Talk about old times. Tell her what's happening in your life. If you are far away, or nearby but busy (or close and not busy, but don't like spending time with your parent), call or e-mail as often as you can. Any sort of contact is better than none. Tell her what's happening with various family members and old friends—Michael just got his braces off, Tammy has a new boyfriend, Brian is applying for a new job, old Ted Wollman finally sold his apartment. Give her all the details, however mundane they might seem.

Include your parent, whenever possible, in family activities. Even if she can't actually participate, she should be there. Or, if she can't be there, let her know that she is wanted, and then take a video of the event for her to watch later. And be sure she has plenty of family photos around her, wherever she lives.

Encourage other family members to stop by for a visit, call, write, or, if your parent is hooked up to the Internet, send her e-mail. Let her know, in any way that you can, that she still has family who care.

FRIENDS, OLD AND NEW

MANY OF YOUR PARENT'S OLD FRIENDS might be just that, *old*. They are deceased, or too disabled to get out, or perhaps they live elsewhere now. Digging up friendships and a social life is difficult at any age, but it seems to be hardest just when you need it most. Your parent might need a little push from you.

Urge her to call an old friend or new acquaintance for lunch, a potluck supper, or a movie. If she can't get out, maybe there's someone she likes who might come visit her. If she is invited somewhere, or even if you're invited somewhere and she's welcome to come along, make the effort to get her up and out, even if mobilizing isn't easy.

> " *My father is eighty-three and has Alzheimer's. Last year, old family friends invited him and me to a Christmas party. My immediate reaction was to leave him home. He is aware of his surroundings sometimes, but often he's pretty oblivious. He's also not terribly mobile. But my sister urged me to take him, so I dressed him up, put on his old holly tie that he always used to wear at Christmas, and got him out the door.*
>
> *I felt like I was making a mistake, that people would stare, that he would embarrass himself, that he wouldn't know what was happening.*
>
> *It turned out that, of course, all these old friends were in their eighties too. One friend of his was crumpled over in a wheelchair with Parkinson's. Several had walkers. Half of them couldn't hear well.*
>
> *They were all so kind and patient with him. He came to life. He didn't remember anyone's name, but he had so much fun. I hadn't seen that spark in his eye in ages.*"
>
> —SALLY R.

If she doesn't know many people nearby, get her to join some club, class, or activity—the League of Women Voters, a painting class, a bridge club.

If she's in a nursing home or other senior facility, check out the activity schedule and encourage her to participate. Even if she doesn't like crafts or lectures, urge her to try some of the activities. Meet people. Get out there.

Many communities have volunteer programs in which volunteers will visit homebound elderly. If hers doesn't, you still might find a volunteer through a service club, senior organization, or religious organization.

Once she makes a friend or two, or if you've found a friendly volunteer, set up standing dates—a card game every Tuesday night, lunch every Thursday—so she doesn't have to think about creating new social events each week.

SPIRITUAL FULFILLMENT

UNLIKE OTHER AGE GROUPS, NEARLY all elderly people consider themselves at least somewhat religious. This may be largely generational. It might also be partly due to the fact that, as a person heads into life's last stages, questions about mortality, the purpose of life, and spirituality often take on greater importance. It might also be that elderly people finally have time for services and prayer.

Whatever the reasons, for most elderly people, the church, synagogue, or other place of worship is the most important source of social support out-side of the family. And, as it turns out, this is a very good thing. Being religious is directly correlated to better physical and mental health. The evidence for this is overwhelming. A number of studies have shown that people who are religious get sick less often, recover faster, and have a greater ability to cope with illness, disability, and loss. They view ailments and disabilities as less painful and less cumbersome than those who are not religious. They clearly have less depression and anxiety, and have a greater sense of motivation, hope, and optimism.

Religion gives people a sense of meaning and hope and a positive attitude. These feelings help them to do more, take care of themselves, and reach out to others. Hopelessness and worry, on the other hand, contribute to heart disease, high blood pressure, stroke, and other disorders.

Religion also offers a large dose of social interaction. If your parent attends services, he is getting out and seeing people, and they are seeing him. He is making and continuing friendships. People ask about his health, notice if he's looking ill, and possibly offer to help in some way. He is then more apt to take care of himself and feel better about himself.

Whether or not your parent practiced a religion in his younger days, he might like to go to church or synagogue, attend a religious discussion group, speak to a member of the clergy, or simply have someone read to him from the Bible or other religious books.

It's quite possible that he may not want to bother you with this, or that he is embarrassed to suggest it, or that he won't think of it unless you suggest it. Encourage your parent to pursue his religious beliefs and explore his faith. Even without a structured, formal religion, he can examine his spiritual views, read about spiritual issues, and rediscover his faith.

REMINISCING

THE NEXT TIME YOUR FATHER DRIFTS back several decades and tells you stories you've heard before, rather than shaking your head in resignation or despair, encourage him to tell more. He's doing something that's enormously healing. Reminiscing allows him to review his life, think through important issues, see his accomplishments, let go of his regrets. It also returns him, temporarily, to a time when he was younger, stronger, more confident, and more capable.

If you can get your parent to tell new stories or flesh out the old ones, reminiscing can be a wonderful experience for you, too. Or your children might like to share this activity with their grandparent. Exploring these details gives you insight into your parent's life and background, and it may be one of the last chances you have to learn about your heritage.

Tape-record your father's tales, because you are sure to forget important details or a tone of voice that made the story his. Ask about his life as well as his views of historical events

he witnessed. What was his childhood house like? What about the school he attended? What were his parents like? How did he travel or dress or cook as a young boy? Why did he choose his

> " *I was doing everything for my mother. I was miserable and she was miserable. She'd say things like, 'Don't trouble yourself,' and 'I'm fine,' and 'I really wish you wouldn't do this.' She felt I was ruining my life for her, which I was in a way, and that made her unhappy.*
>
> *I found a note pinned to a bulletin board in town that a teenager was looking for after-school work. I called her and set her up visiting my mom.*
>
> *It's been amazing. It's like the daughter she never had. They bake cookies together. Well, my mother sits in her wheelchair giving out instructions while Sarah bakes cookies, I should say. They talk about their lives. My mother gives Sarah constant advice about friends and boys and schoolwork. Sometimes she helps her with her homework.*
>
> *I had arranged for Sarah to come by twice a week, but she stops in almost every day because I think she loves this almost as much as my mother does. She's a godsend."*
>
> —JERRY B.

REFUSING TO BUDGE

Your parent's most serious obstacle to social, mental, and spiritual involvement may not be disability or illness, but her own ageist attitudes. If she has always viewed old age in a negative light, then she is likely to believe that she's now too old to do, to learn, to give, or to care.

Of course, this negativity is circular and becomes self-fulfilling. Because inactive, she becomes bored and weak which leads to more feelings of worthlessness and, in turn, more inertia. Over time, the idea of doing something becomes terrifying and/or ridiculous.

Start very small, and focus on her particular interests and needs. If her hands are still dexterous and she used to enjoy sewing, rather than giving her a new McCall's pattern, ask her if she wouldn't mind hemming a skirt for you. If you have found a kind volunteer to keep her company, start with only a very brief visit once a week.

If your parent continues to reject your efforts to get her out, if she is lethargic, is withdrawn, and has no interest in the things she used to enjoy, if she insists on sitting in her recliner and watching reruns all day, it might very well be a sign of depression or early dementia. Talk with her doctor. Get help.

career? What girls did he date? Does he remember the first time he met your mother? What presidential elections were most exciting to him and why? What was life like for him during the Depression? Where was he during World War II?

Get your parent to talk about your ancestors. Draw a family tree together, gathering additional information from other relatives. Find out who your grandparents and great-grandparents were, and what they were like. This is invaluable information that tells you who you are and where you came from. It's something you can pass down to your children and grandchildren.

As your parent talks, let him ramble about subjects he most enjoys. Don't correct him or force him to stay within some chronological order. Just listen, encourage him, and enjoy it.

If your parent can't speak or grows tired easily, he might enjoy hearing you reminisce about his life and family times. You can simply flip through a photo album together as a touchstone to talking about various events in the past.

CREATIVE OUTLETS

EVEN PEOPLE WHO HAVE NEVER shown much interest in art, dance, or music during their younger days can suddenly find a passion for it now that they have time on their hands, losses to grieve, and issues to resolve. Once again, don't predetermine what your parent wants to do, needs to do, likes to do, or can't do.

See if she might be interested in taking an art class or picking up some charcoal pencils and a pad. Perhaps a ball of clay to mold and push around in her arthritic hands, or some shells, trinkets, and scraps to glue into a collage. Drawing, painting, and sculpting help people to release tension, sort through conflicts, and grieve losses. Creativity also taps into an important part of the brain, and the soul, that doesn't get much activity.

Music, too, soothes so much in us. Did your parent ever play an instrument? Would she like to try again? Would she like to listen to a fun new song or old favorite, and dance or just sway to the beat? Research shows that music triggers the release of opiates and endorphins in the body, which help lower blood pressure, improve breathing, alleviate pain, and generally make a person feel good. Dance, even in some limited way, does all this and adds an element of exercise to the activity.

If she doesn't want to "do," maybe she'd like to watch or listen. You might take her to a local play, a ballet, a gallery opening, or a musical. If she can't get out, you might buy a video of a dance, an orchestra, or the life of a favorite artist. Or, she might just like to lie in bed and listen to old show

> " *Dad and I always had what I call a business relationship. We talked about finances and health and practical matters, but never emotions and that sort of thing.*
>
> *Then one day I was visiting him in the hospital and running out of conversation and, for some reason, I asked him about a girl he dated in college. I guess I had heard her name somewhere. Well, his eyes got misty and he started telling me all about being in love for the first time and the college parties and how hurt he was when she left him. He got lost in his past, lying in that bed, with tubes all over the place. He told me about other women he dated, his friends, funny things that happened, and the day he met my mother.*
>
> *He was like a kid, remembering all this stuff. And I was seeing, for the first time in my life, this very human, vulnerable, and youthful side of my father.*"
>
> —ALICIA B.

tunes, songs from her youth, or a favorite composer.

VOLUNTEERING

VOLUNTEERING IS A WONDERFUL WAY for your parent to regain a sense of purpose, which is so enormously beneficial to heart and mind. It will give her a reason for being and caring. It

A RIDE IN THE COUNTRY

If your parent is very frail and doesn't get out much, he will benefit from a change of scene and some fresh air. Even if it takes some logistics to get him into the car, try it. Driving down a country road, by the sea, or along a busy city street may cheer him up considerably. If you don't have time for pleasure trips, take him with you when you run your errands, just to get him out of the house.

will also help her to meet new people of different ages, to take her mind off problems, and to be involved in the community, politics, the arts, children, medical care, women's issue—whatever interests her. Volunteers help in food pantries, tutor children, counsel battered women, assist disaster victims, work in hospitals and prisons, raise money for various organizations, and myriad other things.

Even if your parent can't leave the house or her bed, she may be able to make phone calls or edit letters. If she is in a nursing home, she may be able to give tours, answer visitors' questions, deliver meals or flowers, or visit patients in the infirmary.

If your parent would like to help other older people in the commu-nity—delivering meals, reading mail to people with poor vision, visiting homebound elderly, escorting people to medical appointments or shopping centers, doing minor home repairs, or assisting in a senior center—contact the area agency on aging (see page 628) and ask about Older Americans Act programs or other similar volun-teer programs.

Senior Corps, a federal program, runs several large senior volunteer programs, including the Retired and Senior Volunteer Program (RSVP), Foster Grandparents, and Senior Companions (800-424-8867 or www. seniorcorps.org).

If your parent is a retired busi-ness executive or small business owner, he or she might like to get involved with the Service Corps of Retired Executives (SCORE), which provides free counseling to small business own-ers (800-634-0245 or www.score.org).

To find out about other possibil-ities, call local churches, synagogues, senior and community centers, hos-pitals, libraries, schools, foundations, grassroots organizations, day care cen-ters, fund-raising groups, political campaigns, local museums, theaters, nature centers, the United Way, the Red Cross, or the local chapter of AARP. You should also contact the local volunteer center in your parent's area, which you can find through the Points of Light Foundation (800-VOLUNTEER or www.points oflight.org) or Volunteers of America (800-899-0089 or www.volunteersof america.org).

CROSSING
THE GENERATION GAP

IF YOUR PARENT HAS ALWAYS BEEN good with children, he can, and should, still have them in his life. Even if he never liked them much, he might enjoy them now that he has more time, and less activity, on his hands.

A connection between the young and the old enriches the young, and certainly makes the old feel young again. Your parent might volunteer to help youngsters, or you can set up an arrangement in which youngsters visit him at home or at his nursing home, adult day-care program, or other facility.

Call local schools, day-care centers, Boy Scout and Girl Scout troops, religious organizations, and other groups to find out about ways your parent might either help or be helped.

The Foster Grandparent Program puts elderly citizens to work (for a small compensation) in hospitals, schools, and day-care programs. The participants may help children who have been abused or neglected, may care for premature infants or young children with disabilities, or mentor young mothers and troubled teens (800-424-8867 or www.seniorcorps. org). Some communities also have their own foster grandparent programs, which simply put young children who have no grandparents in contact with elderly people. You can call local organizations or simply call friends and family and see if they know of a

> *My father lives in a nursing home, and he gets very bored and lonely. When anyone visits him, it's as though he won the lottery, he gets so excited. The rest of the time he basically sleeps and roams the hallways and talks to the nurses. He's not interested in any of the games or activities at the home and says all the other residents are 'too old' or half-crazy.*
>
> *I've tried a lot of things, and I think my most successful effort was signing him up as a foster grandparent. This little boy, Tyler, not only visits, but also sends him games and calls when he has homework questions. They've developed a really nice relationship."*
>
> —ELEANOR R.

little boy or girl nearby who could use a grandparent. He can simply take on the role by inviting them over for cookies and cards now and then.

Family Friends, a program run by the National Council on the Aging, trains older adults to work with seriously ill or disabled children (202-479-6672 or www.family-friends.org).

Experience Corps also works with older volunteers, hooking them up in urban schools to serve as advocates for children and to teach them various skills they need in life (202-478-6190 or www.experiencecorps.org).

CREATURE COMFORTS

WHAT HAS COME TO BE KNOWN IN medical lingo as pet-facilitated therapy, or PFT—basically, having a dog or cat—clearly boosts people's emotional states as well as their physical health.

Animals make people feel loved and less alone, and they give elderly people a sense of responsibility. And, since Rascal needs a daily walk, a dog provides a little exercise as well. For someone who is anxious or agitated, stroking a pet is calming. Pets also ease depression.

The findings about pet-facilitated therapy have been so conclusive that federal law now mandates that elderly people living in subsidized housing be allowed to keep pets, so don't let the landlord shoo Patches or Felix out the door.

While a dog or cat provides the most companionship, a bird, hamster, tank of fish or other animal can also ease loneliness and provide entertainment. These smaller, simpler pets are particularly useful if your parent is very frail or confused.

WORKING FOR PAY

IF YOUR PARENT DOESN'T WANT TO work for free and she is relatively able, she may be able to find a job that pays. More and more shops and restaurants, for example, are finding that older people are often more reliable and harder working than teenagers, and some senior organizations specifically look to hire older people. The area agency on aging should know of local employment programs for seniors. Also, look through the want ads or call businesses that may interest your parent—a museum gift shop, a hospital, a clothing store, a movie theater. You might also contact local senior centers to see if they know of such jobs.

LENDING A HAND

IN EARLIER DAYS, YOU MAY NOT HAVE wanted to bother or burden your parent by asking for favors. Well, now is the time to ask. If your parent is bored, give her a project, something that would also help you. Ask her to sort through old photos, write addresses on holiday greeting cards, look something up in the library or on the Internet for you, snap beans, or otherwise give you a hand in your personal or business life. You get a task done, and she feels useful.

EXERCISING THE MIND

IT'S NEVER TOO LATE TO LEARN, EVEN for a very old dog. Call local colleges, community centers, high school extension programs, museums, and senior centers and ask about classes and lectures. If your parent is able, he might learn to paint with oils, cook Italian food, or play the piano. Perhaps he wants to study classical music or learn about modern architecture. He can hear about Malaysia, Mayans, Monarch butterflies, Mars, or Marconi. He might learn about wetlands, fossils, microbes, rain forests, or explorers.

Find out about tours of museums and art galleries, many of which have special programs and prices for the elderly. For his next birthday, buy your parent tickets to the ballet, theater, or opera.

Chronic illness and bed rest can muddle your parent's mind and make him listless. If your father is unable to get out of the house, get him books and lectures on tape, or videotapes from the local library. There are literally thousands of courses and lectures offered on the Internet. Do a search for whatever interests him.

He doesn't have to take it all in— there are no exams. He doesn't even have to take much of it in. But learning gives a person energy, optimism, and pride. And it will take him briefly away from his pain and troubles.

You might make it both educational and social. Make a Friday date to have pizza and watch a documentary, or a group of friends might listen to books or lectures on tape independently, and then discuss them later at a get-together.

TRAVEL AND OTHER EXPLORATION

IF HE'S MOBILE AT ALL, YOUR PARENT can go on a tour—senior citizen or otherwise—to foreign countries or nearby cities, colleges, botanical gardens, and historic sites and monuments. You may even want to join him. (Some tours don't require any walking, if your father needs to ride.)

Most senior centers offer discount trips, from day trips to weekend foliage

SO MANY GADGETS AND GIZMOS

Don't assume that just because your parent is severely arthritic, deaf, shaky from Parkinson's, or blind that he can't do the things he enjoys. In this era of accessibility and technology, there are literally thousands of gadgets, gizmos, and other products on the market that make gardening, sewing, fishing, reading, traveling, bowling, hunting, swimming, and other hobbies, sports, interests, and adventures possible. Search the Internet for your parent's favorite activity, but add the word *disabled* or *accessibility* to the search window. Or see page 131 for some starting points.

tours to full vacations. Colleges and special-interest organizations, like museums, environmental groups, and history clubs, often offer tours for seniors.

Numerous travel agencies specialize in travel for people who are elderly and/or have disabilities. Look on the Internet under "disability travel," "wheelchair travel," or "senior travel," or call a local travel agent and ask for suggestions.

The Elderhostel organization (877-426-8056 or www.elderhostel.org)

> " *The thing my mother loved most was music. The Jewish home where she lived had concerts and even a music therapy class, but she couldn't go because she was afraid of riding in the elevator by herself, and the nurse said there wasn't enough staff to escort her. One day I ran into the woman who directed the program in the hallway. I told her about my mother, and she said she would be happy to bring Mom to and from the class each day. It was such a relief. Her spirits seemed to pick up right away."*
>
> —BARBARA F.

offers an enormous array of trips, tours, and courses for older people. Their staff can suggest trips that might be right for your parent. (One of their repeat participants is 100 years old, legally blind, and in a wheelchair, so don't assume that your parent is too old for this.)

VIDEOTAPES AND BOOKS

IF YOUR PARENT IS LAID UP OR JUST tends to stay in, get her some books and movies. She may not have the initiative to do this for herself, but once she is involved in a good story, she may get lost in it. How about some of her favorite old films?

If she is active, get her to start a book club, with friends gathering once a month to discuss a book they have all read, or she might get some friends together to see a weekly movie at home or in the community room at her residence.

You can get small laptop DVD players. She can use earphones, if she needs the volume particularly loud and doesn't want to bother a roommate.

If your parent has trouble seeing, there are devices that enlarge the words in a book onto a screen. If she can't read, get books with large print or books on cassette or compact disk. Contact your local library or bookstore, both of which should have numerous books on tape and large print books. You can also contact the Library of Congress (800-424-8567 or www.loc.gov/nls) or go to www.amazon.com or www.largeprintbooks.com on the Internet. Sometimes local volunteers will read to older people. For people with hearing loss, the Captioned Media Program (800-237-6213 or www.cfv.org) loans videos with captioning free of charge.

PROJECTS AND HOBBIES

MAYBE YOUR PARENT ISN'T INTO making birdhouses, but what about other hobbies and projects, like gardening, bird-watching, fishing, collecting, model building, or painting?

Think small-scale. If she doesn't want to take care of a full garden, she can have a few small planters in a window. The joy of gardening on a small scale has the same rewards of watching something grow and bloom. If she can't get about, put a bird feeder near the window so she can watch the different birds from a comfortable seat. If her interest grows, buy her a pair of binoculars and a bird guide for her birthday.

Ask what she used to do in her younger days; she might enjoy reviving an old hobby. If she doesn't want to do things on her own, ask at senior centers about hobby clubs, or see if she can round up a few friends or neighbors who might like to explore a new subject or start a project with her.

SPORTS AND GAMES

SPORTS AND GAMES ARE A TERRIFIC way to exercise, meet people, and build some confidence. It might be bingo, bridge, or shuffleboard, or it could be walking, playing golf, cross-country skiing, or swimming. Your father may have to take it easy, but that doesn't mean he can't participate. Some other activities to consider include fishing, horseshoes, darts, bowling, croquet, badminton, archery, miniature golf, or pool. Local gyms, YMCAs, and senior centers may arrange or know of such events, or call the local department of recreation or community center.

SENIOR CENTER ACTIVITIES

SENIOR CENTERS AND ADULT DAY service centers offer elders a place to socialize, talk about the events of the day, attend lectures, go on trips, learn new skills, and, in some cases, find out

SIMPLE PLEASURES

If your parent is severely ill, heavily medicated, or suffering from dementia, it may take very little to entertain him. Children's games, like checkers or Go Fish, an otherwise monotonous task like sticking labels on envelopes, stroking a cat, or listening to the jingle-jangle of children's songs may give his day a boost. What might seem silly to you may engage or even delight him.

about practical matters like estate planning and budgeting. If there is more than one center in the area, your parent is welcome to sign up for classes at any or all of them.

THE INTERNET

WHILE IT DOESN'T BEGIN TO REPLACE real friendship and face-to-face social contacts, the Internet is a powerful tool that can give your parent access to an abundance of information and link her to family, friends, and even a few new acquaintances.

Grandparents can suddenly communicate with children, grandchildren, and friends all over the world with a quick e-mail, a scanned photo, or an Instant Message. If your parent can't get out, it's a wonderful way to bring the world in. If you're far away or at work, it also offers you another way to check in, keep in touch, and otherwise see how your parent is doing.

With the Internet, your parent can pursue lifelong interests or delve into new topics. She can look up her family tree, track down relatives or friends, and read her hometown newspaper. She can learn about foreign places, go back in history, read about a favorite movie star, pursue a hobby, or play games. It will give her a sense of independence and involvement, and keep both her brain and fingers active.

She can also visit "chat rooms" or join online support groups to talk anonymously with others who might share her interests, problems, or concerns. While she should be careful about scams and fraud on the Internet (see page 344), it will open a whole new world to her.

Most libraries, senior centers, assisted-living facilities, and nursing homes now offer Internet access, as do many coffee shops. Otherwise, you might buy your parent a simple and relatively inexpensive computer.

If your parent has trouble navigating the Internet, using the mouse, typing, or is otherwise deterred, many senior centers, libraries, adult education programs, and assisted-living and nursing homes offer Internet classes to the elderly. Several Web sites also offer tutorials (including www.generationsonline.com, www.aarp.org/learninternet, and www.folksonline.com).

Dating, Sex, and Marriage

Your parent may be old, but he's not dead. Just because someone's hair turns white, joints grow stiff, and ears can't hear, does not mean that he or she has no need for intimate relationships, even physically intimate ones. Arthritis, diabetes, hypertension, and hearing loss have not made your parent any less of a person. All people, until their last breaths, need love and intimacy almost as much as they need food and water.

DATING

IT CAN BE UNSETTLING FOR A CHILD, even a fully grown child who is facing his own senior years, to discover that Mom has fallen in love, or that Dad is acting like a teenager around a certain someone. He's ninety-two years old, for Pete's sake. He can hardly see, much less walk. He's got fifteen medical ailments. Someone has to cut up his meat and lay out his pills and help him get his pants on. So what is this about? Is he some kind of pervert? What does this woman want from him? Is she after his money? Isn't this a betrayal of Mom? She was his wife for nearly fifty years, after all.

You may be taken aback if your parent starts dating. In the process of caring for an elderly person, it's tempting to depersonalize her. That is, she becomes a set of medical ailments and physical needs, a pile of bills and a list of home-care workers. She is not a person who starts up a new relationship and gets in a tizzy over a first kiss.

You may also feel that this is somehow disloyal to your other parent, even though he may have died some time ago. (Or maybe he died recently. Remember, your mother might have been losing her husband over a long period and dealt with much of that grief before he was gone.)

Late in life, even very late in life, flirting and dating, touching, and gazing into someone's eyes is heavenly. It provides companionship and feelings of youthfulness, of being alive. Really alive. It boosts self-esteem and gets the old ticker beating. Hooray, hooray! Love and sex are not stripped away at the nursing-home door, nor are residents deprived of their rights to engage in such activities.

SEX

THE WHOLE IDEA OF LOVE AT A LATE age may seem sort of "cute," until you wake up to the obvious: Your parent is staying in the certain someone's apartment. At night. All night. *What are they doing in there?* Ageism hits its lowest point right here with the assumption that people in their eighties and nineties are beyond dating and could not possibly be having sex.

Sex very late in life, if your parent is fortunate enough to have it, is often more about intimacy and companionship than about physical pleas-

> " *Two years after my dad died, my mother met a man, and they began to go to the movies together and have lunch occasionally. She was so nervous about it, like a schoolgirl. I kept saying, 'It's okay. Just enjoy it. He's nice.' I could see her, right before my eyes, becoming young again.*
>
> *They've been together now for several years, maybe three or four. She's bent over with arthritis and he can barely hear or see, but they are so happy together. It's like a whole new life has opened up for her. It makes me feel like there's so much promise, that life doesn't end at eighty.*"
>
> —JENNY R.

ure. Sure, there's a physical need and sometimes a response, but at this wise stage of life, sex tends to be more about caring, closeness, understanding, mutual admiration, sharing, and loyalty. The emotional and psychological aspect takes on greater importance.

Coupled with this, sex is not a bad form of exercise, it reduces anxiety, and it reassures a person that, yes, this old body still functions.

Forgetting your reaction for a moment, the idea of dating, much less having sex, may be frightening and daunting for your parent. She may be guilty of ageism, too. She might think she's too old for such behavior, or that only immoral, lustful women even think about such things. Anyway, it's

> *My mother was widowed after sixty years of marriage, and two years later she met someone and is about to remarry. She's eighty-five and he's eighty. I think it's wonderful. It's darling. I am delighted for her.*
>
> *My sister has met him, and she thinks he has memory problems. She worries that Mom will have to take care of him. Actually, because my sister lives closest to them, she worries that she will have to care for both of them. I don't think we have any say in the matter. This is what Mom wants. It makes her happy."*
>
> —DIANNE D.

been a long time, and her body's not much to look at, and it might not respond the way it once did, and, gee, will she remember what to do?

All of these worries can get in the way of meeting people, becoming intimate, and, finally, having sex. Your father might not function sexually simply because he is so afraid of not functioning. Worry alone gets in the way, and then a spiral sets in, because once someone has "failed," the fear of doing so again becomes an overriding concern.

Your parent might be reluctant to get involved with someone or, once involved, have problems with sex for the same reasons younger people do— boredom, fear, grief, anxiety, fatigue, depression.

Then there are problems associated with age: Sex at an old age usually takes longer, men require more time to become erect, women may require lubrication, and the two might have to find an imaginative position because of sore knees and replaced hips.

One of the major causes of sexual dysfunction, aside from all the psychological ones, is medications and alcohol. Antidepressants, tranquilizers, and a host of other medications, as well as alcohol, can douse desire or otherwise interfere with normal sexual functioning.

Finally, your parent might worry that medical problems, such as arthritis, heart disease, incontinence, or surgery, make it impossible or dangerous for her to have sex. But this simply isn't true. Most obstacles are surmountable. And the benefits certainly outweigh any risks.

(The good news: no interruptions from children, lots of free time, and slower male responses. Also no worries about pregnancy, unless Dad has found someone much younger; men can still make babies late in life.)

Your parent should talk to his or her doctor, but given that most people do not want to raise such issues with their doctors (much less anyone else), and given that many doctors do not know the answers to these sorts of questions, you might alert your parent to some other sources of information. The National Institute on Aging has a short pamphlet on sexuality late in life, and there are several books on sexuality late in life (although many

DATING, SEX, AND DEMENTIA

People with dementia can also fall in love and, yes, have sex. In the early stages, that might be perfectly fine—wonderful, in fact. If your parent is still somewhat competent and seems to know, at least to some extent, what he is doing; if this is consistent with other things he has done in his life; and if there is no abuse or force involved, then it's probably nothing to worry about. Indeed, it's something to celebrate. But later in the disease, when your parent's ability to reason is largely gone, dating raises a number of issues. If you are concerned, talk with his doctor, a psychiatrist who knows about such things, or others involved in his care.

If your parent is inappropriately sexual, see page 519 on ways you might help curb this. If your parent is living among others who have dementia, and someone is making unwanted sexual gestures or advances, talk to the staff of the facility. Urge your parent to keep a distance, and talk to her about how she should respond if this person were to undress, make rude remarks, or make some other sexual advance. Remember, this lack of inhibition is part of a disease, not part of the person.

of these consider fifty and sixty to be "late in life").

Support and encourage your parent. Okay, it's not a subject you're eager to bring up with her. But try to be accepting of any hint of interest on her part. Encourage it. Ease any tension and remind your parent, if possible, that romance and passion are good for the soul.

If you can't say the "s" word, talk about dating instead. Ask her if she misses dating or ever thinks about dating. Does she miss having male company? Would she like to date? If her spouse has recently passed away, encourage her to get out and do things where she'll meet men.

Let her know that there are literally dozens of dating services that specialize in "senior dating." (Unfortunately, because women generally live longer than men, they don't have a large crop of men to choose from, but senior men have their pick. About 60 percent of older women are single, whereas only 20 percent of older men are.)

If your parent shows an interest in someone, let her know that you and other loved ones are behind it all the way. Wouldn't it be nice if your parent were no longer alone? If she had a companion? No, you won't have the control over her that you once had. Yes, there is a chance she will remarry, which might muddle some issues for the family. But what a joy for her if she finds someone to do things with, to share life with, to love.

AND MARRIAGE

YOUR PARENT IS MOVING IN WITH someone or getting married. You may like this fellow; you may not. Either way, all sorts of questions arise. Will he take adequate care of her? Will he now be making decisions about her living situation and guiding her care? Or worse, is she going to end up taking care of him in her last years? What is his health status? Maybe you will end up taking care of both of them! That won't do. And, goodness gracious, how will they sort out their finances?

It's time to talk.

Obviously, you need to iron out your own feelings. Perhaps you don't like this new mate. Perhaps you are worried that you won't see as much of your parent now. You might have concerns about the restructuring of the family, traditions, and other matters. Perhaps you are concerned about your parent's finances and about your own inheritance. Whatever the issues, address them as best you can. Talk openly with your parent.

Remember, she is an adult. You are not her parent. If she is competent, you have no say in this decision. This is her money, her life, and her choice. If she is happy, try to be happy for her. Imagine yourself at her age finding someone who cares for you and for whom you care. Let go of some issues. What matters is her happiness,

not how this arrangement affects you. Try to create new traditions and patterns around this new situation.

Still, don't let love blind you or your parent. Romance and wedding planning are exciting, but when a late-life marriage is in the air, be realistic and get some practical advice. Marriage will drastically affect your parent's living situation, daily habits, other relations, finances, estate, and many other legal issues.

Your mother should talk with an elder law attorney and possibly a financial adviser. Who is going to make medical decisions on her behalf? Who will decide if she needs nursing-home care at some point? Who will handle her assets should she become incapacitated or incompetent? Has she assigned power of attorney to someone? Does she have a living will or a health-care proxy? In other words, will this new spouse make all decisions regarding living, medical care, and finances, or does that authority reside with an adult child or some other trusted person?

Or, what happens when your father has a stroke and his brand-new wife wants to send him off to a nursing home, but you think he should stay in his house with some nursing care? Who makes decisions about life-sustaining medical treatments at the end of his life? Will you have any say?

As for finances, ideally, couples are open about their finances and sort everything out in advance. What are each person's assets, income, expected future income, debts, and other financial obligations? What insurance policies exist, and who are the beneficiaries? How will this affect Medicaid eligibility and eligibility for other services? Will assets be held individually, as "joint tenants," as "tenants in common," or in a trust for someone else?

Because these issues get particularly messy late in life, when people have various accounts, assets, and financial needs, and might also have some cognitive impairment, your parent should sign a prenuptial agreement detailing everything. Any agreement should be updated from time to time, as assets, needs, and relationships change.

If your parent has dementia or is incapacitated and you are worried that this new love is purely out for his wallet, look into obtaining guardianship, get him to put assets into a trust, or at least have him sign a durable power of attorney giving you some authority over his finances.

Once again, the focus is your parent's happiness and choices. Unless real trouble is brewing, it is not about whether or not you approve of or like the situation.

HOMOSEXUALITY

HOMOSEXUALITY WAS NOT CONSIDered acceptable in your parent's generation, but it is becoming far more so now. As a result, many elderly homosexuals who have never revealed their sexual preferences before are suddenly becoming open about it. In fact, they might have been in a heterosexual relationship for years, perhaps unhappily, because they did not want

---

STDs AND HIV

Never too old to have sex, but also never too old to contract sexually transmitted diseases (STDs), such as genital warts, herpes, chlamydia, or hepatitis B. And certainly everyone who is sexually active is at risk of becoming infected with HIV, the virus that causes AIDS. Your parent should talk with a doctor about how to protect himself, or he should at least use a latex condom. For more information about HIV and the elderly, contact the National Association on HIV Over Fifty (617-233-7107 or www.hivoverfifty.org).

---

to admit their sexual preference, even to themselves.

An estimated 10 percent of all elderly people are homosexual. They endure all the same stresses and worries as elderly heterosexuals, plus the added hardship of discrimination. If your parent is in a nursing home or other group facility, the isolation may be compounded.

Again, there are groups and organizations to turn to for help. Many of them are locally based, so the best thing to do is search the Internet for groups in the area. You should also contact Senior Action in a Gay Environment, or SAGE (212-741-2247 or www.sage usa.org).

TIPS FOR DAILY LIVING

Safety First • Preventing Falls • Hygiene
• Dressing • Eating • The Question of Driving
• Useful Gadgets and Gizmos

....

W HO CAN HELP BUT WORRY ABOUT AN ELDERLY PARENT getting through the day, or even part of the day, alone? *What if Dad falls? I don't think Mother should be driving. Is he eating anything? How does she get herself dressed in the morning? Isn't he lonely?* And yet, in this country, more than 1.5 million people over the age of eighty-five live alone (more than 10 million people over sixty-five live alone), and millions more spend at least part of the day on their own. Most of them like it this way; they want to stay in their own homes. And in most cases, it is exactly where they should be. So, if that is what he wishes, do what you can to keep your parent living independently in his own home.

If your father has arthritis, diabetes, fuzzy vision, and mild dementia, it doesn't mean that it's time for a nursing home or that you have to follow him around tending to his every need. You don't want to, and he probably doesn't want you to, either.

Whether your parent lives alone, with you, or in some sort of group facility, you can do some minor renovations, rearrange his home, buy some useful gadgets, and help him change some habits so that he can live as independently as possible, for as long as possible. He can maintain his autonomy and reduce the risk of accidents, falls, crimes, and other emergencies that could cut his life short or make it miserable.

Ask your parent about the details of his day or spend a day with him observing how he goes about his basic chores. Even if someone is around to help him, there might be things that he can actually do for himself. Does he have trouble holding his razor, walking down stairs, heating up spaghetti, or locking the front door? Does he have a way to get groceries or visit a friend? Once you know the day's snags, brainstorm for solutions. (Be sure to involve your parent in this effort.)

There are a number of ways to make cooking more manageable, dressing more doable, exercise more feasible, life less risky, and free time more entertaining. If you need help with a specific problem and don't find a solution here, contact an occupational therapist, visiting nurse, carpenter, or electrician, depending upon the situation. Be sure to check out some of the handy gadgets discussed at the end of this chapter.

Safety First

Bad eyesight, arthritis, poor balance, multiple medications, and other health problems all put your parent at risk for accidents. Look through her house for hazards. Be particularly thorough if your parent suffers from any sort of confusion.

◆ Put a 911 reminder near the phone or designate one button for 911. Keep a clearly written, large-print list of other emergency phone numbers by every phone, or program them into the telephone's memory. The list should include police, fire, ambulance, your home and work numbers, and the phone number of a nearby relative or a neighbor. Don't assume your parent will remember your number, or even 911, if she's injured, burglarized, or in some other trouble. Even the keenest minds can go blank during moments of panic. Because of this, you might also put her street address in clear letters by the phone in case she becomes muddled when talking to emergency crews.

◆ Alert police and fire departments to the fact that your parent is elderly and lives alone. Don't rely on window decals to alert them to her presence. Ask if there are any special precautions you should take.

◆ Make sure that chemicals, harsh cleaners, insecticides, medications, paints, etc. are all labeled with big, clear letters. If your parent gets confused easily, put them out of sight completely.

◆ Check to see that smoke detectors and carbon monoxide detectors all work. Your parent's waning sense of smell makes a smoke detector that much more important, but research suggests that a third of smoke detectors have dead or missing batteries. They should be checked at least every couple of months. Be sure smoke detectors are located on each floor of the house, especially outside bedroom doors. Also, you might want to set off the alarm so that your parent knows the sound and what it means.

◆ Check for easy escape routes, in case of fire. Your parent may not be able to climb out of a window, so look for escapes she could use. Is the back door wide enough for your mother's wheelchair? Is there a back stairway that your father can manage? If possible, hold a fire drill. If your parent might not be able to escape because of a disability, call the local fire department and ask for safety instructions.

◆ Buy a small fire extinguisher that is easy to handle and put it in a clearly visible place, preferably in the kitchen, where fires often start. And instruct your parent in how to use it.

◆ Have any specific medical instructions on an identification bracelet or, at the very least, taped to a wall where medics and other emergency crews will see it.

◆ Have at least two flashlights, with working batteries, ready to use and easy to find if the lights go out. Put one by your parent's bed and one on a kitchen table. If there is a blackout, several large flashlights are safer than candles.

◆ Make sure all bathroom and kitchen outlets contain working circuit interrupters to prevent shocks.

◆ In the kitchen, check to see that all burners and the oven work properly. Be sure that outlets are not overloaded, and that wires don't rest on a hot toaster, for example. Is your mother apt to reach for equipment located above the hot stove, in which case a sleeve or apron string might catch fire? If so, rearrange things.

◆ Because of their thinner skin and slower reactions, elderly people are at risk for scalding. Set the hot water heater so the temperature of the water doesn't rise above 120°F.

◆ If your parent gets cold easily, buy him some good long underwear and turn up the heat. Be careful with space heaters and electric blankets, as they can cause burns and fires.

◆ If your parent has even mild dementia or confusion, you might want to register him with the Alzheimer's Association's Safe Return program, in which your parent is given an identification card and becomes part of a national photo database. Learn more about it through the association (800-272-3900 or www.alz.org).

MEDICAL EMERGENCY IDENTIFICATION

SLIP A MEDICAL IDENTIFICATION CARD into your parent's wallet so in case there is ever an emergency, medical crews will know who he is, whom to contact, and whether he has any medical conditions that require special attention.

You can make one yourself or, in many locations, the area agency on aging distributes free identification tags, to either hang on a chain or place in a wallet. Otherwise, several companies sell them (look under "Medical Emergency Information" in the Yellow Pages or on the Internet). MedicAlert is one of the oldest companies making medical identification bracelets (888-633-4298 or www.medicalert.org).

EMERGENCY RESPONSE SYSTEMS

"I'VE FALLEN AND I CAN'T GET UP" made for an amusing ad, but the message was quite serious. Emergency response systems are worth the investment if you are worried about your parent living alone.

The emergency response system provides your parent with a help button which can be worn as a pendant or on a wrist band. At the response center your parent is identified by a code. If she falls, has chest pains, or needs help for any reason, she pushes the button which triggers her telephone to automatically dial a response center. The center will then call 911 or will phone your parent. If your parent cannot get to the phone, the responder talks with her through a two-way intercom that is attached to the phone. If she doesn't respond to the call or says that there is, indeed, an emergency, the responder then calls an emergency crew.

Dozens of companies now sell emergency response systems. You can find them in the Yellow Pages or on the Internet under "emergency response system," or check with a medical supply store. Or you can ask your parent's doctor if the hospital he is affiliated with offers such a service.

Prices vary, so call several companies. Some sell the system (usually for $100 to $2,000) and then charge a monthly service fee ($10 to $40). Others rent systems (for $15 to $60 a month, after an initial installation charge). Still other companies lease systems for a set time. Renting and leasing are often preferable because you don't have to worry about repairs or a company going defunct or moving. Hospitals and social service organizations sometimes offer the systems for free or at a discount to people living on low incomes.

When comparing systems, ask for details about the staff receiving

WATCHFUL EYES

E mergency response systems are only helpful if your parent can, in a crisis, push the button. There may be instances in which he can't—something happens when he's in the shower or sleeping, or he becomes sick, injured, or confused quite suddenly and doesn't have the wherewithal to sound the alarm.

If your parent lives alone and doesn't have regular visitors, it's advisable to have some other way of knowing if there's trouble.

You can ask a neighbor to alert you if he notices anything unusual (the house is dark in the evening, for example, or your father hasn't been seen walking the dog in the morning). You can ask anyone who sees your parent on a regular basis—the newspaper deliverer, the apartment superintendent, a barber, a rabbi, or a grocery clerk—to contact you if anything seems wrong. (Of course, you should approach only those individuals you and your parent trust completely. You don't want strangers to know that your parent is frail and alone.)

People who deliver meals for meals-on-wheels programs are taught to recognize warning signs (your parent looks pale or shaky or confused, or doesn't answer the door). Also, mail carriers and utility workers are sometimes trained to spot trouble—the mail hasn't been picked up, the lawn hasn't been mowed, the power hasn't been used. Call the local post office and utility company to find out if such a program exists in your parent's community.

emergency calls. Are they available twenty-four hours a day, seven days a week? How are they trained? Do they speak your parent's native language? Find out the company's average response time (if they are not checking their response time periodically, they should be). How often and how does the center test the system to be sure it's working?

Be sure your parent can operate the buttons. Then test the system to see how well it operates within his house and how far he can venture into the backyard, for example, before the system fails.

Ask if your parent can try the system for a trial period or get a money-back guarantee. Find out about warranty, cancellation, service, and repair policies. What happens if your parent cancels a lease arrangement? What happens if the system is faulty? How would it be repaired? What would that cost? What happens if your parent moves?

Shop around. Be sure you are dealing with a reputable company. Find the best system and best value.

Once your parent has an emergency response system, check the batteries regularly. It's no good to have it if it's not working.

Crime Precautions

The elderly are popular targets for criminals because they are easy prey. But there's no need for your parent to lock herself in the house or be afraid to go out. Even if she is physically frail, common sense can protect her from most dangerous situations.

Talk to your parent about the precautions she should take and what she should do in specific situations. Do some role-playing. Going through the motions now will mean quicker and smarter reactions should there ever be a problem. Check with the local senior center or police department to find out about talks on crime prevention. In the meantime:

◆ Let the local police department know that your parent is elderly and living alone, especially if she lives in a small town where the police might pay some special attention to her.

◆ Make sure your parent can properly operate all his home door locks and that he uses them. If he has trouble using a key, he might switch to a coded lock. Get locks that can be opened from the inside without a key, in case he needs to exit quickly.

◆ Install a peephole in the front door. Your parent should not open the door for anyone unfamiliar—a salesperson or repair person—unless she has asked that person to come. She might also invest in an intercom for the front door.

◆ If your parent doesn't already have one, install a security alarm system in his house. Then, make sure he actually uses it. You can also install "panic buttons" by his bed or favorite chair, which he can press to alert the police or any security guards to trouble.

◆ Look into installing outdoor lights that are triggered by motion; they will go on as soon as your parent nears the property—or as soon as someone else does. Several companies also sell remote controls that operate house lights, as well as thermostats, a radio, or a television, from afar. When your parent arrives home at night, he can light up the house and even make it noisy several minutes before arriving, allowing burglars time to escape (and the house time to warm up). You can also install exterior floodlights that can be operated from the bedroom.

◆ Talk with your parent about where and when it is best for him to walk outdoors. There may be certain routes to the store or the park that are safer than others, and particular times of day when he should opt for cabs or buses.

> *My mother was always active. At ninety-six, she volunteered, traveled, read. But when she fell and broke her ankle she was immobile for a couple of months, and that really killed her spirit. She could never get around well after that, and so her mood, her body, everything just went. She died a year later."*
>
> —MEL T.

◆ Your parent should leave diamond rings or expensive watches at home when traveling in cities or in any crime-ridden areas. They attract thieves and pickpockets.

◆ Money and credit cards should be carried in an inside pocket or money belt rather than a purse, which can be snatched. Nevertheless, your parent should always carry a little cash ($20 or $30) with him so he has something to hand over to a mugger.

Preventing Falls

Everyone catches a toe or trips on a step occasionally, but at your parent's age, a minor tumble can have major repercussions. Older bodies break more easily than younger ones, and they don't heal as quickly or as completely. Then, while they are trying to heal, enforced bed rest exacerbates previous medical ills and can cause new ones, such as pneumonia, infections, bedsores, and other circulatory disorders.

One out of every three Americans sixty-five years or older and living in the community (as opposed to a nursing home) has a pretty serious fall at least once a year. (That only includes those that are reported, so the actual number is probably much higher.) In nursing homes, that rate rises about threefold.

Falls often result in fractures of the hip, spine, pelvis, hand, and wrist, as well as spinal cord and brain injuries. A fracture in an elderly person can have dire consequences. For example, half of all older people who fracture a hip never fully recover—they end up needing canes, walkers, or wheelchairs for the rest of their lives. Twenty-five percent of them die within six months of the injury. Furthermore, 40 percent of elderly people entering nursing homes cite falls as one reason for the move; 25 percent say it is the primary reason.

To put all this more simply, falling is one of the most serious health risks facing older people. Preventing falls should be a primary concern for you and your parent.

The problem is that most people do exactly the opposite of what they should do. Afraid of falling, elderly people become extremely cautious and are reluctant to get up and move around. Care providers support this guarded approach by urging the elderly person to remain stationary—*Don't move. I'll get it for you.* Ironically,

HOME MODIFICATION

Your parent's home can be renovated to accommodate almost any disability. In addition to the suggestions listed throughout this chapter, you can do more major renovations to make a house even more accessible—ramps, lower sinks, wheelchair-accessible bathrooms, automatic door openers, etc.

AARP (888-687-2277 or www.aarp.org) has information on how to make a home user-friendly for people with disabilities.

The National Rehabilitation Information Center (800-346-2742 or www.naric.com) can supply information on disabilities, rehabilitation, home modification, rehabilitation equipment, and local organizations.

The National Resource Center on Supportive Housing and Home Modification (213-740-1364 or www.homemods.org), based in California, has information about home modification as well as a database of local programs and contractors who specialize in such work, and will do other maintenance work for seniors at a discount.

this is a surefire way to increase the risk of falls (not to mention making life pretty dull and miserable). Sedentary, your parent will have less strength, balance, and flexibility, and will be more apt to, yes, fall. It's a downward spiral, so try to avoid it.

Furthermore, your parent will become dependent, isolated, and depressed, and have health problems related to his inactive lifestyle, such as constipation, loss of appetite, insomnia, and poor circulation.

The best way to prevent falls is through exercises that help balance, coordination, flexibility, and strength. Urge your parent to get up and move as much as possible. The ancient Chinese art of tai chi, which involves slow and controlled movements, is a particularly good way for elderly people to increase balance and prevent falls. (See page 66 for more on exercise and the elderly—gentle exercises that can be done no matter how old or frail or sick your parent might be.)

Beyond that, find out what, besides weak leg muscles and poor coordination, might be behind any imbalance. Medications, poor vision or hearing, arthritis, depression, confusion, dizziness, circulatory disease, and heart disease can all make someone tippy. Your parent should ask her doctor if she can lower the dose of certain medications, especially sleeping pills, antidepressants, and blood pressure medications. She should also attend to any vision problems, dizziness, circulation ailments, and arthritis.

PRACTICE MAKES PERFECT SENSE

Show your parent what to do in case he falls. Coach him through a practice session: Get him to lie down and then roll onto his belly and push himself up onto his hands and knees. He should then crawl to a piece of furniture that he can use for support while he pulls himself up. Or, he can crawl to a phone and call for help. (Or consider buying a medical alert system.) This drill may sound a little silly, but when people fall, they often become confused and disoriented. If they have practiced what to do in advance, it should come to them more easily when they need to do it.

Your parent should be tested for osteoporosis with a bone-density test. Osteoporosis makes bones brittle and therefore makes falls more dangerous. Medications may be necessary to strengthen her bones. (Men get osteoporosis too, by the way.) Some people who are at high risk wear padding on their hips to help protect them from injuries in case of a fall, although some doctors contend this doesn't help much. But it can't hurt, and it may give your parent the confidence she needs to get out of her chair.

If your parent is stiff or becomes dizzy or wobbly easily, she should practice getting up slowly from a chair and using handrails and other supports as she moves about a room. She should consider getting a cane or walker. Tell her to get over any hangups about thinking a cane makes her look older. Think of it as "cane power" and a ticket to more independence. Once she gets a cane or walker, have her talk with a physical therapist about ways to use the device safely and effectively.

Finally, get rid of anything that might cause your parent to topple—the loose rugs, the tricky half-step, the cups on the top shelf that require a footstool—and add some things that help her maintain her balance—good lighting, handrails, strong arms on chairs.

While everyone with an older parent should be alert to the threat of falls, you need to be particularly cautious if your parent has Parkinson's disease, dementia, poor eyesight, arthritis, or, as we mentioned, osteoporosis. Be wary also if your parent has any injury or disability in her legs, has fallen before, has had a stroke, or is taking medications (or alcohol) that might make her unstable, dizzy, or faint.

ROOM-BY-ROOM PREVENTION

A VISITING NURSE OR AN OCCUPAtional or physical therapist can examine your parent's home for hazards and show you how to reduce risks. If the inspection is done as part of a hospital discharge, Medicare or other insurance policies may cover the cost. But you can also tour your parent's house yourself and look for places where she has to bend, reach, stoop, or step over something. Look for anything that might trip her up or get in her way. While you're at it, if she spends any time at your house or elsewhere, check out those places for traps that might cause trouble.

Here some things you can do to prevent falls:

Floors and Pathways

• Check carpets for worn areas and rips. Tack down any flaps or curled edges.

• Use low-pile, wall-to-wall carpeting wherever possible. Avoid thick-pile carpets.

• Get rid of throw rugs or make sure they have a rubber, nonskid backing on them.

• Use nonslip wax or be sure that wax is buffed thoroughly.

• Make sure floors are even and level. Repair loose floorboards and remove thresholds at doorways.

• Clear hallways and other pathways of wastepaper baskets, footstools, magazine racks, electrical wires, and other small objects.

• If your parent has any hanging plants, be sure she doesn't have to duck to get past them (or reach up on tiptoes to water them).

> "*My father has this little, three-legged pine table in his living room, right by his favorite chair. Every time he got up or sat down, he would lean on the table, using it for balance. I told him a hundred times that the table was wobbly, and that one day he was going to lean on it, fall over, and kill himself. I even bought him a new table one year, but he didn't use it. He's pretty stubborn. He said, 'I've had this table here for forty-five years and I haven't fallen yet. Why would I fall now?'*
>
> *But I think my warning sank in a little, even though he would never admit it. I've noticed that he doesn't really lean on that table anymore. He puts more weight on the chair. He listens if I bother him enough about something. I just have to be a little more stubborn than he is.*"
>
> —SKIP R.

• Install handrails in hallways.

Stairs

• Avoid stairs completely, if possible. This may mean turning a downstairs den into a bedroom or building ramps onto short stairways. You can also buy a lift that carries a passenger up and down stairs in a chair—expensive, but helpful if you can afford one.

MEDICAL ALERT

If your parent has a serious fall and is in pain, don't move her unless you need to restore her breathing or get her away from fire, out of water, or clear from some other danger. Call an emergency crew. Cover her with a blanket if it's cool and assure her that medical help is coming. Continue to talk to her in a calm voice until help has arrived.

• When stairs are unavoidable, each step should be no more than seven inches high and deep enough to comfortably fit a person's foot (11 or 12 inches, ideally). All of them should be the same height and width.

• Be sure handrails are sturdy and extend the full length of the stairs. Handrails should be placed on both sides of the stairs. Don't forget stairs leading to a basement and those by the front and back doors.

• Mark the edges of steps—or any place the floor changes elevation even slightly—with brightly colored, glow-in-the-dark adhesive tape.

• Use nonslip treads on each step. Consider getting rid of carpeting on stairways, as it rounds off the edges of steps and shortens the depth of each step, making footing precarious.

Furniture

• Make sure that chairs are high enough to get out of and into easily, and that they have strong armrests and high backs that can be used for support. If necessary, keep a walker or cane by the chair or look into electric-powered pneumatic chairs that lift a person up, lower him down, and get him in and out more easily. You can also buy wedged cushions that provide a little help in getting out of a chair.

• Likewise, make sure the bed is not too high or too low, so your parent can get in and out easily.

• Get rid of beds and other furniture with nonlocking wheels.

• Furniture legs that curve outward create a tripping hazard. Move such furniture out of any pathway or get rid of it.

• Avoid three-legged tables, which are not sturdy.

• Repair broken or wobbly furniture immediately.

Bathrooms and Kitchens

• Install grab bars near toilets and tubs. Do not let your parent rely on towel bars for support.

• Buy a raised toilet seat, which makes sitting and getting up far easier.

• Attach a wall-mounted liquid soap dispenser in the shower so your parent is not fumbling around picking up bars of soap.

• Install nonslip strips or rubber mats on the floor of the tub or shower.

• Place nonslip strips or rubber-bottom bathmats on the bathroom floor. Keep a nonslip rug or runner, or a rubber mat, in front of the kitchen sink where the floor is apt to be wet and slippery.

• Avoid bath oils, which make feet and hands slippery.

• A shower curtain may be easier to manage than a glass door, but make sure it's hung on a secure rod that is screwed into the wall, not a tension rod. If your parent slips, a curtain on a screwed-in rod will offer better support.

• Your parent or someone else in the household should clean up any grease, water, or other spills right away.

Lighting

• Lighting should be bright and evenly distributed. Older eyes need more light. They also don't adjust quickly to changes in lighting, so avoid having dark hallways that lead into brightly lit stairways, or vice versa.

• Reduce glare by aiming lights at a wall or the ceiling, and use low-glare bulbs and lampshades. If there is a sunny window facing your parent as he uses the stairs, hang curtains or shades to block the glare.

• Make sure light switches are easy to use and easy to reach. They should be placed at the entrance of each room, and at both the top and the bottom of any stairs, so your parent isn't walking through a dark room to get to a light.

• Install a light by the bed so your parent isn't fumbling around at night when she needs to get up.

• Use night-lights in the hallway, the bathroom, the kitchen, the stairway, or anywhere else your parent might venture at night.

• You can install sound-activated lights that go on when your parent gets up during the night and go off after she has stopped moving around. Look for them in catalogs, medical supply stores, hardware stores, or lighting stores.

Other Measures

• Buck fashion. Make sure your parent has comfortable, sturdy, nonslip (i.e., rubber-soled) shoes with low, broad-based heels and wide toes. Sneakers with splayed soles provide a solid base. Avoid sandals and shoes with open heels or toes. Bedroom slippers should have rubber soles. If your mother likes to walk around in her socks, get socks with rubber pads on the bottom.

• Beware of alcohol, which has a pronounced effect in the elderly and will affect balance and reflexes.

• Check the temperature. Both low and high body temperature can make a person dizzy. In general, the thermostat probably needs to be higher than it used to be, even at night, when the thermostat should be around 65 degrees. When temperatures rise, be sure your parent's

FEELING DIZZY

Up to 30 percent of elderly people feel dizzy frequently or regularly, making them even more prone to falls and more apt to avoid the sort of activity and exercise that might help them become more stable. Dizziness can also lead to social withdrawal, loss of independence, and depression.

Dizziness is an imprecise term. A person might feel that the room is revolving, or that she is tilting and unsteady on her feet, or she might feel light-headed and faint, or some other form of dizziness.

While dizziness in a younger person is usually a symptom of a specific disease, in the elderly it is often the result of myriad diseases and impairments. We feel balanced because numerous systems (cardiological, respiratory, psychological, auditory, visual, neurological, psychiatric, and chemical) are functioning and communicating properly. When any of these systems is out of whack, a person can end up feeling dizzy. Medications can cause or worsen dizziness.

Bring this to the doctor's attention. Even if one or two causes are treated, it should reduce the severity of the dizziness. Medications might need altering, antidepressants sometimes help, and certain exercises can reduce dizziness. (Even if they worsen it at first, over time they can help.) People can also be taught to keep dizziness at bay by avoiding certain over-the-counter drugs, not taking excessively hot showers and baths, limiting salt, and learning to rise slowly from beds and chairs.

home is air-conditioned, or at least well fanned. (If she doesn't have air-conditioning, she might need to install a room air conditioner or move to an air-conditioned facility during the hottest part of the day.)

• Organize things so that frequently used items are within easy reach.

• Place telephones in those places where your parent spends the most time—next to the bed, by his easy chair—or get him a portable phone. (But he has to take it with him and not lose it or it will be more trouble than it's worth.)

• Teach your parent how to rise from chairs and beds gradually to avoid light-headedness. She should get up in stages, with two hands planted firmly on armrests or other supports.

• Install grab bars by the closet, so when your parent is dressing, he has something to hold on to for balance.

• If necessary, encourage your parent to use a cane or walker. A doctor should fit it and your parent should be taught how to use it correctly.

• If your father uses a cane, attach a loose wrist strap to one end. Then, if he drops it, it won't fall to the ground and leave him in the precarious position of having to stoop to pick it up.

• In winter in northern climes, your parent should keep a bag of rock salt or sand by the front door so he can toss a few scoops on icy steps. He needs to beware of wet, slippery, or uneven pavement. Tell him to walk on grass or loose snow instead of hard, wet, or icy patches, and to step slowly over slippery surfaces, with his feet apart and his knees slightly bent. (And remember those rubber soles!)

IF YOUR PARENT FALLS

IF YOUR PARENT FALLS AND DOESN'T seem to have broken any bones (no severe pain or difficulty moving), stay calm. Speak to her gently, reassuring her and informing her of what you are doing to help.

If you are able, lift her up using your legs, not your back. This means bending at your knees, getting a good hold, and pushing up with your legs. Hold her under her shoulders; don't pull on a hand or elbow. Likewise, if you need to turn your parent over, pull at her torso, or hip and thigh; don't pull on a foot, leg, or wrist. If you need to turn her around, don't twist your body; pivot by taking small steps.

If your parent is too heavy for you to lift, bring a sturdy table or chair to her so she can lift herself up with your help. Talk to her as you move her, telling her exactly what you are doing so the two of you don't get twisted up and both end up on the floor.

If you cannot lift her up, don't hurt yourself trying. Wait for help to arrive. In the meantime, keep her warm, hydrated, and calm.

Whether or not she is injured, have your parent make an appointment with her doctor so he can determine what caused the fall and can talk to her about ways of preventing accidents in the future. Falls are sometimes indicators that a drug is causing problems or that your parent has an illness such as dehydration, heart disease, stroke, infection, pneumonia, or internal bleeding.

If a fall leads to a fracture, she may be disabled for some time. Be aware of the complications that often accompany this more sedentary time of healing, such as pressure sores, stiffness, and swelling. (See page 249 for more on pressure sores, which are also known as bedsores.)

A physical therapist can go over range-of-motion exercises and stretches she can do to avoid stiffness, maintain her self-care skills, and keep her circulation strong. Contrary to what your instincts might tell you, the more she does, the faster she'll heal.

Bathing and Grooming

Sometimes you, and your parent, have to let go of a few things. Proper hygiene is important, as it prevents infections and makes a person feel good. But keep in mind, a couple of baths a week are fine; sponge baths in between are useful.

If you or someone else is helping your parent bathe and brush:

◆ Grab bars in the bathroom and raised toilet seats make life easier for aching knees and backs.

◆ Buy a chair made for the shower or use a small stool, as long as it's

> *In my mother's era, you took baths. She never used the shower. Ever. But I couldn't get her into the tub. And if I did, she couldn't get up once she got down. I said to her, 'A shower is so wonderful. You don't know what you're missing.' But she absolutely would not do it.*
>
> *Finally, she did try it, not long ago. She had her first shower at ninety-some-years old. I said, 'Isn't this wonderful?' You know, I'm standing outside and she's in there, but I'm holding her and I'm getting all wet. She wouldn't say that she liked it. But she accepted it."*
>
> —MARGARET F.

stable and won't slip (and is waterproof). You can also buy a rubber device that deflates to lower a person gently into the tub and then inflates to get him out again.

◆ Level-style faucets, rather than knobs, are easier to use for arthritic hands. (They are a good idea for door and cabinet handles, as well.)

◆ If your parent is immobile, a sponge bath is as good as a regular bath. Typically, a home health aide will bathe your parent, but if you are doing it yourself, prepare a bowl of warm, slightly soapy water, and with a soft washcloth wipe her down, top to bottom, being sure to get into all cracks and under every fold of skin. Dry thoroughly. You can also buy a rubber basin for washing her hair while she is in a bed or in a chair, or a full-body tub for the bed (which may be a little unwieldy).

◆ It is easier to brush someone else's teeth with an electric toothbrush. Use very little toothpaste. When your parent is quite sick, simply use a wet, soft toothbrush or damp washcloth or disposable mouth cleaner (available in medical supply stores) to wipe the teeth, gums, and tongue.

◆ Finally, medical supply stores, mail-order catalogs, and online stores (see page 131) sell a mind-boggling array of bathroom gizmos, such as a razor holder that attaches to the hand, a dental floss holder for those who have trouble winding the thread around their fingers, and a wall-mounted soap dispenser. You can also buy sponges with long handles, toothbrushes with thick handles, and nail clippers, toothpaste dispensers, mirrors, showerhead attachments, and urinals that are simple to use.

In the Dressing Room

If your parent has trouble reaching the zipper on the back of her dress, managing the tiny buttons on her sweater, or getting her shoes tied, explore the latest line of "easy clothing"

for both men and women—pants with Velcro closures, shirts with snaps, dresses with large zipper handles or ones that pull on from the front and then are sealed with a Velcro closure down the back, large jerseys that pull over the head, shoes that slip on, and skirts that pull on.

But before anyone pays for new clothes, think about ways to make the clothes she already owns easier to use. Buttons can be replaced with zippers or Velcro, and elastic shoelaces turn tie-up shoes into slip-ons. Or check the racks of a shop he or she already likes. Jersey dresses with wide necks slide over

MORE THAN CLEAN—BEAUTIFUL

Good hygiene is important not only for good health (poor hygiene can lead to skin infections), but also for self-esteem. People feel better when they look good. A new hairdo and some makeup may seem unnecessary at this point, but it should improve your mother's outlook. Your father will feel more dapper and proud with a clean shave and combed hair.

Make sure your parent has the proper tools not only for basic hygiene, but also for a bit of primping. Your father may be able to use the toilet safely, but can he open his aftershave? Can your mother manage a powder puff? (She may say that she doesn't care about makeup anymore in an effort to hide her problems, so you have to play sleuth.) Easy-to-open lids and other handy devices should help. Also, find out about local barbers and beauticians who make house calls. Some offer discounts to senior citizens.

Don't forget the little clothing touches that make your parent feel attractive. If your father likes to wear a tie but can no longer tie it, buy him a clip-on tie. Give your mother a colorful silk scarf, which hides humped shoulders, surrounds the face with color, and makes her feel special. (You can tie it permanently so all she has to do is slip it over her head.)

" When my mother's hair started to fall out after the chemotherapy, I didn't think much about it. We all knew it would happen, and she's never been terribly concerned about her appearance.

A friend of hers suggested that she buy a wig. I thought, 'Mom? In a wig? Never!' But sure enough, she bought one and she wears it all the time. She looks pretty good in it, and it's made a big difference in how she feels. She has a lot more confidence."

—DIANA M.

the head, and wrap-around dresses pull on like a coat. Sweatpants and tops are often the easiest (and most comfortable) outfits to wear, and many stores now sell attractive elastic-waist pants.

A few other tips:
• Go a size or two larger, which will help clothes go on easier and offer room for easy movement.

• For sensitive skin, find silky materials or soft knits.

• If your parent has trouble balancing while dressing, consider clothing that can be put on while sitting, such as wraparound or pullover dresses. Unfortunately, those who opt for pants will have to slide the pants on and then

EASY DRESSING

If you want to order new clothes that are designed for people with disabilities, including those who are in wheelchairs or suffer from incontinence, search the Internet (under "clothes for seniors" or "adaptive clothing" or "wheelchair clothes"). There are dozens of manufacturers. If you're having trouble, here are some places to start:

American Health Care Apparel
800-252-0584
www.clothesforseniors.com

Buck & Buck
800-458-0600
www.buckandbuck.com

Caring Concepts
800-336-2660
www.caringconcepts.com

Fashion Ease
800-221-8929
www.fashionease.com

Wardrobe Wagon
800-992-2737
www.wardrobewagon.com

balance briefly while pulling them up. Elastic-waist pants are easier than any with zippers and buckles.

• A variety of gadgets can make dressing easier, such as metallic arms or "grippers" that help pull socks and pants on, devices that pull buttons through their holes, and extra-long shoehorns. (See page 131 for more information.)

What's for Dinner?

Your parent might not be eating well for a variety of reasons, some of them easily solved. Try to ascertain what is hindering his diet, because poor diet can lead to all sorts of medical problems and worsen existing illness, not to mention make your parent feel tired and apathetic. Can he get to the grocery store? Can he open a can? Are his dentures bothering him? Is he having trouble swallowing? Is he worried about paying for food? Or is food simply not interesting to him? Talk to him, or watch him at mealtimes and figure out what is getting in the way of healthful eating, and then search for solutions. (See pages 73 and 658 for information on diet and nutrition.) Here are a few thoughts on making healthful eating easier:

IN THE GROCERY STORE

◆ If your parent can't get to the grocery store, contact local transportation services or a senior center to see if a senior van or volunteer can give her a ride. If transportation is not the issue—if she simply is not mobile—talk to a volunteer service, her religious organization, or perhaps even a neighbor or friend to see if someone might do the shopping for her. Some grocery stores have delivery services.

◆ Once a month—perhaps on a shopping trip with you or with someone else who can help with heavy bags—your parent should stock up on frozen and canned foods, pasta, rice, beans, cereal, and other staples that keep well. (Bread, butter, and meats can all be frozen and used at a later date.) Interim shopping trips he makes on his own can be used for getting light loads of fresh fruits, vegetables, and dairy products.

◆ Buy things that don't keep in small quantities. If your father is shopping for one, he should ask the grocer to break open large containers and give him just two potatoes or a half-dozen eggs. Most will do this readily. He can buy small portions of cheese, cooked meat, a pint of milk, and a half-pound of hamburger so unused food doesn't spoil, or he can get regular portions of some things and freeze small amounts for later use.

◆ "Long-life," or UHT, milk (heated at ultra-high temperatures) costs a little more but can be stored on the shelf at room temperature for up to six months. (Once it is opened, it must

> " *In the weeks and months after my father died, my mother didn't eat much. She couldn't be bothered to make a real meal just for herself. She said she hated eating alone. So she lost a lot of weight, which was bad because she was thin to start with.*
>
> *I taught her how to sauté vegetables in a wok and showed her a few easy pasta and rice recipes— all things she can do in one pot with very little work. Whenever I visit, I load up her shelves and refrigerator with food. She protests a lot, but she eats it. Maybe only because she can't stand to see things go to waste."*
>
> —JENNIFER S.

be refrigerated, and lasts about ten days.) It is perfectly safe, quite tasty if chilled before drinking, and just as nutritious as regular milk.

◆ When buying prepared foods, your parent should read the labels, looking for products with the lowest sodium and fat content. (Canned vegetables often contain sodium and syrup or butter sauces; frozen ones are usually a better choice.) Frozen and prepared dinners are more healthful than they used to be and can be supplemented with a salad, steamed vegetables, or a piece of fresh fruit.

◆ Dietary supplement drinks, like Ensure or Boost, and powdered breakfast drinks are useful now and then, when your parent doesn't feel up to cooking or is not interested in eating. But don't rely on them as a regular staple.

◆ If your mother walks to the corner grocery or has to transport her bags from the bus stop, get her a handcart for toting them.

◆ If money is a concern, your parent should buy low-cost foods, like rice, dried beans, pasta, and frozen vegetables. Look for coupons. Buy food on sale. Find a cost-cutting store. See if there is a food pantry in town. Learn about meal programs (page 141) and whether your parent is eligible for food stamps (page 334).

IN THE KITCHEN

◆ If your parent has stiff joints or weak muscles, there are dozens of aids available—jar openers, spoon holders, lightweight cookware, stirring devices, etc.—to make cooking easier (see page 131).

◆ Replace faucet knobs with levers and small button knobs on cupboards with large horseshoe-shaped knobs.

◆ If possible, update the kitchen equipment. Small toast-and-broil ovens, microwaves, and woks are convenient for single-serving meals, and food processors are helpful for chopping and slicing.

◆ If your parent uses a gas range, make sure the dials are easy to read. If she has poor vision or suffers from mild confusion, mark the "off" position

WHEN COOKING ISN'T POSSIBLE

There are all sorts of programs to ensure that the elderly have access to nutritional food. Congregate meals offered at local community centers, churches, and senior centers are nutritious, social, and inexpensive or free. Even if your parent goes only once or twice a week, you'll know that he's eating well at least some of the time. Some senior centers provide transportation to meals as well.

If your parent can't go out, find out about meal-delivery services, which are also free or inexpensive. (See page 141 for more on meal programs.) If your parent can afford it, she might hire someone to drop off a meal each day or to pack her freezer with a week's worth of homemade food, which should be fresher and more interesting than a delivery service. She can also order frozen meals by mail. (Search on the Internet under "meal delivery.")

clearly with a strip of colored tape. (If she's more severely confused you might have to shut a gas range off.)

◆ Put Lazy Susans in cabinets that are full of small items so your parent has easy access to them, or use pull-out drawers that are easily reached instead of cabinets.

◆ Move utensils, plates, food, pans, and other frequently used items to lower shelves or onto the countertop so your parent doesn't have to reach high shelves or stoop to get things from low places.

◆ Buy your parent a cookbook (large-print, if necessary) with easy recipes that serve just one or two people. Some cookbooks cater to special diets, with low-salt or fat-free dishes. Or, show your parent how to make a few easy dishes, then write down the directions for her. She can add vegetables, beans, tofu, or rice to a can of broth or other soup; toss some tomatoes, cheese, vegetables, or leftover meat into a helping of pasta; fold all sorts of food into a small omelet; or sauté an assortment of favorite foods in a wok.

◆ If you bring food to your parent, make sure that he can easily open and heat whatever you bring. He may just toss it out, not wanting to admit that he couldn't undo the twist-tie on the bag or unwrap the foil.

◆ If you are cooking for your parent, prepare the foods she prefers. She may be much happier with meat loaf, baked beans, and rice pudding than with fancier fare.

◆ Be sure there is a small, easy-to-use fire extinguisher in the kitchen and that your parent knows how to use it.

AT THE TABLE

◆ Make dining social. Elderly people often fail to eat well purely because they don't like to eat alone. Join your parent for meals occasionally, and when you can't be there, urge him to get together with friends. He might enjoy a regular potluck dinner, to which each person brings one simple item, or a regular dinner date with a friend.

◆ If your parent has trouble with fine motor skills, buy him forks and knives with longer, heavier, thicker, or bent handles; glasses with built-in straws; and plates with rims.

◆ Food that doesn't have to be cut up is easier for less dexterous hands, and finger food is often easier for people with dementia, who can be confused by utensils. Finger food might include cheese cubes or string cheese, chicken nuggets, any hors d'oeuvres, small sandwiches, egg rolls, cut-up vegetables and dips, or French toast strips.

◆ Elderly people typically have less sense of smell and taste, so food is often unappetizing to them. To perk up food, rather than adding more salt, your parent should throw in some herbs, spices, extracts, lemon, or garlic, and he should heat food whenever possible, so it gives

MAKE IT SPECIAL

Remember, eating is not just a chore. It is, or should be, an enjoyable part of the day. It should fill the senses and please the soul. There should be rich aromas and interesting textures and wonderful flavors. And it should be social and relaxing. Not every day, perhaps, but some of the time.

Of course, life isn't perfect and your parent's life is far from perfect. But do whatever you can to make meals special, and remember, even small things count. If your parent is able to cook, give her some recipes for simple but elegant meals. Drop off a favorite meal or, if you aren't nearby, send gourmet food by mail occasionally. Many of these just need reheating. Find foods from her home country or from her childhood that she might enjoy or, if she's up for it, introduce her to some new foods.

When your mother dines alone, encourage her to put her dinner on a plate, rather than eating it out of the pan, and to sit down at the table to eat. If she's in a nursing home, eating propped up in bed on an institutional tray, bring over good food, of course. But you might also bring a pretty linen cloth and a small vase of flowers (even fake ones will do) to make dining seem a bit more special.

off more aroma. A variety of textures on the plate—crunchy vegetables, creamy sauces, crispy crusts—also makes a meal more appetizing.

♦ Portions should be small so meals don't look overwhelming. The sheer volume of food may spoil your parent's limited appetite. Several small meals over the course of the day may be preferable.

♦ Be sure his dentures fit properly and that he has no other dental problems that are hindering his eating.

♦ When your family dines together, let your parent eat at her own pace. Have her start before the others sit down, or let the children leave the table while she finishes. If she feels that others are waiting for her, she may quit in midmeal, or worse, hurry and choke on something.

♦ If your parent lives with you, don't enforce "normal" mealtimes. Sometimes, as people grow older, the established routines don't work anymore. Your mother may eat six small meals a day instead of three larger ones. For her nibbling, have healthful snacks on hand such as chopped vegetables, raisins and other dried fruit, popcorn, cole slaw, yogurt, cheese, hummus, meat slices, apples and other fresh fruit, and peanut butter and crackers.

WHEN SWALLOWING IS DIFFICULT

IF YOUR PARENT HAS TROUBLE CHEWing and swallowing, or is unable to feed herself, you or some other caregiver should be more involved.

People who have had a stroke, or have dementia, cerebral palsy, Parkinson's disease, head or neck cancer, or injuries to the head, neck, or chest sometimes suffer from dysphagia, a condition in which swallowing is painful, difficult, or impossible. This puts them at serious risk of malnutrition, dehydration, choking, or getting liquid or food into their lungs and then developing pneumonia. Surgery or medication may help open the passageway. A speech-language pathologist can also teach a person ways to eat. Be sure to talk with your parent's doctor if you notice a lot of coughing or gagging, or if your parent is not eating as he used to.

♦ Your parent should have small meals several times a day.

♦ Get her to eat sitting up, if possible. She should eat slowly, pausing between bites. She should take small bites or sips, and avoid talking while eating.

♦ Semisolid foods, like mashed potatoes and thick soups (without chunks), are best. Pretty much anything can be pulverized into a thick, smooth consistency. A food processor or blender (or even a handheld masher) will grind meat, mash potatoes, and puree vegetables and fruit. Also, try scrambled eggs, oatmeal (banana, cinnamon, or maple syrup add flavor), egg salad, creamed sweet potatoes, bread pudding, custard, applesauce, flavored gelatin, and milkshakes. Honestly, baby food straight

AT HOME, IN THE BEDROOM

If your parent is in bed or in a bedroom most or all of the time, you need to set up his room for days of dining and entertainment, as well as for safety. If you don't live with your parent, many of these things can be done during a visit.

◆ Make sure your parent is situated on the same floor as a bathroom, preferably close to his room. Otherwise, buy a commode for his room. (Medicare will often cover the cost.)

◆ If you have any choice, select a room for your parent that has a large window and a view, or bright, cheery pictures on the wall.

◆ Arrange the room so there is a sitting area for visitors, and for your parent if she's not bedbound— a chair or two, a reading lamp, and a table near a window or in front of a television set, for example.

◆ Place a table near the bed where she can store all the day's needs— magazines or books, pills, a water glass and pitcher, a lamp, a telephone, a radio, writing paper, a clock, a calendar, remote controls, etc.

◆ Set up a television so your parent can watch it easily, and make sure he has a remote control.

◆ Buy a large pillow for sitting up comfortably in bed (most department stores sell cushions for reclining, and medical supply stores have large triangular-shaped foam cushions for propping people up), and supplement this with regular pillows.

◆ If the house is large, put a bell or a baby monitor by the bed so your parent can call for someone if necessary. Or buy a telephone with an intercom so he can summon help. (If he lives alone,

---

from the jar is soft, nutritious, and perfectly good for adults. If you mash foods into an unappetizing-looking lump, use a mold to make it more appealing and garnish it with lemon or herbs.

◆ Thick liquids are easier to swallow than thin ones. Add powdered milk, ice cream, honey, powdered eggs,

pudding, gelatin, or a commercial thickening agent to liquids. Some people can swallow carbonated beverages more easily than noncarbonated ones.

◆ Serve foods that are either hot (120-140°F) or cold (35-40°F), as this will help trigger a swallow reflex.

two), see if a home health aide or a local volunteer can help.

FOOD SAFETY

WHILE MOST OF US CAN TOLERATE hundreds of germs without any ill effects, the elderly, who have weaker immune systems, are vulnerable to the bacteria, parasites, and chemical contaminants in food. They also don't recover easily once they become sick. As a result, you and your parent need to take some extra precautions.

The problem is, this is a time of life when people tend to be particularly bad about food safety. If your parent gets a little confused from time to time, he might forget to put food back in the refrigerator, or forget how long the meat has been cooking (three minutes), or be certain that he just bought that month-old milk. Some elderly people keep the month-old milk and drink it because they don't want to spend money on a new carton. Others don't realize that the milk and other foods have spoiled because their sense of smell just isn't what it used to be.

Here are some food safety tips to discuss with your parent, use yourself when cooking for him, or pass on to any aide or companion who is cooking for him:

◆ Elderly people should avoid raw or undercooked fish, meat, poultry, and eggs; raw or unpasteurized milk or cheese; unpasteurized or untreated fruit or vegetable juice; and (yes, it's true) raw alfalfa sprouts.

make sure there is a phone by the bed.)

◆ Stock some crackers and other nonperishable foods by the bed so you don't have to come running every time your parent wants a snack. You might even buy a miniature refrigerator for his room or load up a cooler with food each morning if you're away much of the day.

◆ You can buy or rent all sorts of equipment to make bed rest more manageable—for example, an electric or manual hospital bed, side rails for getting up or turning over, a trapeze above the bed to grab and pull up on, a hospital-style table that slides over the bed, wheelchairs, and walkers. These items are expensive, but Medicare may cover some of the cost.

◆ Sauces help dry food slide down more easily, and there are endless possibilities: cream, apple, barbecue, gravy, lemon, wine, tomato, cheese, etc.

◆ If you are feeding your parent, never hurry her or thrust oversized bites at her. If you don't have the time (and one meal can take an hour or

MEDICAL ALERT

Common symptoms of food-borne illness include diarrhea, nausea, vomiting, abdominal cramping, and fever. Get treatment immediately, letting the doctor know what your parent ate recently.

◆ Meat and eggs should be cooked thoroughly. Use a clean food thermometer. Cook roasts and steaks to 145°F and poultry to 180°F (so when pierced, the juice is not pink). Ground beef should be cooked through (sorry, no medium rare for your elderly parent), egg whites and yolks should be firm, and fish should be opaque. (In other words, no pink, anywhere.)

◆ When shopping, put meat, fish, and poultry in separate bags so they don't drip and contaminate other foods.

◆ Don't buy food in cans that are dented or bulging, or jars that are cracked or have loose-fitting lids.

◆ Check the dates on food and buy those with the longest shelf life remaining.

◆ Remind your parent to throw out food that is past the expiration date, moldy, or smelly. If his sense of smell is poor, he should mark food clearly with a date when it should be tossed.

◆ Rinse all raw produce in water, without soap. Use a small scrub brush to remove dirt.

◆ Store cut or peeled fruits and vegetables in the refrigerator.

◆ After preparing one food item and before going on to the next, wash hands, cutting boards, and utensils with hot soapy water, especially if raw meat is involved. Better yet, prepare meat on a different work surface. Bacteria from the raw chicken, for example, can easily travel to the salad if the two are chopped on the same surface, or if unwashed hands handle both.

◆ Wash the kitchen sponge in the dishwasher or throw it in the microwave (on high for at least one minute) every other day to kill bacteria. For the same reason, throw the dishtowel into the washing machine (or into the microwave) every few days. When cleaning up an area where raw meat was cut, use paper towels.

◆ Thaw frozen foods in the refrigerator, under cold running water, or in the microwave, not on the counter. When thawing food in a microwave, cook the food immediately after.

◆ When microwaving, turn the food during the cooking time to be sure there are no cool or undercooked spots. Reheat leftovers to 165°F.

◆ Perishable food, leftovers, and takeout food should not be left out for more than two hours (and that's pushing it; in warm weather, stick to a one-hour limit). Throw out anything that has sat at room temperature for more than two hours.

◆ When food will not be eaten immediately, either cover it in foil and put it in the oven at 140°F or higher to keep it warm, or put it in the fridge or freezer until you are ready to reheat it. (It's okay to put warm food directly into the freezer.)

◆ Divide large portions of food into small, shallow containers for future single servings.

◆ Don't forget the water. As with food, your parent will be more susceptible to contaminants. Buy her a water filter or bottled water. (To learn

---

FOOD SAFETY INFORMATION

For more information about food storage and safety, contact the following:

USDA Meat and Poultry Hotline
888-674-6854
www.fsis.usda.gov

FDA Center for Food Safety and Applied Nutrition
888-723-3366
www.cfsan.fda.gov

Government Food Safety Information
www.foodsafety.gov

---

more about the quality of her tap water, visit the Environmental Protection Agency's safe water Web site at www.epa.gov/safewater.)

In the Driver's Seat

Anyone who has followed a snail-paced car or one that darts past stop signs knows that plenty of older drivers shouldn't be on the roads. Studies show that, overall, the elderly have fewer collisions than other age groups, but that is largely because they drive fewer miles. Turn the statistics around, and you find that the elderly have more car accidents and violations per miles driven than other age groups. And accidents are likely to involve fatalities, largely because the elderly are more frail and apt to be more seriously injured.

The problem is that as people age, reflexes slow, joints stiffen, and coordination declines. People generally have a narrower field of vision, are more sensitive to glare, need more light in order to see, and can't follow moving objects well. Illness, such as dementia, arthritis, insomnia, diabetes, depression, and Parkinson's disease, severely compounds the hazards. Many medications also make driving more dangerous, especially sleep aids, antihistamines, strong painkillers, antidepressants, and diabetes medications. Your parent's doctor might be able to adjust his prescriptions to lessen any affect on driving.

And yet, driving is a way of life. Who can forget the exhilaration of turning sixteen and getting a driver's license? It was a ticket to freedom and a sign of maturity. Throughout life, driving gives us independence and autonomy. To give up this mobility, and the independence it represents, can be devastating for your parent. Even if she has no place to go or if ample public transportation is available (which is not usually the case), her driver's license and the car keys are a vital part of her life.

SAFETY
BEHIND THE WHEEL

GO OUT FOR A DRIVE WITH YOUR parent. Be sure there really is a problem and, if so, determine exactly what it is. Is your parent having trouble turning her neck to see behind her? Is she getting caught in intersections while trying to turn left? Is she squinting to see the road in the evening? Once you see what is happening, address specific issues. Here are some ideas to make driving easier and improve safety:

◆ If your parent hasn't had his eyesight and hearing tested recently, he should make the necessary appointments at once.

◆ Urge your parent to exercise—and be sure to include neck and shoulder stretches—which will improve his reaction time, his range of motion, and his attentiveness. Simply stretching his

neck each day by rotating his head side to side and up and down, and circling his shoulders, may help him twist around to parallel park or check oncoming traffic with greater agility and safety.

◆ Get your parent to wear her seat belt, both at the shoulder and at the waist. (Let her know that airbags and shoulder straps are not a replacement for safety belts that go around the waist.) Be sure that she can fasten and unfasten the belt easily. Automotive shops can adjust the shoulder strap so that it is comfortable or reset the belt so it can be more easily hooked and unhooked.

◆ If your parent is small, shrunken with age, or just particularly frail, you might want to consider disabling the airbag, which can come out with such force that it can break fragile bones and blood vessels.

◆ If your parent suffers from dizziness, confusion, or blurred eyesight, all of which affect driving, ask the doctor about ways to reduce these symptoms. They may be caused by untreated illness or inappropriate medications.

◆ Your parent should read all medication labels carefully and talk with the pharmacist or doctor to be sure that a particular medication won't make him drowsy and therefore unsafe on the roads.

◆ Make sure that your parent's car is in good working order, including brakes, defroster, defogger (for front and rear window), battery, wipers, dashboard light, exterior lights, and turn signals. Headlights should be clean and wipers should be replaced periodically.

◆ Install large mirrors and add extra mirrors if your parent is having trouble turning his head to see what's behind him.

◆ There are a number of devices that can solve particular problems. For example, if your mother cannot see clearly over the dashboard, buy a seat cushion at an automotive store. (Don't use a pillow because it might slip.) Automotive stores also sell gadgets to raise the pedals and spinner knobs that can make a steering wheel more responsive for people with limited arm and shoulder movement.

◆ If your parent is buying a new car, opt for power everything brakes, seats, steering, locks, etc.

◆ Be sure that your parent plans trips ahead of time and knows exactly where is he going without looking at a map. Even if it means that the drive takes a little longer, he should take a route that avoids complex intersections or difficult left turns. Whenever possible, he should stick to streets that he knows.

◆ Avoid distractions, like the radio, cell phone, and chatty passengers. All attention should be focused on the road.

◆ Once on the road, your parent should avoid driving:

- at night, dawn, or dusk
- during rush hour
- on unfamiliar routes
- in city centers or on busy streets
- long distances
- in bad weather
- when he's feeling sick, stressed, or tired

◆ If he feels at all sleepy while driving, he should pull off the road and have a short nap, get out and stretch, or stop for coffee.

Meanwhile, begin to wean your parent from his automobile because, chances are, eventually he will not be able to drive. It's easier to do this when he has some time to make the transition. As he is adjusting his driving habits, introduce him to carpools and public transportation or offer to drive him yourself, if possible. Find other friends, relatives, neighbors, or volunteers who are willing to give him a ride occasionally. Do it in such a way that your parent can save face. Make it possible for him to bow out of driving without feeling embarrassed.

By the way, if your parent shuns public transportation because he feels that buses and particularly taxis are too expensive, let him know that owning and operating a car costs nearly $7,000 a year—that's a lot of money to put toward taxis!

WHEN IT'S TIME TO QUIT

THE QUESTION OF QUITTING IS A HOT potato that no one wants to touch. Family members often know that an elderly person is a danger on the roads,

DRIVING REFRESHER COURSES AND OTHER HELP

Your parent can take a refresher course in driving, which will not only help her to be a safer driver and keep her license, but as a bonus will qualify her for a lower insurance premium in most states. AARP (888-687-2277 or www.aarp.org) offers a driver safety course. Senior centers, local AAA offices, driving schools, and the Department of Motor Vehicles should have information about other driving courses in your parent's area.

Some groups also issue information and brochures that you can request or print from their Web sites. The AAA Foundation for Traffic Safety (www.seniordrivers.org) has exercises, driving tips, and a self-exam for older drivers. AARP also has a wide variety of information and guides for older drivers.

but they don't dare do anything about it. They might not want Grandpa driving their children around, but then might look the other way when he's by himself. Taking action is simply too painful and difficult.

What you need to remember is that he is also endangering the lives of others. This is not a time to shy away from confrontation. If your parent is not safe on the roads, you need to act. Immediately.

Unfortunately, you can't rely on the state to monitor his driving. Most states, reluctant to alienate a large population of elderly voters, refuse to retest or otherwise restrict older drivers.

A doctor may be able to determine if your parent should get off the road, which might, in turn, help your parent believe it. But you may have to speak with his doctor to alert him to

the situation. There are also driver assessment booklets available from AARP and the AAA Foundation for Traffic Safety (see the box above for phone numbers and Web sites).

When you confront your parent, brace yourself, because he is bound to be hurt, if not furious. Be sensitive to the gravity of what you are suggesting, and to the implications, both practical and emotional, but remain firm in your resolve. And be ready with solutions to his travel problems—look into public and senior transportation programs, and ask family and friends if they can provide some transportation. If your parent uses his driver's license for identification, call the Department of Motor Vehicles to request a photo ID card.

If all else fails, you can report an unsafe driver to the DMV or your state licensing agency. It's a difficult step, but it may be your only choice. Find out in advance what happens when someone is reported; states have varying procedures. And ask that your name be kept confidential.

(If your parent has dementia, it can work to your advantage in this case. You might disable the car and tell him that it's scheduled to go to the shop. This reasoning could work repeatedly for some time.)

Useful Gadgets and Gizmos

There is no end to the number of useful gadgets and gizmos you can order from catalogs, find in medical supply stores, or view on the Internet, all to make dressing, dining, shopping, reading, walking, gardening, and everything else easier for your parent. From talking thermometers for aged eyes to special fishing gear for stiff fingers, if your parent needs it, someone sells it.

It's worth flipping through some catalogs or browsing through the Internet just to get a sense of what's available. Sometimes, you can duplicate these items with a little ingenuity. (For example, you can make utensils heavier or give them thicker handles by simply padding the handle with weights and tape; you can lengthen an unreachable zipper or a light cord with a piece of ribbon; or you can make a dress easier to wear by replacing buttons with Velcro.)

You can buy lifts that carry a person up stairs, automatic door openers, lights that respond to verbal commands, and ramps for vans.

For cooking, there are all sorts of tea kettles and jug tippers, crumb trays, large bibs, weighted utensils, large-print cookbooks, jar and can openers, and special cutting boards, knives, and electric choppers for easy slicing and dicing.

For bathing, you can buy a variety of stools, chairs, and benches, as well as shampooing basins for the bed. For dressing, there are grabbers that help pull on socks and pull down zippers, special easy-to-wear clothing, and hooks that help do buttons. Long-handled brushes and combs are easy for those who can't reach around easily.

There are phones that allow you to put pictures of friends and family on automatic-dial buttons, and phones with voice-activated dialers. For people who always lose essential items (you might want to buy one of these for yourself), you can get a base unit with buttons that trigger a beeper on corresponding items: keys, eyeglasses, cell phones, purses, wallets, the phone book, etc.

For people who are hard of hearing, there are amplifiers for phones and televisions. For people who have poor vision, there are books on tape, alarms, and large-print everything, as well as devices that send an enlarged image from a book to a TV screen.

For people who have trouble getting in and out of chairs and cars, there are supports and pulleys and ramps.

WHERE TO FIND HELP

To find helpful devices, start by contacting ABLEDATA, a federally funded database of assistive products and manufacturers, which also has "information specialists" on hand to assist you (800-227-0216 or www.abledata.com).

Each state also has a federally funded "assistive technology project," which is dedicated to helping residents get the assistive devices they need. To find the program in your state, contact ABLEDATA or go to the Web site of the Association of Tech Act Projects (www.ataporg.org).

The National Resource Center on Supportive Housing and Home Modification (213-740-1364 or www.homemods.org) focuses on home modification, but also has information on accessibility products on its Web site.

Beyond that, there are literally hundreds of companies, which you can find either in a phone book or through the Internet (search under "disability products" or "assistive devices" or something more specific, like "vision aids"). While we are not endorsing any companies, here are the names of a few larger ones, just to get you started. (Several clothing companies are listed on page 118.)

GENERAL

Functional Solutions
800-235-7054
www.beabletodo.com

Gold Violin
877-648-8400
www.goldviolin.com

Maddak
973-628-7600
www.maddak.com

Mail Order Medical Supply
800-232-7443
www.momscatalog.com

The Wright Stuff
877-750-0376
www.thewright-stuff.com

Independent Living Aids
800-537-2118
www.independentliving.com

RECREATION, HOBBIES, AND SPORTS

Access to Recreation
800-634-4351
www.accesstr.com

MEMORY PROBLEMS

The Alzheimer's Store
800-752-3238
www.alzstore.com

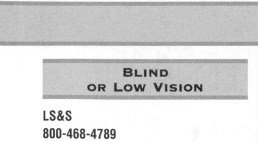

BLIND OR LOW VISION

LS&S
800-468-4789
www.lssproducts.com

National Federation of the Blind Online Store
www.kifwebe.com

National Association for Visually Handicapped
www.navh.org

DEAF AND HARD OF HEARING

Hearmore
800-881-4327,
TTY 800-281-3555
www.hearmore.com

Harris Communications
800-825-6758,
TTY 800-825-9187
www.harriscomm.com

CANES

Canesgalore
800-346-6400
www.canesgalore.com

The Walking Cane Depot
888-399-4870
www.walkingcanedepot.com

And there are dozens of grabbers, turners, levers, and openers to help people reach high items, turn taps or knobs or keys, open jars, or pick up sewing needles.

For the enthusiast, you can buy cardholders and card shufflers, reels that bring in the big fish, or cradles from which to launch a bowling ball. The list goes on and on.

You can also find a number of canes, walkers, and electric scooters for a parent who is weak, stiff, or otherwise finds movement painful or impossible.

Chapter Seven

GETTING HELP

Assessing the Need • Help from Family and Friends
• Community Services
• Geriatric Care Managers

....

YOUR FATHER NEEDS SOMEONE TO COME OVER FOR A FEW hours each week to do some light housekeeping and buy groceries. Or perhaps your mother has dementia and needs intermittent nursing care, as well as a full-time person who can bathe and dress her, feed her, and guide her through the day. Or maybe your parent just needs someone to talk to, a friend. Whatever the needs, you can't possibly do it all, which means that you have to find others who can do it for you.

The sooner you get help, the better. First of all, learning about available services now, even if you don't use them yet, is invaluable. You will know where to turn when you do need help, you can get your parent on any waiting lists, and, most important, you might find you can use some services sooner than you think.

It's tempting to try to do it all yourself, but the most successful caregivers get plenty of help. You want to give your parent your best, but you can't do that if you are worn out and miserable. Getting help will allow you to give her a little more of what only you can give: your love and attention.

Finding the right mix of services and support, not to mention affordable care, will take time. Unfortunately, senior services tend to be a bit willy-nilly, and no one source has all the information you need. Fortunately, there are far more services available than there were a few years ago. Talk to others who have cared for a relative in the same community, and make a few calls to agencies and organizations to find out what is offered locally. Large cities generally have a greater range of services than small towns, but even in rural areas you should be able to find help.

Assessing the Need

Before you sign your mother up for extensive and expensive care, determine exactly what she needs. Write a list and be specific. Does she need help first thing in the morning getting showered and dressed? Does she need someone to shop and cook for her? Or does she simply need a ride to the grocery store? Or would a meal delivery program be just the ticket? Does she need someone to take her to the doctor's office now and then? Someone to keep her company? Someone to clean the house? Or does she need in-home nursing care? Would it help if she spent a few days a week at an adult day-care program, which would provide both supervision and an opportunity to socialize? Does she have cognitive problems that require that you hire someone with special training? Or does she simply have a difficult personality that requires someone have a little chutzpah?

While you contemplate her needs, consider modifications to her home that would allow her to do more for herself. Sometimes minor renovations to the bathroom, kitchen, or stairwell can make life a whole lot more manageable. See Chapter Six for tips on how to make the tasks of daily life simpler and safer for her.

In the end, you might discover that she doesn't require round-the-clock home health aides after all; maybe she'll be fine with an hour or two of help each morning to get her dressed and fed, then she can go to a day-care center during the day, and her dinner can be delivered.

If you are not sure what sort of help she needs, or there is some disagreement in the family about what to do, sometimes an area agency on aging or a local senior center will have a caseworker on hand who can do a formal assessment and guide you in finding help. You can also hire a geriatric care manager to do this.

Help from Family and Friends

When your father needs help, family and close friends may volunteer their services right away. (If family members aren't helping, get after them. See page 170 for more on dealing with siblings.) Use all these helpers as much as possible.

But what about other relatives and less intimate friends? What about your parent's neighbors? What about your own friends? All of these people can supplement the work of volunteers, community programs, and profes-

A REMINDER

Be organized, even if you're facing a crisis, or before you know it, you'll have crumpled brochures tucked in kitchen drawers and illegible notes scribbled on napkins and Post-its. As you learn about community services, develop a filing system with folders for each topic and a master list of all relevant agencies and representatives with their phone numbers and extensions. (Refer to page 16 for a refresher on organization.)

sionals, providing not only practical help but also much-needed emotional support and assurance.

Certainly when others ask if there's anything they can do to help, say yes. Suggest a specific (very small) task they might do. When people do anything out of the blue for your parent, like dropping off a meal or stopping by for a visit, be enormously appreciative and let them know how welcome it is. (They just might do it again.)

You may be reluctant to ask for help, but keep in mind that while people may not readily volunteer their services, they are often more than happy to help out once they are asked. Keep favors very small. Perhaps someone will pick up a few extra groceries for your parent while doing her own shopping, get books or videos at the library once a month, or drop by for a visit every now and then. A neighbor might be willing to take your parent's garbage out once a week when he's hauling out his own bags. A neighbor's child could adopt your parent as a grandparent, or you might pay a local teenager to come by one or two afternoons a week to keep your parent company and help a little around the house. Or maybe a young new mother who's taking time off from work would like to make a little money by delivering lunch and dinner to your parent or stopping by in the afternoon for an hour to play cards or chat.

Don't forget your own friends. If someone is in the same situation, she (or he) might share some of the workload—you check out local day-care and home-care options while your friend investigates Medicaid eligibility and rules. Those who aren't in the same situation might be willing to exchange duties with you in the name of mutual relief and a refreshing change of pace—a friend sits with your parent while you take her children to the mall. Or think about starting a cooperative of people who are caring for aging parents. Not an emotional support group, but a real cooperative—people working together, sharing tasks and trading information. You can begin by posting an ad at the local senior center.

Community Services

Communities establish services for the elderly in response to the demographics and specific needs of the local population. As a result, while all communities offer a handful of basic services to elderly residents, the details of those programs are as different as the communities themselves. Adult day care in one town might be very small, simple, and personal, perhaps with a children's day-care program in the next room, while in another town it is large and professional, and offers everything from medical care to pet care. The funding sources, costs, and sponsors are equally diverse, with services being offered by public agencies, private businesses, churches and synagogues, civic groups,

and charities. In most cases, your parent or your family has to pay for community services, but a few are free and some are subsidized.

The chart on page 138 describes types of services offered in most areas, but you will need to call to get the specifics of what's available in your parent's community.

TELEPHONE REASSURANCE AND VISITORS

MOST COMMUNITIES HAVE A TELEphone reassurance program in which volunteers, often senior citizens, call once a day or once every few days to see how your parent is doing. Some programs will send visitors to her house to provide a little companionship and to check up on her. In either case, the volunteer will ask how your parent is doing and remind her of anything she needs to do. *Did you take your medications this morning? What did you eat for lunch? Do you remember that you have a doctor's appointment this afternoon?* If anything seems askew, the volunteer will alert you or another person who is designated as a contact.

Using such a service should ease your mind and reduce the number of interruptions at work, as well as helping your parent.

The programs are usually run by senior centers, religious organizations, and other public or nonprofit agencies. Sometimes the services are offered by privately owned home-care agencies, in which case there will be a fee.

COMMUNITY SERVICES AT A GLANCE

Type of Help	Services Provided	Average Costs*
Telephone reassurance and friendly visitors	Phone calls or brief visits to check on your parent's well-being	Free or minimal charge
Companions	Companionship, supervision, and some help with meals and tasks	$5 to $20 an hour, some free or subsidized through state-funded programs (live-in: $200 to $700 a week)
Homemakers	Light housekeeping, laundry, cooking, errands, some help with bathing and dressing	$6 to $30 an hour, although sometimes free or charged on a sliding scale
Chore services	Minor repairs and handyman chores	Free or based on a sliding scale, plus materials
Meal programs	Group dining at a community center, or meals delivered to the house	Free or minimal charge
Transportation services	Rides to day care, senior centers, shopping malls, or appointments	Free or minimal charge
Senior centers	Clubs that provide social activities, lectures, meals, and information	Usually free
Adult day services (adult day care)	Supervision, recreation, meals, and some health care and counseling. Transportation is often provided	$50 on average, but can run up to $150 a day; some are subsidized; covered by Medicaid in some states
Case managers and geriatiric care managers	Assessment, guidance, advice, and more	Community agencies may provide some consultation for free or on a sliding scale; if hired privately between $75 to $250 an hour

Prices vary widely depending upon the area and whether you hire workers through an agency.

COMPANIONS

COMPANIONS KEEP YOUR PARENT company, help him with minor tasks, and generally watch over him. But the term is a broad one. Some companions focus on the companionship aspect, while others provide supervision and assistance. Some stop by for an occasional friendly visit, while others work on a schedule. Most companions do not do any serious housework or chores, but they might prepare a light meal, help your parent get dressed, or pick up a few groceries on the way over. While it's great if you can find someone with experience caring for elderly people, finding a loving, caring person who can get along with your parent is your primary goal.

Many communities have free or low-cost companion programs run by a public agency or a private group. Churches or other religious organizations also sponsor companions. Local senior centers often know of companion programs in the area.

Volunteer programs are wonderful if your parent simply needs company. But if she needs reliable and consistent help, you might need to hire a paid companion.

Home-care agencies often have companions (look in the Yellow Pages under "home care"), which is usually the easiest route, but also the most expensive. However, agencies do have advantages (see page 155).

You can find companions on your own in much the same way you would hire a babysitter. Referrals are always

> " After his wife died, my father-in-law went into hibernation. He stayed at home and watched television. My husband said he was fine, but I was worried. He aged so quickly and seemed so lonely. I had him for dinner once a week, but we both work and we have two young boys, so we couldn't do much.
>
> I learned about a companion program and convinced Dad to try it. I think it's really been great for him. Scott, the companion, is in much the same situation as Dad. He's alone and can't get around all that well. He visits two or three times a week now, and they play rummy and have lunch together. Last week they went to a hockey game together, which is something Dad always loved but hadn't done in years.
>
> What's been really interesting, and totally unexpected, is that his health has improved so much. He literally looks twenty years younger."
>
> —LUCY A.

the best bet. Ask friends who have an elderly parent in the area, as well as those who might know about good nannies and sitters. Many of these people care for young and old alike.

If referrals don't get you anywhere, put a classified ad in the local newspaper, or post a sign in a senior center or church or community center. (If you run an ad, leave your telephone

BENEFITS, DISCOUNTS, AND SPECIAL SERVICES

If you put on your sleuthing cap, you may very well find that your parent is eligible for a number of free and discounted community services. Contact the area agency on aging, the Veterans Administration, and the Centers for Medicare and Medicaid. The National Council on the Aging has a Web site, www.benefitscheckup.org, that takes information about location and income and then lists benefits for which a person may be eligible. Also try local senior centers and community groups, the U.S. Office of Personnel Management (for federal employees), the local health department, and organizations aligned with specific diseases and issues.

Beyond government and community programs, businesses often offer special services and discounts to the elderly. See if the library might deliver books, a grocery store might deliver groceries, or a hair stylist might make house calls. Some doctors even make house calls. Whatever the need, it's worth a few calls to see what is available.

number, not your parent's. You don't want to publicize her vulnerability.)

If your parent lives in a senior housing complex, there may be another elderly person, who is perhaps more capable than your parent, who would visit regularly.

Companions cost anywhere from $5 to $20 an hour, depending upon the area and the services provided. (The upper end of the spectrum is for companions hired through an agency and those workers who are simply worth their weight in gold.) Prices for live-in companions vary wildly depending upon who and where; some expect to have a phone and television, meals, use of a car, and/or other transportation expenses.

If your parent only needs a little help around the house, then someone might be willing to provide care and supervision in exchange for rent. If there is a spare bedroom, this arrangement can be less expensive, but it also means giving up some privacy.

HOMEMAKERS

HOMEMAKERS GENERALLY DO MORE physical work and less socializing than companions, but the distinction is faint and largely depends upon the individual. Homemakers do laundry and light housecleaning, prepare meals, and usually will assist with other tasks, such as shopping and helping your parent to bathe and dress. Many homemakers, especially those hired through home-care agencies, are trained specifically in caring for elderly people, and some can teach your parent how to manage certain household tasks on his own. But again, the quality and extent of the service depends upon the individual worker.

In most cases, your parent has to foot the bill, but in some areas, homemakers are available at no charge or on a sliding scale, and paid for by public monies. However, there can be long waiting lists for such services. In some states, under certain circumstances (if, for example, your parent is considered eligible for nursing-home coverage), Medicaid will cover some of the expense of homemakers.

As with companions, if homemakers are not offered through community programs, you can hire one through most home-care agencies or find one by putting an ad in the local newspaper or on a community bulletin board.

CHORE SERVICES

CHORE SERVICE PROGRAMS ENLIST workers, often volunteers, who do minor repairs and odd jobs for elderly residents. Most won't tackle major repairs or renovations, and they might not do regular chores like shoveling snow, but they will usually build ramps, weather-strip windows, put up storm windows, or install grab bars.

Chore services, like visitor and telephone services, are sometimes offered by local nonprofit groups, such as senior centers or churches. Your parent pays for the materials that are needed, but the labor is often free or charged based on need. (Your parent may have to meet some minimum income guidelines to be eligible.)

Try the area agency on aging and senior centers first. The National Resource Center on Supportive Housing and Home Modification (213-740-1364 or www.homemods.org) also has a list of carpenters and handymen who will do home renovations for the elderly at a discount.

MEAL PROGRAMS

IF YOUR PARENT CAN'T OR WON'T COOK for himself no matter how you simplify the kitchen, or if he isn't eating well for some other reason, look into congregate dining and meal delivery programs.

Congregate meals are typically hot lunches served in schools, community centers, apartment buildings, churches and synagogues, senior centers, adult day-care centers or other community sites. Most programs are open to all elderly people, and they often provide transportation to and from the site. The meals meet federal nutrition guidelines, and some programs have kosher, vegetarian, low-salt, diabetic, and other special meals.

Congregate meals usually cost nothing. Some programs request a voluntary contribution based on income, but the average donation is less than a dollar a meal, and many programs accept federal food stamps.

WHERE TO FIND HELP

Services for the elderly are often scattered and uncoordinated, so you'll need to talk to several people before you get a full picture of what's available. To learn about the services in your parent's community, people and organizations you should contact:

The area agency on aging. Begin your search with the agency on aging in your parent's area. The agency can direct you to services and, in some cases, let you talk to a case manager about the specific needs of your parent. Some also offer legal, financial, and family counseling free.

You can find it by calling the Eldercare Locator (800-677-1116 or www.eldercare.gov), or the state unit on aging (listed in Appendix B, page 628). Many agencies have their own Web sites.

Local senior centers. Some centers provide services directly and some sponsor senior advocates who counsel residents about community services.

Senior centers typically offer workshops, lectures, and support groups for caregivers as well, so inquire about all services that are offered.

Discharge planners and care managers. Most hospitals employ nurses or social workers who arrange housing, home care, and community services for patients who are leaving the hospital. Although it is best to contact the planner while your parent is in the hospital (even if she is there for a one-day procedure that has nothing to do with her disability), some discharge planners may offer guidance even if your parent is not a hospital patient. Ask your parent's doctor about this or call the hospital directly.

Employers. See if your workplace (or the workplace of your parent, your spouse, a sibling, or an adult child) has an employee assistance program. Many of these programs provide information, referrals, and counseling to people who are caring for an elderly person. A few companies offer referrals nationwide (very helpful if you live in Tulsa and your parent is in Tucson).

Local organizations. The United Way, Jewish Family Services, the Lions Club, and other community groups, many of which directly fund or offer services, can be good sources for referrals.

Churches and synagogues. Even if your parent is not affiliated with any religious organization, such groups often provide direct help to people of all faiths, or can refer you to programs and services in the area.

National organizations. For virtually every ailment or interest—from asthma to veterans—there is an organization that can guide you to services, refer you to professionals, and provide information. Many, such as the Alzheimer's Association and the Arthritis Foundation, have local chapters that provide services directly. Dozens of these organizations are listed in Appendix A, page 600; additional ones can be found in the phone book, on the Internet, or in the *Directory of Associations,* available in most public libraries. You can also get referrals to national organizations by calling the National Health Information Center (800-336-4797 or www.health.gov/nhic) or the National Rehabilitation Information Center (800-346-2742 or www.naric.com).

Government agencies. The local health department can tell you about free flu shots, health screenings, and other health services for the elderly. The parks and recreation department may direct you to exercise classes for the elderly. The departments of housing and social services may also know about services and programs for the elderly.

Be patient and persistent. Call in the middle of the morning when the lines tend to be freer. But don't give up. The help is often there, and your parent, as a taxpayer, is paying for it.

The Yellow Pages. If you haven't found the help you need, try the phone book. (If you live far away from your parent, bring home a copy from your next visit.) Look under such headings as senior, elder, or aging, or under a particular subject (home care, diaper service, Jewish services, meal delivery). And before you wedge the book back under the phone, look at the first few pages of the White Pages, where emergency numbers, hotlines, and often-used community services are usually listed. You should find information about services for the elderly as well as information about special telephone services for deaf or disabled people, and utility discounts for senior citizens.

211. Many communities have established (and others are in the process of establishing) information and referral lines, which are contacted by dialing 211. Operators are trained to link people to social services and local programs. For more information, try dialing 211 or visit www.211.org.

The best part of all is that the meals are social occasions. If your parent doesn't know people in the neighborhood, the first few visits may seem a little awkward, but eventually he will meet people and become accustomed to this routine.

If your parent can't leave the house, meal delivery programs will bring a hot lunch and sometimes a frozen or cold bagged dinner to his doorstep. These programs, called by a variety of names but generically known as "meals-on-wheels," are often operated by senior centers, religious organizations, or hospitals. Most are free (they have to be free if they receive federal monies), although they will solicit a donation (and they need it badly). Some private groups charge a nominal fee. To be eligible, your parent must be homebound and unable to prepare meals alone, but there is no income limit. As a bonus, the volunteers who deliver the food are usually trained to look for signs of trouble.

To find out about meal delivery programs in your parent's area, call the area agency on aging, local senior center, or go to the Meals on Wheels Association of America's Web site, www.mowaa.org.

If there is no meal program in your parent's community or if there is a waiting list, which there often is, you can order frozen meals from Golden Cuisine (800-886-4084 or www.goldencuisinestore.com) that meet federal nutritional requirements. (These are the same meals that many meals-on-wheels programs drop off as a frozen second meal of the day.)

If your parent wants something fancier and is willing to spend the money, there are numerous companies that will mail slightly more gourmet frozen meals to your parent. Be sure that they meet the nutritional needs of your parent, come in single servings, and are easy to prepare (as in, open, microwave, eat). You can find them by searching online under "meal delivery."

Or, if she can afford it, some cooks and caterers will come to your parent's house and prepare a week's worth of meals. This may not be as expensive as you think, especially because the servings are usually large enough to be stretched into two meals. The senior center may know of such people in your parent's community, or look in the phone directory for private caterers.

TRANSPORTATION SERVICES

IF YOUR PARENT NEEDS A RIDE TO A doctor's appointment, the grocery store, day care, or elsewhere, a number of public and private groups provide door-to-door transportation specifically to elderly or disabled people. The area agency on aging should know about vans, buses, and private drivers who serve elderly residents. Some services pick up groups of people on a set day and take them to a shopping center, for example. Some take elderly people door-to-door for appointments and errands on an on-call basis. Most

BRAINSTORMING OPTIONS

Before you spend a fortune on professional workers, think about more creative options. For example, if there is a spare bedroom in your parent's home, or a den that can be converted into a bedroom, find a college student, a struggling writer, or a young couple who would like to live with your parent in exchange for some help around the house and companionship. Your parent loves Italian? What about a foreign-exchange student from Italy? Call a college housing office, put an ad in the newspaper, or call the local shared-housing program (see page 415).

This type of arrangement may provide less constant or reliable care than a companion or homemaker, but if your parent is still relatively independent, it is usually less expensive than hiring companions and aides, and it can work out wonderfully. It will also make your parent feel less like an invalid (because no one is being paid to watch him) and it may provide greater continuity—it may even blossom into a wonderful friendship.

Another possibility is for your parent to share a companion or homemaker with another elderly person who lives down the block or in the same apartment building, as workers often want a full-time job. A worker could get your mother up, bathed, and dressed, then go to the neighbor's house for two hours to help out there; return to your parent briefly to get her lunch; and then come back in the late afternoon to prepare her dinner. Be sure that the worker can be contacted quickly in case one person suddenly needs her assistance. Or maybe your parent can take in another elderly person and share care and each other's companionship within the one house.

of the vans are equipped to take people in wheelchairs. These community services are usually free, but some groups ask for a donation or charge a minimal fee.

In addition, the local department of public transportation can tell you about bus routes, discounts to seniors, and other special transportation services.

SENIOR CENTERS

SENIOR CENTERS WERE ORIGINALLY established as social clubs for relatively healthy elderly people, but that focus has changed. As the population grows older and more frail, senior centers are serving a more diverse and needy population. Some are still small social clubs that operate out of a church

WHEN YOUR PARENT BLOCKS THE PATH

You've found a reliable homemaker as well as a good adult day-care center, but your mother says no. She insists that she doesn't need help (she forgets that she has set off the smoke alarm three times in the past month), she refuses to go to "one of those places for old people," she wants only you to help her, and she doesn't want strangers in her home. When you persist and send the homemaker over anyway, she throws soup at her and fires her on the spot.

Before you blow your top, remember, her fears are pronounced these days. She may be confused about what is happening. She may feel vulnerable and be desperately afraid of being robbed or hurt by strangers. She may have already lost too much and not be willing to let go of anything else (like her independence and privacy). Or she may be worried that you are abandoning her. And yes, she might be manipulating you. Telling her that her fears are silly won't erase them and may only magnify them. Pushing her to accept services she doesn't want will only fortify her objections.

Encourage your mother to express her fears and concerns, and then acknowledge her worries. If she just seems stubborn, think about what might be behind her obstinacy. Then let her know that you care and that you are doing your best. Finally, be candid about the risks and opportunities the situation presents. Does she realize what could or will happen if she doesn't allow people to help her? Does she understand what she stands to get if she does allow them in—hot meals, a caring companion, and help with all sorts of daily tasks? (If your parent is confused because of dementia, see page 488 for tips on hiring and working with companions and other in-home helpers.)

If the situation is not dire, proceed slowly as you introduce new services. For example, you might introduce a worker in some neutral location, like a restaurant over coffee. Or, start by getting someone to do her shopping

basement, but some are large, publicly funded organizations, housed in free-standing buildings and offering an array of services, including help with chores, volunteer visitors, homemakers, adult day care, recreational programs, meals, health screenings, counseling, exercise classes, lectures, and field trips.

Call and find out what your parent's local senior center offers, because it probably does a lot more than run

or to drop off a meal every afternoon, rather than sending a companion across her sacred doorstep. Find someone who is kind and patient, someone who can earn your mother's trust over time. Once she trusts one person to enter her home, she may be open to more help, more hours, and other workers.

If this doesn't work, or if the situation doesn't allow for such small steps, you might have to leave your parent for a period of time without your help so that she understands the severity of the situation. A day or two without meals or an hour or two in soiled clothing may help her understand that she needs regular assistance, which you can't provide.

If the situation is dangerous or if you can't handle this yourself, consider hiring a geriatric care manager (see page 149) or a social worker from a family service agency who can guide your mother into this new way of life. Many of these professionals are trained specifically to do just that.

bingo games. If nothing else, it should be a good source of information and referrals to local services. Senior centers are usually free and open to all elderly residents of any age, income, or health status.

ADULT DAY CARE

YOUR MOTHER IS WEAK, AND HER memory is fading. She can't get her own meals, she needs help getting to the toilet, and she cannot remember why she called you. You're available during most weekends to care for her, but what do you do the other five days of the week? One answer is adult day care (now known as adult day services; the name was changed for obvious reasons), which provides care and supervision outside the home to elderly people who have physical or mental limitations.

While the programs offer varying services, the sort of thing that happens is this: Your mother is picked up by a van at 8 or 9 A.M., taken to a place where she is fed and cared for by trained staff, and then dropped off at home at 5 or 6 P.M. While at the center, she sees friends, listens to music, has a hot lunch, goes for a walk or does some gentle exercises, and maybe receives some occupational therapy or routine medical attention. Just as important as what she gets, however, is what you get—a break from the work and stress of her daily care.

Most centers accept people with dementia, and many care for people who are so frail that they would otherwise have to live in a nursing home. Some programs have expanded to provide weekend respite care (your parent stays at the center so you get a weekend off), periodic home care, pharmacy and laboratory services, rides to appointments and errands, and, when necessary, alternate housing. The

While I'm at work, I have two companions who come in shifts to watch Mother. One is excellent, and I love her dearly, but Mother is really awful to her. Frances is an articulate, intelligent, retired professional who is doing this work in order to keep active. She is very thoughtful, kind, and sympathetic. Mother was a nurse, and I think she feels resentful and threatened by having this capable person take care of her. She is rude, uncooperative, and mean to her.

The other companion is young and sweet, but, you know, nobody's home. Every day is a new day for her. I have to tell her everything all over again. Mother gets along just fine with her—perhaps because she is so simple.

I spend a lot of time apologizing to Frances and a lot of time explaining things to Susie. I guess there's no perfect solution. Anytime you have someone caring for your parent, there's bound to be some problem."

—Barbara H.

best ones will have waiting lists, so get on this early.

A typical center costs about $50 a day, although prices range from a few dollars up to $150 a day. Clients usually pay most or all of these fees themselves, although in some states, Medicaid covers adult day services.

Some centers are subsidized or publicly owned and can charge a lower rate or assess fees on a sliding scale, and sometimes communities have programs to help with such costs. Given the high cost of home care or elderly housing, adult day services is a bargain at almost any price.

Larger communities often have more than one center, and some cities have dozens of them. Unfortunately, many rural areas have nothing. If your parent has choices, see which center offers the level of care that she needs and then, if there is still some choice, tour the centers. While some are simply supervision in a church basement, most now offer a menu of services.

Ideally, a center should be clean, attractive, well ventilated, and safe. It should allow for some time spent outdoors. The indoors should be arranged to meet the needs of clients—no open door if someone with dementia might roam out, an amply wide bathroom for people in wheelchairs, etc. Activities should actually be interesting (stay away from those that rely on television and bingo games) and manageable for your parent.

Staffing is vital. A program should have a nurse and a social worker on staff, at least one "care provider" for every six clients (or one for every four if the clients are severely impaired and need a lot of assistance), and should provide some minimal training for the staff. But perhaps even more important, the staff should enjoy older people, be upbeat and involved, and interact easily with the clients. This requires a visit or two. Is the staff harried and flustered? Annoyed by client requests? Standing to the side chatting among themselves? Talk to the staff about how they might handle particular issues involving your parent, such as incontinence, aggressive behavior, confusion, immobility, blindness, etc.

Ask for references and contact them, and talk to other clients and caregivers as they come and go from the facility.

If your parent refuses to go, be persistent. Address her concerns and urge her to try it for a few days. People are often surprised at how much they enjoy adult day services once they get used to it. But it can take several tries before your parent reaches the point of acceptance.

To find adult day services, it's best to look in the local phone book, but you can also call the local agency on aging (see page 628) or senior center, or contact the National Adult Day Services Association (800-558-5301 or www.nadsa.org).

Geriatric Care Managers

If you are far away, busy with other things, facing a crisis, wrestling with family members, or just need some guidance and support, a geriatric care manager can counsel your family, assess your parent's situation, connect her to appropriate services,

> " *My mother would just stay in bed, almost all day. I could not get her up to do anything. She would eat and that was it. Day care was the answer to my prayers. I still have a hard time getting her to go each morning, but once she's there, she's fine. She does things and meets people. She's really started coming out of her shell. We've even started playing cards together in the evenings.*"
>
> — Linda K.

and oversee some or all of her care on an ongoing basis.

Care managers (also known as eldercare consultants and case managers, although these terms often refer to people who offer less extensive help) are usually social workers, nurses, or psychologists with training in geriatrics or gerontology. They can handle almost any facet of your parent's care, either short or long term.

You can retain a manager simply to assess your parent's situation and introduce you to community services; to oversee a particular issue, say, finding a good nursing home, dealing with nursing-home staff, or mediating a family dispute; to fill in while you take a break; or to jump in when there's an emergency. A care manager can also take over the whole kit and caboodle—hire, coordinate, and monitor home-care workers, locate community services, work with financial advisers and lawyers, get your parent to appointments, and, an invaluable bonus, offer a sympathetic ear and some reassuring support to you, the frazzled child. In most cases, you can take it a day at a time and expand, reduce, or cancel the service at any point.

Typically, a care manager will meet with your parent, family members, and others involved in your parent's care. He or she will assess your parent's abilities and living situation, confer with doctors, and, depending upon the job, research your parent's financial and legal situation. Then the manager will draft a detailed plan, outlining what services will be provided, when, by whom, and at what cost, specifying the manager's role and fees. All of this should be updated and modified over time, as necessary.

Once the services are in place, the manager should keep you posted on your parent's care and well-being. You should request a written monthly report, a weekly phone call, or some other kind of routine communication.

None of this is cheap. Sometimes the area agency on aging or a local family service organization has case managers who will, for free or on a sliding scale, advise families on various issues, and they might even do an at-home assessment. The services will not be as extensive or individualized, but certainly should be very useful.

Private geriatric care managers, on the other hand, sometimes charge a flat rate for a particular service, which might range from $200 to $2,000, depending upon the task.

Others charge hourly, at anywhere from $75 to $250 an hour. An assessment might last three hours, or it could last ten hours if the manager has to talk to nursing-home staff, numerous doctors, specialists, and advisers. You can minimize costs by helping with some of this. (You can ask the manager to give you a list of jobs, like getting information from the doctor or calling a nursing home about a particular issue.)

Keep in mind that a care manager's fee does not include the cost of services themselves—home health aides, nurses, medical supplies, etc. Plus, geriatric care managers usually charge their usual hourly rate for travel and telephone time.

It's expensive, but if you find the right care manager and you can afford it, it can be well worth the money.

Before you hire a geriatric care manager, check the person's training and experience. They should have some background in social work, nursing, gerontology, or some related field, and, ideally, they should have been doing this for some time. Find out how long the person has been in your parent's community—newcomers won't be as familiar with local services and also might lack rapport with important personnel. Ask how many clients the person is currently serving and whether they limit their caseloads. The fewer clients on a person's plate, the more time and attention she can give to your parent. A care manager with more than forty clients will spend, on average, less than an hour a week considering and monitoring your parent's suituation. Be sure there is backup in place in case the care manager is unavailable. As with other employees, get a written agreement regarding the job description and fees.

Also, if a care manager is finding workers for you, find out if he or she is simply serving as an employment service—hiring people to work and getting a fee for it. Be sure these are the best workers and that you are not paying excessively for them. Listen to a care manager's recommendations, but then check them out yourself, if you can.

To find a geriatric care manager, contact the area agency on aging or the National Association of Professional Geriatric Care Managers (520-881-8008 or www.caremanager.org). Or go on the Internet and search under "geriatric care manager," including your parent's town or state in the search.

Chapter Eight

MORE HELP, AT HOME

Home Health Care • Nurses, Therapists, and Aides • The Hiring Process • Managing the Troops • Respite Care

I F YOUR MOTHER IS ILL, VERY FRAIL, OR CONFUSED, INJURED, or recovering from surgery and needs more than the services described in the previous chapter, health-care workers will come into her home. Such care is often arranged by hospital discharge planners, but you can also use a home-care agency or make arrangements on your own. It's not inexpensive and Medicare rarely covers it, but sometimes community programs help defray the costs. Medicaid might cover these services if your parent would otherwise be in a nursing home.

As before, first assess your parent's needs. Does she need round-the-clock supervision and help, nursing care, or occasional companions? Pinpoint her specific, daily needs. Then determine what level of care she needs and how many hours a day (or week) she needs this help.

Once you have workers in place, you'll have to monitor their work. But you should also let go some and use this time to attend to yourself and your life. When workers are good to your parent, be very good to them; you don't want them to leave you.

Home Health Care

Home health care is classified into two categories, "skilled" and "custodial" care, based on Medicare's definitions. Skilled care refers to more intensive medical care, provided by or supervised by nurses and therapists (physical, occupational, speech). Custodial care means help with bathing, dressing, cooking, shopping, and other daily tasks, which is often provided by health aides and companions.

While home health care is a blessing, it can also be a headache, or in some cases, an outright disaster. You need to hire people carefully and then keep a watchful eye on what is happening in your parent's home. If you find a reliable, trustworthy, and caring home care worker, treat her or him like gold.

NURSES

DOCTORS STOPPED MAKING HOUSE calls some time ago (although some are going back to the old ways; see page 200 for more on house calls), but nurses make house calls routinely these days, and they do much of the work that doctors used to do. They can monitor your parent's health, change dressings, insert catheters and intravenous lines, administer medications, give injections, and perform other medical tasks. They can teach your parent or family members how

" *When my father left the hospital, I took a leave from work and went home to help my mother care for him. It was the most grueling few weeks of my life. We had to be with my father, or within earshot of him, pretty much every minute of the day. We were lifting him, turning him, feeding him, cleaning him, and helping him go to the bathroom. Mom was staying with him at night, too, and she wasn't getting much sleep.*

About two weeks into it, we realized that we needed help. We were physically and mentally fried. We hired a home health aide who came every morning. But even with that, we were still both exhausted. So we hired a companion who came five afternoons a week and stayed overnight three nights a week.

I'm not sure why it took us so long to get help. We should have had all that in place the day he came home from the hospital."

—GLORIA J.

to perform some tasks, and they oversee other workers.

Registered nurses, or RNs, have at least two years of nursing school and are licensed by the state in which they practice. Licensed practical nurses, or LPNs, have at least one year of specialized education and must also be licensed. LPNs work under the supervision of an RN.

HOME CARE AND OTHER HELP

Type of Help	Services Provided	Average Costs*
Home Health Aides	Personal care (bathing, feeding, dressing, toileting, etc.), minor medical care, and light housekeeping	$7 to $25 an hour; may be covered by Medicare
Nurses	Nursing care	$20 to $90 an hour; rarely covered by Medicare; sometimes covered by Medicaid
Physical, occupational, and speech therapists	Training in physical movement, doing daily tasks, or communication	$20 to $90 an hour; rarely covered by Medicare; sometimes covered by Medicaid
Respite care	A break for caregivers, from a few hours to a few weeks	Cost varies widely; may be subsidized or provided by volunteers

Prices vary widely depending upon the area and whether you hire workers through an agency.

While you can hire nurses independently, they typically work for home-care agencies and, under the terms of Medicare, can work in your parent's home only under a doctor's orders.

THERAPISTS

AS PART OF YOUR PARENT'S HOME care, the doctor may recommend that some sort of therapist visit him on a regular basis.

Physical therapists work the muscles and joints to improve mobility, flexibility, and strength, usually after an injury, surgery, or an illness (such as a stroke). They use various exercises, heat, massage, and other techniques to restore mobility.

Occupational therapists train people with rigid fingers, stiff hips, dim vision, or other disabilities to perform daily tasks by working on muscular control and coordination, teaching them new ways to do things, setting them up with special equipment, and making adjustments to the home.

Speech therapists help people who have trouble speaking or understanding speech (because of a stroke or other illness or injury) to communicate again. They can also help people who have trouble swallowing or breathing.

SOCIAL WORKERS AND NUTRITIONISTS

NUTRITIONISTS WILL GET YOUR parent on a diet that is healthful, manageable, and compatible with his medications and any illness that might be affecting him.

Social workers often work as part of the home-care team, counseling clients and their families about social and emotional issues, reviewing the living situation and needs of the elderly person, and referring families to appropriate community services.

These individuals all make house calls, often through a hospital or home-care agency. The cost is often covered by insurance if it is medically necessary and part of a hospital discharge plan of care.

HOME HEALTH AIDES AND NURSE'S AIDES

HOME HEALTH AIDES AND NURSE'S aides are trained to provide "custodial" care—help with bathing, dressing, getting to the toilet, and other personal tasks. Some will prepare meals and do light housekeeping (but only that which pertains to your parent, such as changing and laundering his sheets and tidying his room). Many are trained to do simple medical procedures, such as changing bandages, checking catheters and intravenous lines, taking temperatures, or administering medications, but only under the supervision of a nurse.

Certified home health aides usually have a little more medical training than noncertified home care aides or personal care aides, who may have very little training.

Fees vary, depending upon the experience and training of the aide and the cost of living in the area. Medicare

> *" I used to stay in the house the whole time the aide was there. It was a control thing for me. I felt that I had to oversee everything and that I couldn't trust anyone with my father. I was afraid that if I left, something would happen. Fortunately, I've gotten over that. Now I leave the minute the aide arrives. I go shopping, run errands, or visit friends. A couple of times I took my bills and mail to the library just to be out of the house. It's really an important break in the day for me."*
>
> —GRACE D.

and other insurance will cover the cost of home health aides only when their services are needed as part of a package of "skilled" nursing care.

The Hiring Process

When a member of the local church or synagogue volunteers to call on your mother, you can go on instinct alone. But if you are contracting with an agency or hiring a freelance worker to care for your parent on a regular basis, do some homework. Ask a lot of questions, get referrals, and get any agreement in writing.

You can hire home-care workers either through an agency or directly. There are advantages to either route.

A NOTE ON FINANCES

Home care is expensive, but almost any type of care your parent receives now will be costly, and in many cases, care provided at home or in the community is the least expensive and most attractive option.

Medicare will pay for "skilled" care, which includes licensed nurses and therapists (physical, occupational, speech) and accompanying care that is prescribed by a doctor for medical reasons. The care must be provided by an agency that is certified by Medicare; it must be intermittent, not full time (fewer than 28 hours a week); and your parent must be homebound, meaning that she cannot leave the house without a lot of assistance and gets out only for medical appointments and possibly to go to religious services or to get a haircut. And even then, coverage is limited to 21 days.

Medicare and most private health insurance policies do not cover the cost of custodial care (help with bathing, toileting, dressing, etc.) unless it is an integral part of the care described above, and then only for a short time.

Medicaid coverage is usually more generous than Medicare. While the details vary by state, intermittent home care is typically covered if a person qualifies for nursing-home care. Find out the Medicaid rules in your parent's area early because states have various programs that help cover home-care costs.

Finally, government agencies and charitable organizations sometimes offer subsidies and fees based on sliding scales. The area agency on aging or long-term care ombudsman (listed on page 628) will know more about this.

Whatever you do about home care, consider the nursing-home option early. It's worth looking at what exists and you may want to get your parent's name on any waiting lists, just in case. Also, if your parent's savings are running low, it may be better to apply while she still has enough to pay for six months to a year of nursing-home care. Once she is on Medicaid, she may have fewer choices.

See Chapter Sixteen for more on Medicare, Medicaid, and ways to pay for long-term care.

Most important, if your parent expects Medicare to foot the bill, she must receive her care from a certified agency. Certification also means that the agency and workers meet minimal standards set by the federal government. In most cases, Medicaid services must also be provided by a certified agency, although states have their own rules regarding coverage.

If your parent isn't eligible for Medicare, she might get some financial relief if she hires an agency associated with the local health department, for example, or one operated by a Visiting Nurse Association. Services may be subsidized by public monies or donations, meaning that your parent will pay only what she can afford.

Besides that, agencies make life easier. Their staff will develop a plan, find the right workers, screen them, and then oversee their work. They also provide back-up in case a worker cancels. If an agency offers a full range of services, the care tends to be better coordinated and more comprehensive than anything you can arrange on your own. And finally, agencies have insurance in case of an accident and they handle the paperwork, such as social security and tax forms for employees.

If you hire workers independently, you will pay less and you will have more control over whom you hire and the work that's done. But use caution. Get a number of references and monitor workers carefully. Many unaffiliated workers are first-rate and provide excellent care, but there are scoundrels in the world.

CONTRACTING WITH A HOME-CARE AGENCY

WHAT COMPANY YOU USE DEPENDS, in part, upon whether your parent needs skilled nursing care, and whether Medicare or Medicaid will cover her care.

If your parent is leaving the hospital or has just recently left the hospital, talk with the hospital's discharge planner or social worker about setting up home care. These people are usually pretty savvy to what's available, what's covered, and what's reliable. They will also call and make arrangements for your parent, in most cases. (Keep in mind, however, that some hospitals have financial arrangements with certain health-care agencies, so there might be some bias.)

Otherwise, you can get the names of certified agencies, as well as some quality information, through Medicare's Home Health Compare program (800-633-4227 or www.medicare.gov). You can also ask your parent's doctor, or contact the area agency on aging or the National Association for Home Care & Hospice (202-547-7424 or www.nahc.org), which has an agency locator on its Web site.

If Medicare will not cover your parent's care, there are additional options. You can still use a certified agency (and many have separate arms for less-intensive "custodial" care) or you can find individual workers yourself (discussed later in this chapter). You can also use a noncertified agency. These work very much like certified home-care agencies except that, of course, they are not certified and most do not provide "skilled" nursing care. The National Private Duty Association (317-844-7105 or www.privateduty-homecare.org), has the names of many of these private duty companies on their Web site.

Here are some questions to ask when looking for a home-care agency:

◆ What services does the agency provide? Who is on the home-care team—physicians, nurses, therapists, dietitians, social workers, home health aides, homemakers, companions, volunteers?

◆ What is the cost for these services? Are there a minimum number of hours per week or for each visit? (If your parent only needs help bathing and dressing, which might take an hour or two, will you be charged for a four-hour minimum?) Are there extra charges that might arise unexpectedly? Is there any maximum to how much care will be provided? (Ask to have all agreements, including services to be provided and financial arrangements, put in writing.)

◆ Is the agency certified to receive Medicare and Medicaid reimbursement?

◆ Can it subsidize care for people who cannot pay for themselves? (Government and voluntary agencies, such as a Visiting Nurse Association, often have public or private money to cover some care.)

◆ Can the staff meet the special needs of my parent, whether religious,

cultural, or medical (Alzheimer's, dialysis, diabetes, etc.)?

◆ How does the agency determine what services my parent needs? Will a nurse evaluate him? Will he or she consult with my parent's doctor and my family? (Ask to have a plan of care drawn up and updated as your parent's condition changes.)

◆ How will his care be coordinated? Who oversees workers? Will a supervisor visit regularly? How do I reach a supervisor if there is a problem?

◆ Is someone available 24/7 in case of emergency? Are backups provided when workers cancel or don't show up? (Again, get this in writing.)

◆ Will the same person care for my parent consistently, or will the guards change regularly (which is less desirable, but often unavoidable). If my parent doesn't get along with a particular worker, can someone else be assigned to him? Can we interview two or three aides and select one?

◆ What sorts of training does staff receive, aside from general geriatric care (care for patients with dementia, first aid, communicating with someone who has trouble communicating, caring for a blind person, caring for someone who is incontinent, etc.)? Do you do background checks on workers (such as a criminal check)?

◆ How much say does the family have in the plan of care? How does the client or family file complaints?

PACE, HMOs, AND WAIVER PROGRAMS

If your parent has little money but needs a lot of help, you might be inclined to put him into a nursing home and let Medicaid pick up the tab. But some states have programs aimed at helping just such people so they can stay in their own homes.

Medicaid covers nursing-home bills for people eligible for nursing-home care. But under "waiver programs," states use this money to provide home and community services instead, which keeps people at home and often saves the state money. The state medical assistance office (page 639) or area agency on aging (page 628) will know of such programs in your parent's state.

Programs of All-inclusive Care for the Elderly, or PACE, provide extensive care at home and in the community to those who are nursing-home eligible. The only difference is that these act a bit like an HMO in that the care must be received from a specific site or organization.

Services in a PACE program usually include all medical, social, and rehabilitative services, including transportation, adult day care, rehabilitative therapy, meals, medical care, home health care, prescription drugs, social services, respite care, and, when necessary, hospital and nursing-home care. Services are provided 24 hours a day, every day of the year.

For those who qualify for Medicaid, the services are fully covered. Other people must pay a monthly fee. While not inexpensive ($3,000 a month and up), PACE may be cheaper than paying for services separately.

Unfortunately, there are fewer than fifty PACE sites in the United States to date. To find them, call the area agency on aging, contact Medicare (800-MEDICARE or visit www.medicare.gov), or visit the Web site of the National PACE Association (www.natlpaceassn.org).

A somewhat similar program, called social HMOs or Social Managed Care Plans, is for Medicare beneficiaries, but, unfortunately, is even harder to find. There are only a handful of these programs in the entire country. Again, contact the area agency on aging to learn more about this.

◆ Is the agency licensed by the state and in compliance with all state regulations? (Agencies that provide nursing and therapeutic care must be licensed.)

◆ Is the agency accredited by a trade association, such as the National League for Nursing, which sets standards for the industry? (Accreditation means that an agency has met certain requirements with regard to staffing, training, and supervision, but not all agencies choose to take part even if they meet the requirements, so don't rule out an agency simply because it is not accredited.)

◆ Is the agency insured and bonded (which protects your parent in case of theft or accidents)? Does it provide worker's compensation so you are not liable if an employee is injured while caring for your parent?

◆ Under what conditions can the client or the agency terminate services?

◆ Can the agency provide references? Be specific when you ask for references so you don't talk to a few selected people who were happy with the service. For example, get the names of two clients who live within five miles of your parent, or two clients with dementia who received care within the past month. Then ask these references (clients or their families) specific questions: Did the agency respond quickly to the client's changing needs? Did workers arrive for work on time? Were workers courteous and polite? Was there a need to change workers? And so on.

HIRING INDEPENDENTLY

To FIND A CAREGIVER ON YOUR OWN, get names of workers from the agency on aging in your parent's area; talk to her doctor or a case worker from the doctor's office or the hospital; check with the local senior center; talk to friends and neighbors; and look through the classified ads or put an ad in the paper yourself.

There are registries that will provide you with names of freelance workers and then take a cut of the worker's fee. These are essentially employment services for health-care workers. They are not the same as home care or private duty agencies; workers are not screened or supervised in any way, nor are such registries certified or regulated. While they can be useful, you still need to screen workers carefully yourself, and you will be responsible for any paperwork, filing state and federal payroll taxes, and supervision.

However you hunt, weed through candidates by phone first, finding out what language they speak, what experience they have, what hours they are available, how many months or years they might be able to commit to this, whether they can meet your parent's particular needs, whether or not they smoke, and, if necessary, whether they have a valid driver's license and a car.

When you finally meet someone face-to-face, you will know quite a bit in the first few minutes by watching how he or she interacts with you and with your parent. Is this person respectful, courteous, and well groomed? On time? Easy to get along with? Well versed in the issues of aging and caring for an aged person?

Here are some other issues to consider:

♦ What qualifications does this person have? Many workers will not need qualifications or certification, but if, say, you are hiring a nurse, ask about licensing or call the state's board of nurses to check.

♦ What prior experience does this person have? Does he or she have experience working with the particular problems that affect your parent?

♦ Is he or she physically capable of meeting your parent's needs—can he or she support your parent so he can move from a bed to a chair, for example?

♦ Exactly what chores and services will this person perform, and can he or she perform them?

♦ Depending upon the nature of the work and the employee, you might find out if the worker is bonded (has a bond that will cover any lawsuit that might arise).

♦ You might also do a background check to find out about any criminal record, driving violations, and licenses, and to verify past employment. Ask to see identification so you know that you have the right name. You can then ask the local police department, look through the local Yellow Pages (under "investigators" or "detectives"), or go online to one of the many companies that do such checks (usually for under $25). Do a search under "background check" or "crime check."

Once you select an employee, get a home phone number and cell phone number where he or she can be reached, as well as a home address. Draft a contract, to be signed by both of you, stating the starting date of the job, the days and hours of employment, the job requirements, the pay plus any bonuses or benefits involved, vacation days and time off, and the types of things that would lead to termination.

It all seems very serious and formal until you've had an employee steal from you, get drunk on the job, damage your home, neglect his work, or worse, abuse your parent. If your parent is not terribly alert or able to keep an eye on things herself, all of this is only that much more important.

Managing the Troops

If your parent needs constant home care and you are overseeing that care, it may seem as though you have taken a full-time job as staff manager. You have to ensure that workers show up on time, do what needs to be done responsibly, get along with your parent, and don't leave until they're relieved by the next shift. If this is all happening most of the time, then you are one lucky son of a gun.

We hired what was essentially a babysitter to stay with my father. Kim was about sixteen or seventeen at the time, trying to earn some money over her summer vacation.

One afternoon I arrived when she was leaving—we had a sort of changing of the guards each day—and I realized that she had been crying. I followed her out on the porch, and we had a long talk about how my father reminded her of her grandfather, who had died a few years earlier. Apparently, she had been really close to her grandfather, and she was reliving his death every day. It was very sad, but also very sweet. I had thought of her as a sitter, but after we talked, I saw her as someone who was really sharing this pain with me, someone who really cared about my father."

—GRACE D.

Even if you're used to managing people, it can be an uncomfortable and trying job. Home-care workers perform personal tasks in the most intimate surroundings. Seemingly small mistakes can cause enormous anguish and frustration. *She's always late . . . forgot to remind Dad to take his pills, again . . . smokes in the house . . . argues with me . . . knows nothing about caring for an elderly person . . . thinks she knows everything. . . .*

It is a delicate situation, but open communication and willingness to compromise will help you, and your parent, immensely.

◆ **Keep workers happy.** A worker who is treated with respect and kindness is more apt to treat your parent with respect and kindness. During these tough times, it may be hard for you to think about anyone else's needs, but do what you can. Welcome any worker into your parent's home, make sure she has a place for her belongings, decent food to eat, and, if she is living in or working long shifts, some breaks and privacy occasionally. Be sensitive to her needs and the pressure she faces, both on the job and away from it.

When there is a problem, don't assume it is the fault of the employee, or at least don't lambaste anyone the first time around. There might have been some miscommunication, or maybe she got busy with other things. Offer a gentle reminder. *You are so sweet to bring donuts over here, and with all that's going on I probably didn't make this clear, but Dad's got diabetes, so he really shouldn't eat those. Would you mind terribly eating them before you come?*

When things are done well, show your appreciation. Just saying "thank you" will mean a great deal, but if a worker is exceptional, write a note to her supervisor, give her a bonus, or buy an occasional gift. (People working for agencies don't get paid as much as you might think; the agency takes a hefty portion of the fee.)

When someone is really good and you want to keep her, pay her amply and be sure that she is happy.

◆ **Foster this relationship.** Ideally, you are the silent partner in this relationship. In most cases, it is less important that you like a home-care worker than that your parent and she get along.

Encourage this budding friendship from the start. Tell the worker about your parent—what makes her tick, what she used to be like, what will win her over, and what could infuriate her. And tell your parent about the worker—who she is, where she comes from, what she does and why she does it. Then, step back and let them get to know each other.

If your parent is thrilled to see you leave and a worker arrive in the morning, don't be jealous, be grateful.

◆ **Make it easy.** Whatever tasks need to be done, make them as manageable as possible. Confer with the aide or companion or whomever on what would help—perhaps an alarm that goes off when your parent needs to take medications, or a higher toilet seat so there's not so much lifting, or some soft music to ease agitation. If a family member is giving a worker trouble, protect

WHEN YOUR PARENT CAN'T BE PLEASED

If your parent has lofty expectations, if he is never pleased with any worker, resents the fact that he has to be cared for, and takes it out on a worker, stay calm. Again.

Find out what's really going on. Is this worker no good, or is your parent the problem? If it's your parent, it may be that he is just miserably unhappy and feeling that life is hard. Although you may be sick of hearing about it, let him air his hostility, fears, and hurts. Your calm reaction and willingness to listen will get you further than arguing. Once he's stated his case, explain to him—slowly and clearly but firmly—that while this situation may not be ideal, it is the only option. Remind him that you are not abandoning him, that you will continue to see him and care for him.

Talk with the worker as well. Help her understand your parent's situation and feelings. Help her to see that this is not personal, that it is not about her (although it seems that way). Encourage her to be flexible and have a sense of humor. And beg her to please put up with some occasional wrath. Tell her to call you if she needs to let off some steam, and be sympathetic when she does. (See page 146 for more on parents who get in the way of getting help.)

EMERGENCY INFORMATION

 Anytime someone is working in your house or you have volunteers or other outsiders helping with a parent's care, be sure that all important information and phone numbers are readily available.

◆ Post emergency numbers—for fire, police, ambulance, and poison control—in large red writing near all phones.

◆ Have a list of important numbers by the phone that is most often used and be sure it's legible. This should include your home, work, and cell phone numbers, as well as numbers for other family members. List the doctor or doctors involved in your parent's care, the local pharmacy, the hospital, and names and numbers of helpful friends and neighbors. You might also include numbers for a repair person and heating, electrical, and plumbing companies.

◆ Have a fire extinguisher easily accessible in the kitchen and be sure any worker knows how to use it.

◆ Any special medical information that might be needed by emergency crews should either be on a medical bracelet on your parent or written and displayed prominently. If your parent has a living will or at-home Do Not Resuscitate order, be sure that is also readily available.

◆ Display your parent's phone number and street address near a phone, in case a worker needs to pass that on to emergency crews. (In a state of panic, people can forget such information.)

◆ Be sure any worker knows where to find emergency medical supplies, secondary fire escape routes, breaker boxes, and water shut-off valves.

---

her. Give her the tools to do her job well, because if you take care of her, she will take better care of your parent.

◆ **Communicate clearly.** Be direct and open from the start. Talk with this employee about your expectations and

your parent's needs. If necessary, give him or her a detailed description of the duties and a daily schedule so there are no misunderstandings about what is involved in this job. And make any house rules clear—regarding smoking, noise levels, food consumption, alcohol consumption, or anything else that concerns you or your parent. Do it diplomatically, as a list of reminders, not orders.

Then let the worker give you her list of needs and preferences as well—what tasks she will do, what she won't do, when she likes to take breaks, how she likes to handle problems. Even if she doesn't express any needs, asking shows that you care.

If there comes a time when your parent or you want things done differently, raise the subject right then, because the longer you wait, the more difficult it will be to institute change. Likewise, ask that workers be candid with you about their problems or frustrations.

◆ **Compromise.** No one is going to care for your mother in exactly the way you think she should be cared for. No one is going to give her the attention, devotion, and individual care that you would give her, or that she deserves. And no one is going to treat her home the way you or she would. All of which means that you have to accept a standard that is considerably less than perfect and learn to ignore a few minor errors or irritating habits.

Try several people if necessary, but be ready to compromise, or you will be hiring and firing in rapid succession. The aide may be watching television when you think she should be tending to your parent, but if your parent likes her, and she is doing a reasonably good job, hang on to her.

> " *My mother is now on Medicaid, but I supplement the pay of the two women who take care of her. They earn so little and they work so hard. They are incredible with her. Vicky will wash Mom's hair, not because it needs it, but because Mom enjoys it so much. Kathy will stop at the store on her way to the house in the morning to pick up anything Mom needs. They really are wonderful. They are almost like family. And because of them I can stay in my own apartment and continue working. So I pay them extra and do anything else I can to keep them happy."*
>
> —Jacqui L.

◆ **Monitor the work.** If your parent is able and alert, then he can supervise his own care. But if he isn't, it's important that you make unannounced visits occasionally.

If you are using a care manager, you still need to stay apprised of how things are going. In theory, a care manager oversees everything for you, but it's important that you have a hand on the reins as well. Monitor the care to see if it meets the goals of the plan the manager has drafted.

If you can't drop in and your parent isn't alert enough to monitor his own care and relay information to you, ask a friend or neighbor to check in from time to time, or see if there's

WHEN THERE IS TROUBLE

Serious problems are rare, but they happen. A worker mistreats your parent, steals from him, or gets drunk on the job. The best protection is prevention— don't leave jewelry or money lying around, for example. In other words, don't tempt fate. Rule number two: Trust your instincts. If you think something's not right, there's a good chance it isn't.

Be alert to any sign of possible physical abuse, such as unexplained bruises or wounds, and to indications of emotional abuse, such as a parent's unusual fear or nightmares.

If your parent is confused, she may make accusations that are false because she is paranoid or anxious. Try to confirm her complaints, and, if you determine that she is inventing problems, reassure her that you understand her fears, but that she is safe. If her accusations continue, even if they are untrue, find another worker with whom she is more comfortable.

If Medicare covers your parent's care, and you feel that a home-care agency is not giving your parent proper care or is withholding care, contact the Quality Improvement Organization in her state. Medicare contracts QIOs to be sure that patients receive quality care. You can find the local QIO through Medicare (800-633-4227 or www.medicare.gov).

When you suspect serious trouble and have reason to think that your suspicions are valid, act immediately. Dismiss the worker and call the area agency on aging to find out how to report abuse, neglect, or exploitation.

Depending upon the problem, you may want to contact a local elder abuse hotline, Better Business Bureau, consumers' affairs office, or licensing agency. Notify the bank if the problem has to do with your parent's accounts. If you are working through a home health agency that is certified by Medicare, you can file complaints with the state Home Health Hotline, which might be listed in the phone book, or you can get the number through Medicare (above).

a volunteer who might do it (call the area agency on aging or senior center).

If you think there may be trouble, consider buying a webcam (sometimes called a grannycam or nannycam), which is a small camera, often mounted high on a wall, which allows you to videotape a room in your parent's house. You can arrange it so that you can go onto the Internet and view a room directly. (Remember, however, that you are only seeing one part of one room; lots of things can happen beyond the eye of a camera. Also, this may create some mutual distrust and make the worker uncomfortable.)

◆ **Use common sense.** Don't leave valuables or cash in sight or even in obvious places. Keep alcohol, narcotics, and any dangerous substances locked away. Don't give a worker access to your parent's bank account or wallet

Respite Care

Anyone with hands-on responsibility for a frail parent needs a break occasionally, if not regularly. Start using respite care as soon as possible. You will need it before you think you do. You also need to get your parent accustomed to other caregivers before he is deeply established in a routine that includes only you.

Respite is a broad term that may mean having someone come over one evening a week so you can go out for dinner, but it typically means moving your parent temporarily to a nursing home or other facility, or hiring ample help for a week or two while you go on vacation, deal with a family emergency, or simply escape the day-to-day rigors of caregiving.

You might believe that you are the only one who can oversee your parent's care. You may be afraid that

> *I have decided to take a week off by myself. I am going to a little cottage near a lake. I haven't told Mum yet, but I feel no guilt at all.*
>
> *At first it felt like a ruthless decision. I thought I should keep being here for her. Or, if I took some time off, I thought I should visit friends or do something with my grandchildren. But the pressure has been intense. I feel so time-bound, so scheduled, as if my life is just about the needs of other people. I really want a week to myself, for me, not for anyone else. Just to look at the water and clear my head. That's my gift to myself."*
>
> —ANN S.

if you leave, your mother will have a stroke or your father will hate you for "deserting" him. You may worry that if you move your parent temporarily or have someone replace you for a few days, everything will fall apart. You may worry, and he may not like it, but you need to do it.

Ask the area agency on aging about respite programs, or call nursing homes, which sometimes provide respite care. Veterans' hospitals may also provide respite as part of your parent's regular medical care. Some adult day services also offer respite care.

Medicare covers respite when it is part of hospice care, but not in most other cases. If the kind of care your parent needs is too costly—and it can be quite expensive—talk to family, friends, and neighbors. People are often willing to help out for a brief time. Between community programs and family ties, you should be able to put together a schedule so you can take a break.

WHEN USING RESPITE

◆ Leave detailed, written instructions about your parent's medications, meals, and habits, even if you have discussed each item thoroughly with any staff or workers ahead of time.

◆ Leave a list of all emergency phone numbers, and at least two backup contacts.

◆ Show respite helpers where to find the emergency medical supplies.

◆ If you are an integral part of your parent's day, try a brief trial of leaving him with someone before heading off for any extended trip.

◆ Have a backup plan. Companions and aides can cancel just when you are about to drive away. Talk to other family members who might step in if your parent is deserted, and make sure a home-care agency guarantees that your parent will be covered during your absence.

◆ Don't be talked out of this break, even if your parent says or hints that her life is over or you are being selfish. She will survive your absence.

Chapter Nine

THE INNER CIRCLE

Working with Siblings • A Family Meeting
• Dealing with a Spouse • The Sandwich Generation
• Balancing Career and Caregiving

....

C ARING FOR AN AGED PARENT CAN STRENGTHEN SOME
relationships—you may find a new appreciation for your
husband or develop a closer bond with your sister—but it
can drive a sharp wedge into others. Unfortunately, the people we
are closest to, the ones we have known the longest and the most
intimately, are also the ones who can most infuriate and hurt us.
Perhaps we expect too much or give too little or just know each
other way too well. Maybe we are too much alike or too deeply vested
in the issues. Whatever the reasons for it, at no time is this dynamic
more apparent than during times of stress, when we need more from
each other, yet have less to offer.

Your involvement in your parent's care is likely to affect all
your relationships. Siblings who may have been at the fringe of your
life are now smack in the center. A mate who may not be able to
fully understand what you are going through may feel neglected.
Children want time that you simply don't have to give right now.
At work, bosses and colleagues offer a valuable diversion from
your parent's care, but they create yet another layer of stress as you

struggle to balance the demands of the job with the demands at home.

To some extent, you have to accept that things are going to be a bit rocky for now. These other people in your life will survive without your full attention. (Remember, you are not responsible for everyone's happiness.) The most important thing you can do right now for any relationship is to keep the lines of communication open and your priorities intact.

Working with Siblings

Your mother is hospitalized with a broken hip, and the doctor suggests that she be moved into a nursing home. Your sister drives up for the weekend, one brother flies in, and a second brother doesn't make the trip, but tells you to keep him posted. Over the weekend, the three of you make repeated visits to the hospital, meet with a discharge planner and nursing-home administrators, and then gather in the evening at your family home, exhausted and distraught.

Tempers are short. Opinions are strong and divided. After several confrontations, disagreements and misunderstandings, spells of silence, tears, and angry words, you find a residence for Mom, but by the time everyone departs, no one is speaking.

When a parent becomes ill, sibling relationships are tested, and even friendly alliances can become volatile. Old battles thought to be dormant reemerge, and new conflicts arise.

Reunited, perhaps at a family home, siblings often revert to childhood roles and behaviors, and they compete, just like in old times, for Mom's affection or Dad's praise. You're full-grown adults now, perhaps with full-grown children of your own, but old patterns and labels are hard to shake. One is bossy, one is the black sheep, one is the martyr, one is the princess, one is the mischief-maker, one never helps, and one always does the bulk of the work (whether anyone wants her to or not); one was closer to Mom, and the other was closer to Dad (or thinks she was).

Discussions are heated and opinions are strong because these relationships are complex, but also because the matter at hand—your parent's health and happiness—is one that everyone cares deeply about. One sibling approaches everything matter-of-factly, one is pure emotion, and one may not be able to accept what is happening at all. She refuses to believe that Mom is as sick as you say or that Dad needs help. Relationships are further strained because one sibling, inevitably, takes on far more work and responsibility than the others.

If your parent's needs are pressing, don't try to resolve old conflicts now. You can't possibly come up with the emotional reserve needed for it, nor should you divert so much of your attention to something that can wait. Your parent needs you now, and her care should be everyone's primary concern. Acknowledge the tensions and find ways to work around problems that are getting in the way of your parent's care.

ADAPTING TO NEW ROLES: A PRIMARY CAREGIVER

OFTEN, WHEN A PARENT GROWS FRAIL, one sibling gravitates toward the role of primary caregiver and takes on the majority of the work. This person may be closest to her parent geographically or emotionally. She may be the one who always takes charge, the one with the most time to give, or the one who typically takes care of others. (And, yes, she is usually a she.)

However this role is established and for whatever reasons, it can make everyone in the family uncomfortable. The primary caregiver may be resentful because she is doing more than her share, and the others may feel shut out.

If you are the primary caregiver, get your siblings involved right away. You may feel that you can handle your parent's care, and that no one else can do it as well as you can. And early on, there may not be all that much to do. But those reins can become very heavy, very quickly. If you don't share

HELPING THE WELL PARENT

When one parent is the primary caregiver for a sick or frail parent, you need to support and care for the healthier of the two. Helping her will then enable her to give her best to her spouse. And it may help her to stay well so you don't end up caring for two ailing parents. See page 62 on caring for the well (or somewhat well) spouse.

them now, you may find yourself stuck with them later, when they are unmanageable.

In addition to the sheer work involved, this can be a lonely undertaking. You need siblings to share the decisions, the worries, and the stress. And you need their support. If you are frazzled, weary, and resentful, you can't give your parent the kind of care he needs. If others chip in and perhaps even support you, you can then give your best when you are with your parent.

Plus, your siblings need to be involved, and your parent needs her other children. As close as the two of you might be, she gains from all of these relationships.

Be honest, but nonaccusing, when you approach siblings for help. You may think it's obvious that you're overworked

WHEN SIBLINGS WON'T HELP

If a sibling refuses to help in your parent's care, urge and prod. Hold a family meeting (see page 174). Get a counselor, social worker, or other professional involved. Find ways that this sibling can help that are manageable for him or her. If your brother's relationship with your mother is tense, give him jobs that don't require that he actually spend time with her (i.e., finances, research). If his relationship with you is the problem, you may have to step away and let him help in his own way, without your involvement.

At some point, however, you need to stop wasting your breath. If a sibling absolutely will not help no matter how you plead, this is his or her decision. Your sister might not be able to accept that your parent is sick or dying. Or your brother might have such a complex and painful relationship with your father that he can't begin to deal with any of this. Or maybe your sibling is terribly busy with other things, or simply self-involved. Drop it. And try to be understanding and forgiving. Your sibling has his reasons—ones that you may never understand—and, in the end, he will have to live with this decision. Let go of it; move on to more productive tasks.

By the way, be forewarned of a common occurrence that those in the field call "the brother from California syndrome" (or from Massachusetts, if you live on the west coast). It goes something like this: One or more children are deep in the trenches, dealing with an aged parent regularly. In sweeps a sibling from far away for a brief visit (often a brother who has some vague knowledge of medicine or law). Sizing up the situation quickly, he criticizes his siblings for all that they are doing wrong and directs them on what should be happening instead.

This does not go over well. But if you know it's coming, it might be easier to deal with. Don't bother arguing. Just nod, let him know how much you appreciate all his insight, and take him to the airport on time.

and they are not helping, but your siblings might not realize what is involved and all that you do. They may not think that you need their assistance, or that you want them involved.

Or, they simply might not know how to help. Sometimes siblings feel that they would be interfering, or they may not want to take directions from you, or they may not agree with the way you are handling things, so they stay away.

Explain your feelings. (Use "I" instead of "you" sentences, as in, "I feel overwhelmed," rather than, "You never help.") Explain what you do and what you need help with. Before you assign any tasks, ask how and where they might be willing to step in.

If you want their help, you have to listen to their opinions and let them do things their own way. You have to be willing to compromise.

When siblings do help in any way (even if it's not *your* way), be appreciative. Thank them for giving you a break or taking over a duty or listening to your gripes.

Over time, if you continue in the role of primary caregiver, be sure to listen to your siblings' concerns, hear their opinions, keep them informed, and let them help in any way they can. Whether or not they're able to express it, your siblings care and need to be kept up-to-date.

Sometimes the problem is not that siblings won't help, but that the primary caregiver won't relinquish duties. Even those who complain bitterly that no one helps sometimes have trouble letting go when push comes to shove. You (or your sibling) need to think long and hard about what it is that is keeping you from letting go. What are you afraid might happen if others do this job? And what are you trying to achieve by doing it all yourself—a new relationship with your parent, everyone's admiration, immortality for your parent? You need to separate the realistic goals from the unobtainable ones. Then, you should pick out the jobs that you most want to keep, and let go of the others.

SECONDARY CAREGIVERS

IF YOU ARE NOT THE PRIMARY CARE-giver, maintain your own relationship with your parent by visiting, calling, or writing regularly. Offer whatever help you can and stay involved.

When there is a problem, when you feel shut out or ignored or don't like the way your sibling is handling things, talk to her. Be sympathetic to her situation and credit her for all she is doing, but then explain what you are feeling or what you think should be done differently. Be clear, but also respectful. The primary caregiver might not be your favorite sibling right now, but this is a huge undertaking, and she is under a lot of stress. In fact, she may be living and breathing this task. It's hard for her to worry about you or see beyond her own problems. So be gentle and understanding.

In many instances, the best way to help your parent is to support this sibling, the primary caregiver. Even if you don't always agree with her, acknowledge the work she is doing, let her blow off steam, and give her a break from her duties whenever you can.

If you have no interest in helping your parent directly (or even if you do), you might offer to help the primary caregiver herself—do her taxes this year if you're a financial whiz, pick

> " *My brother refused to believe that my mother had dementia. I would tell him specific things that she did and how impossible things were becoming, but he always came up with an excuse for her. And then he would tell me that I was the one with the problem, that I was being overprotective.*
>
> *I brought Mom to his house one Saturday. I knew that the only way he would realize what was happening was if he saw it for himself, if he spent some real time with her. When we arrived, I told him that I had to go out of town and left Mom with him for the night. I didn't give him an out.*
>
> *When I came back for her the next day, he took one look at me, and for the first time in my life, I saw my brother cry. It was very sad, and I felt sorry for him. I understood—he really hadn't wanted to see it. But I had to do it. I needed his help and his support. I couldn't handle it alone any longer."*
>
> —Terry B.

up groceries for her, watch her kids, treat her to a massage.

If you live on the opposite coast, you may see things more clearly from a distance (but, then again, you may not), but the primary caregiver is the one living with this, caring for your parent regularly, and giving up an enormous amount along the way. She knows quite a bit about your parent's care. Mostly, she needs your loving support. If you are living far away or rarely involved for some other reason, and you have suggestions, make them gently. Very gently.

A FAMILY MEETING

No matter how you feel about your siblings, get your family together, either informally after a holiday meal or for a structured meeting, with an agenda and perhaps even a family or geriatric counselor. Such a gathering will enable all of you to take a hard look at your parent's situation, hear your parent's views, make plans for the future, and dole out responsibility for specific duties. If caregiving duties are already doled out and horrendously lopsided, this is an opportunity to make things more even.

Such a meeting also provides a forum where each person can air his or her views, learn what others are feeling, share much-needed emotional support, and devise a way to work as a team—if not in harmony, then at least under some sort of temporary truce.

The first meeting may be a little rough if you and your siblings don't get along (or even if you do). The room may be filled with concern, discomfort, and fear, unfriendly ghosts of the past, as well as love and a desire to help. Siblings will have their own agendas, axes to grind, hidden resentments, viewpoints, fears, and needs. They may be mired in grief, denial, or anger. They may be confused by their role, both in the family and in this new task. They may not be able to accept what is happening or to listen to others.

Don't give up. This is the beginning of a process. Just getting together and acknowledging that your parent's situation needs attention and that you need to work together is in itself an accomplishment.

If getting together is physically impossible, organize a telephone conference call. Or, have a private "chat room" for your family on the Internet, which is not ideal, but can be helpful when siblings have particularly bitter relationships. Writing provides a little more distance, and is more sterile, than direct communication.

◆ **Who comes.** It's important to keep your parent centrally involved in any discussion about his care and his future. It is his life, after all, and no one likes to be instructed on how to live. There are, however, situations in which a parent might not be present at a family meeting, at least not at the first one.

Obviously, if your parent is extremely ill or confused, he won't be able to attend, although you should keep him abreast of what's happening and get his thoughts and views, if at all possible. You also may want to hold one or two meetings without him to iron out differences or simply talk more freely about particular issues.

It's best to limit participants to siblings and anyone who is integrally involved in your parent's care (a grandchild, a parent's sibling, a regular aide,

AN ONLY CHILD

An only child does not have siblings to argue with, which is wonderful, but he also has no siblings with whom to share the worries, decisions, and responsibilities. If you are caring for a parent on your own, talk with a counselor or join a support group. Make time for close friends. Find others who understand your situation. You need someplace where you can express your concerns and perhaps get some advice and insight from others.

a trusted adviser). You might also have a lawyer, accountant, geriatric care manager, or some other professional present. But try to keep the number small and manageable.

Family members who cannot attend can participate by conference call. Those who say they do not want to get involved or that they have nothing to offer should be urged to come anyway. They should know what is happening, may have some valuable suggestions, and might be (should be) persuaded to help. In other words, don't take no for an answer unless the reasons are extremely good.

◆ **A moderator.** If everyone's cool and calm and the issues are straightforward, you can pick a moderator from the family. But if yours is like most families, and emotions are high and the issues complex, find an outsider to moderate who can guide the discussion, make sure everyone has a chance to talk, and encourage people to listen to each others' perspectives.

An outside moderator should be a neutral party, someone who is not related to the family and who is good at mediating disputes—a member of the clergy, a hospice counselor, a social worker, or a geriatric care manager. Someone who is well versed in geriatrics and the issues of parentcare is preferable. (Or, if you are dealing with a particular financial or legal issue, you might want to ask a lawyer or financial adviser to moderate.)

The area agency on aging should be able to direct you to a social worker or family mediator (800-677-1116 or www.eldercare.gov), or you can find a family therapist in the phone book or a geriatric care manager through the National Association of Professional Geriatric Care Managers (520-881-8008 or www.caremanager.org).

◆ **An agenda.** Though it may seem awfully formal, having an agenda will make it clear why you are meeting and help keep the conversation on course. Sometime before the meeting, have each sibling write down the topics that he or she wants to discuss. A moderator or a sibling who's been chosen in advance to organize the meeting should incorporate these suggestions into a manageable agenda.

Don't try to settle everything in one or two meetings, or you will become tired and cranky and the discussion will rapidly deteriorate. Prioritize issues and set a time limit on the meeting. (As for what might be on an agenda, see page 178.)

◆ **Advance research.** If necessary, get family members to research certain issues in advance of your meeting. For example, one sibling might look into financial and legal matters while another checks out community resources and housing options. Then, when you do meet, you'll know some of the options and have a better idea of what needs to be done.

◆ **Some guidelines.** To make sure everyone is heard and the meeting accomplishes what you want it to, agree upon some guidelines in advance. Ask others for suggestions or adapt the following guidelines to suit your needs:

1. No one is allowed to dominate the meeting. If you don't have a moderator to direct and focus the discussion, agree that each person will talk for no more than, say, five minutes at a time—and use a timer, if necessary.

2. When someone is speaking, others must listen without interrupting. Listening, and really digesting what others have to say, is an essential goal of these meetings. If you get nothing else accomplished, be sure that you all hear each other's views. If people have trouble absorbing what others are saying, ask each to briefly repeat the last speaker's message before taking his turn.

3. Each person should use sentences that begin with "I"—speaking only about his own opinions, feelings, and actions—and avoid finger-pointing statements that begin with "you."

4. Since your parent's care is the reason for this meeting, all discussions should relate directly to this subject. Steer away from old arguments and debates that are not relevant or helpful. If there are particularly touchy issues floating about that are simply unresolvable, then state clearly at the bottom of your agenda a list of issues that are *not* to be discussed.

♦ **What to discuss.** You are having this meeting to discuss one thing: your parent's current needs and future care. Everyone needs to be clear about the facts and the issues. What is your parent's diagnosis and prognosis? If there is confusion about your parent's health, get his doctor or a nurse to briefly outline the situation in a note to the family. Don't assume everyone is operating with the same information. It's best to spell it out so you all know what is what.

What are the biggest concerns right now—where your parent should live, how she will pay her bills, whether she should have a particular test or operation, her day-to-day care and survival, loneliness and depression?

(Remember, keep your parent front and center through all of this. If he is present, make sure he voices his concerns and opinions. If he is not present, keep his needs, not everyone else's, at the fore.)

> " *My mother lives with us, and my two sisters got very resentful because I was telling them when they could visit her. I didn't want them just dropping in whenever they were in town. It's invasive, and I'm not the world's greatest housekeeper. Besides, I hoped they would plan their visits when I couldn't be home so Mom wouldn't be alone. I would say, 'I have a class on Tuesday and Thursday, and it would be helpful if you could visit then.' But they got indignant and accused me of trying to keep them away from her. It got so that we were hardly speaking to each other.*
>
> *When Mom needed more help, I spoke to a social worker at the hospital, and she asked everyone to meet with her. When we started to explain how we were feeling without yelling at each other, everything seemed so simple and sort of childish. I think we were all worried about Mom, and taking it out on each other. We have a lot more understanding of each other now. There are still sparks sometimes, but we've really pulled together as a family."*
>
> —CAROL G.

Once you've got a handle on the situation, determine exactly what needs to be done. Make a detailed list of all jobs—researching community services, touring nursing homes, meeting with

FAMILY MEETING AGENDA

◆ What are your parent's current health problems and her physical and cognitive limitations?

◆ What are her current needs, in terms of day-to-day help and care?

◆ Are there ways to rearrange and renovate her house to allow her to do more for herself?

◆ What services are needed in her home, or from the community?

◆ Is her current living situation working out, or should she move? What options are available?

◆ What is her financial situation? Can she pay her bills? Can she afford the services she needs? Is she eligible for, or nearing eligibility for, Medicaid?

◆ What, exactly, needs to be done at this point? Make a detailed list.

◆ Which tasks can each person take on? Make a list of assignments.

◆ What might be enjoyable for your parent? (Your parent might *need* someone to deliver meals, but she might *enjoy* visits from grandchildren, daily walks, books on tape, etc.) Who can do some of this?

◆ Beyond helping your parent, how will each person help and support the primary caregiver?

◆ What care, services, housing, and financial assistance might your parent need in the future? Is there anything that can be done now to prepare? Who might help with this?

◆ When will you meet or communicate next?

◆ Finally, create a plan, in writing, detailing schedules and assignments, and make copies for each person.

◆ At the end, each person might talk briefly about his feelings about all this, any fears, resentment, grief, etc. (This can be helpful and supportive in a family that is relatively close, but if there are tensions, keep this brief and avoid delving into conflicts.)

lawyers, contacting a geriatric care manager, doing housework, transporting your parent to the doctor, paying bills, and filling out insurance forms. If your parent needs regular care, make a schedule of what needs to happen each day.

Talk about your parent's finances—how her bills are being paid, insurance, benefits, etc. Create a budget, detailing her income, assets, and expenses, and then talk about how to fill holes in the budget.

Then talk about the future. What lies ahead? What does the doctor say about her future health and care? Will your parent need community services? Will she need more help at home? Will she need to move? Can she pay for her future health care and other bills? Does someone need to research Medicaid, discounts, subsidies, special programs for low-income people, and other financial options?

Include in your list of things that need to be done the job of spokesperson —someone to represent your family when conferring with professionals. This person will not control any aspect of your parent's care; she will merely serve as the family's voice. She should, for example, talk with your parent's doctor, asking any questions that siblings might have, and then relay information to the others. Communicating with one spokesperson is far easier for professionals, and it reduces the risk of misinformation and misunderstandings. The spokesperson may or may not be the same person for each issue— one may be the medical liaison while another deals with lawyers. (If your family is large, create a telephone chain so the spokesperson doesn't have to make all the calls or use e-mail to communicate.)

Then, you've got to start dividing up the duties . . .

♦ **Dividing up the duties.** Quite often, one person will shoulder a disproportionate share of a parent's care, but one of the main goals of this meeting is to even things out as much as possible. Anyone already carrying a heavier load has to let go of some of it, and others have to pick up some slack. (You might have to use more community services and home care to relieve an unmanageable situation.)

Once you have a list of tasks, make assignments. Start by letting people volunteer for jobs. You never know what someone wants to do, feels they would be most equipped to do, or couldn't stand to do. Your brother may be uncomfortable with the idea of bathing or dressing your mother (and your mother might be uncomfortable with that, too), while another sibling simply has no mind for business matters. Let people pick tasks, and then work out what's left.

Be leery of excuses. *I live too far away. I'm too busy with the children. I'm not good at this.* Everyone can do something. Siblings who live far away can handle bills, research local agencies by phone, and offer the primary caregiver occasional respite. Those with young children can cook meals for your parent, get prescriptions filled,

" Last time I visited my mother, my husband came with me. I got a sinus infection while we were there and spent a lot of time in bed, so he was in charge. Each day, when he went off to read the paper, Mom would come down and say, 'Now don't let me disturb you, dear. Keep on reading.' But then she would talk and talk and talk at him for hours.

I wouldn't have wished this on him, but in retrospect I'm relieved that he had that experience. Now he can understand why I come home from these visits feeling so exhausted."

—CARLA P.

pick up groceries, and fill in from time to time. Even siblings who have cool relations with this parent need to help. They don't have to love her; they just have to be responsible adults.

Keep in mind, everyone has different commitments in life, and they weigh those commitments on their own personal scale. Don't decide that one sibling should take on the lion's share of the work because he or she doesn't have the responsibilities that you do. Perhaps a sibling has made a conscious decision not to have children because she wants time for her painting. That doesn't mean that she must now give that up to care for your parent just because you opted to have children.

Similarly, each sibling has a unique relationship with your parent. One may feel duty bound to a parent she adores, while another is not only distant from this parent, but feels angry and resentful toward her. It's the same parent, but a very different relationship. This will mean a very different perspective when it comes to offering help.

Once you agree upon a division of labor, make a detailed schedule of who will do what, when, and where. Make sure everyone involved has a copy. Then, give your plan a trial run. In a few months, reconvene to discuss how things are working, to reassess your parent's needs, and to make any necessary adjustments to your plan.

Significant Others

If you have a strong and supportive relationship with a spouse, it will be an enormous help to you now. A spouse who listens, empathizes, and takes on some additional household responsibilities is a godsend and deserves huge thanks. On the other hand, whatever problems exist in the relationship will be exacerbated now. A parent's care often causes marital rifts, some of them deep.

If your parent needs you for the short term, your spouse will have to make do without you for a time. You may not be with him physically or you may be absent emotionally. Either way, your parent's care is a priority, and

WHEN RELATIONSHIPS ARE ESPECIALLY ROCKY

You might be wishing that you were an only child right about now.

When you just can't get along, you and your siblings need to find a way to care for your parent without stepping on each other's toes. You may have to schedule visits so you don't run into each other, for example. Or you may need to hire a geriatric care manager to assess the situation, divide duties, and cast the deciding vote when you can't agree on the best course of action.

It may be tempting to simply go about your day without speaking, and for some families that might work. But in most cases, the chill between you will be detrimental to your parent, and to each of you personally. You and your siblings should avoid battlegrounds, but you do need to communicate about your parent's care.

While it's not easy—not at all easy—make a concerted effort to let go of certain issues. If an age-old fight has kept you from speaking to your sister for years, try to get beyond it. The issue won't disappear, but put it aside for now. Identify your common goal (your parent's care) and focus your energies on that.

You might find that communicating by e-mail is easier, providing distance and a chance to edit your thoughts (and do edit them before hitting "send").

A geriatric care manager who is trained in both counseling and gerontology can be enormously helpful in these situations. He or she can act as intermediary, keep discussions on track, and provide a calming force. Care managers with a background in family therapy or psychology may be particularly helpful when tensions are high.

However you handle the specifics of your relationships and your parent's care, resist the temptation to elbow a sibling out who wants to be involved.

Each grown child has a unique and important relationship with a parent. Accept and allow these other relationships. Make room for them to work in their own particular way. It may seem that your sibling is harsh on your mother or emotionally distant from your father, but this is their relationship. It has formed over many years. It is what it is for reasons you may never understand. You are not going to change it, nor should you try.

> *I live with my mother and needed help. At our first family meeting, everyone agreed to pitch in, but to be honest, it didn't work. So finally, when I couldn't deal with it anymore, I left home.*
>
> *It's hard to admit that I did that, but it got results. I told them, 'I'm not going back home until there's a written schedule and it's adhered to.' Of course, then they all had to pitch in. Once they realized exactly what was going on, once they lived it and saw what I was dealing with, they were willing to help. We made out a schedule, and most of the time it works."*
>
> —LINDA K.

you both have to make compromises, at least for now.

However, if your parent's care becomes a long-term and all-consuming undertaking, if you are absorbed by her needs for more than a few months, do not jeopardize your marriage. It is too important. Your parent will have to do with less of you because your spouse, even if he (or she) doesn't say so, needs a little more of you. Here are some approaches that should help during this time:

◆ **Clarify who's responsible.** Is each of you solely responsible for your own parents, and not at all responsible for your spouse's parents? Is the woman responsible for both sets of parents?

(Of course not, but this assumption is made with frightening regularity.) Should a spouse be expected to give up his weekends, vacations, or evenings to join you when you visit your parent? Or should a spouse give up the pleasure of your company because you believe you should be at your parent's side during every free minute you have?

These perceptions will vary enormously from couple to couple. Talk about them. Don't make assumptions or hang on to unspoken expectations. Come up with an agreement.

In general, your parent is your responsibility, and you can't expect your spouse to take on your family duties. But you *can* reasonably expect him to support you through this period, offer a shoulder to cry on and a sympathetic ear, and take on some extra household and child care duties to ease the pressures you face.

◆ **Communicate.** Relationships are complex. Parentcare is stressful. And men and women really do come from different planets.

It's likely neither of you truly understands what the other is going through, needs, or feels. Talk about it. As always, use sentences that begin with "I" instead of those blaming sentences that begin with "you." Small misunderstandings can expand into large ones if not attended to. Talk.

◆ **Be clear about how your spouse can help.** Don't assume that your spouse knows how to help, but is simple refusing to, the cad. He may want to help, but truly not know how.

He may offer advice, only to find that it triggers an argument. Unable to "fix things" for you, he feels inadequate and resentful.

Don't expect your spouse to read your mind or know what you need. Tell him, in concrete terms, what you need from him, whether it is emotional support and understanding or more tangible assistance. *I need to stop by Mom's house two nights a week. It would be great if you could shop and make dinner on those days.* (Of course, if you leave dinner in his hands, you have to be accepting of what he considers to be "dinner." You might be eating a lot of pizza.)

◆ **Consider his feelings.** Your spouse will certainly be affected by the stress you are under and the changes in the household. Not only is he getting less of your attention, but he's got to cope with your bad moods, burned dinners, and sudden interest in alcohol. If he has been your soul mate in the past, he may feel shut out because he can't share your anxiety and grief.

A spouse may be afraid that if he voices his own needs or opinions, he will appear selfish or unsympathetic. And no matter what is happening with you, he will have his own grief to deal with. He may be reminded of the loss of his parent, forced to think about his parents' future, or haunted by his own aging process.

With all that you are dealing with, it's hard to think about someone else's sadness or anxiety—or the reasons someone might not be as helpful

> *When my mother-in-law became sick, I started visiting her, fixing her meals, making sure that she was all right. I guess it's my nature to take care of people. But then I became resentful. I don't really like her—she is very critical—and I had my own parents to take care of. I couldn't hide my resentment, and it caused regular spats between Steve and me.*
>
> *Finally, I told him that I was glad to help, but that I would not be responsible for her care. I was firm about it. I explained what I would and would not do.*
>
> *He was incredibly understanding. He didn't realize that I had been feeling any of this. Through our conversation, he began to realize that he'd been denying the whole thing about his mother and dumping it on my shoulders.*
>
> *I still visit her, but not nearly as much, and usually with support from him, which is all I really wanted in the first place."*
>
> —ROSE M.

or supportive as you'd like—but try. Encourage your spouse to talk about his feelings. And give him the time and the space to vent them.

◆ **Make time for your mate.** When a parent's care is chronic, don't forget to take time out for a dinner

KEEPING SANE AT HOME

If your parent's care consumes a great deal of your time and emotions, call a meeting of your own immediate family—your spouse and children. A planned discussion, rather than talking about it here and there, over the laundry or TV, will be more productive.

Follow the guidelines outlined for family meetings earlier in this chapter. Let each person talk about what he or she feels, and then discuss how everyone can work together and support each other, assigning specific chores and duties if necessary. When the issues are knotty, a family counselor, found through a mental health center or a family doctor, can be helpful.

with your spouse, quiet walks together, occasional getaways, and other spouse-type stuff (sex). Make time not simply for heavy talks, but for play, shopping, relaxing, laughing, and simply staying in touch. These dates may not seem like a priority at the moment, but they are vital to your marriage as well as your own mental health. (It's understandable that you might not want to have sex right now, but your spouse might be taking that as a personal rejection. Talk about this too, if possible.)

◆ **Be appreciative.** Even if the help you receive is minimal, thank your spouse for it. He (or she) may not be doing anything more than putting up with your stress and busier hours. Thank him for it. He'll be more likely to help in the future. Positive reinforcement works.

The Sandwich Generation

Your parents are elderly, your children are still children, and you are being pulled by both ends of the age spectrum. Each day you face a dilemma: Do you take Dad to his doctor's appointment or get your son to school on time? Do you visit your mother or watch your daughter's soccer game? When the day is done, there is practically no "you" left, just the echoes of all the people who need you.

The dual demand of child and aging parent is so common that it has its own names—"the sandwich generation," "women caught in the middle," "the caregiver crunch." For working moms, the dilemma might better be called "the impossible dream."

Having children around when a parent grows frail actually has some benefits—a child can pitch in and help, and a grandparent might enjoy a child's company—but it can also leave you feeling torn, guilt-ridden, and irritable. (What else is new?)

It is vital that you are organized, very, very organized. Think ahead about what might come. Learn about community services and housing options *early*. And always, always, always have a Plan B. Keep a list of available sitters and companions up to date.

Don't let your child get lost in the commotion, slipping down your ladder of priorities until he is hardly on it anymore. Address his needs and concerns, and be sure that your parent's crisis does not compromise the quality of your relationship with him.

◆ **Be honest.** Children, even very young children, can understand much more than we give them credit for. Certainly a child of any age feels the stress in the household and your anxiety.

Talk to them. Tell your children what is happening, what you are feeling, why you are sad, and why you don't have as much time for them. Keep it simple, especially if they are young. Then, encourage them to ask questions, and answer their questions directly. If a parent is dying, talk about that as openly as you can, too. (For more on children and grief, see page 576.)

◆ **Take time to listen.** Don't assume that you understand a child's concerns. Let her tell you about them. Children respond to illness in unexpected ways and worry about issues that adults may not even consider. For example, a child may be wondering if she is going to have to give up her bedroom if Grandpa moves in, she may be worrying more about your health than about a grandparent's health, or she may be concerned that Grandma's ailment is contagious.

Your child may not open up on your schedule, so be ready and attuned. When you sense that a child wants to talk, stop what you are doing. Get off the phone, put the dinner on hold. A child might not "save" his emotions for later, when you are free.

When he does open up, no matter what he says, be careful not to make him feel that his emotions are wrong, trivial, or silly. And let him know you've really heard him and that you take his concerns seriously.

◆ **Set aside time for them.** In your bulging schedule, planning a trip to the zoo may seem like a joke, but it's not. Spend some time, just the two of you (or five of you), doing something, *anything*, unrelated to Grandma. If you can't go to the zoo, take a short detour on the way to the grocery store and go to the park or a toy store, even briefly. Have a lunch or dinner date, perhaps going out with just one child. Or, if you have to make a long car trip, take a child with you and turn it into a special occasion.

◆ **Let him help.** If a child shows any interest in helping with your parent's care (or even if he doesn't), give him a job to do. Keep your requests reasonable. Even a toddler can stroke Grandma, carry her blanket to her, or draw a picture for her. Children want

> *My father has been quite frail for three years, and I feel angry sometimes that my children aren't seeing the man I knew. I tell them what he used to be like, but they just see this very weak person who needs a lot of peace and quiet.*
>
> *Last time we were there, the kids were playing in the garden, and he said, 'When the hell are you going to leave? This noise is too much.'*
>
> *I don't know whether to bring them up next summer when I go. It's hard on him and hard on them."*
>
> —JANE C.

to be included in family life and will be proud of how they help (even if they gripe while doing it).

◆ **Let her refuse to help, too.** Younger children may be eager to help, but older children, especially adolescents, may want to keep a distance. They may be uncomfortable with their grief or sadness, or feel "grossed out" by aspects of your parent's care. Or they may be preoccupied with what they consider to be more important aspects of life—friends, parties, music, or sports. While these priorities may seem skewed to you, they are a normal and necessary part of teenage development. Urge teenagers to understand the importance of family and responsibility, but allow them to be teenagers, too, even if it means distancing themselves some from you and your parent's situation.

◆ **Get at the cause of bad behavior.** Children have an uncanny ability to pick up on stress. Your stress makes them stressed, and that makes them cry and whine and run in circles (if they are young), or slam doors (if they are older).

Children also misbehave to express their own pain, jealousy, and confusion. Sometimes, if the only way a child can get your attention is by doing something bad, then that is what he is going to do. For him, an angry reaction from you is better than no reaction at all.

Remember that you are the adult here. Your child is far less able than you are to deal with all these emotions. Spending time with him and talking openly should fend off some problems. But when there are outbursts, remain calm and try to understand the root of the problem. Don't condone his behavior, but allow some of it. Everyone needs a little forgiveness right now. If things become unmanageable or worrisome, talk with a family counselor or a child psychologist.

◆ **Show your children your younger parent.** If your parent is very sick, confused, or grumpy, pull out some old photos or, better yet, some home movies. Show your children what Grandpa used to be like in his younger and stronger days. You might tell them stories of things you used to do together. Help them to understand who this man is and what he means to you. Help them to separate the sickness from the person.

CLUB SANDWICHES AND SUPER HEROES

TODAY, MORE AND MORE CAREGIVERS are not only taking care of children and parents, but grandparents as well, turning the simple sandwich into a triple-decker.

The sandwich can only be called a hero for those taking care of an assortment of parents, in-laws, or aunts and uncles, grandparents, stepparents, or other aging, frail people. Just as they get Mom settled in a nursing home, and Dad set up at adult day care, they get a call about an aunt or a father-in-law who needs help. The pile-up is beyond anyone's dreams (or worst nightmare), and an overwhelming task takes on colossal dimensions.

It's time for some serious restructuring and a lot of help. You are no longer a daughter, granddaughter, niece, stepdaughter, or daughter-in-law. You are a general. And this is war.

Gather the troops. Call in the reserves. Enlist volunteers. Assign duties. Use each and every community service available. There's no room for emotion right now. This has to be handled quickly and effectively. Forget guilt. Just do what you can to get the job done.

Take each person's situation, one at a time, and formulate a plan of action. What are their needs? What services are available? Who can help and how? Unload all extra duties.

If you can afford one, find a geriatric care manager or case manager who can help you now (some work for government or public agencies and charge little, if anything). You don't necessarily need a full-service care manager, but you do need someone to help you identify community services and draw on any and all benefits to which your parent/aunt/in-law/grandparent is entitled. This is especially important for those relatives who live far away.

You are no longer a sandwich. You are now, officially, a hero. But you are not a hero because you take it all on, taking care of everyone in reach and out of reach. You are a hero because you know how to take action, delegate jobs, and take advantage of all services that are available.

Well done, soldier.

The Working Caregiver

You are sitting in your office and the phone rings. It's your father. His speech is garbled and he seems confused. You're worried, but you have a meeting with your boss in ten minutes. What do you do?

Your mother goes to adult day care until five o'clock each day, but you don't get off work until six. What do you do?

The hospital just called. Your parent broke her hip. She's in intensive care. Decisions need to be made. Even if you leave work now, you wouldn't be at the hospital for several hours (if, that is, you can get a plane ticket on such short notice). What do you do?

When a parent needs help, many caregivers cut back their work hours, some end up quitting their jobs, and some change jobs. Most continue on, but many jeopardize their jobs and futures by leaving early, taking calls at work, coming in late, and missing days of work. When they are at work, they are so exhausted and preoccupied that they are barely present. Before you veer off your career track or quit your job, think long and hard about your options.

◆ **Plan, plan, plan.** Regardless of your parent's health, plan ahead. Be prepared. When you work, it is vital that you are always prepared, always one step ahead.

Be sure that you have the names and phone numbers of several people on whom you can call. Your father's not answering his phone? You'll need the number of a neighbor, friend, or volunteer who can run over and check on him. (Be sure a key to his house is hidden someplace so you can direct this person on how to get in.) Your mother's water pipe just burst and water is flooding into her living room? Have the name of a repair person (or two) who lives near her. Better yet, have the name of an electrician, plumber, carpenter, and mechanic. Know the number for any security alarm company with which she deals. Have a master list of emergency numbers, including her doctor, accountant, lawyer, bank, and the people mentioned already, at your workplace or in a briefcase. Take it with you on any business trips.

Also, be sure your parent has signed a durable power of attorney and power of attorney for health care.

And do all that research early—long before you think you might need it—because you just never know, and you won't have time to do it when a crisis strikes. Find out about services in your parent's community—transportation, adult day care, home-care agencies, volunteers, companions, homemakers, etc. Learn about assisted living, nursing homes, and other housing options. You don't want to be sitting at work, with no idea of what's what, when you get a call from the hospital saying that your parent needs to move into a nursing home. If you know which residence is best, half your work is done. (See Chapter One for more on planning ahead.)

◆ **Plan some more.** If you know that your parent is likely to need you in the near future—if she is ill and the doctor says she could have another stroke any day, for example—talk with your boss and take responsibility for making provisions to get your job done if you are suddenly called away.

◆ **Set priorities.** Write a list of everything that you need to do, and then scratch some items from it. Or at least, put a few things on the bottom of the list, then prioritize. What has to be done, what can be put off, what can be forgotten?

◆ **Enlist help.** This is no time to be the martyr. You can't do it all, so accept it. Get help! Talk to relatives, friends, and neighbors about how they might pitch in. Find volunteers who can check on your parent regularly or when a crisis strikes during work hours. Use community services, big and small, as soon as you need them. Sign up for meal delivery, book delivery, grocery delivery, garbage pickup, homemaker services, adult day care, and anything else that might ease the strain.

This help doesn't have to be directly aimed at your parent. You need help, too. Get others to pick up your son at school, pick up groceries, drop off meals, return videos, or just lend a supportive ear.

♦ **Contact the human resources department.** Many large companies and some smaller ones have personnel who can provide information about eldercare and community services, or they are hooked to a service that provides national referrals and counseling. Some companies offer flexible hours and job sharing. Others sponsor support groups, seminars, and information fairs on eldercare.

♦ **Organize your time.** Make a schedule of your day, and look for ways to be more efficient. Are there errands that can be skipped, or done in the morning or during breaks at work? Can your week be better organized? Can you shop for a week's worth of food in one hit? Can you do some research while sitting in the dentist's office? Can you get up earlier, watch less television, or use your lunch break more efficiently?

> ## DISCRETION AROUND THE WATER COOLER
>
> At work, be careful what you say to whom. It's fine to use eldercare services offered by the human resources department. It's fine to talk to your boss about changing your schedule. But you don't want to stand around the water cooler or coffee maker griping about your parent's needs, and all the time you spend at work dealing with her care.

♦ **Keep your roles separate.** Sometimes it can't be helped, but making phone calls or searching the Internet on company time is a risky habit if you want to keep your job. Make phone calls during a lunch break or in the evening whenever possible.

♦ **Yes, once again, take care of yourself.** The boss is yelling at you, your spouse is tired of all this, your children are whining, and then, well, there's your parent. You are on the right path for a nervous breakdown or at least a good case of the flu.

Take ten minutes out each day for stretches, deep breathing, meditation, or even just a quiet moment alone. If you work for a large company, there might be a support group for caregivers within the business. Find the time to go because it will help you to

THE FAMILY AND MEDICAL LEAVE ACT

Under the 1993 Family and Medical Leave Act, employees must be offered at least twelve weeks of unpaid leave to care for an ill family member—a parent, spouse, or child (but not a grandparent or the parent of a spouse). The Act applies only to businesses with fifty or more employees. An employee must have been with the company for at least one year and must have logged at least 1,250 hours in the previous twelve months (about twenty-four hours a week) to be eligible for leave.

The Act mandates that:

◆ If possible, employees must give thirty days notice that they are taking a leave.

◆ Employees (except for those in the 10 percent of highest-paid positions) are entitled to get their old job back, or a post with equivalent duties, benefits, and pay.

◆ Employees are entitled to their full health benefits while on leave. However, an employer can demand to be paid back for insurance premiums if the employee quits the job at the end of the leave.

◆ Leave can be taken in bits and pieces—a few days or even a few hours at a time—if the employer and employee both agree on the arrangement.

◆ An employer can require that vacation or sick days be used at the beginning of the leave.

---

be more productive and patient. (You might also find an online support group, although face-to-face is best.)

◆ **Set down rules.** If your parent or a health aide calls you at work regularly (several times a day is definitely "regularly"), set down firm rules about when you can be interrupted and under what circumstances. It sounds cold, but it's better to be clear than to be annoyed with your parent and reprimanded by your supervisor.

◆ **Set limits.** When you are working, this is critical. Set realistic expectations for yourself, particularly in regard to your parent's care. You cannot do everything for her, so define what you can and will do, and what you can't and won't do. (See page 44 for more on setting limits.)

◆ **Let go of some things.** So your house is a mess, the garden's unkempt, you haven't put photos in a photo album for more than three years, and heaven knows your clothes are getting a bit shabby. Forget it. The cobwebs can wait. If you are a perfectionist, be less perfect. Focus on what's really important. Weeds can be attractive.

◆ **Have a Plan B.** Always, always, always have more than one plan in place, more than one name and number to call. If your parent is dependent upon a companion who comes each day, have the name of a second one or an agency that can send someone over on a moment's notice. If you rely on your parent's neighbor to keep an eye on things, get the name of someone else who can run over when there's a crisis and the first neighbor isn't answering her phone.

◆ **Hook your parent up to the Internet.** If your mother calls you at work ten times a day, teach her how to use e-mail. She can contact you to her heart's content, and you can read it when you get a chance.

NEGOTIATING WITH YOUR BOSS

MOST PEOPLE ARE HESITANT TO speak with a boss about family responsibilities, and really, you'll have to use your own judgment here. It will depend upon your boss and your relationship with him or her. In most cases, bosses would rather know what's going on and work out a plan than have you sneaking out early and coming in late with no explanation.

Bosses want employees to be happy, sure, but their number one concern is getting the job done. So when you talk to a boss about changing hours, taking time off, or other work arrangements, couch it in terms a boss can appreciate.

Rather than telling a sob story and asking your boss to help you, come up with a plan and then pitch it to the boss. (*I'll leave at 3 P.M., but come in at 7 A.M., when it's quiet and I can get more done.*) Work out all the details in advance and then explain why your plan will be at least as good as the current way of operating and perhaps even better. (You might want to draft a written proposal, outlining the plan, before you meet.)

As you sell your idea, be sure to keep the focus on your professional goals and the goals of the company, rather than only on your personal needs. And let the boss know that you are committed to this job.

Propose a trial period, which gives both you and your boss a chance to test this arrangement before buying it.

A COMPANY PLAN

IF YOUR WORKPLACE HAS A LARGE pool of employees who are caring for an elderly relative, talk with company executives about flexible hours, a shorter work week, and job sharing. More and more companies are allowing such arrangements, as so many employees now care for elderly people and children. Many companies also provide support groups, information, referrals, and counseling, and a few even offer financial benefits to help cover some costs of eldercare.

Some have contracts with eldercare consulting firms, which provide referrals nationwide (given that so many employees care for parents who live far away), along with counseling and caregiving guidance. Some of the more established consulting companies include LifeCare Inc. (800-873-4636 or www.lifecare.com), Ceridian's LifeWorks Services (800-729-7655 or www.myceridian.com), and Child & Eldercare Insights (440-356-2900 or www.carereports.com). Or contact AARP (888-687-2277 or www.aarp.org) for information on how companies can develop eldercare services for employees.

Making arrangements for caregivers is good business. By making life manageable and supporting these workers, the workers and the companies will be more productive.

Nationwide, between 15 and 25 percent of the work force, perhaps more, has some responsibility for an elderly person, and many workers have significant duties, spending twenty to forty hours a week caring for an elderly relative. Eldercare costs U.S. businesses billions of dollars a year in lost productivity. But studies show that with company support (referral services, flexible hours, etc.), employees are less apt to use their business phones for personal calls, arrive late or leave early, call in sick, use drugs and alcohol, or have financial problems. (When approaching executives, don't lay all this on too heavy, or they may start screening job applicants and hire orphans only.)

Find out what other companies in your area or in the same industry are doing and use them as role models. Employers often respond to competition.

DOCTOR DO'S AND DON'TS

Rx for the Elderly • A Good Doctor • A Geriatric Checkup • An Informed Advocate • Alternative Medicine

A LTHOUGH YOU MAY BE DOING THE LION'S SHARE OF THE work, seeing your parent through her senior years is a team effort. And a key member of that team is your parent's personal physician.

Whether your mother is having regular appointments with an orthopedist, a cardiologist, and hematologist or a series of tests and treatments for an advanced stage of cancer, she needs one primary physician at the helm. One doctor should keep track of all of her ailments and medications, refer her to specialists when necessary, and then coordinate her care so that treatments for one problem don't aggravate another—a serious and all-too-common problem in the medical care of elderly patients.

She also needs to be an informed and outspoken patient, or if you are handling her health care, you need to be an informed advocate for her. That means familiarizing yourself with her symptoms and any treatment options, being sure the doctor gives her problems ample attention, participating in decisions, and then helping your parent to actually do what needs to be done. It means being willing to ask questions, seek second opinions, and when your parent's medical care is not satisfactory, find a new doctor. Once your parent has a trusted physician and you become comfortable in your role as her advocate, your work and your worries will be much lighter.

Rx for the Elderly

Old bodies are different than younger ones, so they require different medical care. For starters, the fragility of the system means that an otherwise treatable illness may be life-threatening, a common disease may cause uncommon symptoms, and a recommended dose of medication may produce dangerous side effects. A drug that a young person can use without difficulty can cause confusion, incontinence, or blurry vision in an older patient. Withdrawal and apathy in an older patient may not signal depression, but stroke or heart disease.

The sheer number of diseases and symptoms involved complicates the medical care of an elderly person enormously. For example, when heart disease, diabetes, arthritis, and dementia are all at play, it's hard for even the best doctor to know exactly what's causing what and which treatments will be most effective and cause the fewest side effects. A doctor caring for an older patient can't simply mend a broken ankle; he or she needs to recognize that the patient has fallen because her vision is waning or because the combination of her arthritis medication and her heart pills is making her dizzy.

A doctor caring for your parent should have plenty of experience with the elderly, and should think holistically. That is, he or she should look beyond the immediate symptoms or test results and consider the entire package—the patient's other ailments and treatments, as well as her housing arrangements, exercise regime, diet, daily habits, social supports, and perhaps even her financial situation, because each of these plays a role in her general health and good medical care.

If you have concerns about the care your parent is receiving or think she might benefit from a more thorough exam, think about having a full geriatric assessment (see page 201).

A Good Doctor

Just as children see pediatricians, who specialize in caring for the young, your parent needs a doctor who is familiar with the ailments that are

BEWARE OF AGEISM

Ageism—prejudice against old people—is rampant, even among doctors, social workers, and other professionals who routinely deal with the elderly. They expect old people to be frail, confused, depressed, and incontinent, so they don't do anything to change the situation. They fail to treat ailments or address loneliness or worries. *What does he expect at his age?*

Of course, many of the ailments, as well as some of the physical and mental decline, that are common in old age can be treated. And at any age, patients deserve respect and serious attention to their medical problems.

Beware of ageism in yourself, in others, and even in your parent, who may feel that he is just a worthless old man. Encourage him to get proper medical care, to do the things he loves, to make friends and pursue hobbies. Your parent should do all this despite his age—and perhaps because of it.

common in old age and savvy about the symptoms, treatment regimes, and side effects that are unique to elderly patients.

While it is useful to have a doctor who specializes in geriatrics, it is by no means essential. Good general practitioners and internists are perfectly capable of caring for your parent, especially if they have a lot of experience with elderly patients. If your parent has a primary doctor whom he trusts, he may not need to look any further. But if he is hunting for a new primary doctor, or even if he needs to find a specialist to treat a chronic ailment, a number of issues are worth considering.

♦ **A matter of instincts.** The healing process starts in the mind. If your parent becomes very sick, she will fare better in the hands of someone who instills confidence in her. For this reason, choosing a doctor is partly a matter of personality. A good primary doctor should be one whom your parent trusts and feels comfortable with. It should be someone with whom she can communicate easily. If your parent doesn't like a doctor, but can't quite explain why, help her to find someone else.

Gut instinct is less important when you are looking for a specialist who will treat a specific medical problem. Then, credentials and experience should receive more weight.

♦ **Open and honest.** Open, two-way communication is essential. The doctor should be honest about your parent's health and prognosis and should explain, in simple terms, the necessity for and the results of all tests. Your parent or you should be informed of all treatment options. The doctor should be willing to admit when he or she is uncertain about something or when answers simply don't exist.

Likewise, your parent should feel free to ask questions, even those that may seem silly, and to talk openly about any delicate matters or embarrassing symptoms.

◆ **A credential check.** Take a look at the prospective doctor's background—medical school, residency training, board certifications, and any other qualifications. You can learn about these either by asking the office secretary or by doing a background check on the Internet. You can search under "doctor credentials" for one of

the many sites that does this. (A few of the sites include HealthGrades at www.healthgrades.com, America's Top Doctors at www.americastopdoctors.com, and the American Medical Association at www.ama-assn.org.)

◆ **Beyond credentials: experience.** A Harvard degree does not always a good doctor make. More important than specific credentials is the doctor's experience in treating elderly patients and in dealing with the problem that plagues your parent, whether it's Parkinson's disease or diabetes. If your parent's doctor is not a geriatrician, find out what percentage of his or her practice is devoted to truly elderly patients (define *elderly* because it's not

THINK PREVENTATIVELY

Prevention is the most important and most ignored aspect of medical care. For the elderly, who cannot bounce back from an illness or an injury as easily as their younger counterparts, prevention is critical.

But prevention may not have been part of your parent's upbringing. He may come from the school of if-it-ain't-broke-don't-fix-it. In other words, don't see the doctor unless something is drastically wrong, and don't make adjustments to diet or the house until there is some real reason to. All this means that you may have to do some gentle but forceful persuading.

Make sure your parent's living situation is as safe as possible, see that he is eating healthfully, urge him to get a little exercise, encourage him to be mentally active, and keep after him to have regular physicals, eye exams, and dental checkups. He should also have a one-time pneumococcal vaccine to fight pneumonia, and he should get an influenza shot each fall, as elderly people are highly susceptible to the flu. Either can be life-threatening for an elderly person.

sixty-year-olds) and, in particular, what percent is devoted to elderly patients with your parent's ailments.

◆ **Financial considerations.** You or your parent also need to find out whether a particular doctor "accepts assignment," which means that he or she accepts Medicare's predetermined fees as full payment for services. If not, and if the doctor charges a higher fee, your parent will have to pay the difference out of her own pocket (unless she has Medigap insurance; see Chapter Sixteen for details on Medicare and Medigap). Before making an appointment, ask the office secretary about the doctor's policy. To find a "participating physician" go to www.medicare.gov, call 800-MEDICARE, or look in the *Medicare Participating Physician/Supplier Directory*, found in libraries, social security offices, area agencies on aging, and senior citizens' organizations. (Be aware, however, that the directory might not be up to date, so it's always best to call the doctor's office and ask.)

Likewise, if your parent is part of a managed care plan through Medicare or other insurance, the doctor must be included in the plan. If your parent sees a doctor outside the plan, say, for a second opinion or to see a specialist, she may have to pay extra.

◆ **Affiliations, associates, and emergency backup.** Check whether a doctor has admitting privileges at a respected hospital, or the hospital nearest to your parent. And, if the doc-

tor is in a group practice, find out whether your parent will see this particular doctor only, or whether he may be assigned to whoever is available that day. Is the doctor available on an emergency basis? Some stick to a nine-to-five schedule. Does he or she have an associate who covers during vacations? Does he or she have a wide range of contacts with other doctors in case it is necessary to make a referral (for instance, the doctor might be associated with a large hospital or medical school)?

◆ **Location.** Is it relatively easy for your parent to get to the doctor's office? Is there ample parking? Is it on a bus route, or is there a van service that will take her there? Likewise, will your parent have to go someplace out of her way to have tests and lab work done? A smaller doctor's office might send her far way to have tests done, while a larger office or one that is within a medical center might just send her down the hall.

◆ **A shared philosophy.** If your parent wants aggressive medical care at all costs, or instead feels strongly about hospice care and not having extraordinary treatments at the end of life, the doctor needs to know this. Your parent should find a doctor who respects—and will uphold—her wishes.

Likewise, if your parent is interested in alternative medicine, she needs a doctor who knows something about this or at least doesn't discount it.

WHAT TO BRING TO THE DOCTOR'S OFFICE

Before going to the doctor's office for a checkup, you or your parent should gather all pertinent health insurance cards—Medicare, Medicaid, Medigap, or other identifying health insurance documents—and make a list of all relevant medical information as well as any questions you have. (It's often difficult to remember these matters once an exam begins.) The doctor will need to know about:

☐ Past illnesses or injuries, tests, hospitalizations, and surgeries.

☐ Any current symptoms—dizziness, fatigue, confusion, swelling, bleeding, nausea, weight loss or gain, bowel or bladder problems, personality changes. When did they begin and how? Were they sudden or gradual? It is helpful if you or your parent ranks these concerns in order of their importance rather than mentioning them vaguely or with equal emphasis.

☐ Medications taken in the past and those being used currently, including prescription and over-the-counter drugs as well as diet supplements (also diet aids, nicotine gum, vitamins, laxatives, decongestants, sedatives, eye or nose drops, medicated creams, patches, etc.). You might have to search your parent's medicine cabinets and drawers to compile a complete list.

☐ Allergies or sensitivities to medications or other substances.

☐ Daily eating, sleeping, toileting, and exercise habits.

☐ Eyeglasses, hearing aids, dentures, or other such devices.

☐ Any obstacles faced in daily life—problems with bathing, getting dressed, balancing the checkbook, climbing stairs, communicating clearly.

☐ Family history of physical or mental illness (including parents, siblings, grandparents, children, and blood-related aunts and uncles), which can provide clues to hereditary risk.

☐ Information about tobacco, alcohol, or other substance use.

☐ Prior exposure to heavy metals or chemicals (usually in a workplace).

☐ Names and phone numbers of previous doctors who might have your parent's medical records.

HOW TO FIND
A GOOD DOCTOR

You or your parent can find a good doctor by talking to friends, relatives, or colleagues. Or you can get a recommendation from a trusted gynecologist, pediatrician, or another medical professional. If you happen to be visiting a geriatric unit in a hospital, ask the nurses about local doctors who are particularly good with elderly patients.

Local medical societies and hospitals can give you the names of doctors from their lists of members and employees. (Tell them that you are looking for a board-certified geriatrician or a family doctor who treats a lot of elderly patients.) Most public libraries, social security offices, area agencies on aging, hospitals, and senior citizens' groups have directories of doctors, such as the *Directory of Medical Specialists* and the *American Medical Association Directory*. You can also do a search on the Internet under "find a doctor"; many organizations and companies do this. For doctors who accept Medicare as full payment, go to www.medicare.gov.

Once you have a list of potential doctors, call and ask the receptionist or nurse some questions, and take note not only of the answers, but of the person's courtesy and helpfulness, or lack thereof. It's worth asking if you can speak briefly with the doctor. (Some doctors will, although most won't.) Generally speaking, if the doctor can't schedule a routine physical within the

next two months, it means he or she is popular, which is good, but it also means that she or he is overbooked. Your parent might want to find someone else.

" Mum has one general doctor, who is what I would call a social doctor. He's kind and he's sweet-looking, but he is not a help. He has missed so many things it's amazing. When she was in the hospital after her hip operation, he was going to let her go home without night nurses even though she couldn't get out of bed. Then last fall, he failed to realize that she had severe congestion in her lungs. He'd prescribed diuretics for her, but he never checked to see whether or not she was taking them. He's not thorough at all. He just reassures her and says, 'You're doing splendidly.'

She says, 'I know he isn't a good doctor, but I can't leave him. He's been Dad's doctor and my doctor for too long.' I can't push her to do anything once she's made up her mind. It just means that we have to keep closer tabs on her health and keep pressing him when we think something is wrong. Once I called to see when he would be on vacation and then made an appointment for her during that time just so another doctor in the practice would examine her."

—SUSAN W.

HOUSE CALLS

Some doctors have returned to days of yore and have begun making house calls. If your parent is simply too frail to make the trip to a doctor's office, as many very elderly people are, this is an enormous boon.

While many doctors make house calls occasionally, usually to friends or perhaps to a long-time patient who lives nearby, a few (albeit very few) are now making this a formal part of their practice. Some are even turning it into a full-time practice. Medicare has provisions for this, covering slightly more than it would for a visit to the doctor's office.

You are most apt to find house call physicians in larger metro areas, or in very small rural areas where the doctor knows everyone by name. But the number of physicians who will make house calls is growing.

If your parent cannot get out, or if going out is so overwhelming that it takes hours for her to get out and then days for her to recover, it is worth asking her doctor if he or she is willing to make a house call, or if a physician's assistant or nurse might visit. If not, contact the American Academy of Home Care Physicians (410-676-7966 or www.aahcp.org). If no visiting doctors are listed in your parent's community, call the home-care doctor who is nearest and ask if he or she knows of any doctors in your parent's neighborhood who will visit her at home. The discharge planner at the local hospital or the area agency on aging might also know of doctors or physician's assistants who make house calls.

A Checkup

A physical checkup of an elderly patient should include:

◆ **The body**. An elderly person needs most of the same tests that would be part of any checkup—blood pressure, temperature, weight, and blood and urine tests, as well as any necessary screenings and special tests that are required because of a particular illness, risk, or symptom. In addition, the doctor will look for ailments that are common in the elderly (arthritis, weight loss, thyroid problems, heart disease, etc.). He or she should also review your parent's medical history and medications, as older people often take a number of drugs that are not appropriate.

Unlike other routine physicals, however, geriatric exams should also focus on physical ability and function. A doctor will check your parent's legs for rashes or tenderness, but he or she should also be concerned about gait and dexterity. With a few quick tests, the doctor can find out if your parent can reach, bend, walk, turn, sit down, and get up without difficulty; hear what's being said; pick up a spoon; or read his own pill bottles.

♦ **The brain.** The exam might include a quick test of your parent's cognitive abilities and mental state. Elderly people who are in the earliest stages of dementia can usually compensate for mental lapses with family members, but it's not so easy to cover things up in an exam. And it's helpful to get a diagnosis early.

To check your parent's cognitive abilities, the doctor might, for example, ask her to think of three items and then recall them a minute later, or have her count backward from 100 by sevens. If there is any question about her mental abilities, the doctor will conduct a more comprehensive exam or refer her to someone else for further evaluation. (The exam and follow-up tests are described on page 466.)

The doctor should also ask about any past psychiatric care and your parent's current mental state, including moods, fears, and anxiety. If there is any suggestion of depression, an anxiety disorder, or other mental illness, the doctor might refer your parent to a geriatric psychiatrist for further evaluation.

♦ **The person.** The doctor, a nurse, or a social worker should ask about your parent's eating, sleeping, exercising, and toileting habits. Someone should also inquire, at least briefly, about her housing situation and social supports. Such information will alert a doctor to possible ailments, such as depression, insomnia, incontinence, or malnutrition, and uncover practical problems and potential risks. If your mother isn't eating, does she need to be put in touch with a meal-delivery service? If she lives alone, is she at risk of falling or having other accidents?

If your parent needs social services, the doctor's office may be able to refer her to some. If not, you may have to consult a social worker or case manager.

A GERIATRIC ASSESSMENT

BECAUSE THE MEDICAL CARE OF THE elderly can be so complex, many hospitals and clinics have established geriatric assessment centers (also called geriatric evaluation units). In these centers, a geriatrician heads a team of medical specialists (neurologists, psychiatrists, rheumatologists, etc.), nurses, social workers, physical and occupational therapists, case workers, and dietitians, who address all facets of your parent's health and life. Studies suggest that for very frail or incompetent patients, such comprehensive care can mean fewer accidents, less illness, longer lives, and greater independence.

While some of these centers provide primary medical care, replacing the family doctor, most act as consultants in cases where the patient has dementia, multiple ailments, difficult-to-diagnose symptoms, or a lot of problems managing at home.

Patients are typically referred to a geriatric center by their personal doctors, but you or your parent can make an appointment directly if you have nagging concerns that aren't being answered by his doctor, or if you believe that he needs more comprehensive care than his doctor can offer.

A geriatric assessment lasts anywhere from three hours to several days (although it can be broken up and done in pieces over several visits) and includes a detailed physical, neurological, and mental exam, as well as evaluations by social workers and nurses who will talk with your parent, and perhaps with the family, about your parent's daily life and future. The team will provide counseling as well as practical help, hooking your family up with local services and housing options.

Geriatric centers are usually found in big medical centers or hospitals in large cities, although some are now opening elsewhere. To find one, ask your parent's doctor or call hospitals in the area.

Check with Medicare and other insurance about the possibility of covering a geriatric assessment. They might cover at least some of the cost, which can run from $200 to more than $1,000.

A SEAT IN THE BLEACHERS— OR BEHIND HOME PLATE?

What if your father doesn't want your input or help? What if he doesn't tell you about his medical care or doesn't listen to your advice? As maddening as it may be for you, as long as he is competent, he has the right to manage these issues for himself—up to a point.

If you are concerned about your parent's choice of doctors, express your concerns and offer your assistance. Mention that there have been advances in geriatric medicine, and point out the benefits of having a doctor who knows about these advances. Likewise, if you are concerned about a medical problem, urge him to talk to the doctor about it.

If he blocks your efforts and the issue isn't dire, you may have to back down. But when you think the problem is serious—your mother fainted while walking to the car, she has become uncharacteristically contentious and disoriented, or she has occasional but acute chest pains—you have to be more aggressive. Urge her to call her doctor. But if she doesn't, call the doctor yourself. She can't be helped if no one knows what's happening.

An Informed Advocate

A good doctor is only part of the medical care team; the patient must play an active role as well.

Normally, your parent and his doctor will have their own relationship, which you will have little, if any, part in. But as your parent grows frailer or more confused, you will become his advocate, if not his spokesperson. The medical world can be confounding and intimidating to an outsider, but be bold.

◆ **Ask questions.** If you are overseeing your parent's medical care, or even if you are on the sidelines, don't hesitate to ask questions. If your parent is handling her own care, remind her to ask questions and to write down the answers. Don't be embarrassed that you don't know exactly what the liver is, where it is, or what it does. Don't pretend that you know what an abscess, an antigen, or a fistula is, nodding your head agreeably as the doctor races on. Ask, ask, and ask again. It's important that you, if not your parent, really understand the issues.

Write down any questions that occur to you prior to an appointment and then give them to the doctor so he or she can allot time for them and address the most critical problems first.

If you have questions or concerns that can't wait until the next visit—*Is she supposed to take the new medication*

IN THE EXAMINING ROOM

If you stay with your parent during any segment of the exam, stay in the background. Be careful not to answer questions addressed to him because, quite often, the doctor is not simply looking for an answer, but is observing how your parent responds. You also need to give your parent and the doctor a chance to develop some rapport. If possible, wait until after the exam is over to add any information that may have been omitted.

---

with dinner or before going to bed? Is this dizziness my parent's complaining of serious?—call. Don't be intimidated or worry about whether the question is important enough. The doctor may not be able to talk to you, but an assistant should be able to answer your questions, and, if necessary, the doctor will get back to you later.

◆ **Take notes.** Every time you talk with a doctor or nurse, have a pad handy and take notes. It's easy to forget specifics when you are upset. If your parent is still in charge, encourage her to take notes, or ask the doctor to write down any diagnosis or specific instructions. This will be helpful for your parent, who may not remember the details, and it allows

CHANGING DOCTORS MIDSTREAM

 Small disagreements or doctor-patient tussles can often be remedied by talking about them (or writing a letter, if that's easier), but when the problem is insurmountable, urge your parent to find another doctor. Thank the first one for his or her time, but explain that your parent has found someone with whom she feels more comfortable.

People are often reluctant to switch doctors, no matter how dissatisfied they are, because they are embarrassed or afraid of hurting the doctor's feelings. But most doctors understand that different patients have different needs. Anyway, your parent's medical care is far more important than someone's momentary feelings.

If a doctor implies that you are ungrateful for his or her past devotion, or that the care your parent receives elsewhere will be of a lower standard, don't let it affect your decision.

---

her to relay any important information to you or others helping in her care. *He said I had some kind of bowel problem, oh, what did he call it? Irreversible? Irrational? I don't remember. Something to do with the bowel.*

◆ **Do your homework.** When the doctor hasn't explained the facts clearly or your parent gives you only partial information, do a little research on your own. You don't have to look up every study ever done on Coumadin, but find out what blood clotting is about, what the drugs do to prevent it, what they shouldn't be mixed with, and what side effects are possible. Now, with the Internet, such research is pretty easy to do.

Be sure that your resources are reliable, and don't trust sensational articles from popular magazines or advice from friends. Ask the doctor if there are any brochures or other literature about your parent's condition that you might read. If you don't have a computer at home, go to the library and use the Internet there (see page 206 for specific sites), or consult a medical encyclopedia or drug handbook for consumers.

◆ **Be a keen observer.** If you are involved in your parent's medical care and you see her regularly, keep a mental note of her moods, habits, and complaints. A minor fall, a dull pain, or changes in weight, sleep habits, or moods can all indicate a serious medical problem and should be brought to the doctor's attention. Your parent may not alert the doctor to the problem—she may not be aware of the change, she may not want to talk about it, or she may not remember to talk about it. So the doctor has no way of knowing what is going on without your intervention.

◆ **Keep records.** Maintain an updated list of all your parent's medications (prescription medications as well as nonprescription ones), including the dose, the date that she began and ended any medication, and any adverse side effects from medications; any allergies; the names, addresses, and phone numbers of all doctors seen; special dietary needs; and the dates, places, and reasons for any hospitalizations or surgery.

◆ **Use one spokesperson.** If your parent can't oversee her own medical care, one person should be chosen to be the family spokesperson. He or she should be in contact with the doctor's office and then relay information to others. Of course, it's important that your family spokesperson is sensitive to the concerns of siblings and can communicate easily with them.

◆ **Get a second opinion.** Even if your parent's doctor is terrific, get another opinion on any serious matter, particularly when surgery is recommended. Another doctor will either offer new options or be able to reassure you that this is the best way to proceed.

Because a doctor may be reluctant to disagree with a colleague, seek out the second doctor on your own if possible. You are more apt to get an unbiased opinion and different viewpoint, as doctors tend to recommend people who share their medical philosophy.

◆ **Use caution when comparing.** Don't give too much weight to the tales of other people who had a similar illness. A stroke is not a stroke is not a stroke, particularly when it happens in an elderly body. So don't second-guess the doctor just because Aunt Ashley was cured when she had these same symptoms.

◆ **Be a team player.** While you should be a staunch and persistent advocate for your parent, you also need to work with the doctor and other health professionals. Be open about your concerns and questions, but also be patient and understanding. Doctors work under enormous pressures, and there are limitations to what they can do.

◆ **Understand the process.** Medicine is as much an art as it is a science. Your parent's doctor doesn't know everything, because everything isn't known and because each person is different. No one test or treatment is likely to provide "the cure" or "the answer"; it is all part of an ongoing process.

Your desire for clarity, answers, and action may push a doctor to act in ways that are not in your parent's best interests. A doctor might, for example, prescribe a potent drug simply to appease anxious family members who want something done. A linear "cure" mentality is apt to lead to disappointment, and it also

QUICK ACCESS TO MEDICAL INFORMATION

 The Internet is loaded with medical information (as well as caregiver support). But be careful. Some of it is useful, a lot of it is simply an effort to get you to buy a product, and some of it is misleading or false. And when it comes to medical issues, the Internet may give you far more than you ever needed or wanted to know. Be a mindful consumer. Only use sites of reputable organizations, which means large foundations, medical associations, government sites, medical journals, or other established organizations. Beware of any site trying to sell something. Check the source and the date of any information. If you are not connected to the Internet, the public library should have access.

Some good starting points for medical information are:

◆ Healthfinder (www.healthfinder.gov), created by the U.S. Department of Health and Human Services, provides information on a wide range of health issues from various public health agencies, professional groups, universities, and journals.

◆ WebMD (www.webmd.com) has a vast array of articles for the general public and should answer any questions that Healthfinder did not. If you want more detailed information, WebMD's sister site, Medscape (www.medscape.com) is geared toward clinicians and other health-care providers.

◆ Most illnesses and disabilities have their own associations or organizations, and corresponding Web sites, such as the Alzheimer's Association, the Arthritis Foundation, the American Cancer Society, etc. To find organizations linked to a particular issue or illness, contact the National Health Information Center (800-336-4797 or www.

---

might distract you from your parent's more important day-to-day care and comfort.

◆ **Get a medical power of attorney.** A medical power of attorney, or health-care proxy, is a legal form that gives you or some other person the authority to make medical decisions on your parent's behalf if, for some reason, she cannot make them for herself. This document is easily obtained from Last Acts Partnership (800-989-9455 or www.lastactspartnership.org) and everyone (including you) should have one.

health.gov/nhic). For information about less common ailments, contact the National Organization for Rare Disorders (800-999-6673 or www.rarediseases.org).

◆ The above Web sites should give you what you need, but if you're hungry for more, the National Institute on Aging and the National Library of Medicine have paired up to provide health information that is specific to seniors (www.nihseniorhealth.gov).

◆ If you want to get more technical, you can access the entire database of the National Library of Medicine, known as Medline, at www.nlm.nih.gov.

◆ The *Merck Manual of Geriatrics* is for doctors, but it is full of good information, and the entire manual, which is regularly updated, is available at www.merck.com.

Be sure your parent's doctor has a copy of this and any other advance directives (such as a living will). Your parent should talk with her chosen proxy at some length about her priorities, preferences, and feelings about medical care, especially medical care when death is near.

Complementary and Alternative Medicine

Although many forms of alternative medicine are based on ancient medical practices, it is not the stuff of your parent's generation.

Much of it is a waste of time, some of it is downright dangerous, but many unconventional approaches are effective, so it is certainly worth looking into. Just use reason and caution.

Alternative medicine is, as the name suggests, treatment that is used in place of conventional practices; complementary medicine is that which is used at the same time as conventional treatment. "Integrative medicine," which is probably the best approach, is the use of conventional medicine in conjunction with any unconventional treatment that is widely thought to be safe and effective.

Complementary and alternative medicine (known in some circles as CAM) includes acupuncture, herbal treatments, imagery, homeopathy, chiropractic, osteopathy, massage, hormones, and dozens of other approaches (like juice therapy, oxygen therapy, and sound therapy). Much of it stems from ancient practices that have been used for thousands of years in China and India—the Chinese therapy qigong, the Japanese therapy Reiki, and the Indian system of ayurveda, all of which emphasize the body's energy and balance.

These approaches have gained enormous popularity recently because people have become disenchanted with traditional medicine; they have taken more control over their health care and want a more holistic approach. Perhaps more than anything else, CAM has attracted a following because claims of success and promises of hope (whether true or not) are so alluring.

There is little solid scientific data on the value of such practices, although some studies have been completed and many more are now underway. But anecdotal evidence along with preliminary studies suggests that many of these practices are safe and some are effective.

A sampling of the more popular techniques and treatments are discussed briefly here, to give you some idea of what's available. You can find more information by contacting the National Center for Complementary and Alternative Medicine at 888-644-6226 or www.nccam.nih.gov or by searching through other respected medical books and Web sites.

NOTE: Be very cautious when using any complementary or alternative medicine. Your parent should always check with his doctor before adopting any integrative medical regimen, not necessarily to get the doctor's support of a particular therapy, but to make sure that it won't interfere with his ongoing medical care or cause troublesome or dangerous side effects. For example, certain herbal medicines are potent drugs and may be hazardous if used with your parent's current medications. Ginkgo can cause bleeding when people are already taking blood-thinning drugs. St. John's wort can interfere with antidepressant medications and chemotherapy. Kava has been linked to liver disease. Your parent should absolutely tell the doctor if he is considering taking or is taking any supplements. Also:

◆ Your parent should never rely on an alternative medicine practitioner for a diagnosis. Always check back with the primary doctor.

◆ Older bodies typically don't tolerate things as well as younger bodies do, and the confluence of medical ailments makes treatment complicated. In other words, use extra caution when trying an alternative therapy on an older person.

◆ Just because something seems to work for a friend does not mean it will work for your parent.

◆ Learn the credentials, training, and fees of any practitioner. You can ask your parent's primary doctor for a recommendation or contact professional organizations. Some large medical centers have CAM centers or clinics.

◆ Finally, be forewarned that most CAM must be paid for out of pocket. Insurance coverage is usually very limited. Medicare covers some chiropractic services and may add coverage for some other CAM. Medicaid rules vary by state.

SUPPLEMENTS

SUPPLEMENTS USED TO REFER SIMPLY to vitamins and minerals, basically a one-a-day tablet. And many vitamins and minerals are critical to good health, particularly at your parent's age. But now the word *supplement* refers to a broad array of amino acids, herbal products, animal tissues, and questionable ingredients usually given in pill or liquid form, but often loaded into drinks, water, bars, and candy.

Just because something is "herbal" or "natural" does not in any way mean that it's safe. As noted earlier, many are quite toxic, and others interact poorly with conventional drugs. So, again, read the literature and check with your parent's doctor first.

Supplements, or "nutraceuticals," as they are sometimes called, are virtually unregulated. Manufacturers do not have to prove that products are effective, or even safe. They can make all sorts of outlandish and unproven claims on advertising and labels. They can even say that wild claims are "scientifically proven" when they are not.

So don't believe what you read on these labels. The promises are grand and full of hope, but disregard them. Read up on any supplement from reputable sources, talk to your parent's doctor, and buy only from large, established companies.

Having said all that, there is evidence that a few supplements are safe and seemingly effective. For example, glucosamine, which comes from the shells of certain shellfish, and chondroitin sulfate, which is largely made from shark cartilage, have been shown to be effective in easing the pain of osteoarthritis. These compounds are found naturally in the body and are thought to play a role in cartilage formation and repair. Likewise, zinc, along with vitamins C and E, beta carotene, and copper, seems to slow progression of age-related macular degeneration.

Again, talk with your parent's doctor about the use of supplements.

ACUPUNCTURE

ACUPUNCTURE, WHICH ORIGINATED more than two thousand years ago, is one of the oldest and most popular medical procedures in the world.

In this therapy, trained practitioners insert extremely fine needles into particular points in the body. It is usually painless but can cause a slight tingling sensation. The theory is that the human body has an energy called *qi* (pronounced "chee"), which regulates the body's spiritual, emotional, physical, and mental balance. *Qi* moves about the body on "meridians." By stimulating points along these meridians, the acupuncturist tries to restore balance and keep a person's *qi* flowing smoothly.

While western doctors have not discovered physical evidence of these meridians, many theorize that acupuncture triggers the release of natural painkillers and "uppers" in the body.

In any case, it works for many people, particularly when treating acute pain, and nausea due to chemotherapy. It also appears to be somewhat effective in treating asthma, addictions, arthritis, and insomnia, among other things. Increasingly, traditional doctors are pairing up acupuncture with traditional pain medications and finding that they can use a lower dose of the medications.

Most states now have standards in place for certification and licensing of acupuncturists. Many medical doctors are also now being trained in acupuncture. Be sure to find a trained and respected acupuncturist who uses disposable needles (otherwise, there is a risk of infection).

Acupressure is similar to acupuncture, but the practitioner uses fingertips to apply pressure rather than inserting needles.

CHIROPRACTIC

CHIROPRACTIC MEDICINE IS CLEARLY one of the most popular forms of alternative medicine, making it seem almost mainstream. The theory behind chiropractic medicine is that misalignments (called "subluxations") in the skeleton, particularly in the spine, interfere with the work of the nervous system and the body's natural defenses. When the scaffolding is adjusted, the body can begin to heal itself. It is an ancient practice dating back at least two thousand years.

Chiropractic is particularly useful in treating ailments in the muscles, joints, and bones, such as neck pain, headaches, strains, and arthritis. Evidence suggests that it is as effective at treating low back pain as conventional medicine. (Of course, some studies also suggest that doing nothing is also as effective; that is, the pain eventually goes away by itself.)

Chiropractors usually have four years of specialized training and get a D.C., or Doctor of Chiropractic, degree. Many insurance companies, as well as Medicare and, in some states, Medicaid, offer at least some coverage for chiropractic treatment.

HOMEOPATHIC

AS WITH SO MANY OTHER FORMS OF alternative medicine, homeopathy rests on the idea of a life force or vital force present in the body. When this force, or energy, is out of balance, people become sick. When it is put back into balance, the body can begin to heal itself.

Homeopathic remedies are usually *extremely* diluted amounts of plant, mineral, or animal substances that would, in larger amounts, cause the very illness that is being treated, or at least cause the symptoms of that illness. The idea is that this kick-starts the body's own defense mechanisms.

Treatments are generally tailored to individuals, which means that the first visit is apt to be a long one, as the practitioner comes to understand the individual and the ailment.

Homeopathy was discovered in Germany in the late 1700s, a time when two of the most common medical treatments were bloodletting and purging. It was an effort to take a less violent approach to treatment, and to use the body's own potent resources to heal itself.

Homeopaths take a variety of routes to get their training, including correspondence courses. Most, however, are licensed in something else—medicine, naturopathy, chiropractic, acupuncture—and offer homeopathy as well.

While scientific studies have not proven much, if any, effect from most homeopathy, millions of people use it in this country, and it has been integrated into the national health systems of numerous countries.

BIOFEEDBACK

BIOFEEDBACK MEANS JUST WHAT IT says: You get feedback on what's happening to you biologically. Then, you gradually learn to control it. And it works extremely well for many people. People can watch their heart rate and learn ways to slow it. Likewise, they can reduce their blood pressure, ease muscle tension, calm breathing, and alter skin temperature.

The feedback comes either through a machine or, depending upon what the person is trying to control, directly from the body. Generally a person is hooked up to a device that would, for example, detect electrical signals from certain muscles. When the muscles are tense, an alarm goes off. Eventually, the person relaxes his or her muscles

> " *I wouldn't say that my mother is into alternative medicine—she doesn't try anything terribly radical. But when she was diagnosed with cancer I bought her a couple of books on diet and nutrition. She started taking vitamins. She also started reading books about emotional states and healing—Bernie Siegel stuff. I think it has helped. She is stronger both physically and mentally. I can see the change in her. It makes her feel like she still has some control, like she can take charge and really fight this thing herself."*
>
> —DIANA M.

without the help of the machine. While a variety of medical practitioners offer biofeedback, you can get a referral to a certified practitioner from the Biofeedback Certification Institute of America (303-420-2902 or www.bcia.org).

It is a useful way to control stress and fear, and is often used to treat depression. For some individuals, biofeedback can alleviate tension or migraine headaches, improve incontinence, ease chronic pain, treat insomnia, control blood sugar levels in diabetics, and lower high blood pressure. Some studies suggest that biofeedback might also be effective in treating gastrointestinal disorders, such as nausea, vomiting, abdominal pain, and bloating.

VISUALIZATION

VISUALIZATION, ALSO KNOWN AS guided imagery, can be very helpful for elderly people, particularly those who are in chronic pain, anxious, worried, or depressed, and those who are near death.

In one form of imagery, the person imagines a relaxing scene or situation. For example, he or she might imagine herself lying on the beach, the warmth of the sun touching her skin, the steady sound of the waves, the weight of her body as it sinks heavily into the soft sand, etc. Putting oneself into this other place, entering it completely with the mind, relaxes the body and relieves anxiety, tension, and pain.

In another type of visualization, a person imagines his body healing itself, imagines weak areas growing stronger, important nutrients entering the bloodstream, or strong immune cells fending off an enemy infection. The mind might not be able to instruct the body directly, but because this sort of thinking fosters a sense of control and power, it helps a person feel better and perhaps heal.

MASSAGE

MASSAGE FEELS GOOD AND CAN BE therapeutic, as it relieves tension, which helps to reduce stress and ease pain. However, for an elderly person who is not comfortable with physical contact—and many from this generation are not—this will not be relaxing.

If your parent is game, a massage makes a nice gift. Many massage therapists make house calls. Be sure, however, to check with your parent's doctor first, to make sure this is okay for your parent. Massage might release an embolism, causing stroke. Alert the therapist to sore areas or brittle bones.

Massage can be light or firm, rubbing or pounding, squeezing or kneading. Some massage therapists use electric vibrators to massage muscles. Others use hot stones.

THERAPEUTIC TOUCH

IF YOUR PARENT DOES NOT ENJOY physical contact, therapeutic touch is still an option (although many elderly people would still be unhappy about even this). A session of this might make a nice gift as well, especially if your parent is living alone or in a nursing home.

Therapeutic touch is based on the notion that the hands of these therapists have a healing force. The therapists usually don't touch the client, but rather slide their hands two to four inches above the skin (or clothes; a person does not have to undress for this). In doing so, the healer identifies energy imbalances and corrects them.

Whether energy is actually rebalanced—or perhaps having a gentle, slow-moving, peaceful person focus her attention on your body is in itself calming—therapeutic touch does seems to reduce anxiety, increase relaxation, and reduce pain.

MEDITATION

YOUR PARENT MIGHT POOH-POOH the idea of meditating, but research suggests that meditation is great for both body and soul.

Meditation is really just conscious relaxation. It means paying attention to one's breathing, relaxing the muscles, and clearing the mind of all the rubbish that consumes it. Once someone is successfully meditating, his breathing becomes deep and regular, and his mind is detached from the problems of daily life. It is useful for anyone, but it's particularly effective in treating stress, pain, hypertension, and heart disease, and is thought to strengthen the immune system. Caregivers as well as their aged parents can benefit from meditating.

Unlike some other therapies, it takes practice and motivation to master it. While there are teachers who teach it, videos can guide someone through the steps.

A WORD OF CAUTION

Beware of any claims of quick fixes and medical breakthroughs. Certainly, ads claiming to restore hearing, revitalize skin, reverse baldness, stop aging (millions of these), and strengthen memory may be tough to pass by. But pass them by you must.

These are the snake-oil salesmen of yesterday, preying on people's deepest fears and adversity. They promise to cure whatever ails you, whatever might pique your interest and sell their product.

Medical discoveries take place over time and, once made, still must be proved, disproved, tested, and retested. If you or your parent hears about something that sounds promising, ask the doctor about it. But don't pin your hopes on a cure that sounds too good to be true. It probably is.

THE BODY IMPERFECT:
PART I

*A Muddle of Medications • Vision • Hearing • Sleep
• Dehydration • Skin Problems • Dental Care*

Y OUR OVERRIDING CONCERN RIGHT NOW MAY BE STROKE, cancer, dementia, heart disease, or some other life-threatening illness, and understandably so. But don't lose sight of your parent's seemingly more mundane complaints, such as blurry eyesight, incontinence, and restless nights. Doctors will attend to severe illness, but they often ignore these other ailments. And they need attention. In fact, for your parent, these problems may be more troublesome day-to-day than any serious disease. His poor hearing may distance him from people he loves, his itchy skin may keep him awake at night, and his crippled knees may prevent him from doing the things he most enjoys.

Be careful not to pass off these complaints as unavoidable aspects of old age. *That's what happens at eighty-six. What do you expect?* Certainly, many ailments are more common in old age, but that doesn't mean they are untreatable or less worthy of attention. Your father isn't suffering because he is old; he is suffering because he is sick. The fact of the matter is that something can be done about almost all of his symptoms. Some are preventable, most are treatable, and a few are curable. And life with any disability can be made more manageable.

The information supplied here is not meant to replace the advice of a doctor, but if you are aware of the problems, the symptoms, and some remedies, you can alert the doctor and brainstorm for solutions. You can also make changes around your parent's house and in his daily life to keep him comfortable and independent for as long as possible.

Understanding what your parent is up against—why he doesn't remember what you said (he didn't hear it), or why he is so grumpy (he is in pain)—should also give you more patience and compassion as you try to help him now.

ON THE LOOKOUT FOR SYMPTOMS

Problem	Signs of Trouble
Overmedication	A cabinet filled with prescriptions from multiple physicians; confusion, drowsiness, or agitation
Vision loss	Squinting, pulling back to read small print, failing to notice stop signs, trouble following sporting events or driving at night
Hearing loss	Saying "what?" a lot, constantly turning the volume up, staring vacantly while others talk
Insomnia	Complaints of fatigue, long periods spent in bed, frequent naps, wandering at night
Hyperthermia	Sweating, dizziness, nausea, or, in severe cases, hot and dry skin, rapid pulse, and confusion
Hypothermia	Lethargy, confusion, paleness, shallow breathing (even in normal temperatures)
Skin problems	Unusual-looking moles; itchy, cracked, red, or irritated skin
Mouth ailments	Pain, dry mouth, difficulty chewing

A Muddle of Medications

The thought of your father as a druggie may seem absurd, but take another look in his medicine cabinet. A prescription for pain, a blood thinner, a little something to help him sleep, a pill to aid digestion, medication to lower his cholesterol, a pill for his memory, and something for his arthritis. It's not uncommon for an older person to make weekly visits to the pharmacist; the average elderly person is taking more than six medications at any one time.

This would be risky in any person, but it becomes particularly worrisome in an elderly person as they have a variety of health problems, and frail, older bodies do not tolerate drugs in the same ways young bodies do. Changes in hormones, body fat and water content, metabolism, blood flow, stomach acids, and kidney function all affect the way bodies absorb, use, and discard drugs. Drugs that work well in younger patients might not be appropriate for older patients (and, unfortunately, few drug studies include truly old patients). And pills that your parent took at sixty might not be right for her at eighty.

Given the number of drugs and illnesses involved, the fragility of the body involved, the lack of oversight and the likelihood for error (taking the wrong medications or failing to follow directions), the chances of troublesome or dangerous side effects are enormous. Misuse of medications can cause serious health complications, even death. It can easily worsen an existing illness or cause new problems.

And yet, inappropriate drug use among the elderly is referred to as "the nation's other drug problem"—it is almost epidemic.

The reasons are numerous. Doctors overprescribe, fail to stop medications that are no longer needed, prescribe doses that are too high for an elderly person, prescribe drugs that are completely inappropriate for an elderly person, or prescribe drugs in dangerous combinations. Because so many doctors are involved, simple lack of communication is often to blame. Doctor A is not aware of what doctors B and C have prescribed.

Elderly patients are also to blame. They fail to give their doctors a complete medical history that includes all the medications that they are taking. And, perhaps the biggest problem of all, elderly people commonly don't take medications as directed. They discontinue a regime before it has run its full course, forget to take a medication, or skip doses to save money or to avoid side effects. Studies suggest that more than half of elderly people do not take their medications as directed.

If you are involved in your parent's medical care, ask questions when a new drug is prescribed. Keep careful records of the drugs she takes—the names of the drugs, the reason for them, the dates they are started and stopped, side effects, and instructions.

If you are not with her on a regular basis, be sure your parent or some other care provider is keeping records.

Then, if your parent has a new symptom or says she just doesn't feel like herself, look back in these records to see when she began taking any new medications and alert the doctor. Side effects common among the elderly include restlessness, dizziness, poor balance and falls, sedation, loss of memory, confusion, blurred vision, depression, constipation, abdominal pain, changes in sleep habits, inconti nence, tremors, and skin problems, such as rashes and unusual sensitivity to the sun (causing burns, blisters, or swelling).

THE INFORMED CONSUMER

WHEN A NEW MEDICATION IS PRE-scribed, your parent or some caregiver should get full information from the doctor and pharmacist and write it all down. (Be sure, too, to write down the correct spelling of the drug and its brand name.)

Questions about medications for the doctor:

◆ What is this drug supposed to do? Is it treating the cause of the problem or only the symptoms? If it's the latter, is there any way to treat the cause?

◆ Is there another way to treat this problem, such as with a change in diet, exercise, or lifestyle?

◆ Is it safe for your parent to use this with the other medications or supplements she now uses?

IN A NURSING HOME

If your parent is in a nursing home, be particularly vigilant about her medications. Nursing-home residents take even more medications than other elderly people, and there is evidence that many of these drugs are unnecessary or inappropriate. Given a resident's even frailer health and generally lower weight, this is very dangerous.

Be sure that your parent is not being oversedated as a way to dull aggressive or difficult behavior. Antipsychotics are dangerous and not terribly useful in nonpsychotic people, but are often used, particularly when a person suffers from dementia. They can cause sedation, dizziness, restlessness, and confusion, as well as a muscular disorder that causes tremors, called tardive dyskinesia, which is often irreversible.

◆ What is the proper dose for someone my mother's age? (Because the elderly tend to be sensitive to drugs, they should start at very low doses—often one-quarter to one-half of that given to a younger or larger person—and then the dose can be gradually increased as needed.)

GOOD MEDICINE

◆ Be sure your parent has one doctor overseeing her medical care and that he or she has a complete list of *all* medications and supplements your parent takes, including prescription drugs, over-the-counter (nonprescription) drugs, vitamins, herbal remedies, eye or ear drops.

◆ This list of medications should be reviewed regularly.

◆ Always get a doctor's okay before making any change in a medication routine. Your parent should not take more of a drug to increase the effect or stop taking a drug because she feels better or is experiencing some side effect.

◆ Make sure any doctor who sees your parent knows about any allergies he might have.

◆ Your parent may be taking medications, especially over-the-counter medications, such as antihistamines or sleeping pills, out of habit, unaware that these may be dangerous for him. If the pills are addictive, he may need help from the doctor. Find out which ones should be stopped or at least taken in lower doses.

◆ Keep pills intended for emergencies in a place where they can easily be found by your parent, you, or some other caretaker.

◆ Never let your parent take a friend's pills, even if he has the same symptoms as the friend.

◆ If your parent has missed a dose or two of medication, call the doctor or pharmacist to find out what to do, rather than blindly returning to the original routine.

◆ What time or times of day should she take it?

◆ How should she take it? Does she need to take it with food or drink? Or should she avoid any particular foods, drinks, or activities while taking it?

◆ What are the possible side effects or allergic reactions one should watch for or be aware of? What should I do if my parent has a bad reaction? (There are usually trade-offs to be made when treating elderly patients—for example, your parent may need to take a drug that worsens her confusion in order to get rid of the far more troubling hallucinations she is suffering. Weigh all the pros and cons with the doctor.)

♦ Don't crush or break a pill without first asking the pharmacist. You might destroy a coating designed to protect the stomach, or upset the long action of a time-released medication.

♦ Don't leave pills out where a child can get them. More than one-third of all incidents of children poisoned by prescription drugs involve a grandparent's pills. Be particularly careful if your parent gets drugs in vials without childproof caps.

♦ Throw out drugs that are old—as a general rule, after one year. (Over-the-counter drugs now have expiration dates on them. Prescription drugs usually don't, but the pharmacist will mark the bottle if you ask.)

♦ How long does it take for this drug to have an effect, and how will she know if it's working? Is there a goal (a particular blood pressure, for example) that she is trying to achieve? Should she continue to take it even after she feels better? If not, when should she stop taking it? Your parent or you should check regularly with the doctor to find out if the drug is still needed or if the dose can be lowered.

♦ What if my parent misses a dose?

♦ Is it habit-forming? Will it be difficult for her to stop taking it?

♦ Is there an alternative that requires fewer doses each day (which might then be an easier regime for your parent to follow)?

♦ Are there remedies that might counter expected side effects (such as stool softeners for constipation or the active cultures in yogurt to fight yeast infections)?

Questions for the pharmacist:

♦ Is there a generic version that is just as good, but less expensive?

♦ How should this medication be stored? (Away from light? In the refrigerator?)

♦ If your parent has trouble swallowing, is there a way to get it down more easily? Can she get this medication in liquid form, can the pills be crushed, or can a capsule be opened and the powder mixed with food to make it easier to swallow?

♦ If she has trouble seeing, does the pharmacist have large-print labels?

♦ Can she get the medication in easy-to-open bottles (rather than those with childproof caps)?

♦ What is the expiration date?

♦ If it is a new prescription, is it possible to fill just half of it, to be sure there are no adverse effects, before paying for the entire prescription?

◆ Can you review the directions for me?

Before you leave, check that this is actually the right medication. Read the label and be sure both the patient's name and the drug name are correct. Some medication names differ by just a letter, and busy pharmacists have been known to dole out the wrong drug.

KEEPING TABS ON COMPLIANCE

MOST OF US HAVE TROUBLE REMEMbering to take medication, especially if the pills have no immediate effect, if the symptoms they're treating are already gone, or if they have unpleasant side effects. For the elderly, who are apt to be using multiple drugs simultaneously and who may tend toward forgetfulness anyway, noncompliance is a serious problem.

If you are in the role of watchdog or caretaker, there are a few things you can do to improve your parent's habits. First, impress upon her the importance of following the prescribed routine in order to treat the illness completely and avoid complications.

Next, buy her a pillbox, not a pretty little one, but a serious pillbox

DAILY MEDICATION SCHEDULE								
		MORNING						
MEDICATION NAME / DOSE	SPECIAL INSTRUCTIONS	7	8	9	10	11	12	

with multiple compartments for different drugs and separate labels indicating the time of day each is to be taken. Large pillboxes, which hold daily doses for the entire week, are useful if you are filling the boxes for your parent during a weekly visit. You can find an assortment of pillboxes in medical supply stores and large pharmacies.

Put the pillbox, or pill bottles if you forego the pillbox, in a place where your parent will see them and be reminded to take them. For example, pills to be taken at bedtime might be placed on the toothbrush stand, and those to be taken in the morning, on the breakfast table. Then be sure to label each bottle in clear, dark letters: "Take one with breakfast" or "Take two before bed."

You can also stick notes to the refrigerator or bathroom mirror or on her lunch tray, reminding her to take pills.

When more than one person is dispensing your parent's medications, or your parent simply needs a little more organization, make a large chart, something like the one below, and mark off when a pill is taken. If your parent is in charge and has trouble reading the pill bottle labels, color-code the chart, matching the color of the bottle or pill with a similar color

		AFTERNOON				EVENING					
1	2	3	4	5	6	7	8	9	10	11	12

on the chart (*blue pills at two, white pills at six, pink liquid at ten,* etc.).

If your father forgets because of dementia or another illness, it is best if someone actually sees him take his medication.

You can buy an array of pill-related paraphernalia—pillboxes, reminder alarms, organizers, dispensers, watches, and even reminders that work with handheld computers—at pharmacies, medical supply stores, or online.

If worse comes to worst, call your parent (or have someone else call him) at pill time and have him take his medicine while you wait on the phone. If you're willing to spend the money (about $45 a month), Verbaprompt is a telephone system that reminds people to take their medications (www.verbaprompt.com).

SAVING MONEY ON MEDICATIONS

MEDICATIONS CAN BE SO WILDLY expensive that older people skimp on their doses or skip treatments completely—obviously a very bad idea. Others forgo groceries or other necessities to pay for medications. There are ways to save.

See page 355 for a description of Medicare's drug plan and what it will cover, along with information about various Medigap and Medicare Advantage plans, some of which offer some drug coverage.

Beyond that, many states, communities, organizations, and pharmaceutical companies have programs to help elderly people with the cost of prescription drugs. Far more people are eligible than use the programs, so it's worth checking to see if your parent might fit the bill. There are also commercial programs that have no eligibility requirements and charge only a nominal enrollment fee, but then offer drugs at a discount.

The easiest thing to do is to look at the database for prescription drug assistance programs online at www.medicare.gov or call Medicare at 800-MEDICARE. It will tell you what programs your parent is eligible for in her area, as well as provide information on Medicare and Medigap policies, special discounts for government employees and veterans, and commercial discount providers with no eligibility requirements.

You can also learn about discount programs through these Web sites: www.benefitscheckuprx.com (of the National Council on the Aging), www.helpingpatients.org (of the Pharmaceutical Research and Manufacturers of America), and www.rxassist.org (of Volunteers in Health Care).

Several major drug companies have banded together to offer discounts to Medicare participants with lower incomes through something called the Together Rx Card. Your parent simply shows the card with the prescription and receives a discount of 15 to 40 percent. To find out if your parent is eligible (income levels vary by state, but it was about $30,000 for a single person in 2004), call 800-865-7211 or visit online www.togetherrx.com. Other

HYPERTENSION

Your parent doesn't need to wait for the doctor to tell him that he has high blood pressure, or hypertension, to start doing something about it. Most older people have it, and the lifestyle changes one should adopt in order to lower blood pressure—stop smoking, lose weight, exercise, consume less fat and cholesterol, cut back on alcohol, cut back on salt—are good for everyone.

High blood pressure means that the heart is working hard, too hard, to force blood around the body. This undue force increases the risk of stroke and heart disease, as well as kidney disease, blindness, and other diseases. A blood pressure of 140/90 mmHg (millimeters of mercury) or higher is too high.

To learn more about lowering blood pressure and generally taking care of oneself, see Chapter Four. If lifestyle changes alone don't do the trick (and be sure to give these a wholehearted effort first), your parent's doctor will prescribe drugs. Often two or more are needed to bring blood pressure down significantly. Be sure your parent takes these as directed and, if he has trouble with side effects, see if the doctor can't modify the dose or the drug.

drug companies, as well as large pharmacy chains, offer similar discount cards through their own programs. If your parent buys a particularly expensive drug routinely, call the company directly, or contact the Pharmaceutical Research and Manufacturers of America for information (800-762-4636 or www.helpingpatients.org).

Your parent can also order drugs through online or mail-order companies, which are often cheaper than the local pharmacy, especially when you order in bulk. There are dozens of such companies, most good, a few bad. This is a perfectly acceptable and safe thing to do. In fact, not only are the drugs often cheaper, but ordering online is convenient because your parent doesn't have to leave the house. But use caution and common sense. Compare several to find the best deal and the most reputable company.

The easiest way to find out if a Web site is run by a licensed pharmacy is to check for a VIPPS certification seal (Verified Internet Pharmacy Practice Sites), which means that the National Association of Boards of Pharmacy has approved it for online sales. (You can check a company's licensing or get a list of VIPPS pharmacies online at www.nabp.net.) Companies that sell online should require a prescription from a doctor, should verify that prescription, and should have a registered pharmacist available to answer questions. AARP (888-687-2277 or www.aarppharmacy.com) also has a prescription drug discount plan for members.

Other ways to save:

◆ See if there isn't a generic version of the drug. Generic drugs are just as effective and safe as their brand-name counterparts and usually much cheaper.

◆ Shop around. Pharmacy prices vary widely, even within one area. While it's wonderful to have one pharmacist who has a record of all the medications your parent takes, it might be cheaper to have a few sources. One supplier may have the lowest price on asthma medication, but another may have less expensive Prozac. Comparison shop any time she gets a new prescription.

◆ If a particular prescription is not included in your parent's drug coverage plan, ask the doctor if an equally effective drug is on the list of covered drugs. If not, see if the doctor might get an exception granted from the insurer.

◆ Ask the doctor about splitting pills. Sometimes, if your parent needs a dose of 40mg of a particular drug, it is cheaper to buy the pills in 80mg tablets and split them in half. (Your parent should not split pills and take less than directed. She should also ask the pharmacist if it's okay to split pills well in advance or if they need to be taken as soon as they are split.)

◆ Ask about free samples. Some doctors will dole out a small supply of free samples to help patients with expenses.

◆ Find out if a larger prescription might cost less. Often a bottle of fifty pills is cheaper than a bottle of twenty-five. Be sure they will keep, however.

◆ When starting a new prescription, ask the pharmacist to fill just part of the prescription. Then your parent can see if the drug causes any adverse reactions before she pays for the entire prescription.

◆ If your parent is in a nursing home, keep tabs on the cost of medications—both prescription and over-the-counter drugs. Many nursing homes charge wildly inflated rates—sometimes two or three times what a drug would cost elsewhere. If that's the case, demand the right to buy your parent's medications yourself.

◆ Associations and foundations connected to specific illnesses (Alzheimer's, Parkinson's, arthritis, etc.) often know of ways to get drugs pertaining to that illness at a discount.

Vision

When your mother squints and then stretches out her arm in order to make out the numbers in the phone book, it is probably because she has presbyopia. Presbyopia commonly sets in around age forty, when the lens of the eye becomes more rigid, making it hard for people to see close objects or small print. In most cases, presbyopia is easily remedied with a pair of reading glasses or bifocals. Magnifying glasses from the local drugstore are fine if the condition isn't complicated by other factors.

But there are a number of more subtle changes in vision that typically occur later in life, changes that your parent may not be aware of, but that will make life much harder for her. For example, older eyes can't see well in dim light, are more easily blinded by glare, and can't refocus quickly from near to far, or from light to dark. They also don't discriminate easily between colors and contrasts, such as the edge of a step, and they have trouble following moving objects, such as cars on the highway. Even if your parent insists that her vision hasn't changed, assume that it has and try to compensate wherever you can around the house. (Some tips are offered on pages 226 and 227.)

Older eyes also frequently suffer from excessive tears because they are more sensitive to wind, temperature changes, and light. Eyes can also get teary because they are overly dry, or because of something more serious, like an infection. Floaters, those tiny specks that seem to drift across the field of vision, can become annoying in old age. They cannot be wiped away; they are actually inside the eyeball. If they are bothersome, your parent should talk to an eye doctor, as floaters can be a sign of a more serious problem, like retinal detachment.

> " *When my mother's vision began to fade, she became quite depressed. She always loved to read, but that became more and more difficult until finally she couldn't do it at all. She started listening to the radio and watching television up close. But she missed her reading terribly.*
>
> *It was a nurse at the home who set her up with books on tape. She has a good tape player, and each month she receives a stack of tapes in the mail. She listens for hours, and the funny thing is that she has expanded her reading repertoire. She used to just read mysteries. Now it's political books, biographies, racy romances, classical books, everything. She listened to a book last month about World War II planes, and she was telling us all about them. She's like a kid again, learning all this stuff.*"
>
> —MEL T.

EYE DISEASES

IN ADDITION TO THE NORMAL VISION changes that happen with age, there are four eye diseases that frequently afflict older people:

◆ **Cataracts.** More than half of people over age sixty-five have cataracts, although in most cases the symptoms are mild. With age, areas in the transparent lens of the eye become cloudy,

MAKING THE WORLD MORE VISIBLE

◆ Brighten the house, especially in stairways and places where your parent reads. Older people need nearly three times as much light as younger people. A 75-watt bulb placed one or two feet away is usually fine for reading, but try different intensities to see what's most comfortable for your parent. (A reading light should be positioned behind the shoulder on the same side as your parent's better eye.)

◆ Decrease glare by covering shiny surfaces and avoiding waxy floors. Aim lights at a wall or ceiling to create indirect light. Add blinds or curtains to windows that tend to be filled with bright sunlight.

◆ Distribute light evenly, because old eyes have trouble refocusing when going from light to dark.

◆ Get your parent some sunglasses with 100 percent UV (ultraviolet) protection to cut down on glare and to protect her eyes from future damage.

◆ Put night-lights in the bedroom, hallways, and bathroom, as your parent's night vision may be poor.

◆ Use reflector tape or colored tape on the edges of stairs to make the steps easier to see.

◆ Make sure light switches are accessible at the entrance to all rooms.

◆ Install lights that are triggered by dusk.

◆ Your parent might buy a larger television or perhaps a black-and-white one, which is sometimes easier to view.

◆ Buy lubricating eye drops, sometimes called artificial tears (not saline solution or eye drops for redness), available in most pharmacies.

hindering vision, especially if the cataract is in the center of the lens.

Having cataracts is a little like viewing the world through a pair of fogged-up goggles, but the change happens so gradually that your parent may not realize anything is wrong. At first, he may simply have trouble doing things, and then become frustrated and embarrassed. Even mild cataracts can dull night vision and make the eyes extremely sensitive to glare and bright light, which make driving at night dangerous. Again, your parent should have regular eye exams.

Dryness, a common problem, makes eyes itch, sting, and burn. (If dry eyes persist, your parent should see an ophthalmologist, as chronic dryness can lead to more serious problems.)

◆ Check your parent's medications and then follow up with a call to the prescribing doctors' offices if you are concerned. Certain medications can disturb vision or make eyes dry.

◆ Review your parent's driving habits and urge him to avoid highways and night driving.

◆ Wear bright colors when you visit if your parent's vision has grown quite poor.

◆ Write notes in big, clear letters with a black-ink, felt-tipped pen.

◆ If your parent's vision is very faint, encourage her to touch things— hold your hand, feel your face, or explore a new object with her hands.

Sometimes a person can get by simply by using magnifiers and stronger lighting. But at some point, if the cataract interferes with everyday activities, surgery may be necessary. Cataract surgery is a relatively simple and painless procedure. More than 90 percent of patients experience dramatic improvement. The surgery is accomplished in less than an hour, usually in a hospital clinic or doctor's office, and your parent can return home the same day.

The eye takes about a month to heal fully and several more weeks to adjust. In the meantime, your parent can resume his regular daily activities, including driving, reading, and working, although he may have to wear large dark glasses to protect his eyes.

◆ **Glaucoma.** People usually don't experience symptoms of glaucoma until the damage is done—a good reason to get your parent to the eye doctor regularly! An eye doctor can detect the problem early and treat it. But untreated, glaucoma can lead to partial or total blindness that cannot be reversed.

For a variety of reasons, fluid inside the eyeball fails to drain adequately. It builds up until it squeezes the optic nerve in the back of the eye. Over time, the nerve is damaged irreversibly. This leads to vision loss or blindness. Glaucoma tends to run in families and is more common among African Americans, people with diabetes or previous eye injuries, and people who have used steroids over an extended period of time.

When the trouble is spotted early, medications (oral medications or eye drops) can stop or slow the damage. If your parent is given medications for glaucoma, it is critical that she continue to use them even if she doesn't notice any change in her symptoms.

When medications aren't working, doctors often recommend surgery to repair the eye's drainage system. Laser surgery, which can be performed in less than twenty minutes and is painless and often successful, is often tried before more traditional surgery is used.

◆ **Macular degeneration.** Or, more precisely, age-related macular degeneration, known as AMD. It is a disease of the retina, a thin layer of cells lining the back of the eye, which converts visual images into electrical impulses and sends them on to the brain. AMD occurs when the macula, the part of the retina responsible for seeing fine details in the center of the field of vision, breaks down or degenerates. This slowly creates a blind or fuzzy spot in the center of one's vision. Straight lines might seem curved, and printed words may look disjointed.

Macular degeneration usually affects both eyes (sometimes one at a time) and worsens steadily until the blurry area at the center of the field of vision completely blocks out, say, several words on a page—the very words the person is trying to read.

Most people have what's known as the "dry" form of AMD, which comes on slowly and is caused by deposits in the macula. The "wet" form is less common and more severe. Small blood vessels leak into the eye. Eventually, a person can lose all central vision. Age-related macular degeneration is the leading cause of severe vision loss among people over sixty.

Your parent should get medical help early. While there is no cure, there are treatments that can slow the dis-

---

MEDICAL ALERT

 Even in the absence of symptoms, the American Academy of Ophthalmology recommends that people over sixty-five have their eyes examined every two years, or more often if a person has an eye disease, a family history of eye disease, or another risk factor, such as diabetes.

Your parent should see an eye doctor immediately if:

◆ Her vision becomes blurred or distorted, or she complains of "seeing double"

◆ She sees flashes of light or halos

◆ Her eyes are sore, swollen, or leaking unusual amounts of discharge

◆ She has wandering or crossed eyes

◆ She loses her peripheral vision or her vision in one eye

◆ She becomes acutely sensitive to light and glare

ease. Research suggests that certain supplements (vitamins C and E, beta-carotene, zinc, and copper) can slow the loss of vision, but your parent should talk to his eye doctor and his primary doctor before taking any supplements. In some cases, laser surgery is helpful.

Once the damage is done, he should consult a low-vision specialist. With the low-vision aids that are available today and some motivation, your parent should be able to read and continue to do other activities he enjoys.

✦ **Diabetic retinopathy.** Blood vessels in the retina of the eye leak, blurring vision and, if left untreated, cause blindness. The longer someone has diabetes, the greater chance he has of developing this disease. The best prevention is proper care of the diabetes and annual eye exams. Laser treatment or surgery can often improve vision and slow the decline, but only modestly.

LOW-VISION AIDS

THERE IS A VAST ASSORTMENT OF low-vision products available that can make the world more visible—from magnifying glasses and large-print calculators to computers that talk and magnifiers that transfer the words in a book to a computer screen. These products can be found in some medical supply stores, through company catalogs, or online (search for "low-vision aids" and you'll find dozens of companies, or try some of the companies listed on page 132). Both the

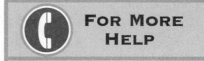

FOR MORE HELP

National Eye Institute
301-496-5248
www.nei.nih.gov

....

National Association for Visually Handicapped
800-677-9965
www.navh.org

....

National Federation of the Blind
410-659-9314
www.nfb.org

....

The Glaucoma Foundation
212-285-0080
www.glaucomafoundation.org

....

American Macular Degeneration Foundation
413-268-7660
www.macular.org

....

Lighthouse International
800-829-0500
www.lighthouse.org

National Federation of the Blind (www.nfb.org) and the National Association for Visually Handicapped (www.navh.org) have online shops. An eye doctor or other low-vision specialist should also be able to guide your parent to appropriate aids.

Many companies have special services for people who are totally or partially blind. For example, some telephone companies offer dialing aids, free operator assistance, and a list of special products to people with vision or hearing disabilities. Other companies may be willing to send catalogs, bills, or newsletters in large-print format.

Large-print books, magazines, and newspapers that are printed in

18-point type like this,

for example, are a godsend. The local library should have some, and others can be borrowed through an interlibrary loan.

Large bookstores, as well as online bookstores (www.amazon.com, www.barnesandnoble.com) have most top-selling books in large print, as well as audio books on cassette or CD. The National Association for Visually Handicapped (212-889-3141 or www. navh.org) has a lending library of large-print books. You can also make articles or documents more readable for your parent by duplicating them on a photocopy machine that enlarges the original.

The National Library Service for the Blind and Physically Handicapped (800-424-8567 or www.loc.gov/nls), which is part of the Library of Congress, lends audio books and magazines on cassette, as well as the equipment needed to play them, all for free. Postage is also free when returning equipment, tapes, or disks. Anyone with poor eyesight or a physical handicap that prevents him from holding a book or turning a page is eligible for these services, through the local library.

Hearing

Hearing loss among the elderly is a silent epidemic, so to speak. Estimates suggest that more than a third of people over sixty, and half of those over eighty-five, have significant hearing loss. But how many of these people have their hearing checked, visit hearing specialists, or wear a hearing aid? Very few. Which means that thousands of older people are walking around with little or no idea of what others are saying, even though help is available.

Loss of hearing can have a dramatic impact on your parent's life, more so than loss of vision. As Helen Keller put it, blindness cuts people off from the environment; deafness cuts them off from other people. Over time, poor hearing can make your parent withdrawn, irritable, and depressed.

Furthermore, it's dangerous. Your parent might not be able to hear fire alarms, oncoming cars or honking horns, emergency sirens, dogs barking, or other alerts.

Hearing loss goes untreated, in part, because doctors rarely screen for it and patients don't discuss it. Your parent may think that it's just a part of aging, or that you are just an incurable mumbler. Even if she recognized the problem, she might not want to wear a hearing aid. (Today's aids are barely visible; they work better than older models; and there are many other ways to help with hearing problems.)

Hearing loss also goes undiagnosed and untreated because it develops so gradually that the loss is almost imperceptible. People don't suddenly realize that they can't hear and call the doctor. Instead, they turn up the television, ask to have things repeated, and misunderstand the occasional comment.

With time, however, conversation becomes a chore, not a pleasure, and the person begins to withdraw and lose self-esteem. Depression is twice as common among people with hearing loss. In some cases, loss of hearing leads to delusions and other psychotic symptoms.

If your parent is saying "What?" a lot, or nodding without any understanding of what has been said, urge him to have his hearing checked by his doctor, or get his doctor to recommend an otologist or otolaryngologist (doctors who specialize in disorders of the ear). Sometimes the problem can be treated—for example, if an infection, earwax, or another obstruction is found. Assuming the problem is not curable, your parent should then see an audiologist, who will measure his hearing and suggest solutions.

Hearing loss can be addressed both by changes in the way people communicate (see box, page 233) and by the use of various types of aids. Technology being what it is, the menu of choices is growing daily. An audiologist can talk to your parent about his lifestyle and needs, and then discuss options that might be best for him. An audiologist should continue to work with your parent until he finds a reasonable solution.

Because this can be a sensitive subject, approach it gingerly. Ask your father if he thinks there is a problem, rather than telling him that there is one. And avoid criticism or accusations. *You never hear what I'm saying. You are deaf as a post.* Explain what he is missing by not dealing with his hearing loss and what he stands to gain by addressing it. Urge him to at least talk to an audiologist to get the facts and to learn what the options are. If he insists that he doesn't have a problem, that others mumble, don't fight it. *Perhaps I'm not speaking clearly and I need to work on that. Let's approach this together.*

PRESBYCUSIS

MORE THAN 90 PERCENT OF HEARING loss is the result of presbycusis, also referred to as sensorineural hearing loss or nerve deafness. Noise, diet, hypertension, infections, illness, head injury, genetics, and just plain time can all play a role, but generally presbycusis is thought to be a normal part of aging. People don't lose volume as much as they lose clarity, so again, they aren't aware that they are losing their hearing. Your father may be able to hear you just fine; the problem is that he can't understand you. Higher-pitched sounds, in particular, can become fuzzy (making it harder to understand women and children), and consonants, such as "s," "f," and "z," may be indistinguishable from one another. Your mother might ask you to repeat yourself, and when you do so in a louder voice, she says, "Don't shout! I'm not deaf, you know!"

Sensorineural hearing loss also makes it difficult to filter out background noise, so your parent may have more trouble hearing a conversation in a room full of people or if the television is on.

TINNITUS

TINNITUS CAUSES A RINGING, BUZZing, clicking, or hissing sound in the ear, which is not simply annoying; it can hinder hearing and make it almost impossible for some people to get through the day. It is caused by loud noise, medications, illness, allergies, and hearing loss itself.

If your parent has tinnitus, or suspects it, she should see her doctor to see if it is due to treatable causes. If it's not treatable, an audiologist can help find ways to alleviate it. Often, several approaches work better than just one.

A tinnitus mask fits on the ear and emits a "white noise" to drown out or soften the humming. Or your parent can create her own white noise by listening to the static of a radio or fuzzy television channel on low volume. "Bedside maskers" are little boxes that do basically the same thing. Or better yet, buy her some nature tapes of ocean waves, birds calling, crickets chirping, or the wind blowing, which will not only help soften the buzzing, but might also help her relax.

Relaxation techniques to reduce stress (which seems to worsen tinnitus) and biofeedback, in which a person learns to control certain bodily functions by becoming familiar with them, can be very helpful. Some medications are also used to alleviate tinnitus.

If other hearing loss is involved, then a hearing aid can ease the hearing loss and also, by amplifying other sounds, ease some of the tinnitus.

Finally, antidepressants are sometimes needed to ease some of the depression and anxiety that often accompanies tinnitus.

HELPFUL GADGETS

THERE ARE OTHER WAYS TO ENHANCE hearing. Systems can amplify televisions, radios, telephones, mobile phones, answering machines, pagers, computers, and almost anything else that involves noise. Some work with hearing aids; some are used without.

Special alarm systems are most important, and anyone can use them; they do not involve hearing aids. These include alarms for doorbells, telephone ringers, clocks, smoke detectors, carbon monoxide detectors, and the like. Some products provide a visual signal, such as flashing lights (and you can make them flash in different ways to differentiate the phone ringing from the doorbell buzzing, for example); some provide a tactile signal, such as a vibration; and others simply amplify the sound. If you do nothing else, be sure your parent can hear his smoke and carbon monoxide detectors.

MAKING THE WORLD MORE AUDIBLE

- Sit or stand within three feet of your parent when talking to him. (Don't yell to him from the kitchen.)

- Face your parent when you speak and be sure he is looking at you before you begin speaking. (And make sure his good ear is aimed in your direction.)

- Sit in the spotlight. There should be ample lighting, and it should be aimed at you, the speaker.

- Don't put your hands over any part of your face.

- Turn off the television, the running water, or other background noise.

- Speak clearly. Don't try to talk to your parent while you are eating, chewing gum, or smoking. Enunciate clearly, but don't exaggerate your lip movement, as that can make it difficult to read lips (which we all do a little, even without formal training).

- Speak loudly, but don't shout, because it will only make your words more difficult to understand. Increase your volume slightly, without raising your pitch.

- Use simple and direct sentences. When you are asked to repeat something, rephrase it. Different words may be easier for your parent to grasp.

- Use body language (touching, pointing, nodding) and lots of facial expression.

- Introduce the subject matter before starting a conversation. "Dad, about Thanksgiving. . . ." If you switch topics midway through a conversation, make that clear: "Okay, now let's talk about your friend Ralph. . . ."

- If you go to a restaurant, ask for the quietest table. Avoid tables near the kitchen or near bands or stereo speakers. Better yet, choose restaurants that are quiet or go at off times.

- Do not ignore the person with hearing loss, or talk about him, or for him, as if he were not present. This will only make him withdraw more and stop trying to understand.

- Whether or not your parent wears a hearing aid, he can also consult a speech therapist who can provide further tips to make the world more audible.

Your parent might also look into text telephones, which allow phone conversations to be typed, and closed-captioning television, which puts the words in text at the bottom of the screen and is available on all new TVs with screens larger than 13 inches (diagonally).

While many of these sorts of gadgets can be purchased online or through catalogs, it's best to buy any complex or expensive device in person, so your parent can get expert advice, see and discuss the options, and possibly even try out a product. Once he knows exactly what he wants, he might be able to find it online at a cheaper price, but he should check the return policy. Other items, such as vibrating alarms or amplifiers for a phone or television, are safe to buy from any reputable company.

ASSISTIVE LISTENING DEVICES

BASICALLY, THESE DEVICES AMPLIFY a desired sound (a person speaking in a restaurant, actors in a movie or play, a speaker at a lecture, a sermon, etc.) while reducing the volume of the other noise in the room. By placing a microphone close to the sound source, the device focuses on one sound while filtering out others.

Some are designed for close, one-on-one communication, while others are meant for distance, such as a movie theater or auditorium. Some are designed to be used alone; others can be used with a hearing aid or cochlear implant, improving the performance of the aid. (Don't let your parent think that a hearing aid is all he needs; the combination of hearing aid and a listening device can greatly improve hearing.) Many of the ones that are used in conjunction with a hearing aid require that the aid have a special switch called a "T-switch."

Some listening devices are simple, hard-wired affairs: a microphone for the speaker and a headset for the listener (or the sound can be delivered directly into a hearing aid). These are good for close proximity and intimate settings. Then there are three kinds of wireless systems, which are primarily used in theaters, lecture halls, and large places of worship. They include FM systems, which are like miniature radios; inductive loops, which transmit sounds using magnetic fields; and infrared systems, which use invisible infrared light to transmit sound. Most places that have such systems advertise it, or you can call and ask.

HEARING AIDS

THE MOVE TO HEARING AIDS, WITH all the stigma that is attached to them, may be a tough one. Your parent may resist this with his heels dug in. But don't give up easily because hearing aids will reconnect him to his world, his friends, family, and interests.

If your parent tried hearing aids in the past, got frustrated, and dumped them in the toilet, urge him to try again. The technology has changed a great deal and there are types—digital circuitry, implantable, programmable, telecoil, etc.—that work far better than those of yesterday.

Start by having him get his hearing checked to be sure there isn't a treatable problem—an infection or obstruction. (This is also helpful because now some of the onus of discussing hearing aids is on the doctor.)

While you plead and prod, be sympathetic to your father's distaste for this idea, his insistence that they don't work, or his concern that he'll look like an old man. Explain that many hearing aids today are barely noticeable. Explain to him that he looks older and more conspicuous when he's constantly asking people to repeat themselves, leaning forward with a hand cupped behind his ear, and missing entire conversations.

Once your parent agrees to try a hearing aid, his doctor should recommend someone to fit it for him—usually a certified audiologist, who has a graduate degree in hearing impairment, or a licensed hearing aid dealer, who has less training, but usually plenty of experience. Be sure your parent sees someone who is experienced and reputable and will spend a lot of time with him, because he will be extremely frustrated if a hearing aid is not properly fitted or suited to him.

The specialist should do a complete exam, including hearing tests and evaluations, and then discuss various kinds of hearing aids. He or she should take time to listen to your parent and understand his particular needs, as the best hearing aid for one person is not necessarily the best for another. Sometimes, an audiologist will let a person try a couple of options to see which one works best for him.

FINANCIAL AID

While a few insurance policies cover the costs of testing and even some part of the cost of a hearing aid or cochlear implant, most don't. As a result, many older people (as well as younger ones) don't buy the devices or choose a cheaper but less effective aid.

Help is available. Some civic and community organizations will help cover the cost of a hearing aid if your parent can't afford it. The Alexander Graham Bell Association for the Deaf and Hard of Hearing Web site (www.agbell.org) has a list of organizations that offer financial assistance, or you can call Self Help for Hard of Hearing People (301-657-2248) and an operator will tell you about organizations in your parent's area that offer financial assistance. You might also check with local civic organizations, the local senior center, the area agency on aging, and other community and religious organizations.

> *One night I took my mother to see a show in New York, figuring that even if she couldn't hear everything, she would enjoy the colors and lights and dancing. They had these plug-in amplifying headphones, and it was a miracle. For the first time in years, she could hear everything. She lit up. From then on, she went to the theater every chance she could."*
> —WILL B.

Models range from tiny ones that fit snugly, and almost invisibly, inside the ear canal, to ones that fit in the outer ear, to larger ones that curl around the outer part of the ear. While the smallest models are less visible, they sometimes have tiny control knobs that can be challenging for stiff fingers. Most hearing aids sold today are extremely small, in part because today's technology is so advanced.

The least expensive hearing aids simply amplify sound—all sounds. More expensive aids have microchips that allow the user to switch settings, depending upon the situation—a crowded restaurant, a quiet conversation, a large theater. Digital aids, which convert sound waves into digital signals, actually analyze the environment and reprogram themselves automatically. These are the most expensive aids, but they also offer the most precision and least feedback, or whistling.

Implantable hearing aids, which are particularly useful for people with mild to moderate hearing loss from nerve damage, don't tend to cause the whistling and distortion that sometimes come with traditional hearing aids, and they reduce occlusion—the feeling that you are hearing through a tunnel or can. Sound is generally clearer and more natural, and there is less interference from background noise. However, they are expensive, costing several thousand dollars (although some regular hearing aids cost that much).

The implantable aids are composed of a tiny magnet, which is implanted near the bones of the middle ear, and a sound processor, which is worn in the ear canal or behind the ear. The implant procedure is done with local anesthetic and takes about thirty minutes.

When buying any hearing aid, your parent should shop around because prices and service vary. While price is a pivotal factor, don't forget to shop for good service—personal attention, adjustments, warranties, repairs, and maintenance for the life of the aid. The aid should come with at least a thirty-day trial period, during which your parent can return the device with a full refund (most suppliers will charge a minimal service fee, and often costs for testing as well as any custom-fit parts are not refundable).

MAKING THE ADJUSTMENT

GETTING THE RIGHT HEARING AID IS only half of the battle. Now your parent needs to grow accustomed to wearing a piece of plastic in or around his ear, and to figure out the dials.

Most difficult of all, he has to adjust to a cacophony of new sounds. Unfortunately, a hearing aid is not like a pair of glasses. Your parent will not walk out of the hearing aid shop, suddenly have clear hearing, and say, "Wow, this is great!" A hearing aid not only makes the world louder; it can also make it sound hectic and distorted. Hearing aids are not like human ears; they don't selectively tune in one noise and tune out others.

Because it can be so hard to adjust to a hearing aid—and even harder late in life—and because a lot of hearing aids aren't fitted properly in the first place, nearly a quarter of the people who buy them end up not using them.

But if your parent gets the right device and some training, goes back for readjustments when necessary (and it's often necessary), and then can be convinced to wear it for, say, three to six months to get used to it, it is likely that he will adopt it for good and it will change his world.

Give him a lot of encouragement and support during this period, and try to be understanding. If he doesn't like his hearing aid, urge him to go back and try a different one or see if the one he has can be adjusted.

When whistling or ringing is a problem, which it commonly is, it's usually because the microphone is picking up noise, or feedback, from the amplifier inside the ear. Your parent should talk to the audiologist about ways to reduce the noise. If he changes

FOR MORE HELP

American Speech-Language-Hearing Association
800-638-8255
www.asha.org

Self Help for Hard of Hearing People
301-657-2248
www.shhh.org

American Tinnitus Association
800-634-8978
www.ata.org

National Institute on Deafness and Other Communication Disorders
800-241-1044
www.nidcd.nih.gov

American Academy of Audiology
800-222-2336
www.audiology.org

American Academy of Otolaryngology—Head and Neck Surgery
703-836-4444
www.entnet.org

hearing aids, he will need time to adjust to a new sound, as each hearing aid is different.

Your parent should not hesitate to go back to the specialist and discuss any problems he is having. Any good dispenser of aids will not only fit your parent with a hearing aid, but will then spend time making sure it's the right one and training him to use it correctly.

COCHLEAR IMPLANTS

FOR PEOPLE WHO ARE PROFOUNDLY deaf, cochlear implants can be the answer. However, they require surgery, they are very expensive (more than $50,000), and they require some training while the person learns to interpret the sounds created by the implant.

A cochlear implant is made up of three parts: a microphone, which picks up sound; a speech processor, which converts sound into electronic signals; and a receiver, which sends the signals to the brain. The microphone is worn behind the ear; the processor is about the size of a beeper and is carried in a pocket or slipped onto a belt; and the receiver is a disk about the size of a quarter, which is surgically implanted under the skin behind the ear.

While hearing aids amplify sound, implants actually compensate for damage to the ear, replicating what an ear normally does—convert sound waves into electrical impulses and send them to the brain, where they are recognizable. Still, an implant does not replicate that process perfectly, and the sound is not what it would be normally.

Sleep

Sleep, wonderful sleep. It's an elusive state for many older people. More than a third of people over sixty-five have trouble getting to sleep and staying there.

It's not that old age changes a person's need for sleep—Dad might be napping because he needs more sleep than he used to, or waking up at 5 A.M. because he needs less. Most people, at any age, need at least seven to eight hours of sleep each day. But after age forty, and certainly after sixty, people typically spend less time in the deepest stages of sleep. Their sleep is lighter, and they wake up more easily during the night. Some people do not even realize that they are waking up; they drift in and out of sleep without any recollection of it, and then don't understand why they are so tired the next day.

In addition to age-related changes in the body's sleep-wake cycle, pain, illness, depression, stress, grief, hormonal changes, inactivity, and poor diet are all to blame for disrupting normal sleeping patterns. So are drugs, especially diuretics, drugs used to treat Parkinson's disease, certain antidepressants, antihypertensives, steroids, decongestants, painkillers, and asthma medications, as well as caffeine, tobacco, and alcohol. Dementia, which upsets a person's 24-hour clock, can drive wake-sleep patterns even further out of kilter.

If your parent complains of insomnia, be sure her assessment is correct. Sometimes elderly people have misconceptions about sleep, believing they need more than they do. If your parent is bored, she might rather be asleep than awake, and consequently spends a lot of time in bed. The best indication of whether she is getting enough sleep is how refreshed and rested she feels when she wakes up.

If she is truly suffering from insomnia, whatever the underlying cause, it can plunge her into a downward tailspin. Worrying about sleep is the surest way to stay awake. Alcohol, sleeping pills, and going to bed too early—all intended to make resting more restful—just make matters worse.

Sleeping pills require special caution because they can have such dire effects on an elderly person. Yet the elderly use them disproportionately, consuming more than 25 percent of the sleeping pills sold in this country. Sleeping pills (including over-the-counter ones) should be used only as a last resort, for no more than several days at a time, and always under a doctor's guidance. They can cause confusion and anxiety in elderly people, especially when taken for long periods of time or in conjunction with other drugs. (It is possible for an older person who is using sleeping pills to become so disoriented that he is misdiagnosed as having dementia.)

SLEEP DISORDERS

THE ELDERLY ARE PRONE TO A number of sleep disorders, among them:

◆ **Restless leg syndrome and periodic limb movement disorder.** The former causes a person's legs to feel fidgety, tingly, and sometimes eager to run or move, just as he is

> " My Mom, who's always been one of the most chipper, upbeat people I know, became very depressed last fall. She was lethargic and mopey and didn't want to go out with her friends. On one visit I brought up the subject of her granddaughter's upcoming wedding, knowing she'd been looking forward to it for a long time. She sort of shrugged and said she'd go, 'If I'm still around.' That was so uncharacteristic of her that I urged her to see a doctor.
>
> He took her off the blood pressure pills that she'd been taking since she was sixty-five—that's about eighteen years. He said that age had changed her body chemistry so he changed the medication and greatly reduced the dosage. And sure enough, as soon as her medication was adjusted her spirits returned to normal. Not only did she get to the wedding but, as usual, she was the life of the party!"
>
> —LORETTA R.

trying to fall asleep, or after any prolonged period of inactivity (like sitting on a plane or bus).

In periodic limb movement, the limbs jerk involuntarily after a person has fallen asleep, disturbing rest but not waking the person fully. The movements last for only a few seconds, but they can recur often, every thirty seconds or so. (Periodic leg movements may disturb a spouse's sleep as well,

TIPS FOR A GOOD NIGHT'S SLEEP

There is no standard recipe for success, so get your parent to explore several approaches and see what works for her. Beyond the measures suggested here, she should talk with her doctor to see if there are any medications or illnesses that might be interfering with her sleep.

◆ Stick to a routine of going to bed and getting up at the same time each day, which will help regulate the body's clock.

◆ A pre-bed ritual, such as bathing, reading, or listening to music, may help your parent unwind and get her body in the mood for sleep. (She should not discuss stressful topics, play competitive card games, or watch upsetting late-night television just before bed.)

◆ Exercise, the elixir for so many problems, is a great antidote for insomnia. A brisk walk in the fresh air in the morning or afternoon is sure to help with sleep problems. Exercising near bedtime, however, may only worsen the insomnia.

◆ Stay awake. Seems like odd advice, but resting all day makes sleeping at night that much more difficult. Limit napping to no more than thirty minutes each day. Naps taken around the middle of the day—at about 2 or 3 P.M.—are the most refreshing. If your parent is nodding off in the late afternoon or early evening, this will interfere with a good night's rest. (Find out if she is dozing off in front of the television without realizing it.)

◆ Your parent should use the bathroom right before going to bed and try not to drink a lot of fluids late in the evening.

◆ Reserve the bedroom for sleeping and sex. Your parent shouldn't be getting in bed at 8 P.M. to read or watch television for an hour before turning the light out. She should wait until she is ready to sleep before she goes to bed.

◆ Make the bedroom conducive to sleep. It should be dark (but leave a night-light on if she's apt to get up in the night and might be confused), cool, and quiet. When noises are unavoidable, include some "white" noise, like a fan or the soft hum of radio static, to cover up more intermittent noises.

◆ The bedroom should feel safe, comfortable, and familiar. If your parent is in a new bedroom, fill it with familiar objects, photos, and mementos. Make sure she has a supportive, comfortable mattress and good pillows.

◆ Comfortable, loose-fitting sleepwear will help.

◆ Check all medications. Ask the doctor to review your parent's drugs to see if any might be affecting her sleep patterns. If so, see if the medication can be taken earlier in the day, if the prescription can be changed, or if the dose can be reduced.

◆ Dinner should be light, low-fat, and not excessively spicy, and it should be served several hours before bedtime. It's fine for your parent to have a snack before bed if she is apt to be awakened by hunger. A warm glass of milk just before climbing under the covers helps some people sleep.

◆ Tobacco, alcohol, and caffeine all interfere with normal sleeping patterns. Caffeine, which is a stimulant, is obviously a very bad idea in the evening. And even though a drink helps people relax, it also keeps them from falling into the deepest phases of sleep, and it causes them to wake in the middle of the night as the effects of the alcohol wear off. Nicotine is also a stimulant.

◆ Buy your parent a relaxation tape or teach her some mind-relaxing techniques. For example, ask her to close her eyes and imagine herself lying on the beach or some other favorite spot. In a slow, calm voice, tell her to smell the salty air, listen to the gentle rhythm of the waves, and feel the warmth of the sand against her body. Have her take deep, slow breaths as she feels the sun warming her skin and relaxing each muscle and joint— first her toes, then her ankles, legs, lower back, stomach, chest, shoulders, and eventually the muscles of her face. You can do this over the phone if need be, but with time, she should be able to do it for herself.

◆ When sleep doesn't come after, say, fifteen or twenty minutes, or if your parent is wakeful in the middle of the night, she should get up and read or knit or do something else, rather than lie in bed worrying about sleep.

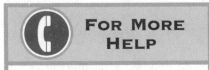

FOR MORE HELP

The National Center on Sleep Disorders Research
301-435-0199
www.nhlbi.nih.gov/about/ncsdr

....

The National Sleep Foundation
202-347-3471
www.sleepfoundation.org

....

Restless Legs Syndrome Foundation
507-287-6465
www.rls.org

....

American Sleep Apnea Association
202-293-3650
www.sleepapnea.org

so both your parents may be tired during the day. If so, they should move into separate beds.)

It's not clear what causes these syndromes, but they do have a genetic component. So if your mother is affected, you might well be, too. Caffeine, iron deficiency (anemia), and certain diseases also seem to play a role.

Caffeine should be limited and any iron deficiency should be remedied. Massaging the legs before bed, putting either hot or cold compresses on the legs, or taking a warm bath can help. Exercising during the day is always beneficial. Relaxation techniques before bed can help ease the

fidgets. While severe cases of restless leg syndrome can be treated with medications, drugs should be a last resort and used only under the supervision of a doctor.

When restless leg syndrome is accompanied by periodic limb movement, as it often is, and the person is not helped by other methods, doctors sometimes prescribe something called "transcutaneous electric nerve stimulation," in which electric stimulation is applied to the legs for fifteen to thirty minutes just before going to bed.

◆ **Sleep apnea.** For various reasons, some people stop breathing for several seconds or even a couple of minutes, often repeatedly through the night. The sleeper is jarred awake as he gasps for a breath, but the awakenings are so brief that he usually isn't aware of them.

Obstructive sleep apnea, which is most common in overweight men, is often caused by an obstruction in the airway—the muscles in the throat relax and block the airway—so that air cannot flow out of the nose or mouth.

In a less common type of sleep apnea, called central sleep apnea, the brain fails to regulate breathing properly during sleep.

In some cases, people stop breathing twenty or thirty times per hour, leaving them exhausted the next day. They often have headaches in the morning and, with time, can develop high blood pressure, depression, irritability, and memory problems. It also seems to increase the risk of heart attack and stroke.

The most obvious symptoms are loud snoring and daytime fatigue. To get it diagnosed with certainty, however, your parent should visit a sleep clinic. Sleep specialists have a number of ways of treating apnea, including weight loss and banning the use of alcohol, tobacco, and sleeping pills (which make it more likely that the airways will collapse at night). Pillows can be used to keep the sleeper on his side, rather than his back.

Treatment commonly includes the use of an air pressure gadget that the sleeper wears at night. A mask is worn over the nose, and air is forced into the nasal passages to prevent the airway from closing.

Dental appliances are sometimes used to reposition the lower jaw. In extreme cases, doctors may recommend surgery to remove excessive tissue and increase the size of the airway.

YOUR SLEEP

IF YOUR MOTHER LIVES WITH OTHERS, her lack of sleep can affect everyone in the household. She may keep others awake at night if she is pacing, tossing about, or watching television. She may be grumpy, distracted, depressed, and increasingly susceptible to illness as her immune system tires out.

Try the tips on pages 240 and 241. Then, buy yourself some earplugs and be sure your parent's room is set up so she can get whatever she needs—

a lamp and a glass of water on the night table, a commode by the bed, etc. (You don't want her wandering around the house looking for a cup.)

If nothing helps, you may have to put your needs above hers. As a caregiver, you are pushed to your limit during the day; you need your sleep at night. Talk to the doctor about the possibility of getting sleeping pills for her. While it's not ideal and careful monitoring is required, it's sometimes necessary to give an elderly person sleeping pills so the rest of the family can sleep. If this is not medically advisable, consider hiring someone to cover for you during the evenings, or you may have to start looking into other housing options for your parent.

Temperature Regulation

Older people can become severely chilled simply sleeping in a cool room, or dangerously overheated in temperatures that the rest of us find quite comfortable.

Much of the problem is biological. Older bodies have less protective fat and aren't as adept at constricting and dilating blood vessels, or shivering and sweating. Disease can further weaken the body's ability to warm itself or cool itself. Also, in certain situations, an elderly brain, especially if it's confused, may fail to get the message that the body is too cold or too hot. As a result, your parent might

RECOGNIZING A TEMPERATURE CRISIS

WARNING: Hyperthermia and hypothermia are both medical emergencies that require immediate medical attention.

Signs and Symptoms	What to Do
Hyperthermia Heat exhaustion: 　Clammy, pale skin 　Heavy sweating 　Dizziness 　Weakness 　Nausea 　Headache 　Cramps 　Chills 　Rapid, shallow breathing 　Swelling of ankles and feet	Get your parent to a cool room or shaded area. Make him lie down, with his feet raised about 12 inches. Remove or loosen clothing and sponge his forehead and body with cool (not cold) water. Give him water, preferably with a little salt in it, or a drink like Gatorade. Do not bring his temperature down too quickly. Call the doctor.
Heatstroke: 　Hot, dry, red skin 　No sweat 　Rapid pulse 　Body temperature above 104°F 　Unconsciousness or confusion	Call an ambulance immediately. While waiting, keep your parent in a sitting position. Sponge him off and wrap him in a cool (not cold), wet sheet. Give him plenty of water. Do not bring his temperature down too quickly (because it can cause a heart attack) or overcool him.
Hypothermia 　Listless or drowsy 　Pale complexion 　Confusion 　Slow, shallow breathing 　Slurred speech 　Stiff movements 　Shivering (but not necessarily) 　Weak pulse 　Body temperature below 95°F 　Finally, unconsciousness	Call the doctor or 911 immediately. While you are waiting (turn off any air conditioner or fan, of course), turn up the heat, or move your parent to a warmer room. Do not warm him too quickly. Get him into sweaters and a hat and under blankets, or lie close to him and share your body heat. Do not rub him, however, as you might actually injure him. Offer warm (not hot) fluids. Do not let him go to sleep.

stay out in the hot sun for a danger-ously long time, or fail to use a blanket on a cool night.

Some of the problem is also practical. A person with a physical disability or a painful ailment may not want to pull himself up out of a chair to get a sweater or to move into another room that's cooler. Or, in an attempt to save money, your parent may keep the thermostat low or forego air conditioning.

So when the snow is falling or the mercury rising, remind your parent to dress accordingly and protect himself. When you are nearby, be aware of his comfort.

As a summer day heats up, give him plenty of cool drinks and keep physical activity to a minimum. If he doesn't have an air conditioner or fan, look into getting one. Contact the area on aging or local senior center about programs to help people pay for room air conditioners. Otherwise, create as much ventilation as possible by opening windows and doors. Keep direct sunlight out with curtains or shades. If his apartment is hot, your parent should spend the hottest part of the day elsewhere—in an air-conditioned library, mall, or other public place.

In winter, his house should be kept no cooler than 68°F, even at night. Be sure there are plenty of blankets, slippers, sweaters, long underwear, and hats on hand. Your parent might wear a light hat to bed, as body heat escapes through the head, especially when a person's hair has thinned.

Hyperthermia (when the body's temperature gets too high) and hypothermia (when it gets too low) are both medical emergencies. They are particularly worrisome in people who have dementia, stroke, or other neurological disorders, thyroid disorders, Parkinson's disease, diabetes, or cardiovascular disease, or are taking medications that make the body's temperature fluctuate. So be on the alert for symptoms.

Dehydration

Normally, when a body is low on fluids, the kidneys go into an emergency mode and hold on to water, and the brain screams out, "I'm thirsty. I need water." But older kidneys are less efficient at conserving fluids, and the brain may not be getting these messages of thirst, especially if a person·suffers from dementia. Even when the message does come through, a person with mobility problems might decide that a trip to the tap is not worth the effort.

As a result, an older person can become dehydrated easily, and grow confused, tired, light-headed, and faint as his body dries out, yet he may still be unaware that he needs water. Over time, ignoring the body's need for fluids can cause bowel problems, kidney trouble, urinary tract infections, and even delirium.

Get your father to keep a glass or bottle of water (or some other non-caffeinated fluid) nearby at all times, and to make a point of sipping from it as often as possible. Eight glasses of fluid a day is the usual recommendation, but four to six will do. Unless the doctor wants your father to cut down on fluids for medical reasons, it is not possible for him to drink too much water.

Make sure that he isn't limiting his drinking because of incontinence. Consuming less water won't help; it will only cause new problems.

Skin Care

Skin announces the onset of old age with cracks, wrinkles, and spots long before any of us are ready for it, but usually the sags and blemishes are simply ego deflators, caused not by age but all that time in the sun. When we become quite old, however, skin problems can be more serious.

The three most common skin problems facing the elderly, aside from skin cancer, are itchiness, fungal infections, and bedsores. Older skin is thinner and less oily, so it tends to be drier and more susceptible to bruises, infections, and rashes. When injured, it doesn't heal as quickly as it once did, and minor irritations can become seri-ous wounds. All of this means that your parent's skin needs extra TLC.

Itchy, dry skin is the most common skin complaint, especially in the winter when the air is less humid. It may not seem particularly important in the overall scheme of things, but severely itchy skin (known as pruritus) can be horribly annoying and, over time, it can make your parent irritable, and weary from lack of sleep. Here are some ways your parent can ease the dryness and the itch:

◆ Take fewer showers or baths (two or three a week is fine) and keep them short and not too hot. Water and heat draw moisture away from the skin. Hot water is more irritating than warm.

◆ Use a minimal amount of soap, which removes the skin's natural oils. Avoid deodorant and perfumed soaps, which contain chemical irritants. Instead, use glycerin soap with cleansing cream, such as Dove, Basis, or Tone, and then rinse well.

◆ Avoid scrubbing harshly. Use a soft cloth or natural sponge instead of a brush or rough washcloth.

◆ Moisturize. After a bath or shower, your parent should pat his skin dry gently, leaving it moist, and then immediately apply a moisturizer to lock in moisture. Find a moisturizer with petrolatum high on the list of ingredients and avoid moisturizers that contain alcohol, which dries the skin. (Your father may not be in the habit of using lotion, but buy an unscented one and give him a nudge.)

◆ If your parent takes baths, she can add colloidal oatmeal, or cornstarch to the tub water.

◆ Apply pure petroleum jelly to very dry areas after a bath or shower. Your parent might wear pajamas, socks, or something else to protect clothing or sheets from the grease.

◆ Keep sheets and clothing clean. All new clothing should be washed before wearing. Avoid bleaches, fabric softeners, and heavily perfumed detergents, which can irritate skin. Rinse clothes well.

◆ Get your parent to wear cotton, which is less irritating than wool or synthetic clothing.

◆ A humidifier can put a little moisture into dry winter air. But change the water daily and keep the unit clean, as it can breed bacteria and other germs.

◆ Be sure your parent drinks lots of fluids.

◆ Steer him away from alcohol, spicy foods, tobacco, and caffeine.

◆ If itching becomes severe, try calamine lotion, cold compresses, or cortisone creams. Urge your parent to control his scratching (short fingernails and/or gloves will help), which may only aggravate the itch.

◆ If your parent's itching or dryness is severe and doesn't let up, or if itching becomes a nervous habit and is causing sores and bleeding, be sure he sees his doctor or a dermatologist.

Fungal infections can crop up if your parent's immune system is weak or his circulation poor, if he has diabetes, or if he takes antibiotics or corticosteroid drugs.

Fungus grows in warm, moist pockets of the body, like armpits, genitals, the scalp, the mouth, and the spaces around nails and between toes. It causes itchy, cracked skin, which can become infected. If your parent has a fungal infection, she should talk with her doctor. In the meantime, to prevent or help get rid of fungal infections:

◆ Keep skin clean and dry. Use a hair dryer on a cool setting to dry hard-to-reach places.

◆ Wear loose cotton clothing, including underwear and socks (synthetics don't let air circulate as well). Avoid pantyhose.

◆ Change shoes and socks once or twice a day and, if possible, wear sandals or shoes made of mesh or woven fabric that lets air circulate.

◆ Use over-the-counter antifungal cream or powder.

Shingles, or herpes zoster, is a disease of the nervous system that affects the skin. It is caused by the same virus that causes chicken pox. Small amounts of the virus sit dormant in the nervous system for years and then, because of a weakened immune system, stress, or illness, the virus is revived.

The virus travels along the nerves toward the skin, causing fatigue, headaches, and chills several days before the disease is visible—symptoms that can lead to misdiagnosis. Then, as with chicken pox, small blisters appear, but usually only on one patch of the skin, not over the whole body. When the blisters open, shingles can be extremely painful, and the skin can continue to be sensitive for two to four weeks after the blisters have healed. In older people, scarring may ocur.

Antiviral drugs should be started immediately, as they can affect both the severity and duration of the outbreak. Corticosteriods and aspirin will often ease the symptoms, as will a cool compress. Some studies suggest that the practice of tai chi, which helps a person relax, increases a person's immunity to shingles. A vaccine is under study.

Skin infections are common in older people who are ill and quite frail, especially those who have poor circulation, diabetes, or edema. The two most common skin infections—cellulitis and erysipelas—often start at the site of a scratch or wound, and grow into a red rash that is tender and warm to the touch. Erysipelas is often found on the face, has well-defined

ON THE ALERT FOR SKIN CANCER

 Blemishes, warts, freckles, skin tags (tiny, flesh-colored or brown flaps of skin), red dots, moles, and other markings are part of old age. Most are harmless results of sun damage and the aging process, but keep a watchful eye, especially if there is no spouse around who can check your parent's body.

Any moles or other markings that appear suddenly or grow rapidly, are larger than one-quarter of an inch across, bleed or look unusual (for example, pearly round spots, gritty red patches, or irregularly shaped dark moles) could suggest skin cancer and should be seen immediately by your parent's doctor or her dermatologist.

A skin exam should be part of every physical, but since some doctors overlook this, it's worthwhile to ask if he or she will inspect your parent's skin. If anything seems suspicious, the doctor will refer your parent to a dermatologist. If your parent has a history of skin cancer, she should see a dermatologist regularly.

If you provide any hands-on care (and therefore routinely see your parent's skin), be sure to keep an eye out for suspicious moles and bring them to the attention of the doctor.

borders, can cause flulike symptoms, and can lead to serious eye problems as well as blood poisoning or clotting. Either type of infection requires a doctor's immediate attention.

Skin reactions to medications include swelling, burning, itching, blisters, allergic reactions such as hives or rashes, and a heightened sensitivity to the sun (unusual burning or staining after being in the sun). The doctor may be able to change the medication, lower the dosage or, at the very least, treat the reaction. Such reactions may occur after your parent has stopped taking a medication, so keep those medication records handy.

Whether or not she is using medications, your parent should forgo lengthy sunbathing and should wear a strong sunscreen (SPF 15 or higher) anytime she is in the sun for more than a few minutes. (Of course, this precaution applies to everyone, no matter what his or her age.)

PREVENTING BEDSORES

BEDSORES ARE A THREAT ANYTIME your parent is confined to a bed or a chair. The elderly are particularly susceptible to bedsores because their skin is thin and their circulation weak. Continuous pressure on a bony area, such as the heel, elbow, the back of the head, or buttocks, blocks the flow of blood, which damages the skin and tissue below and causes redness, blisters, or open sores. Here are some ways to prevent them:

◆ If your parent is bedridden, he should be repositioned every hour or two, or should shift himself regularly if possible. Move him gently because even being pulled across the sheets can harm his tender skin. Use pillows to raise his heels or elbows off the bed, or to relieve the pressure on his buttocks, hips, and knees.

◆ Get your parent to stand up, sit in a chair, or move about if he can. If he can't, get him to wiggle his toes, flex his arms, jiggle his legs, and rotate his neck — whatever movement is possible—to keep the blood flowing. This should help prevent not only bedsores, but also blood clots, which can form when the body is still.

◆ Be sure your parent's skin is clean and dry, as moisture adds to the risk of bedsores. His sheets should be changed regularly, especially if he is incontinent or sweaty.

◆ Use an egg-crate foam mattress on top of the existing mattress to cushion your parent's body and relieve the pressure of his own weight. More elaborate options include waterbeds and air-filled mattresses.

◆ Elevate his head only slightly, because when the head is raised high, it puts pressure on the back.

◆ Pads of sheepskin will help protect elbows, heels, and other vulnerable areas. You can also buy small trapezelike gadgets that hold the feet up off the bed. (Avoid doughnut-shaped cushions, which cut off the blood supply to the skin that's suspended in the center of the cushion.)

◆ Gentle massage will stimulate circulation (and is wonderful for physical and emotional comfort). But don't massage areas that have become slightly red, because the friction can damage the skin even more.

◆ At the first sign of any redness, alert a doctor or nurse. Untreated, bedsores can become infected and life-threatening.

TLC FOR LEGS AND FEET

◆ Rest with the legs elevated. Avoid long periods of standing or sitting with the legs crossed or folded.

◆ Wash feet daily with mild soap and warm water, rinse and towel dry, being sure to dry between the toes.

◆ Rub lanolin or cold cream into dry feet or skin.

◆ Keep feet warm and dry. Wear shoes made of a material that lets air flow (cotton, mesh, or real leather) and use cotton or wool socks—no synthetics, please. Change socks as often as necessary to keep feet dry and clean.

◆ Be sure your parent is wearing the right size shoe, as feet often expand with age. Shoes should have low or no heels, firm soles, and preferably a wide cut across the toes.

◆ Use thicker socks instead of heating pads and water bottles to warm up cold feet.

◆ Walking or other exercise, foot massages, and leg massages all improve blood flow.

◆ A warm foot bath is soothing for the soul as well as the soles.

◆ Keep toenails trimmed, straight across, to avoid ingrown nails.

◆ Never cut or shave off corns. Over-the-counter medications may help, but they can also burn the skin, so use them cautiously. Small, doughnut-shaped pads can relieve some of the shoe pressure on corns. If they reappear, consult a doctor.

◆ Check feet regularly for cuts, infections, bumps, discoloration, bruises, and other signs of trouble.

◆ If your parent has diabetes, her feet will require special attention, as diabetes affects blood flow and puts the feet at extra risk of infections.

Arms, Legs, and Feet

◆ **Stasis dermatitis.** When a person has poor circulation, fluids often accumulate in the limbs and slow the usual back-and-forth flow of nutrients and waste, causing swelling. The skin becomes cracked and discolored with reddish-brown patches or itchy purple dots, and varicose veins may appear.

If your parent has these symptoms, she should see her doctor because the problem can become severe. Treatment involves reducing pressure in the veins by using support stockings, elevating the legs, and, in some cases, using ointments to reduce the itching.

◆ **Varicose veins.** The bulging blue veins that squiggle down your mother's leg can be painful. They are not, however, dangerous. Veins become distended because the valves that are supposed to keep uphill-flowing blood from draining downhill don't work. Instead, blood headed for the heart flows back down the leg. Your mother should avoid standing for long periods of time and lie down whenever possible with her feet elevated. Support hose (available from a medical supply store) should also help.

◆ **Foot troubles.** After seventy or eighty years of pounding, stamping, and stomping, feet get pretty worn out, but caregivers and doctors alike often neglect them. Goodness knows, they aren't much to look at. But without proper care, the various calluses, corns, bunions, infections, and other sores that develop can become severe and make it difficult and sometimes impossible for your parent to get around on his own two feet.

◆ **Peripheral artery disease.** The blocked arteries of the heart that everyone talks about can also occur in the legs. In fact, atherosclerosis of the legs is extremely common, extremely dangerous, and typically not diagnosed or treated in the elderly. Sometimes a person feels pain in the calf area when walking, or there is discoloration of the legs or feet, or sores that fail to heal, or numbness and coldness in the leg or foot. Usually, however, there are no symptoms at all. But when fatty pieces in the arteries of the leg come loose and travel up to the heart or brain, it can cause a heart attack or stroke.

Risk factors include old age, cigarette smoking, diabetes, high blood pressure, and obesity. Treatment usually begins with exercise, smoking cessation, and weight loss, when necessary. Foot care (see box on page 250) is important. Medications may be necessary.

Teeth and Mouth

Just because your father is old does not mean he has outgrown the dentist's chair. In fact, older people are at more risk than ever of oral cancer,

MEDICAL ALERT

Red or white spots, sores or lumps in the mouth, difficulty chewing or swallowing, or bleeding that does not go away within two weeks should be checked by a dentist, as they can be an early sign of oral cancer.

and people over sixty-five have more tooth decay than other age groups. Furthermore, studies now suggest that brushing, flossing, and visiting the dentist regularly can reduce the risk of heart disease. Bacteria in the mouth can apparently enter the blood stream and wreak havoc in the heart.

Trouble arises for all sorts of reasons. Elderly people often produce less saliva, which is needed to cleanse the teeth. (Dry mouth, by the way, is not a normal part of aging. It is the result of disease, medications, or medical treatments. So if your parent complains of dryness or you notice it, she should talk with her doctor about causes and ways to improve salivary flow.) Some people have problems brushing properly and flossing if they can't see well or have difficulty moving their arms, hands, or wrists. Also, with age, the gums shrink, exposing vulnerable areas of each tooth to potential infection or decay. All of this puts your parent at greater risk of dental problems.

Your parent should see the dentist at least once a year. Dental problems are not only painful and dangerous, they can also make chewing difficult, which can lead to poor nutrition. You or your parent should be sure to alert the dentist about any health problems your parent has, medications she is taking, or treatments she is receiving. Some medications, for instance, don't mix well with the painkillers, antibiotics, and anesthesia used by dentists. She should also alert the dentist to any pain or sores, or problems she has with swallowing, chewing, or dryness.

Wearing dentures is no excuse for skipping checkups or ignoring dental hygiene. False teeth, like glasses, need to be checked and refitted, and the gums, tongue, and insides of the cheeks still need some brushing to kill bacteria and keep the breath fresh.

Here are some tips on caring for your parent's mouth:

◆ See that your parent visits the dentist at least once a year. If he doesn't have a good one, find a dentist with experience in treating elderly patients (some medical schools have postgraduate training in geriatric dentistry).

◆ Be sure he uses toothpaste with fluoride, which helps prevent decay, and brushes at least twice a day. And floss. Don't forget the floss!

◆ If your parent is having trouble managing a toothbrush, elongate the brush by taping a sturdy wooden or plastic stick to it, or enlarge it by attaching a rubber or plastic foam ball to the handle.

◆ An electric toothbrush is sometimes easier to use, but have the dentist or dental hygienist show your parent the best way to use it.

◆ Buy flossing gadgets with handles. They're easier to manage.

◆ If your parent's mouth is dry, ask his doctor if medication might be to blame. Maybe the dose can be lowered or the prescription changed. (Diuretics, antihistamines, antihypertensives, antianxiety drugs, antidepressants, antipsychotics, and drugs for Parkinson's disease all slow the flow of saliva.)

◆ Dry mouth can be relieved temporarily with sugarless candies or gum. Lip lubricants are a must, and chips of ice or sips of water will also help. Citrus fruits wet the mouth but also rinse it in harmful acid, so limit the oranges.

◆ If you brush your parent's teeth for him, ask the dentist or dental hygienist to show you how. (Again, using an electric toothbrush is easier.)

◆ If your parent has trouble swallowing, or if he is confined to bed, skip or limit the toothpaste because he may choke on the foam. Just use a wet brush, or simply wipe his teeth and gums with a damp cloth.

◆ If your parent has recently converted to dentures, he might find eating easier if he has food that is easy to chew, bite-sized, and not sticky.

If you're gasping for air because your father has bad breath, you need to decide just how big a problem it is. Be sensitive. The odor may be caused by his medications or illness, so he may not be able to do anything about it.

If you can tactfully broach the subject, let your parent know that better oral hygiene can help kill some of the germs that cause bad breath. Your parent should brush the roof of his mouth, his tongue, and the inside of his cheeks, in addition to his teeth. Most breath mints and mouthwashes merely cover up odor, but gargling should help, as it loosens mucus lodged at the back of the throat.

Chapter Twelve

THE BODY IMPERFECT

PART II

Bones and Joints • Incontinence • Constipation
• Other Digestive Disorders

S OMETIMES EVEN FAIRLY SERIOUS HEALTH PROBLEMS DO NOT get the full attention of a busy doctor. Or they may not be mentioned to the doctor if your parent is embarrassed about them or believes they can't be treated. Your father may assume that achy, stiff joints are a condition he has to live with. Your mother might be ashamed of her incontinence and so, keeps it a secret. Or your parent might not realize that constipation is treatable. Again, most of these ailments can be treated, and adjustments to your parent's house and daily habits should make any remaining symptoms more bearable.

Learn the warning signs. If you suspect anything is wrong, urge your parent to talk with the doctor. If she denies there's anything wrong, let her know that if she ever had such a problem, she is not alone, and there are treatments. When the problem is severe or affects others (immobilizing arthritis, paralyzing depression, or incontinence), consult the doctor yourself. Your parent may not care if his illness is treated, but you do.

ON THE LOOKOUT FOR SYMPTOMS

Problem	Signs of Trouble
Osteoporosis	Few symptoms until a bone is broken; risk factors include being a woman, old age, a family history of the disease, being thin, smoking, not exercising, and early menopause
Osteoarthritis	Painful joints; achy, stiff movement, especially first thing in the morning
Incontinence	Stains or odors, wet sheets, reluctance to go out
Diabetes	Fatigue, weight loss, blurred vision, itchy skin, frequent urination, thirst, sensations of tingling or numbness, confusion, depression
Anemia	Fatigue, headaches, chest pains, confusion, and, in some cases, a sore tongue

Bones and Joints

The human skeleton may look like a fixed, immutable frame, especially when it's hanging in a biology classroom, but skeletons are living organs that change with diet, exercise, body chemistry and, yes, age.

No matter what else ails your parent, you need to be aware of his body's scaffolding, because when it breaks, the rest of the structure can quickly collapse. Older bones don't heal easily, and your parent may be laid up for months, putting her at risk of circulation problems, bedsores, pneumonia, lung complications, and death.

OSTEOPOROSIS

WITH OSTEOPOROSIS, HEALTHY BONES look like termite-eaten pieces of driftwood, and they can break very easily. It is primarily a woman's ailment because after menopause, when the production of estrogen slows, bone loss occurs rapidly. Women also start out with thinner bones and they live longer, so they are more affected.

But your father is not immune to osteoporosis. As testosterone levels drop, bones lose mass. In fact, about a quarter of people with osteoporosis are men. Unfortunately, old age, along with the changes and inactivity that typically accompanies it, whittles away at the bones of all older people.

Over time, the body's frame can become so brittle that tumbling off a step or tripping on a bathroom rug is all it takes to break a wrist, hip, or other bone. Breaking a hip is serious business. Somewhere between 15 and 25 percent of elderly people who fracture a hip die within a year of their accident, and another 25 percent lose their independence and require long-term nursing care. The bones of the spinal cord can also collapse and compress from osteoporosis, causing deformity and crippling back pain.

The odds of your parent having osteoporosis are staggering. Half of all women and a quarter of all men will fracture a bone due to osteoporosis in their later years. Thirty-two percent of women and 17 percent of men break a hip by the time they are ninety, and osteoporosis is largely to blame.

Spotting Osteoporosis

There are virtually no symptoms of osteoporosis until a bone is broken, which is why it is known as a "silent disease." Stooped posture and a decrease in height, however, often accompany spinal osteoporosis.

A number of factors increase a person's chances of having the disease: old age; being a woman; having a thin body or small frame; a family history of osteoporosis; a diet low in calcium throughout life; a sedentary lifestyle; early menopause (before age forty-five); the absence of estrogen replacement therapy soon after menopause; habitual smoking; and excessive drinking. For reasons that are unclear, Caucasian and Asian American women are far more prone to the disease than are African American women.

Because there are now a number of treatments available to fight osteoporosis, the National Osteoporosis Foundation recommends that all women over sixty-five have their bone density tested. The recommendation is less clear for men, although many doctors argue that men should be routinely tested after age eighty. The tests are expensive, however. Medicare and many other insurance policies cover the cost for elderly women, and for men only when it is deemed medically necessary.

A bone density test is a good idea, but risk alone merits preventative steps—and simply being old is a risk. But if your parent needs convincing, have her talk with her doctor. A look at her medical history and a physical exam, along with some professional advice, should help her understand the importance of prevention and treatment.

Combating Osteoporosis

The best time to fight osteoporosis is long before it sets in, by exercising regularly, getting plenty of calcium and vitamin D, avoiding cigarettes, and keeping alcohol use under control. In fact, prevention of osteoporosis actually begins in childhood, when bones are developing, by getting plenty of calcium, vitamin D, and exercise.

But the battle is not lost at age seventy. With all sorts of new drugs on the market, along with lifestyle changes and precautions, people can strengthen their bones and prevent fractures, even late in life. But do the work now, before there is an accident.

◆ **Exercise.** Frail people, especially those worried about falling, tend to stay sedentary, safely propped up in the living-room chair. But that is absolutely the worst thing to do.

Walking, swimming, riding a stationary bike, lifting weights, and other exercise all strengthen muscles and bones; the bones actually get thicker and stronger. Most important, though, is that exercise enhances balance, coordination, and reflexes, which reduces the risk of falling.

An exercise regime should involve muscles throughout the body. Weight-bearing exercises (in which one is holding up his or her own weight, like walking), as well as weight machines and weight lifting, are all excellent ways to fight osteoporosis. In one study, very frail nursing-home residents put on an exercise regime dramatically increased their muscle strength and even their bone mass in just ten weeks. Practicing tai chi, which improves balance, has been

> *My mother started going downhill after she fell three years ago and broke her hip. Before that she had been very active, going up to Maine for the summers and going into the city on weekends. But the fall slowed her down tremendously. She lost her gusto for life. It's a constant effort to restore her confidence."*
>
> —KEVIN B.

shown to be particularly helpful in reducing falls. (For more on exercise, see page 66.)

◆ **Calcium, vitamin D, and healthful eating.** Ample calcium and vitamin D decrease the rate of bone loss, and reduce the risk of fractures by nearly 30 percent.

Experts recommend that elderly people get 1,200mg (milligrams) of calcium and 400 IU (international units) of vitamin D each day. Some recommend that women who are not taking any estrogen need even more: 1,500mg of calcium and 800 IU of vitamin D a day. Your parent should talk with her doctor.

To meet this requirement, a person would have to drink at least a quart of milk each day, so before your mother goes on a milk binge, buy her some calcium supplements with vitamin D, which helps the body absorb the calcium effectively. Supplements are particularly important for those who get

MEDICAL ALERT

If your parent faints, nearly faints, or has dizzy spells, get her to her doctor. While fainting may be caused by something simple, such as reduced blood flow to the brain due to advanced age or medications, it can also indicate more serious conditions. Any form of dizziness needs to be evaluated.

little calcium in their diet and little sun exposure, such as nursing-home residents during the winter months. Exposure to the sun is necessary for the body to make vitamin D.

Of the many calcium supplements available, calcium citrate causes fewer problems (like constipation) and is more easily absorbed into the body. Your parent might also be able to increase calcium and vitamin D at least somewhat through her diet and then need to take less in a supplement. (For more on calcium and a list of some high-calcium foods, see pages 660–661.)

Adequate vitamin K intake is also important, as it is associated with decreased fracture risk. Keeping sodium (salt) to a minimum also seems to help reduce calcium loss. Newer research suggests that too much retinol, a form of vitamin A, can actually increase the risk of fractures.

◆ **Smoking.** Easier said than done, but nevertheless, your parent should give up cigarettes, which weaken bones. (See page 80 for more on this.)

◆ **Fall prevention.** Even people without osteoporosis can stumble and break a bone. So regardless of your parent's bone density, her house should be made "fall-safe." That means ample lighting, well-secured rugs, marked stairs, sturdy handrails, and some non-skid shoes, among other things. (See page 108 for tips on preventing falls.)

◆ **Drugs.** A number of new drugs are now available to either prevent or treat osteoporosis. The field is evolving rapidly, and newer drugs are expected to come on the market. Your parent should talk with her doctor about these and other options.

Bisphosphonates, which include alendronate (Fosamax) and risedronate (Actonel), slow bone loss and increase bone density. Bisphosphonates have been shown to reduce fractures in postmenopausal women by more than 50 percent.

Calcitonin (Miacalcin and Calcimar), a synthetic version of a hormone that is naturally produced by the body, increases bone mass in the spine. It is not thought to be as effective as bisphosphonates or estrogen replacement therapy, however.

Raloxifene (Evista) is a "selective estrogen receptor modulator," which means that it strengthens bones just as estrogen would, without affecting the breasts and uterus. So it doesn't cause many of the unwanted side effects of estrogen, such as vaginal bleeding, breast tenderness, or increased risk of breast cancer. (It may cause hot flashes in some women.)

Teriparatide (Fortéo), a parathyroid hormone, actually triggers new bone formation and increases bone density in postmenopausal women (and men). It is taken as a daily injection, is quite expensive, and used only for very high-risk patients, as there may be serious side effects.

Estrogen therapy helps combat osteoporosis, but it is now known to increase the risk of heart disease, stroke, and breast cancer, especially when taken for any prolonged period. Furthermore, estrogen therapy is most effective at stopping bone loss in the first few years after menopause (when bone loss is most rapid). Starting it at eighty or ninety is not as effective.

Nonestrogen treatments should be tried first, and estrogen, with or without progestin, should be used only at a low dose for a short period of time, and only by women with severe osteoporosis.

Sometimes estrogen therapy is combined with the drugs described above when a person has extremely low bone density or continues to lose bone. Your mother should talk with her doctor and make a decision based on her family history, health risks and personal preference. Estrogen is generally not advised for men.

Finally, ask the doctor about any drugs your parent might be taking that actually cause bone loss. In particular, glucocorticoid steroids can be to blame. These are found in some medications for arthritis, asthma, seizures, and insomnia.

ARTHRITIS

ARTHRITIS IS NOT A SINGLE DISORDER, but a general term referring to sore or swollen joints. The word actually encompasses about a hundred different diseases, all of which should be treated early, so look for the warning signs: swelling, redness and pain at the joint, stiffness, especially in the morning, and restricted range of motion. If any of these symptoms last for more than two weeks, your parent should see her doctor.

Managing Arthritis

Most types of arthritis cannot be cured, so the aim of treatment is to alleviate pain and increase mobility. If your parent's arthritis is severe, she should talk to a specialist, such as a rheumatologist or orthopedic surgeon.

Some ways to ease arthritis include:

◆ **Nonmedical treatments.** Warm baths and heat pads can relieve the pain and stiffness, while cold packs can reduce swelling and numb pain. (Your parent should try both and see what feels best.) Also, gentle massage can help.

While rest is important during a painful attack, exercise in the interim can prevent joints from stiffening, increase range of motion and mobility, and ease inflammation and pain.

ARTHRITIS: THE COMMON VILLAINS

Osteoarthritis, or degenerative arthritis, is almost universal after age sixty-five, particularly among women, although some people have few or no symptoms. The cartilage in joints, a cushion that allows bones to glide easily back and forth without friction, becomes thin, cracked, and frayed. The joint is painful and movement is limited. It is most common in the joints of the hands, hips, knees, feet, and back.

Severe osteoarthritis can make everyday life exasperating and discouraging. Every movement hurts, and simple tasks, like buttoning a blouse or holding a fork, are challenging, if not impossible. Sometimes a hand will curl and twist into a deformed shape, and might develop knobby lumps, called osteophytes (which look more painful than they actually are).

Osteoarthritis has a number of causes. When it strikes the hands or hips, it tends to be genetic, whereas osteoarthritis in the knees seems to be at least partially due to the strain of obesity. The disease can also be the result of injuries or overuse.

Rheumatoid arthritis also affects women more than men. The body's immune system launches a misdirected attack and injures healthy tissue in the joints. The disease usually begins with an allover achiness, stiffness, and fatigue. The joints become stiff, swollen, red, warm, and painful, especially first thing in the morning. The feet and the hands—particularly the fingers—are often the first joints affected, but over time the disease can spread to elbows, knees, hips, and other joints. Usually the joints are affected symmetrically. That is, the same joints on both sides of the body are hurting. In some cases, pea-size lumps grow under the skin, and the joints become deformed. Rheumatoid arthritis is one of the most difficult types of arthritis to control. It is critical that it be diagnosed and treated early, before bone and cartilage are damaged.

An exercise program should be comfortable, not overly strenuous, and, preferably, recommended by a doctor or physical therapist. Weight-bearing exercises (in which a person carries his or her own weight, such as running, walking, dancing, hiking, or tennis) are recommended, although exercising in a warm pool is often easier on stiff joints. Tai chi also seems to be extremely helpful for people with arthritis, both in terms of easing pain

Gout and pseudogout, two of the most excruciating types of arthritis, occur more often in men than women. In gout, uric acid, which usually drains out of the body with urine, builds up and forms sharp crystals in the joints—often in the big toe, but also in the ankles, elbows, wrists, hands, or knees. In pseudogout, it is crystals of calcium pyrophosphate that collect, and the disease usually affects the large joints (knee, shoulder, hip).

This assault on the joints happens suddenly, lasts for about two or three days, and then slowly fades over a week or two. The joint becomes painful, stiff, and swollen. The skin around the joint becomes dark red and very tender. Even a light brush with the bed sheets can be agonizing. Gout is sometimes accompanied by fever.

The person often has another attack within a year and may experience several more episodes in following years, although some people have just one or two attacks and are never bothered by symptoms again.

and increasing motion. (Check with the local chapter of the Arthritis Foundation for special classes, or order their exercise video for people with arthritis. See page 66 for more on exercise and the elderly.)

If your parent is heavy, losing weight will also ease the burden on her joints. People with gout or pseudo-gout should avoid alcohol, poultry, and organ meats, such as liver and kidneys.

◆ **Handy gadgets.** Canes, walkers, and splints will give your parent support and a little more mobility. Shoes with shock-absorbing insoles can reduce pain. Jar openers, toothpaste dispensers, large-handled flatware, faucet grippers, and other such devices that help people with arthritis can be found in many large pharmacies and in medical supply stores, or they can be purchased through catalogues or over the Internet. (See page 131 for more information.)

◆ **Drugs.** Aspirin and its relatives, ibuprofen and acetaminophen, are typically used to relieve the aches of aged joints and muscles. (By the way, "extra-strength" or "arthritis-strength" aspirin are simply larger doses of plain aspirin.) Acetaminophen (e.g., Tylenol) appears to be the best choice as it works as well as aspirin, but causes fewer side effects. Your parent should not begin any drug regimen without the approval of her doctor.

When acetaminophen doesn't work, sometimes aspirin, ibuprofen, or more powerful, prescription versions of these drugs (known as nonsteroidal anti-inflammatory drugs or NSAIDs) are useful. These drugs block the production of prostaglandins, the source of pain and swelling. However, NSAIDs can produce side effects,

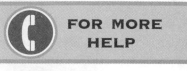

FOR MORE HELP

Arthritis Foundation
800-283-7800
www.arthritis.org

National Institute of Arthritis and Musculoskeletal and Skin Diseases
877-226-4267
www.niams.nih.gov

National Osteoporosis Foundation
800-223-9994
www.nof.org

including ulcers, sodium and water retention, heartburn, vomiting, diarrhea, and headaches. Newer NSAIDs, known as COX-2 inhibitors, may cause fewer side effects.

When NSAIDs don't work, corticosteroids, which are a form of cortisone, a hormone produced naturally by the body, also reduce swelling and pain. Corticosteroids, however, are potent and are usually prescribed only for brief periods.

When osteoarthritis affects the knee, hyaluronic acid can be injected into the area around the knee joint to replace fluids and ease pain.

Glucosamine and chondroitin sulfate, which are found naturally in the body, and form and repair cartilage, appear to be useful in treating mild osteoarthritis. They are made from shellfish shells and shark cartilage, and sold as dietary supplements in health food stores and many pharmacies. Your parent should confer with his doctor before trying it. (Use caution if your parent has diabetes, as glucosamine is a form of sugar; if your parent is taking blood thinners, be aware that chondroitin sulfate thins blood; and, of course, skip it if your parent is allergic to shellfish.)

Rheumatoid arthritis is treated in a number of ways. What's known as "disease-modifying antirheumatic drugs," or DMARDs, are usually the first line of defense, as they slow the disease process and ease pain and stiffness. "Biologic response modifiers" are sometimes used in people with moderate rheumatoid arthritis. Gold compounds and penicillamine, which take two to six months to work, are older drugs that are not used often, but can be helpful in people who cannot tolerate the other drugs.

Gout and pseudogout are treated with NSAIDs, or the drug colchicine, which can sometimes prevent a full-blown attack if taken early. Doctors also try to reduce the level of uric acid in the body with drugs (such as allopurinol, sulfinpyrazone, and probenecid) or, if a large joint is affected, by withdrawing fluid from the joint and injecting corticosteroids to reduce inflammation.

◆ **Physical and occupational therapy.** Physical therapy increases movement, strengthens muscles, and helps people learn new ways to use their joints. Occupational therapy trains people with limited motion to manage everyday tasks. Both are often helpful in conjunction with other treatments.

◆ **Surgery.** If your parent is otherwise healthy, a doctor may recommend surgery to replace a badly damaged joint with an artificial one or to repair damaged cartilage. Be aware that such surgery is a major undertaking, especially if your parent is old or very frail. Ask the doctor about arthroscopy, a less invasive procedure that requires only local anesthesia and usually no hospital stay.

Incontinence

You've just noticed a large stain on your father's pants or a distinctive odor coming from your mother's bedroom. There is a moment of shock. A wave of sorrow. Then the question. *What do I do now?*

It's understandable that you're upset, but try to shake off any disgust or embarrassment. The great shame of incontinence is not the problem itself, but the stigma associated with it and the woeful lack of open conversation. You need to talk with your parent about this. It's a tremendously difficult subject, and you may meet with resistance or denial, but talking is the only way to ease the humiliation and begin to find solutions. And there are solutions.

Be gentle, sympathetic, and tactful. Find a time when others will not overhear or interrupt you. Let your parent know how common the problem is (up to 30 percent of elderly people are completely or partially incontinent; more than 50 percent of those in hospitals or nursing homes are incontinent), and that help is available.

Once the problem is acknowledged, get your parent to a doctor who will give the situation the attention it deserves. You may have to advocate with special persistence here. One study showed that 35 to 50 percent of doctors did nothing when told that a patient was incontinent. If your parent's doctor is not helpful, she should see a urologist, gynecologist, gastroenterologist, or geriatrician. Some geriatric care centers have special clinics devoted to incontinence.

Urinary incontinence is almost always treatable with exercise, bladder training, surgery, and other techniques. Bowel incontinence is a more difficult problem, and far more upsetting psychologically for both you and your parent, but it too can be treated in many instances, and it can always be made more manageable.

Although incontinence can cause infections and depression, it is not as much a medical crisis as it is a social one. Not only will it make your parent feel embarrassed, ashamed, and disgusted, it can lead to withdrawal, isolation, depression, and, because it is so hard on caregivers, institutionalization. You and your parent will fare much better if you each have a thick social skin and a ready sense of humor, as well as determination to find adequate medical care.

URINARY INCONTINENCE

NORMAL BLADDER ROUTINES RUN amok for all sorts of reasons—infections, prostate troubles, hormones, diabetes, dehydration, immobility, surgery, weakened or damaged muscles, and medications. Constipation can cause urinary incontinence if it puts pressure on, or otherwise irritates, the muscles of the bladder. Stroke, dementia, and delirium can also lead to incontinence if the brain isn't sending or receiving bladder or bowel signals normally. How incontinence is treated depends in part on what type of incontinence your parent has.

Managing Urinary Incontinence

Quite often, incontinence disappears on its own. When it doesn't, a doctor's first task is to treat any underlying problem—infection, obstruction, or illness. The doctor should review your parent's medications, as some can worsen incontinence (such as diuretics, tranquilizers, sedatives, drugs for Parkinson's disease, psychotropic drugs, antihistamines, and calcium-channel blockers).

After that, the best attack is a nonmedical one—bladder exercises, bladder training, and regular toilet scheduling. These techniques require commitment and practice, but they are quite successful in treating stress and urge incontinence in particular. About 20 percent of patients are cured, and almost all the rest are helped significantly.

◆ **Kegel exercises.** These exercises require no gym outfit and no sweating, just commitment. Kegel exercises strengthen the ring of muscles around the urethra, the exit tube from the bladder, and are particularly useful in treating stress incontinence. The exercises entail squeezing the muscles of the vagina and anus. Your mother can get the feel of where the muscles are by stopping the flow while she is urinating. (She should not be tightening the muscles in her legs, fanny, or stomach, which are not involved in bladder control.) A nurse or physical therapist can help her learn.

She should do these squeezes (holding each for several seconds) after every visit to the toilet, and at other times throughout the day, for a total of one hundred to two hundred squeezes each day. For stress incontinence, your parent should get in the habit of squeezing these muscles before lifting, sneezing, coughing or, if possible, laughing.

Kegels can be done discreetly while watching television, reading, lying in bed, or even sitting in a restaurant. However, like other workouts, they require dedication. It usually takes at least one month of doing Kegels before any real effect is noticed. Once there's some improvement, your parent should continue the routine to maintain bladder control.

◆ **A schedule.** Have your parent keep track of when she urinates or leaks for a couple of days, and then make a schedule that gets her to the toilet just before she typically needs to use it. She might sit on the toilet, say, every two hours whether she thinks she needs to or not. (Bathroom trips shouldn't be scheduled too frequently, as that can actually cause urge incontinence if the bladder learns to hold only small amounts of fluid.) Your parent might also stick to a schedule of fluid intake—a glass of orange juice at 7 A.M., a glass of water at 10 A.M., and so on.

◆ **Bladder training.** Once your parent schedules bathroom trips, she might be able to extend the time between bathroom trips. In bladder training, a person gets on a schedule of going to the toilet at set intervals, and then slowly lengthens the time between visits. Your parent should increase these intervals until she can wait two or three hours. To practice, your parent should empty her bladder completely, and then suppress any urge in between scheduled trips by relaxing or diverting her attention. ("Holding it" during these intervals can strengthen the muscles around the urethra.)

◆ **Biofeedback.** Used in conjunction with exercises, this technique can be very helpful, especially for stress and urge incontinence. The patient is hooked up to a device that informs him how well he is contracting and relaxing his sphincter, detrusor, and abdominal muscles—all involved in bladder control. People can also use a diary to track their progress. With this information as a guide, the person practices ways to manipulate these

> *My mother got up from her chair in the living room to go in to dinner, and I noticed this spot on the cushion. She is a fastidious woman, and I think she was unaware that anything had happened. She had developed fluid in her abdomen from the cancer, and it was putting pressure on all of her organs, so maybe that triggered the incontinence.*
>
> *I thought, 'Am I going to have to tell her, or will she notice it herself and try to hide it from me?' I wasn't offended by the problem. I was more worried that it would be just one more encroachment on her dignity. I really hurt for her."*
>
> —RUTH S.

muscles and gradually gains better control over them.

◆ **Bedpans and commodes.** If your parent has trouble getting to the bathroom because of a physical disability or urge incontinence, put a commode, bedpan, or urinal by his bed or chair. Or, if it is possible, have him sit or sleep near a bathroom that is not used by anyone else in the family.

◆ **Dietary changes.** Limiting caffeine and alcohol should improve continence, and some studies suggest that avoiding spicy foods, tomatoes, and imitation sweeteners may help, too.

TYPES OF INCONTINENCE

Transient incontinence comes on suddenly and acutely. A person who has never wet his pants starts having accidents, often because he can't physically get to the toilet, or because of an infection, delirium, depression, medication, constipation, or alcohol use. The incontinence is almost always reversible and may even disappear on its own.

Stress incontinence primarily affects women. They laugh, cough, strain, exercise, sneeze, or pick up a heavy box and, oops. The culprit: The ring of muscles around the urethra, which usually holds in urine, is loose, often as a result of bearing children and the hormonal changes of menopause. As a result, small amounts of urine leak out when a woman exerts even the smallest pressure (or "stress") on the bladder.

Urge incontinence is characterized by a sudden and urgent urge to urinate—so sudden that there is not enough time to get to the toilet. The bladder may empty on cue—when someone hears water running or touches water, or when he drinks a small glass of water. Bladder contractions run amok often because of damage to the nerves of the bladder, spinal cord, or brain, caused by Parkinson's disease, Alzheimer's disease, stroke, spinal cord injury, or diabetes. In reflex incontinence, a close cousin of urge incontinence, the bladder releases with no warning at all.

Overflow incontinence occurs when the bladder is always full, and excess urine dribbles out. It is often seen in men with prostate troubles. When the prostate gland, which surrounds the urethra, is enlarged, it can block the passageway so urine can't drain out

Obesity also plays a role in some cases, so you might urge your parent to lose weight.

Your parent should not drink less in order to urinate less. This will cause dehydration and can make her incontinence worse, as highly concentrated urine may result in infections.

◆ **Medications.** In conjunction with exercises and training programs, certain drugs (and there are quite a number of options) can be used to stop bladder contractions, strengthen the resistance of the urethra, or help relax muscles when emptying the bladder.

◆ **Electrical stimulation.** The muscles of the urethra can also be strengthened by short doses of electrical stimulation. Electrodes are

normally during toileting. Instead, the bladder remains full, causing minor leaks throughout the day.

Overflow incontinence is also seen in people who have diabetes, spinal cord injury, and other disorders that block the urethra or prevent the bladder from contracting normally. The buildup of urine can cause bladder or kidney infections if the disorder is not treated.

Functional incontinence is usually caused by physical limitations that prevent a person from getting to the toilet in time. Conditions that hinder mobility, such as severe arthritis or stroke, are often to blame.

Mixed incontinence, when two types of incontinence occur together, usually occurs in women. Stress and urge incontinence are the most common combination.

placed (temporarily) in the vagina or rectum to stimulate the contraction of the urethra muscles and stabilize overactive muscles. This is useful in cases of stress or urge incontinence.

◆ **Implants, plugs, patches, and other devices.** Doctors have had some success injecting collagen, silicone, or other materials into or around the urethra to narrow the opening and help control urination. A stiff ring, called a pessary, can be inserted into the vagina to put pressure on the urethra and reposition it. There are also patches and plugs, somewhat like a tampon, that are helpful for stress incontinence.

◆ **Surgery.** Although a last resort, surgery is sometimes necessary to clear obstructions (for example, an enlarged prostate), to reposition the bladder (in cases of stress incontinence), or to repair or replace the urethra.

◆ **Pads, diapers, and catheters.** These should be used only when all else fails, or for trips and other occasions that require extra security. Besides being uncomfortable, demoralizing, and inconvenient, diapers can worsen incontinence if the person learns to rely on them and stops exercising his bladder muscles. Over time, the body can become desensitized to its own messages. (This is especially true when a person is in the early stages of dementia.) Diapers can also lead to skin irritation and infections.

Nevertheless, when necessary, adult diapers can be lifesavers.

Which of the many varieties to use depends on your parent's own situation and comfort. For minor leaking, a menstrual "maxipad" or a similar pad that's made to absorb urine may be adequate. It's less bulky than a diaper, but offers less protection.

Disposable adult diapers that are "super-absorbent" are thinner than others but still hold quite a bit of fluid. Washable diapers are often cheaper, but don't hold as much fluid and are not

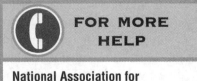

FOR MORE HELP

National Association for Continence
800-252-3337
www.nafc.org

Simon Foundation for Continence
800-237-4666
www.simonfoundation.org

National Kidney and Urologic Diseases Information Clearinghouse
800-891-5390
www.kidney.niddk.nih.gov

International Foundation for Functional Gastrointestinal Disorders
888-964-2001
www.aboutincontinence.org

as convenient. Disposable liners or pads that fit into a washable outer pant may offer the best of both worlds.

Whenever your parent wears diapers, take steps to avoid skin infections and rashes. Your parent should not sit in wet or dirty pants for any longer than absolutely necessary. The crotch must be thoroughly cleaned at every diaper change with mild soap and water and then dried with a cotton towel. A small amount of moisturizer—no powders—helps prevent irritation. Boxes of "wipes," which are handy, along with diaper rash

ointment, can be found in the baby section of grocery stores, department stores, or pharmacies. Use diaper rash cream if necessary, and call a doctor if the irritation doesn't go away in a day or two.

A catheter is absolutely the last step, and generally not a good way to deal with incontinence because infections are so common. A catheter is basically a tube that runs from the bladder into a storage bag that hangs from a bed or is attached to the leg and hidden under pants or a skirt. Your parent is most apt to need a catheter while confined to a bed or wheelchair.

A catheter can be inserted into the bladder permanently by a nurse, or inserted according to a schedule by your parent. There are also catheters that attach to the genitals (a condomlike device for men and a somewhat less useful suction gadget for women). Catheters are often used for overflow incontinence, or for brief periods after surgery or injury. Beware of infections. Catheters need to be changed regularly.

BOWEL INCONTINENCE

BOWEL INCONTINENCE IS A LESS common problem, but a far more troubling one. If your parent is immobile, bed-ridden, or mentally impaired, and you have to change diapers yourself, it may become more than you can handle. Changing diapers and protecting the house against damage is an enormous task, both physically and emotionally. Don't be hard on yourself. Try the treatments and approaches discussed here and talk with your parent's doctor. Bowel, or fecal, incontinence can be treated in most people, if not eliminating the problem completely, then reducing "accident" significantly. If nothing works, you might need to get outside help or even begin to look into assisted-living or nursing-home care.

Be very gentle with your parent. Virtually nothing is more shocking, mortifying, and embarrassing than this. Let her know that this is the result of a medical problem, that it is not her fault, that it is not anything she should feel ashamed of. Let her know that you and her doctor will work with her to get beyond this or at least make it manageable.

Oddly enough, the most common cause of bowel incontinence is constipation. When the bowel is blocked, liquid leaks around the obstruction. Diarrhea is also a common cause of fecal incontinence in elderly people, as they are less able to hold on to soft or liquid stools. Bowel incontinence can also be caused by surgery, medications, illness, childbirth, injury to the anal muscles or the nerves around the rectum (often from straining or prolonged laxative use), dementia, stroke, diabetes, and severe depression.

Treating
Bowel Incontinence

Any severe constipation or diarrhea needs to be treated immediately. If the incontinence remains, the doctor should search for other causes.

A high-fiber diet can help control bowel incontinence by restoring regularity, although in some cases a low-fiber diet is used to reduce stool volume. Also, try the suggestions for treating urinary incontinence—setting schedules, exercising muscles, using commodes—as many are useful in addressing bowel incontinence as well. It's sometimes helpful to get a person to sit on the toilet about half an hour after breakfast, when the bowels are typically stimulated.

A method of biofeedback, in which a balloon is placed in the rectum and the person learns muscle control by watching the results of his efforts on a monitor, is often successful in treating bowel incontinence.

When muscles aren't working properly—the person feels the need to go but can't hold on or get to a bathroom in time—electrical stimulation (using painless electrical currents to "exercise" muscles) can help strengthen the sphincter muscles.

When nerve damage numbs the normal sensations of an approaching bowel movement, enemas or suppositories can be used to empty the bowels on a schedule.

Several drugs are also useful in reducing the number of "episodes." For example, stool-bulking agents can firm up loose stool.

When all else fails, some surgical procedures can help. A torn or damaged sphincter (the ring of muscles around the anus) can be repaired surgically, an artificial sphincter can be implanted, or the rectum can be repositioned.

BETTER BATHROOM HABITS

◆ Clear a path to the toilet. If possible, make sure your parent has a private bathroom, so it's always available.

◆ Place night-lights and/or reflector tapes along the path to the bathroom to avoid stumbling around at night.

◆ Make sure your parent can use the toilet with ease. Install grab bars, buy a raised toilet seat, and put the toilet paper within easy reach.

◆ Get your parent to wear clothing that's easily removable (skirts or elastic-waist pants, Velcro or snap closures instead of buttons, knee-high stockings instead of pantyhose).

◆ If the toilet is far away or shared, buy a commode, bedpan, or hand-held urinal. Get a portable urinal for traveling.

◆ Make sure your parent empties his or her bladder before going to bed.

◆ When in a new place, locate the bathroom immediately. Avoid situations where there are no bathrooms, such as buses or shops without public facilities.

◆ Choose seats in restaurants, airplanes, theaters, etc. that are near a bathroom. Call in advance and plan the seating so you don't have to make a fuss when you arrive.

◆ Use waterproof liners (disposable or washable) under bed sheets, in the car, and on your parent's chair. You can find these at a medical supply store. Or buy waterproof crib sheets, which are sold with other baby supplies, or place a

Constipation

After about age seventy, many people become concerned about their bowels. If they don't go to the bathroom for a day or two, they worry that they may explode. The truth is, not everyone needs to move his bowels every day. In fact, once every three days will get your parent through the week just fine. So if he constantly complains of constipation, but has no symptoms other than irregularity, urge him as gently and tactfully as you can not to worry so much about it.

True constipation—when bowel movements are difficult or painful, and a person has gas, bloating, and a sore, tender belly—is miserable. And if left untreated, it can become extremely serious (and may be a sign of some

plastic shower liner inside a folded sheet and lay it across the middle of the bed. (A shower liner alone is too slippery and may cause your parent to fall.) Never put rubber next to your parent's skin. It's not only uncomfortable; it can cause reactions and severely irritate the skin.

✦ To reduce odors, have your parent deposit soiled clothing in a small pail, equipped with a lid and a deodorizer, placed in an inconspicuous spot in the bathroom.

✦ A fan and an open window, whenever possible, will reduce odor problems. So will an open box of baking soda. Baking soda will get rid of odors in carpets and upholstery, too. Believe it or not, a cut onion left in a room will absorb odors without leaving its own smell—try it!

other disease). A doctor should be consulted if the home remedies listed in this section fail to work.

Constipation may be the result of a number of underlying and treatable conditions. Aging itself leads to changes in physiology that make constipation more common. Beyond that, a variety of illnesses play a role. For example, hormonal problems, such as a thyroid disorder, can disrupt normal habits.

Irritable bowel syndrome (also known as spastic colon or irritable colon syndrome) can cause both constipation and diarrhea. Hemorrhoids or any other sore near the anus can make a person resist the need to go to the bathroom, as can surgery in the abdominal area, though this is usually a temporary problem. Damage to the digestive system from cancer, nerve disorders, Parkinson's disease, diabetes, and other illnesses can harm the digestive tract in such a way that bowel movements become difficult. Immobility after surgery or simply a very sedentary lifestyle can also cause constipation.

Severe constipation, when bowels become impacted, requires medical attention as toxins can seep into the bloodstream. If enemas or suppositories don't work, doctors may have to remove the obstruction manually or, in extreme cases, surgically

Treating Constipation

• **Fiber, fiber, fiber.** A good diet, for bowels and everything else, is packed with green, leafy vegetables, fresh fruit, and whole-grain breads, pasta, and cereals. Fiber, particularly wheat bran, is great for treating and preventing constipation. A high-fiber cereal eaten regularly is a quick fix, but it shouldn't replace more varied and natural sources of fiber. (See page 658 for more on fiber and diet.) If your parent decides to eat high-fiber cereal or use fiber supplements, she should begin slowly, as taking a large amount suddenly may leave her doubled over with stomach cramps. Any initial bloating and gas

> *I guess we all wish for the same thing—that our parents will be independent until they die. Then you could help them with a few practical things, like going shopping or taking care of the house, and you would include them in family affairs, and that would be it. You wouldn't have to hear about every bowel movement, which is the level I am at with my mother. I don't really want to take care of my mother's bowel movements. I'd rather just take her shopping."*
>
> —Barbara F.

should go away within a few days. (She should talk with a doctor before taking fiber supplements; in some cases, fiber is not the best route.)

On the flip side, a diet of high-fat meats and dairy products, eggs, and rich desserts and other sweets, or a routine of eating processed foods (which tend to be low in fiber) can all contribute to constipation.

• **Water, water, water.** Fiber works to aid regularity by absorbing fluids and thereby softening feces. But it can't work in a dry environment. Although, eight glasses of water a day are recommended, four to six will help keep things moving. Soda, juice, or herbal tea work as well as water, but drinks containing alcohol or caffeine won't help at all.

• **Exercise.** Any form of exercise will help keep bowels regular, along with its many other benefits. Your parent needs to get out for a walk or do some stretching. Talk with the doctor about exercises and movements that your parent can do, even from a bed or chair, or call a physical therapist. Any exercise, no matter how little, is better than none. (See page 66 for more on exercise.)

• **Bathroom routines.** When it's time to go to the toilet, it's time to go. Make sure your parent doesn't "hold it," ignore the urge, hurry, or wait for a more convenient time and place. If your parent is in a new place, which can throw off her daily ritual, she should go at the same time of day she normally does and also stick with her regular diet as much as possible.

• **Medications.** Narcotics, antacids, antispasmodic drugs, antihistamines, antihypertensive agents, antidepressants, and tranquilizers can all cause constipation, as can some dietary supplements and a host of other drugs. Talk with the doctor about lowering the dose of any drug you suspect is causing a problem, or about changing or stopping the medication.

• **Easy on the laxatives.** Your parent should use laxatives sparingly and only for short periods of time, as they can worsen the problem. Up to 75 percent of elderly people use laxatives, many of them daily. But contrary to what the ads suggest—that with laxatives, your parent will stroll along breezy seasides or bound over tennis nets—laxatives, when used routinely, can interfere with nature so severely that, over time, the body forgets how to operate on its own. Enemas are equally problematic. So use them with caution or with a doctor's advice. Stool softeners soften hard stools, but don't necessarily treat the constipation; their lubricants may also hinder vitamin absorption. Sugarless candies that contain sorbitol are a relatively safe "laxative" worth trying.

Other Digestive Disorders

MEDICAL ALERT

Blood in stools, dark or oddly colored stools, a sudden change in bowel habits, or pain in the lower abdomen should be reported to the doctor immediately. Also, be sure that your parent has an annual colon exam.

♦ **Diarrhea.** Severe or chronic diarrhea always requires medical attention. But an occasional bout of loose bowels is not a serious problem, though psychologically it can be upsetting.

Diarrhea is the body's way of getting rid of toxins in the digestive tract. It can be caused by bad food, laxatives, antacids, diuretics, antibiotics, chemotherapy, anxiety, or intestinal disorders. Milk and other dairy products can also cause diarrhea in people who are lactose intolerant. Most of the time, the problem disappears fairly quickly on its own.

If it is severe or chronic, or if there is blood in the bowels, diarrhea may be caused by colon cancer, infection, diabetes, severe constipation (when liquid flows around the blockage), or other serious problems that need immediate medical attention.

♦ **Difficulty swallowing.** Dry mouth is a common reason for swallowing difficulty (also known as dysphagia), but the problem can also be caused by weakened throat muscles or disorders such as dementia, cancer, or stroke, which disrupt the signals to and from the brain that control swallowing. Dysphagia is common among the elderly, particularly among those in nursing homes.

Keep an eye out for clues such as coughing, gagging, drooling, belching, and the like, while your parent eats. He might complain of having a "lump in his throat." Check to see if he has trouble swallowing only certain types of foods (for example, liquids and not solids).

Consult a doctor. Unchecked, swallowing difficulties can lead to malnutrition, starvation, choking, or pneumonia (because fluid gets into the lung). A doctor will first try to determine what is causing the problem and, if possible, treat that. A speech therapist might be able to teach your parent exercises to improve his swallowing skills. Some drugs are helpful, although surgery is needed in some cases.

MEDICAL ALERT

 If diarrhea is severe or lasts for more than a week, contact your parent's doctor. In the meantime, it is important that your parent's body be replenished with salt and water. Mix one quart water, a teaspoon of salt, and four teaspoons of sugar (the sugar helps the body absorb the salt). If this mixture is unpalatable, try adding fruit juice instead of sugar, or try a drink with electrolytes, or some plain water along with something salty, like pretzels. Your parent should, if possible, drink up to a pint of this liquid every hour (but ask the doctor, as some elderly people should not drink as much of it) until the diarrhea has subsided. Over-the-counter antidiarrheal medications are not always advised, as diarrhea is a sign that the body needs to rid itself of bacteria or other toxins.

Soft, moist foods and those accompanied by sauces may go down more easily than dry foods or thin liquids like juice or water. They slide down the throat easily, and yet still have enough substance to trigger the swallowing reflex. Urge your parent to sit upright while eating, to eat slowly rather than wolfing down food, to take tiny bites, and to avoid chatting while eating or gulping a drink before a bite of food is chewed and swallowed completely. Sometimes a small change in the tilt of the head can help. (See page 123 for more tips on helping your parent eat when she has problems swallowing.)

◆ **Heartburn.** Medications, chocolates, fried foods, spicy foods, rich foods, caffeine, tobacco, and alcohol may all contribute to the burning pain in your parent's chest, a searing just behind the chest bone that is sometimes mistaken for heart disease. The pain may become worse when your parent leans forward or lies down, as the esophagus fails to close completely and acid flows upward from the stomach.

If certain foods seem to trigger the trouble, obviously your parent should avoid them. Also, he should eat smaller, more frequent meals rather than large meals; eat several hours before bedtime or before lying down at all and elevate his head at night; and avoid tight clothing. Antacids can be helpful, but if this is not enough, he should talk to his doctor about other options, as there are stronger drugs that can help. Some people require surgery.

◆ **Indigestion.** Indigestion, or dyspepsia, is often a Thanksgiving Day problem, caused by overindulgence at the dinner table—eating too much or too fast, or eating rich or spicy foods. But persistent indigestion can also be a sign of a digestive tract disorder, like an ulcer or gall bladder disease. It is usually characterized by heartburn, nausea, vomiting, bloating, and discomfort. Again, a change in diet should solve the problem, but if it doesn't go away, consult the doctor.

♦ **Ulcers.** When the protective lining of the stomach fails to do its job, digestive acids, which break down food in the stomach, can eat away at the stomach lining, creating raw, painful sores called peptic ulcers. In most cases, ulcers are caused by bacteria (*H. pylori*) in the digestive tract, which destroy the mucous coating the walls of the stomach and the duodenum, a short tube leading out of the stomach and into the small intestine.

Ulcers are also caused or worsened by long-term use of aspirin, ibuprofen, and other so-called nonsteroidal anti-inflammatory drugs (NSAIDs). In very rare cases, they are the result of cancer. Stress and spicy foods are no longer thought to be culprits, although they don't help once an ulcer has formed.

Ulcers are common in the elderly, and they can be extremely serious, as they can cause internal bleeding, a blockage in the intestinal tract, and other complications. If you think your parent may have an ulcer, alert her doctor.

Symptoms include a burning or gnawing sensation in the stomach, bloating, and/or nausea that comes on several hours after eating and is relieved by eating, drinking milk, or taking antacids. Sometimes a person is awakened by vague pain and discomfort in the middle of the night (two or three hours after dinner). Symptoms may come and go for several weeks.

The most effective approach is to kill the bacteria with antibiotics, while taking other drugs to reduce the amount of stomach acid and protect the stomach lining. Unfortunately, this can mean taking up to twenty pills a day. Fortunately, the treatment lasts only a week or two.

Patients should also stop using any NSAIDs and forego smoking, caffeine, and alcohol. Meals should be small and frequent. Antacids are helpful, but they must be used with care as some contain large amounts of sodium, and they can interfere with the absorption of other drugs.

♦ **Diverticular disease.** Diverticula are small sacs that develop along the lining of the intestine for reasons that are not clear, although lack of adequate dietary fiber seems to play a role. The presence of these sacs is called diverticulosis, a very common ailment in elderly people. Half of all people over sixty-five have it, but only about 20 percent of them have any symptoms—cramps, bloating, constipation or diarrhea, and pain in the lower abdomen. Usually the symptoms disappear with some rest, a diet high in fiber, plenty of liquids, and, if these don't succeed, antispasmodic drugs or antibiotics.

RX FOR CHOKING

I f your parent has trouble swallowing, be prepared with a little first aid. Learn it in advance, so you're ready.

If he is choking on food or another object, do nothing as long as he is able to speak, cough, or breathe at all.

If your parent is unable to breathe (in which case he may be silent, appear panicked, or grab at his throat), perform the Heimlich maneuver. First, stand behind him, wrapping your arms around his chest. Make a fist just below the rib cage and above the navel, and clasp that fist with your other hand. With a quick, strong thrust of your hands, pull inward and upward four times. (Not so hard as to break his ribs, though.) Repeat this thrusting motion until the food is dislodged.

If the person is horizontal, place one hand just above the navel in the middle of the abdomen. Place the other hand on top of the first hand and press in with a quick thrust. Repeat.

If this fails, call for emergency help and begin artificial respiration. For more information on the Heimlich maneuver and other first-aid techniques, call the local chapter of the American Red Cross.

Diverticulitis is a far more serious problem that requires immediate medical attention. In this case, sacs become inflamed, often because stool gets stuck in the intestine, causing an infection or perforation. Diverticulitis causes pain, fever, and stiffness of the abdomen and can lead to a number of complications. It is treated with antibiotics, intravenous fluids, and, in some cases, surgery.

◆ **Hemorrhoids.** Hemorrhoids can ruin an otherwise good day. Straining puts pressure on the veins around the anus, which distend outward and form small, painful protuberances. Hemorrhoids can also develop internally, in the lower part of the rectum. They are often itchy and painful, and they may be bloody (which will be the only sign when they are internal). Older people may be at greater risk if they sit for long stretches of time, are constipated, or vomit, cough, or sneeze fiercely and repeatedly.

Usually fiber, fluids, and time will relieve the problem. Over-the-counter hemorrhoid creams, warm baths, "baby wipes," petroleum jelly, ice packs, and cold witch hazel can ease the pain and itching. A doughnut-shaped pillow may make sitting more comfortable, but it should be used only for short periods, as it can cause pressure sores. Stool softeners will make defecating less painful. Heavy lifting and straining should be halted. If hemorrhoids persist and are severe, they can be removed or shrunk by several methods, all of them pretty simple.

Be aware that rectal bleeding is not always due to hemorrhoids, can be very serious, and should always get the attention of the doctor.

◆ **Pruritus ani.** Harsh soaps, deodorants, perfumes, aggressive wiping of the anus, synthetic underwear, fungal disease, and topical drugs used to treat other anal disorders (lidocaine, benzocaine) can all cause intense itching of the anus. It is treated by addressing the cause, throwing out the underwear and strong soaps, and wiping more gently with hypoallergenic, scentless baby wipes. Petroleum jelly can help, but hydrocortisone cream is most effective.

◆ **Gas.** Intestinal gas can be unpleasant for both you and your parent, but it is normal and not life-threatening. As with constipation, older people sometimes become overly concerned about gas because they have some preconceived notion of what is "normal." (Tell your parent that a study has shown that men ages twenty-five to thirty-five pass gas ten to twenty times a day.)

Where does gas come from? Usually from swallowing air while eating, or from the production of bacteria in the bowels. It can be eased by avoiding dairy products, as lactose intolerance is common among the elderly. Other dietary culprits include beans, legumes, raisins, broccoli, cauliflower, brussels sprouts, bran, cabbage—all those high-

fiber, low-fat foods that are so healthful. Rather than cut out these good foods, have your parent cut down on them, and put up with a few bad odors.

While gas certainly can cause stomach pains and bloating, it is the ego that usually gets hurt. Elderly people often have little or no control over when or how gas is released. Your parent may embarrass herself, and you, but try to ignore it, cover for her, or joke with her about it.

◆ **Anemia.** Anemia is a blood disorder, not a digestive tract disorder, but it is listed here because it can be caused by digestive or dietary problems. It is common among the elderly, is often undiagnosed, and can have serious consequences.

When a person is diagnosed as anemic, it means that his red blood cells, which carry oxygen around the body, are damaged or in short supply. Anemia, once known as "tired blood,"

SHOTS

 Your parent should absolutely, without a doubt, get a flu (influenza) vaccine every year. The flu can be deadly in frail, elderly people. She should get a shot each year between September and mid-November, before the flu season begins. And because you are taking care of her, you should get one, too.

Everyone seems to know someone who got a flu shot and then got the flu. That might have happened, but the illness was not a result of the shot. Flu shots are made from dead flu viruses and cannot cause the flu. They can cause a bit of redness, soreness, and swelling at the site of the shot and sometimes a low-grade fever or headache for a day or two.

The shot is not foolproof. Your parent might still get the flu. However, the symptoms and duration and risk of death will be greatly reduced. (People who are allergic to eggs should talk to their doctors, as the vaccine is grown in eggs and can cause a severe reaction.)

Medicare and most insurers cover the cost of flu shots. Senior centers and local health departments often offer flu shots.

Be alert to early signs of the flu—chills, fever, dry cough, stuffy nose, muscle aches, headache, and fatigue—as there are medications that can reduce the severity and length of the illness, but they must be taken within forty-eight hours of becoming sick.

Check your parent's vaccination records and be sure she's had a pneumococcal pneumonia vaccine. While this is only needed once in a lifetime (usually after age sixty-five), the Centers for Disease Control and Prevention recommends that people who received their shot more than five years ago and were younger than sixty-five should have it again.

Your parent should also be sure she's up to date on her tetanus and diphtheria vaccines, which should be administered together every ten years. If your parent has never had chicken pox, measles, mumps, or rubella, she should be sure she is vaccinated against those as well.

makes a person feel old and tired—even older and more tired than he already feels. This is why it's often not treated—it looks largely like a bad case of old age. But it can make life cumbersome for your parent, limiting his ability to do simple physical tasks and possibly shortening his life.

Anemia can also cause headaches, shortness of breath, irritability, apathy, cold hands and feet, chest pains, swelling, confusion, dizziness, depression, and, in the case of iron-deficient anemia, restless legs at night, and a sore tongue.

A simple blood test is all it takes to see if your parent suffers from anemia, so it's worth asking your parent's doctor to do such a test.

Iron-deficient anemia, the most common type of anemia found in the elderly, is often caused by internal bleeding, which is often due to ulcers, cancer, hemorrhoids, and other problems in the digestive tract. Other types of anemia may be caused by chronic infection or inflammation, kidney or liver disease, cancer, or folate or vitamin B-12 deficiency.

The doctor should determine the cause and treat any underlying disorder. A diet high in iron might help (meat and poultry, especially the liver, kidneys, and other organs, egg yolks, dark green leafy vegetables, dried fruits, and dried beans and peas), although iron supplements or injections are usually necessary.

♦ **Diabetes.** Noninsulin-dependent diabetes (also known as adult-onset or Type 2 diabetes) is more common in older people who are overweight and inactive. Eight percent of people over sixty-five and up to 25 percent of people over eighty-five have diabetes, a condition in which the body loses its ability to regulate glucose, a simple sugar that acts as fuel.

The pancreas makes insulin, a hormone that regulates the use of glucose in the body. When the body doesn't make insulin or doesn't use it effectively, glucose builds up in the blood, causing an array of problems.

Early signs of the disease include fatigue, weight loss, blurred vision, and sometimes itchy skin. While younger diabetics experience thirst and frequent urination, these symptoms may or may not be present in older people. Instead, they may notice other symptoms, such as tingling in the feet or numbness, confusion, or depression.

If your parent has such symptoms he should see a doctor right away, because diabetes must be carefully managed. Untreated, it can lead to serious trouble, including stroke, blindness, heart disease, kidney failure, nerve damage, unconsciousness, and coma.

The first line of treatment is a controlled diet (devised by a dietitian), exercise, and, when necessary, weight loss. Insulin therapy is often necessary, as is medication—sulfonylurea agents—which stimulate insulin secretion.

If your parent has diabetes, he will need special attention to his feet (check daily for sores, blisters, infections, and heavy calluses, and report any problems to the doctor), skin care (keep it clean, use moisturizers, and take good care of any cut, scratch, or bruise), and oral hygiene (talk with the dentist about avoiding infections).

For more information about diabetes, contact the American Diabetes Association (800-232-3472 or www.diabetes.org).

Chapter Thirteen

MATTERS OF THE MIND

Depression • Anxiety Disorders • Delirium

G ROWING OLD IS NOT EASY, AND AT TIMES IT IS DREADFUL, but it does not, by itself, cause depression, anxiety, or other mental illness. Despite all the losses and disability they face, most elderly people adapt pretty well. Indeed, many find joy and peace in these final years.

When sadness turns into despair, when simple worries become paralyzing, when your parent no longer finds joy in the things she used to love, it is time to seek professional help. Hopelessness, unremitting grief, surliness, and constant worry are not "just a part of growing old." People don't suddenly become depressed because they turned eighty. These are signs of trouble.

In elderly people, physical illness and the medical treatments that accompany them often lead to mental illness. It makes sense that hearing loss and incontinence are associated with high rates of depression because these problems are isolating. But heart attack and stroke are also precursors of depression. It would seem that something else is happening, that some physiological change has occurred that makes otherwise resilient people unable to bounce back.

The reverse is also true. In the elderly, mental illness can cause physical ailments. For example, studies suggest that about half of all complaints of gastrointestinal pain in the elderly—heartburn, diarrhea, nausea, constipation, gastritis, etc.—have a psychological component. That is not to say that these problems are invented. They exist. They are real. But they are caused, at least in part, by anxiety, paranoia, or other mental distress.

Now throw into this mind-matter muddle the death of a spouse, the loss of mobility, and the loss of independence, and you've got yourself an interesting question. What caused what and which came first? The physical illness, mental illness, or environmental factors? What do you treat, and how do you, as the grown child, help?

Depression

Your father doesn't want to play bridge anymore, and he won't even look at a crossword puzzle. He turns down his favorite mint chocolate Girl Scout cookies. He dresses in the same clothes every day and refuses to go out. "What's the point?" he says, staring vacantly at the television set. "I'm just an old man. I'll be dead before you know it." Then he calls you by the wrong name and goes to bed.

You may think that he's just being ornery, causing you untold worry and exasperation, but in truth he may be suffering from depression.

Studies suggest that up to 15 percent of people over sixty-five suffer from some degree of depression. In nursing homes, that rate jumps to somewhere between 30 and 50 percent.

What's alarming, however, is not the number of elderly people who are depressed. What's alarming is that the majority of elderly people suffering from depression are never diagnosed or treated. They wade through old age carrying this unbearable weight until they die (which is usually earlier than it would have been had they been treated).

Depression is ignored in the elderly for all sorts of reasons. They themselves ignore the blackness that has overcome them because they were brought up during a time when depression was considered to be a weakness, a character flaw. They think they should be able to control it themselves.

Perhaps even more distressing, depression is missed because family members assume that being antisocial and grumpy, losing weight, and sleeping at odd hours is just part of growing old. But, of course, depression is not normal at any age.

Depression is also overlooked because the complex stew of illness, medications, and grief that commonly affects elderly people complicates any diagnosis. In the elderly it is often triggered by an illness, particularly heart

ON THE LOOKOUT FOR SYMPTOMS

Problem	Signs of Trouble
Depression	Withdrawal, apathy, crying, hopelessness, changes in weight or sleep habits, vague physical complaints
Anxiety disorders	Excessive worry or fear, agitation, insomnia, muscle tension, irritability
Delirium	Inattentiveness and severe confusion that come on fairly suddenly, often accompanied by grogginess or anxiety
Dementia	Confusion, chronic forgetfulness, and other mental lapses that get progressively worse. (See Chapter Twenty-One for a full discussion of memory loss and dementia.)

disease, stroke, certain cancers, chronic lung disease, arthritis, vitamin B-12 deficiency, Alzheimer's disease, and Parkinson's disease. It can also be triggered by, or worsened by, medications, particularly blood pressure medications, anti-ulcer medications, muscle relaxants, steroids, and drugs for Parkinson's disease.

Many of the symptoms of depression—fatigue, apathy, weight loss, confusion, change in appetite—can easily be attributed to an existing illness or ongoing treatment. *Well, he just had a stroke and it's changed him completely.* It doesn't occur to anyone that the symptoms are pieces of a treatable psychiatric disorder.

Meanwhile, the patient, engulfed by despair, does not follow prescribed treatments for his heart disease or arthritis, does not take care of himself, and fails to show up for medical appointments, thereby derailing all efforts at recovery. The physical illness gets only worse, as does the mental illness.

Such neglect is a shame because depression is virtually always treatable with medication, counseling, or both. Untreated, it increases the risk of stroke and heart disease, and reduces a person's ability to recover from surgery, infection, and illness. It causes confusion and exacerbates dementia. It reduces a person's incentive to care for himself, as we've mentioned, and lowers his energy level. In an attempt to self-medicate, a depressed person may abuse alcohol or drugs. With time, depression causes irreversible brain damage. And, of course, it can lead to suicide.

In a nutshell, depression will make these "golden years" miserable for your parent and everyone around him.

Know the signs of depression, and if you have any concern at all, get your parent medical help. You have to be on your toes because, as noted, the signs are often baffling. Not only might the depression be tied to a serious disease, but elderly people with depression may not complain of sadness, anxiety, or hopelessness; instead, they talk about physical symptoms—an upset stomach, backache, headache, sleepless nights, fatigue, or memory loss.

Understandably, you (as well as the doctor) might be busy wondering about biological causes of the complaints and looking for treatments for the stomach pains and insomnia, rather than suspecting depression. In a person who has numerous health problems, it can be extremely difficult to tell where one thing ends and the other begins.

The loss of a loved one or a series of friends, as well as a move to a nursing home, can cause untold grief, which, unabated, can evolve into a full-blown depression. It can be difficult for a layperson to separate grief from depression. In general, once grief lasts for more than two months, it is considered depression. But when losses pile up—a spouse dies, a friend dies, your parent's arthritis gets worse, he moves into a nursing home—there is no starting point for this artificial clock.

Ask your parent's doctor about the possibility of depression. If the doctor doesn't take this seriously—doctors can be biased or ill-informed—get an opinion from another doctor or a psychiatrist, preferably one with some background or experience in geriatrics.

Even if your parent doesn't meet the strict psychiatric criteria for depres-

> " My father had to be hospitalized twice because of severe infections in his feet. We were all so concerned about his diabetes and his infection that at first we failed to see the real problem: depression. Because he was depressed, he wasn't taking care of himself. He wasn't controlling his diabetes, he wasn't eating well, and he didn't call anyone when he first noticed trouble. I guess he figured it didn't matter."
>
> KATHERINE S.

sion—if he is just mildly depressed, perhaps a bit lethargic or unusually restless—he should still seek help. Mild depression like this usually sorts itself out with time, but counseling, support, and other treatments are available and can be very helpful. Just be careful that a doctor doesn't prescribe antidepressants needlessly, as they can cause serious side effects.

DEPRESSION AND DEMENTIA

YOUR FATHER MAY BE CONFUSED and forgetful, leading you to fear the worst. But before you call the Alzheimer's Association, have him evaluated by a doctor. Depression is often mistaken for dementia and therefore left untreated.

Of course, the complications don't end there. Depression is often coupled with dementia, particularly in the earliest stages of dementia. Between 20 and 40 percent of people with dementia also suffer from depression.

Finally, mild depressive symptoms—lack of energy and initiative, social withdrawal, loss of enthusiasm, and generally sitting around and not wanting to do anything—are sometimes not depression at all, but an early sign of dementia.

Have your parent evaluated as soon as possible. If he has dementia, you both need to know. If he is suffering from depression, regardless of what else is happening with him, it should be treated. Even when depression coexists with dementia, treating the depression will alleviate some of the confusion (albeit not permanently). For more information on dementia, see Chapter Twenty-One.

DEPRESSION, DELUSIONS, AND HALLUCINATIONS

SEVERE DEPRESSION IN THE ELDERLY is sometimes accompanied by delusions—beliefs that are simply not true. For example, a person might be certain that someone is following him or reading his mind, that someone loves him or is being unfaithful, or that he has an illness or deformity that he doesn't have. Older people who are depressed might also have hallucinations—seeing or hearing things that don't exist.

Antipsychotic medications are useful in treating delusions and hallucinations. Electroshock therapy is also effective in these cases.

APPROACHING THE SUBJECT

DEPRESSION IS NOT A MOOD; IT IS A medical illness. The chemistry in the brain has changed and needs rebalancing. Why it comes on is not clear. Loss, fear, boredom, worry, loneliness, and stress all play a role. Some people inherit a genetic vulnerability to depression. Personalities developed early in life—low self-esteem, poor coping skills—play a role as well. Medications, illness, hormonal and biological changes, inactivity, poor diet, and, as mentioned, a move to an institution, can all contribute to depression.

Of course, the mere suggestion that your parent see a psychiatrist, or even his own doctor, about a mental health problem may be pooh-poohed or it may make your parent furious. Make it clear that depression is a biological illness that can be treated; it has nothing to do with personal will or strength. You don't even have to use the word *depression*. Simply explain that diagnosing and treating "whatever this is" will help him remain independent; failing to treat it will certainly lead to more dependence, illness, and disability.

If he still won't budge, tell him that it would be a great relief to you if he at least spoke to a doctor about it. Tell him that you won't stop hassling him until he does it. Or get a trusted doctor or member of the clergy to initiate a discussion with him about his depression. Or, talk to the doctor yourself about it.

If the prospect of seeing a psychiatrist makes your parent uncom-

DEEP IN DEPRESSION

 Brief bouts of sadness and grief are normal, and most people with very mild depressive symptoms get better on their own. But if your parent has several of the following symptoms for more than two weeks (or more than two months after a major loss or move to an institution), press his doctor for action or get him to a psychiatrist.

- Dejection and sadness without any apparent cause

- Feelings of hopelessness, helplessness, guilt, and worthlessness

- Lack of interest in activities that were once considered enjoyable

- Social withdrawal

- Unusual restlessness, irritability, or hostility

- Frequent crying spells, weeping, or tearfulness

- Change in appetite or weight

- Insomnia or change in sleep habits

- Fatigue and lethargy

- Lack of concentration, forgetfulness, indecisiveness

- Excessive worry about finances and health

- Vague complaints of physical aches and pains

- Decline in grooming and personal hygiene

- Increased use of alcohol, drugs, or tobacco

- Talk of death or suicide

fortable, a family doctor who is savvy in such matters can treat the depression. But be sure the doctor takes this seriously; don't be deterred by a physician who tells you "it's natural at his age." No one should have to live with the deep pain of clinical depression.

TREATING DEPRESSION

THE FIRST STEP IN TREATING DEPRESSION in the elderly is to identify any underlying cause or contributing factors (medications, dementia, vitamin deficiency, etc.). Next, most experts recommend a multipronged approach of therapy, antidepressants and lifestyle changes. Do not rely on drugs alone. Indeed, if the depression is not severe, your parent should try therapy and lifestyle changes before starting on drugs, as these prescriptions can cause confusion and other serious side effects in elderly patients.

◆ **Antidepressive drugs.** A variety of antidepressive drugs are effective in treating depression with only minor side effects. These drugs increase the levels of certain chemicals in the brain, called neurotransmitters (because they "transmit" messages between nerve cells). Depression is often the result of an imbalance in these chemicals.

In general, when treating older patients, doctors rely on a type of antidepressant that raises the level of the neurotransmitter serotonin, called selective serotonin reuptake inhibitors, or SSRIs. These drugs (which include common brand names such as Prozac, Paxil, Zoloft, and Celexa) are less apt to cause confusion, drowsiness, or dizziness.

Antidepressants need to be taken for four to eight weeks before they are fully effective and, because recurrence is common, they are often continued at a low dose for at least six to twelve months after the symptoms of depression have subsided. Depending upon the severity of the depression and the number of episodes, a doctor might recommend that your parent stay on a medication for several years.

If a medication causes unpleasant side effects or, after several weeks, does not seem to be helping, your parent should alert his doctor. Sometimes a person needs to try a different antidepressant; sometimes a combination of medications is necessary.

Be sure your parent sticks to any regime. Skipping medications or stopping early may make them ineffective and lead to relapses of depression.

◆ **Psychotherapy.** Sometimes therapy alone can treat depression, especially if the depression is mild. Drug treatments are usually more effective if they are coupled with counseling. The drugs relieve the severity of the depression, bringing a person out of the pit of despair, but they do not resolve any issues that might have contributed to the depression. Therapy, individually or in a group, will help your parent address these problems.

Be sure your parent finds someone whom she trusts and feels comfortable with. She might have to try several therapists before she finds the right fit. Then encourage her to stay with it for at least ten weeks, preferably longer.

More and more people are receiving counseling by phone, especially in rural areas and when people are so disabled or frail that they cannot leave home.

◆ **Electroconvulsive therapy.** When depression is severe or psychotic, and antidepressants and counseling don't help, electroconvulsive therapy, or ECT, can be very effective. It seems to be particularly successful in treating severe depression in elderly patients.

We've all heard horror stories about ECT, but the procedure has been fine-tuned and is considered to be an effective, fast, and safe way to reverse depression. It usually works faster than drugs, but the effects don't last as long. (Medication will sometimes help lower the rate of recurrent bouts of depression.)

In the procedure, a patient is given anesthesia and a muscle relaxant. A padded electrode is then placed at the temple. A small machine sends an electric pulse through the electrode and into the brain until the patient has a minor brain seizure. The seizure triggers neurons to release chemicals that are necessary for a healthy, functioning brain. People often need six to twelve treatments over the course of a few weeks.

The procedure is not painful, but there is a risk of mild memory loss. Most memory problems caused by the treatment subside within a month or two. However, ECT is usually a poor choice for a person with dementia or certain other medical conditions. Your parent, or you, should discuss all the pros and cons with the doctor. Understandably, the idea may frighten your parent (and you), so by all means, get a second opinion.

◆ **Lifestyle.** Exercise, social activities, sleep, community involvement,

GETTING HELP

Because mental illness is so complicated in the elderly and is often linked to illness, medications, and issues that are specific to elderly people, you should look for a psychiatrist (or psychotherapist, for therapy) who has a good deal of experience in dealing with elderly clients. Ask what percent of the practice is clients over sixty-five. Ideally, it should be at least 25 percent. Some psychiatrists are certified in geriatric psychiatry, although they are few and far between. You can get a referral from the American Association for Geriatric Psychiatry (301-654-7850 or www.aagponline.org).

intellectual stimulation, a good diet, and an understanding and loving family will not, by themselves, cure true depression. However, they are extremely potent in easing the pain and then keeping it at bay. Those patients who take care of themselves and have support and encouragement from friends and family always fare better than others.

Be sure your parent gets good medical care. Keep an eye on his diet, exercise, sleep, and other lifestyle issues. Gently encourage him to get back into activities that he once enjoyed, to come to social gatherings, and even try new things.

Creative outlets can be helpful for some people. Drawing, painting, sculpt-ing, and other art forms can help people unload deeply held emotions and understand their own needs. Likewise, dance and music can help release stress and ease feelings of hopelessness.

But remember, when a person is depressed, he cannot "snap out of it" any more than he can snap out of cancer or Parkinson's disease. This is not "just the blues"; it is an illness. Although your impulse may be to try to propel your parent out of this despair, avoid urging him to "cheer up" or to "look on the bright side." Attempts to convince him that life isn't so bad, or to help him see that others are worse off than he is, will only send the message that this is something he can control, and because he is not controlling it, he is a failure.

Listen to his concerns and acknowledge his fears and misery. Let him know that you are there for him, that you care, that you want to help. *I know you feel horrible. We're going to get through this thing together.* Be patient with any irritability, sullenness, or criticism that might come your way. This is largely the disease talking (or refusing to talk), not your parent.

◆ **Other supports.** Your parent might find strength in support groups, either in person or online. Talking to others who struggle with the same issues can make a person feel less alone. Pastoral counseling and spiritual support can also be enormously helpful. Having a pet can be a powerful elixir for depression, as well as for anxiety and other mental illnesses.

◆ **Unconventional medicine.**
There are numerous alternative or complementary therapies, many of them rooted in Chinese, Indian, and Native American cultures, that can be useful in alleviating depression and anxiety. Most take a holistic approach, believing that bodies need to be balanced physically, mentally, and spiritually. They include acupuncture, massage, meditation, yoga, tai chi, breathing exercises, herbs, and other methods to relieve tension and bring the body into balance.

Some people use certain herbs, vitamins, and minerals (riboflavin, magnesium, and thiamine) in treating depression as well as anxiety. There is little scientific evidence on whether this helps or not.

Biofeedback seems to be more helpful in treating anxiety than depression, but some studies suggest it may be effective for depression as well. In biofeedback, a person learns to control their bodily reactions—muscle tension, heart rate, breathing, skin temperature—to stressful or upsetting situations. Guided imagery, or visualization, which involves going into a deep state of relaxation, is often used to treat depression, addiction, and anxiety.

For more information about such approaches, contact the National Center for Complementary and Alternative Medicine, a branch of the National Institutes of Health, at 888-644-6226 or www.nccam.nih.gov. (See page 207 for more on alternative therapies.)

> *After my father moved into the retirement home, he didn't want to do anything. Nothing seemed to please him. He stayed in his room most of the time, refused to see people, and just didn't care about anything. When I suggested that he get help, he became angry.*
>
> *Finally, I couldn't stand it anymore. I marched into his room and told him to get in the car, and I took him to the geriatric psychiatry unit at our local hospital. I've never been forceful with my father, but something just got to me. I couldn't bear to see him like that.*
>
> *He had ECT for several weeks, and now he's in a day program where he meets with the psychiatrist and goes to a support group. I have to say, it's made a difference. He's not jumping about, all excited about life, but he's definitely better."*
>
> —ELEANOR R.

Anxiety Disorders

Has your mother always been a worrywart, or have her anxieties reached new heights? While elderly people are often more cautious (with good reason), about 5 percent of the elderly suffer from a psychiatric ill-ness known as generalized anxiety dis-order.

The defining symptom is exces-sive, daily worry about several issues that lasts for at least six months. The worry or dread is so great that it gets in the way of daily activities. It is usu-ally accompanied by a number of physical reactions, including agitation or restlessness, irritability, exhaustion, insomnia, difficulty concentrating, and muscle tension. Other symptoms sometimes include shakiness and trem-bling, dizziness, shortness of breath,

nausea, hot and cold flashes, frequent urination, and an exaggerated response when startled. A person with an anx-iety disorder is also apt to be extremely vigilant and edgy.

As you know by now, nothing to do with the elderly is simple. There are several ailments that are often mis-taken for anxiety disorder, including hyperthyroidism, and heart or lung diseases that cause palpitations and/or shortness of breath. Also, anxiety and agitation may be symptoms of delir-ium, depression, or dementia, not an illness in its own right. It's possible,

SUICIDE

Suicide is more common among people over the age of sixty-five than in any other age group. The suicide rate among white males over the age of sixty-five is five times that of the general population. White males over the age of eighty are especially prone, with rates soaring above all other age and racial groups. The main reason for suicide: untreated depression.

If your parent talks about harming himself or dying, get help immediately. Do not assume that since he just saw his doctor, he must be safe. Of elderly people who commit suicide, 75 percent have seen their doctors within a month of killing themselves. Many saw their doctors on the same day.

Your parent might resist help, saying that he's fine or he'll handle it himself. Rather than nudging gently, you have to be assertive and forceful. Contact his doctor. Or for more immediate help, go to the hospital emergency room. Remove pills, knives, and other weapons from the house.

If you are concerned about suicide and your parent refuses to accept help, you might have to get what's known as a certificate of involuntary commitment from a judge, psychiatrist, or other physician. This forces your parent to have a brief psychiatric evaluation (which can sometimes be done in the home), and may result in institutionalization for a period.

too, that your parent is reacting to justifiable fears (for example, running out of money or being mugged) and has no psychiatric disorder. By contrast, in an anxiety disorder, the fear far exceeds reality and is unabated when the cause of fear is addressed.

Generalized anxiety disorder is usually caused by some combination of legitimate concern or fear, genetics, disease, medications, caffeine, vitamin B-12 deficiency, and withdrawal from alcohol or sedatives. Dementia is one of the most common causes of anxiety among the elderly. Unfortunately, extreme worrying, sometimes accompanied by attacks of sheer panic, causes a person to withdraw. People then fail to recognize that dementia is at the root of the problem.

Obsessive-compulsive disorder, classified as a type of anxiety disorder, is also relatively common among the elderly, especially elderly women. A person has intrusive and unwanted thoughts, often about something silly, scary, or disgusting, and strong urges to do something repeatedly that eases the obsessions.

Other anxiety disorders include phobias—particularly agoraphobia, which is an intense fear of public places, and claustrophobia, a fear of enclosed spaces—and panic disorders, in which the anxiety comes on suddenly and forcefully.

Obviously, any contributing factor (medications, disease) should be addressed. Treatment also includes counseling to deal with specific causes of concern, family support, biofeed-

FOR MORE HELP

National Institute of Mental Health
866-615-6464
www.nimh.nih.gov

National Foundation for Depressive Illness
800-248-1265
www.depression.org

National Alliance for the Mentally Ill
800-950-6264
www.nami.org

Depression and Bipolar Support Alliance
800-826-3632
www.dbsalliance.org

American Association for Geriatric Psychiatry
301-654-7850
www.aagponline.org

back, and relaxation techniques. See the previous section on treatments for depression, especially those paragraphs concerning psychotherapy, lifestyle changes, unconventional medicine, and other approaches, as these are all extremely useful in treating anxiety. Don't underestimate the value of family support, exercise, meditation, yoga, tai chi, pets, music and art, massage, and other unconventional treatments. Medications can be critical, but they are only one part of the puzzle and should not be the only tack taken.

Antianxiety drugs (preferably shorter-acting ones) should be used only in severe cases because they can cause side effects such as depression, speech trouble, and memory loss. Valium, Dalmane, Librium, Nembutal, Seconal and related drugs should not be prescribed for older people.

Delirium

Delirium is very common in the elderly, but it is, unfortunately, usually unrecognized or misdiagnosed. It is most common among hospitalized elderly, although as people are sent home sooner from the hospital, delirium is moving into nursing homes and private homes. Nearly 20 percent of people over seventy are delirious upon entering the hospital; at least 10 to 20 percent become delirious during their stay.

Delirium can resemble depression, dementia, or even anxiety, but it differs from them in that it typically comes on suddenly and severely, over the course of a few hours or days, and the most notable symptoms are extreme confusion and inattentiveness.

A person with delirium may not be able to follow even a brief discussion, or he may fall asleep in the middle of a conversation. He may suddenly have no idea what is happening, may not recognize familiar faces, or may not know where he is. While most older patients with delirium become quiet and sleepy, some become anxious and restless. In severe cases, they hallucinate and panic.

The most common trigger is surgery. Between 15 to 25 percent of elderly people become delirious after elective surgery, but far more—perhaps as much as 65 percent—become delirious after emergency surgery.

Delirium can also be the result of medications, especially when a new medication is started, a dose is changed, or a medication is stopped. Psychoactive drugs, such as sedatives, antidepressants, opioids, and anticholinergic drugs (as well as many other prescription and nonprescription drugs) are all likely culprits.

Illness, such as stroke, heart failure, or internal bleeding, can precipitate delirium, as can a move to a new environment, dehydration, infections, blindness or deafness, alcohol withdrawal, or severe urinary or fecal incontinence or retention.

People who are already compromised by dementia, Parkinson's disease, stroke, or tumor are at the greatest risk, as are very frail elderly people who do not have the reserves to deal with illness or surgery.

DIAGNOSIS AND TREATMENT

AS WITH DEPRESSION, WHEN DELIRium goes unrecognized or is misdiagnosed, the cost is high. Unchecked, delirium often leads to other serious medical problems, even death. The sooner it is identified, the easier it is to treat.

As the person who best knows your parent, you may be the first to spot the symptoms. Anytime you notice a significant change in your parent's behavior, alert a doctor or nurse immediately and ask about the possibility of delirium.

Since it's often not possible to identify a single cause, doctors attack delirium on many fronts. Any infections or illnesses need to be treated, and over-the-counter drugs should be stopped or, if that is not possible, the dose reduced.

The doctor should also take steps to prevent bedsores, urinary and fecal problems, malnutrition, and other problems that often accompany delirium. Be wary of any attempt to use sedatives or physical restraints to control your parent, as this will most likely only worsen your parent's state.

You play an important role in the treatment of your parent so, if you can, stay nearby. A calm and supportive environment is essential in easing the symptoms. Assure your parent that he is safe and try to keep him calm. Help reorient him by speaking softly and by surrounding him with familiar objects. Put clocks and calendars where he can see them. Make sure he has his glasses and hearing

> " While my mother was in the nursing home, she became very confused and started to act oddly. She refused food and water and would wander about like she didn't know where she was.
>
> I was more concerned than the nurses were, so I was the one who called it to the doctor's attention. He said she was delirious, and he put her through dozens of tests. They found that she was dehydrated, had a urinary tract infection, and was taking too much of an antipsychotic drug. As soon as they adjusted the dose and dealt with her other problems, she returned to normal, or at least to what was normal for her"
>
> — GLORIA C.

aids. Keep movement at a minimum, lighting dim, and the noise level low. Night-lights are sometimes helpful so your parent doesn't become confused if he wakes up in the dark.

Delirium, once properly diagnosed, is usually reversible, but there might be some residual confusion for a few weeks.

Chapter Fourteen

ON THE FIFTH FLOOR

*Entering the Hospital • Tests, Surgery, and Treatments
• Dealing with Staff • Your Role as Advocate
• Comfort on the Fifth Floor • When You Are Far Away
• Preparing for Discharge*

N O MATTER WHAT HOSPITALS DO TO LOOK MORE
welcoming and genial—with large plants in the lobby,
colorful prints on the walls, friendly volunteers at the
door—it never works. Hospitals are scary, especially when you
enter them late in life, when the reasons for going tend to be
serious. For your parent, entering the hospital means enormous
risk and loss of control. He may be dreading a diagnosis, fearful
that he won't be able to return to his own home, or fearful that he
will never leave this place at all.

Your parent needs plenty of love and reassurance now. She also
desperately needs a strong advocate, someone who will communicate
with doctors and nurses; stay informed about tests, treatments, and
other procedures; and make sure she is getting proper care. Mishaps
and mix-ups occur frequently in hospitals, where patients are weak,
contagions run rampant, and staff is overworked and undertrained.

If your parent is confused or too sick to speak for herself, then
your involvement and your physical presence—or the presence of

other friends and family—is essential. Someone needs to be sure she's getting the right medications, getting proper meals, being rotated to avoid bedsores, etc.

However, if you've been caring for your parent on a full-time basis for some time, this hospital stay might also be a much-needed break for you. Keep close tabs on her care, communicate regularly with the nurses, but get others to spend time with her now so you can take advantage of this break. Get family members and friends to rotate watches, or consider hiring someone to stay with your parent for some part of the day. Then, when you are not at the hospital, get your mind off your worries, spend time with friends, and catch up on your sleep. You need it.

Choosing a Hospital

A doctor can work only in those hospitals where he or she has admitting privileges, so there may be little choice in selecting a hospital if your parent is committed to a doctor. Also, her Medicare plan or other insurance might require that she go to doctors and a hospital within a network. However, if there is a choice about which hospital to use and some preparation time, she, or you, should carefully select both the doctor and the hospital.

Most important, choose a doctor who has a lot of experience with this particular procedure, surgery, or treatment, and a hospital that specializes in it. If it's a common procedure, like bypass surgery or a hysterectomy, then the surgeon should have performed close to a hundred such surgeries in the past year. (If it's a less common procedure or your parent lives in a rural area, the number will be lower.)

Generally, large medical centers associated with a university have high-caliber specialists, dedicated clinics, and more sophisticated technology than small community hospitals. Thus, they have higher volume and more experience with many procedures. They are also generally more equipped to treat unusual ailments and perform risky procedures.

But large-scale can also mean that patients get less attention and TLC than they might in a smaller hospital. So if a particular surgeon has privileges at more than one hospital, your parent might be happier in the smaller hospital. (Surgery at a not-for-profit community hospital may also be as much as 25 percent cheaper than at a private hospital.)

> " *My father always went to the same hospital, but when I called 911, the ambulance took him to a different hospital. Here my father was in a strange place, with a new doctor who didn't know him at all, who didn't have any personal relationship with him.*
>
> *It took me more than a week, but I finally got them to move him. They kept saying that he was too weak to make the move, that he was fine where he was. But I knew that he wasn't. I knew that this was an unfamiliar place for him.*
>
> *He was moved, and he died about two weeks later. But I know that he was more comfortable in a familiar place, with doctors and nurses who knew him and where his friends could visit him easily. He couldn't tell me so, but I believe that I did the right thing."*
>
> —CHRIS D.

Another issue to consider: Teaching hospitals train young doctors, using patients as teaching models, which can be disconcerting and, when five or six young doctors are standing around the bedside, embarrassing. However, physicians-in-training ask a lot of questions, which bring important matters to the attending doctor's attention.

Veterans Affairs hospitals are sometimes unwieldy and top-heavy with bureaucracy, but since they are often associated with a university hospital, the medical care is quite good. In any case, they are inexpensive. (The Department of Veterans Affairs, 800-827-1000 or www.va.gov, can tell you about eligibility and benefits.)

In an emergency, your parent may have to go to the nearest hospital— one where her doctor may not be able to treat her. But once she is out of danger, she can usually be transferred.

Do some homework. Talk to others. Find a surgeon and hospital with a good reputation. Some hospitals now put out "report cards," but these are often difficult to obtain and only moderately useful. There are also Web sites that provide quality reports on health-care facilities that accept Medicare, such as www.healthgrades.com.

Entering the Hospital

The hospital will want a variety of information before your parent is admitted, including name, address, Social Security number, phone number, birth date, name of next of kin, and Medicare, Medicaid, and other health insurance numbers. They will ask about advance directives. And they will need to know what medications your parent takes, what allergies she has, and information about previous hospitalizations and injuries.

Among the forms your parent (or you, if you are acting on his behalf) will be asked to sign is a blanket consent form, which basically says that the hospital can do whatever needs to be done while he is under its care. Don't be alarmed. These forms are routine. The staff still needs a patient's consent before undertaking any measures beyond emergency procedures, but most hospitals won't admit patients unless they sign this form. If signing it makes you uncomfortable, add a note before the signature that says, "I'm signing this only so that my parent can be admitted to the hospital."

If you know in advance about the hospitalization, ask if the paperwork can be done early so your parent doesn't have to deal with a lot of questions on an already tense day. Also, see if someone can drop you and your parent off at the hospital so she doesn't have to wait while you park.

If your parent is alert and may be in the hospital for some time, go ahead and ask if there is a choice in rooms, because once your parent is assigned to a room, the staff will be reluctant to move her (it requires a lot of paperwork, as well as physical work). If there is any choice, ask for a bed near a window. Natural light and a view—even if it's a view of a rooftop—can boost the spirits. You should also ask about roommates, privacy, and anything else that concerns your parent. She may not be given a lot of choice, but it's certainly worth asking.

At the same time, inquire about a telephone and television, as it can take a day or two to get these services up and running. If this will be a long

DON'T FORGET

Be *sure* that your parent has signed a living will, describing her wishes regarding end-of-life care, and a health-care proxy, authorizing someone (usually a family member) to make medical decisions on her behalf.

You should have these documents in hand, copies should be filed in her medical chart, and her doctor should be well aware of them.

Even if this hospitalization is routine, be sure these papers are signed. Many older patients become briefly delirious after surgery, even routine surgery, and can't make decisions for themselves. And of course, something unexpected can always occur. You will need them if there is any dispute about your parent's medical care.

It is important that you also talk with your parent about her thoughts, priorities, and wishes concerning aggressive medical care and palliative care at the end of life. Then talk with her doctor about how you might carry out her wishes, depending on the circumstances. See pages 383 and 522 for more on these issues.

PACKING THE BAG

There is little that your parent really needs in a hospital and anything valuable should stay at home. A hospital bag might include:

◆ Hearing aids, eyeglasses, dentures, cane, or walker

◆ A supply of her regular medications, along with a list of her medications, their dosages, any allergies, and medical history

◆ Copies of pertinent legal documents, such as a living will, a health-care proxy form, or other advance directives

◆ Slippers with rubber soles

◆ Socks, preferably with rubber soles

◆ Robe and pajamas or nightgown (short-sleeved or sleeveless, for easy access)

◆ Toiletry items, including toothbrush, toothpaste, deodorant, shampoo, soap, razor, lip balm, and moisturizer (check about whether the hospital allows electrical devices)

◆ A clock and a calendar

◆ Crackers, dried fruit, cereal, or other nonperishable foods, if diet allows

◆ Ear plugs

◆ A telephone credit card number and a small amount of cash for vendors—no more than $20

---

stay, find out about other amenities as well, such as newspaper delivery, barber and hair stylists, Internet access, book and magazine carts. Patients often don't know about these services unless they ask for them.

PREPARING FOR DISCHARGE—IN ADVANCE

AS SOON AS YOU KNOW YOUR parent's prognosis, talk with the hospital's discharge planner, especially if you think your parent may have difficulty returning to his former life after he leaves the hospital. The discharge planner will help you prepare for your parent's return home, lining him up with community services, home care, and medical equipment, or making arrangements for him to move into a rehabilitation center, nursing home, or other living situation. All of this planning takes time, and you want everything to be in place when your parent is ready to leave the hospital.

Sometimes it's helpful to talk to the discharge planner even if you think your parent will be just fine returning to his own home. First of all, he might not be as fine as you'd hoped. Second, discharge planners often have a wealth of information about community services and supports that, if they are not needed now, might be needed in the near future. Use this service while it's at your disposal and you're there, wandering hallways in search of a cup of coffee.

Tests, Surgery, and Treatments

Studies suggest that up to one third of all medical procedures are unnecessary. But it also has been found that older patients often receive too little treatment. On the one hand, doctors tend to overprobe and overscan because they are fearful of malpractice lawsuits, enamored of technology, or baffled by a profusion of unusual symptoms. On the other hand, doctors fail to order certain tests or treatments for the elderly because they don't understand the complexity of an older body, don't see the signs of trouble, or don't see the point of treating certain symptoms in a very old person. (This is ageism!)

How are you to know whether your parent is getting too much or too little? Honestly, you can't, but you can impose safeguards by asking plenty of questions, making informed decisions, and getting a second opinion whenever you have doubts. A second, and

> " When the two of us brought my father to the hospital, my sister asked about the room selection, and I was completely embarrassed. It didn't occur to me that there would be a choice, and I thought she was being frivolous and pushy. But just as I was searching for something conciliatory to say, the woman at the admitting desk said that she could arrange for Dad to be in a private room with a window, even though his insurance covered only a semi-private room. It had to do with their occupancy level. Boy, I learned my lesson."
>
> —KATHERINE S.

even third, opinion is always a good choice. Medicare covers most costs of second opinions and any extra tests required, and, when there's dispute, a third opinion as well.

Also, be sure that Medicare, Medicaid, or other insurance will cover the cost of a procedure and all related expenses. What, if anything, will *not* be covered? If the procedure is not covered, find out what this procedure will cost, in total, in advance.

QUESTIONS TO ASK

OF COURSE, YOU'LL WANT TO BE TACT-ful and considerate, but be sure to ask questions like the following (and write down the answers you are given, as you might forget things):

GUILT, AGAIN?

Remember, your parent is not in the hospital because of something you or anyone else in the family did or failed to do. Don't torture yourself with guilt. *I knew I shouldn't have left her alone. . . . I should have told the doctor he was having chest pains. . . . I shouldn't have taken him out yesterday. . . .*

Life is so clear in hindsight, but there really was no way you or anyone else could have predicted this accident or illness. And doing things differently might not have changed the outcome; in fact, it might have led to a worse problem. This hospitalization is not anyone's fault, so focus your valuable energy on taking care of your parent now, and leave the guilt and blame behind.

◆ Why is this test/treatment/surgery recommended?

◆ How and where will it be performed? How long will it take? How long will it take for my parent to recover?

◆ Is it absolutely necessary? What happens if this is not done?

◆ What will this test tell us, and where will we go from there? (For example, if the doctor is not going to do surgery in either case, why bother with the test?)

◆ What are the potential risks and benefits of this procedure? How might it affect my parent's health and lifestyle?

◆ What other options are there, and what are the risks and benefits of each?

◆ How much will it cost? Is it covered fully by Medicare, Medicaid, or my parent's private insurance?

◆ Can other doctors who are treating my parent use the results from this test or blood sample so it doesn't have to be repeated?

◆ Are there other approaches my parent might try first before undergoing this treatment or procedure, such as changes in diet or exercise, to correct what ails her?

◆ Are any experimental treatments available, and what are the risks and benefits of those?

PREPARING FOR SURGERY

IF YOUR PARENT IS GOING TO HAVE surgery, you or she should talk with the surgeon whom her doctor has recommended and find out his or her credentials and experience—in particular, how often he or she has done this procedure.

Find out how soon and how often the surgeon or your parent's doctor will visit your parent after the surgery and note how to reach each of them if there is a problem or question. Learn about the anesthesiologist's qualifications (is he or she a long-time doctor or just out of training, for example) and make sure he or she will meet with your parent before the surgery, as anesthesiology can be very risky in an elderly person.

If the surgery is exploratory, find out what the doctor expects to find and what he or she might do about it. (Does your parent need to sign a consent form now so the surgeon can do what may need to be done?)

Ask the surgeon about possible complications and their symptoms, and what can be done to avert them. Elderly patients who undergo surgery are at high risk of heart and lung complications, blood clots and delirium. In the case of delirium, those who are forewarned of its possibility fare better than those who are unprepared.

In teaching hospitals, residents (doctors-in-training) often perform surgery, which is not ideal, but might be acceptable as long as your parent's surgeon is close at hand to monitor every move. (The doctor won't usually tell you that he or she is not actually performing the surgery, so you have to ask.) If the idea doesn't sit well with your parent or you, ask the doctor to perform the surgery personally.

WHO ARE ALL THOSE PEOPLE IN WHITE COATS?

Who is checking your parent's stitches? Who is that new young man reading your mother's chart? Who are all those other people in white coats that go by the name "doctor"?

"Attending physicians" are doctors with admitting privileges to a hospital, like your parent's personal doctor. Members of the "house staff" have medical school degrees but are still in training and are not yet certified in a specialty. The house staff is composed of "interns," who are one year out of medical school, and "residents," who are two, three, four (and sometimes more) years out of medical school. Residents perform medical procedures, including surgical procedures, while interns perform less technical tasks and are usually overseen by residents.

Teaching hospitals also have medical students who observe the house staff for the most part, but also perform some minor tasks. They, too, wear white coats and, in some hospitals, are called "doctor," although they do not have medical degrees.

You and your parent are unlikely to know who's who, but feel free to ask.

66 *Sometimes we encourage families to help do things, like feed the patient—either because the person eats better when someone familiar helps, or because the family is going to take this person home and will have to do these things there. We want them to get comfortable with it.*

But some families feel put out by that. They feel like they are being asked to do the nurse's work. It's a challenge for the nurse to say, 'No, I'm not trying to get out of work. This is really better for the patient.' It's a very fine line."

—GAIL W., R.N.

If your parent is having one-day, or ambulatory, surgery, it is best if the procedure is done in a hospital, or in a clinic or office near a hospital, in case there are complications. Be sure that your parent has an escort to and from the clinic.

Before any surgery, you or your parent should talk with the doctor about the aftermath. What sort of attention will she need during her recovery? What medications will she need to take? What kind of pain will she be in and how will that be addressed? What other problems should she expect or hurdles might she face? How mobile and functional will she be once she is discharged? What services might she need after surgery? What will she need to do to minimize ill effects?

Will there be any long-term pain or disability associated with this procedure?

WHERE'S HER DOCTOR?

YOUR PARENT'S PRIMARY DOCTOR may relinquish control once your parent enters the hospital. Usually this is because a specialist is now overseeing her care, or because her doctor focuses only on office-based care. Sometimes doctors prefer, or insurance plans or hospitals require, that a hospital doctor (sometimes called a "hospitalist") oversee patients' care in the hospital.

If this switch is disconcerting, talk with your parent's doctor. It may be that he or she can remain involved. At the very least, her new doctor should be in close communication with her original primary care doctor.

At the Nurse's Station

In the hospital, a doctor will continue to oversee your parent's medical care, but it is the nurses who will tend to his needs and, to a large extent, monitor his health. The nurses are usually the ones to notice if a medication is having bad side effects, if your parent has a new symptom, or if his mood or mental abilities have changed. Nurses know a lot about medicine and often understand a good deal (often more than the doctor) about individual patients. The nurse also acts as a liaison to the other

PRIVATE-DUTY NURSES, AIDES, AND COMPANIONS

Hospital staff do not have time to give each patient the attention he or she may need. Another set of hands is invaluable, especially if your parent needs help eating or getting to the toilet, for example. And another set of eyes to watch for mishaps and neglect can be life-saving.

If you can't be with your parent as much as you'd like, hire a companion or find out if there is a volunteer program in the community or the hospital.

If your parent needs more professional care, you can hire a private-duty nurse or a nurse's aide. This is expensive, however, and insurance is not likely to cover it. The hospital staff can refer you to private-duty nurses, a home-care agency, or a visiting nurse association.

Licensed practical nurses and nurses' aides have less training, but are also less expensive, than registered nurses. A health aide has even less expertise but he or she can monitor your parent's medications and care and help with personal tasks.

Two guidelines to follow if you decide to hire additional help for your parent in the hospital: First, be sure the person you hire knows exactly what you expect her to do, as the hospital is not supervising her work; you are. Second, make it clear to the hospital nurses and other personnel that this is no reflection on their work.

hospital personnel, including social workers, therapists, and escorts.

Unless your parent is in the hospital for a very brief stay, make an effort to get to know the nurses who care for him. Learn their names and build a rapport with them. In the hospital, they are your best allies. You need them on your side in order to assure that your parent receives the best care.

◆ **Show respect.** No matter how urgent your concerns may be, no matter how unraveled you feel, avoid the urge to bark orders. *I don't want my mother waiting for her pain medication. She was supposed to get it at two o'clock!* Protect your parent, guard her rights, and advocate firmly on her behalf, but treat the staff as friend, not foe. Recognize the pressures that nurses and other staff are under. When there is a problem, work with them to find solutions. When you treat them with respect, they will be far more willing to treat you and your parent with respect.

If you do lose your cool, and most likely you will, apologize later.

" *The rehabilitation therapist got very frustrated with my dad because he wasn't cooperating. But he wasn't cooperating because he didn't know what the hell he was doing. He has dementia and he gets anxious and ornery when things are new or when people push him to do things he doesn't want to do.*

I learned that at some point, it's the habit of the rehab people to stop trying. I guess they deal with people like this all day long and it gets to them after awhile. I told the therapists that I understood it probably was demoralizing for them, but also how grateful we'd be if they could keep trying with my dad. I had to cajole and encourage and push to get them to keep working with him, but they did stick with it and Dad did, finally, go along with it."

—JACQUI L.

◆ **Ask questions.** Don't withhold important questions and comments for fear of "bothering" the nurses. Most nurses do not consider questions or comments from family members a bother. Nurses are sometimes helpful at explaining things that the doctor didn't make clear. And your questions may bring an error or an oversight to their attention.

◆ **Provide information.** Be sure the nurses know about any allergies or sensitivities, any other medications your parent is taking, and any symptoms she may have. If you are worried about something in particular, tape a large note by the bed—"Mrs. Parker is severely allergic to all seafood." Also, be sure the nurses know about any special needs, habits, quirks, or preferences that will help them care for your parent. They are usually open to reasonable requests.

If your parent has dementia, has become extremely crotchety in her old age, or can't communicate, tell the nurses what she used to be like, or bring in a couple of photos of her in her younger days—skiing, lecturing, dancing, mothering, or just posing—and put them over her bed. Let people see the person behind the illness.

◆ **Lend a hand.** Your assistance, even with little tasks, makes life easier for everybody—your mother gets better care, you feel useful, and the nurse or aides are relieved of another chore. If your mother needs water or tea, if the juice on the floor needs to be wiped up, if she needs help bathing or feeding herself, take care of it. If you're spending hours on end at the bedside, you might even be helpful to the patient in the neighboring bed.

◆ **Kindness counts.** Anxiety can make you forget all the usual social niceties, but thoughtfulness can be enormously important to an overworked nurse, aide, or orderly. When things are done well, when an extra task is undertaken, express your appreciation.

If your parent is going to be in for a long stay, go a step further. If you bring cookies to your parent, bring some extra for the staff. If one person has been especially thoughtful, send a small gift (a fruit basket, some flowers, or an assortment of nuts or soaps).

Kindness to the staff is especially important if your parent is withdrawn, confused, or a bit of a curmudgeon. It's hard for nurses and aides to be pleasant or helpful when a patient is uncommunicative or rude. You have to make up for your parent's behavior by being especially kind. Remind the staff that your parent's attacks are nothing personal and keep letting them know that you appreciate what they are doing.

Your Role as an Advocate

Unfortunately, hospitals are not safe havens, not in the least. In fact, a hospital is one of the most dangerous places to be. Because doctors and nurses frequently work at, or beyond, capacity, mistakes are made and patients are neglected. And because, by the very nature of the beast, germs are rampant, people contract infections and illnesses they didn't have when they walked in.

You can't eliminate all the risks, but you can reduce them significantly simply by being aware and vigilant. The information given here is not intended to frighten you, but simply to alert you.

MEDICAL MISHAPS

It's shocking how often a patient is given the wrong medication (it should have gone to the patient in the next bed), the wrong treatment, or, yes, treatment to the wrong part of the body (it was the left knee, not the right, that required surgery).

Iatrogenic diseases, namely, those diseases that are caused directly or indirectly by doctors, are a serious hospital problem. An injury or ailment may be caused by a doctor's neglect or incompetence, or it may be the result of acceptable medical care. For example, a necessary treatment for one illness may cause another less serious illness. The elderly are at high risk of iatrogenic disease because their medical care tends to be so complex.

The single most important thing you can do is ask questions. This forces the doctor or nurse to think about what he or she is doing. *Why is my parent getting this medication? Is this treatment necessary? Are you sure those pills are for my parent?*

CONFUSION, DELIRIUM, DEPRESSION

Elderly patients who show no signs of confusion at home may become disoriented, argumentative, and forgetful in the hospital, and those who already suffer from dementia often become more muddled.

Illness, a new environment, medications, and surgery all take a toll on the mind as well as the body. Confusion

> *My mother started talking about a high school friend of hers, a woman she hasn't seen in at least fifty years. Here I was, thinking my mother was very sick and these might be our last moments together. I wanted her attention. I said, 'Mom, why are you doing this?' but she looked up at me as though she didn't have any idea who I was.*
>
> *I was so crushed that I left. I walked the halls for a while and tried to calm down. I was so hurt and angry. I felt betrayed. Then I spoke to this wonderful nurse who helped me realize that I had to take what I could get, that being angry or trying to force her wouldn't help either of us. So I went back in and I just sat there and stroked her hair and listened to her ramble. I learned to meet her wherever she was, not where I wanted her to be."*
>
> —CAROL P.

and anxiety typically appear or grow worse at sundown, when the body is tired and the light is dim. This phenomenon is so common among elderly patients that doctors have a term for it—*sundowning.*

Bring in familiar objects and family photos, and leave on low lights at night. Lots of visits and physical contact will reassure your parent and reduce confusion.

If your parent becomes confused or agitated, remain calm because your mood will affect his. Reassure him that he is safe. Do not argue or disagree with him. *Yes, it is nice here in your office.* Keep conversations simple. Don't ask a lot of questions. And provide lots of reminders. Tell him patiently what day it is, where he is and why, and say the name of anyone entering the room. *Dad, your daughter, Sally, is here to see you.*

If confusion is acute; if your parent suddenly becomes agitated, inattentive, or unable to recognize familiar faces; or if he hallucinates, bring this to the doctor's attention immediately. He may be suffering from delirium, which can be a medical emergency. It often follows surgery, but illness, infection, medications, and changes in the body's chemistry can also trigger it. Treatment includes reducing or discontinuing certain medications and creating a calm environment.

Be on the lookout, too, for depression, which is common in hospitalized elderly patients, especially if they stay in the hospital for more than a few days or suffer from heart attack or stroke. Because you know your parent best, you are in a position to notice personality changes or mood swings. If you suspect depression, talk with his doctor or a hospital psychiatrist.

FALLS AND RESTRAINTS

WHENEVER YOU VISIT YOUR PARENT, take a look around the room for things she might trip over—furniture on wheels, chairs without arms, waxy floors. Fix what you can (for example, buy a rubber runner for the stretch between the bed and the toilet, take the faulty chair out of the room) and, if she is well enough, make her aware of the dangers. Tell her not to lean too heavily on the pole holding her intravenous drip, and show her how to lower the bed and raise the head end so she can rise out of bed more easily.

To guard against falls and to keep patients from pulling out tubes, meandering away or crushing a delicate injury, hospital staff sometimes restrain patients either physically, with arm bands, vests, or full body straps, or chemically, with sedatives, tranquilizers, and other drugs. Be aware of restraints because they are not necessary in most cases, and in some cases they are dangerous.

Be sure you know what sedating drugs your parent is being given and why. Also, if your parent is being physically restrained, ask the doctor if it is absolutely necessary. (Restraints themselves can cause injuries and accidents;

TRUTH TELLING AND DECISION MAKING

Your parent should be given clear and honest information about his health, and he should be involved, to whatever extent possible, in all decisions about his care.

Although people commonly try to "protect" patients from the truth by downplaying the severity of an illness or outright lying about it, this dishonesty does nothing more than isolate and scare people. It does not protect them. It does not give them hope. It does not make the truth go away. Patients always know, at least on some level, what is happening. Silence, deception, and lies only make it worse.

If the doctor tells you more than he tells your parent and you are uncertain about how much to tell her, then say that. *Mom, I spoke to the doctor about your illness. Do you want to talk about it? How much do you want to know?* Be gentle and go slowly, allowing her to stop you at any point along this path. But give her the option of hearing the truth and making decisions.

If your parent cannot speak for herself, or if her mind is in a fog, assume that she can hear and understand what is being said in the room. Again, speak clearly and honestly with her about what is happening. She might not understand it all (then again, she might), but she will be aware of the respect that is being offered her.

" *My father spent so much
time in bed that the nurses
and I thought it would be good for
him to sit up in a chair for a while
each day. But he was so weak that
he would just fall onto the floor
unless he had some support.*

*This strap, it's a seat belt really,
works quite well. He doesn't stay
in the chair long, but at least it's a
change. I don't think it's dangerous
or confining for him—I think it's
freeing in a way because it allows
him to get out of bed."*

—SASHA L.

they are not as useful as people
expect.) Discuss risks, benefits, and
alternative solutions. If restraints are
unavoidable, you can usually get
permission to remove them while you
are visiting, or the staff may free your
parent if you hire a companion to sit
with him.

BEDSORES

ALTHOUGH THE NURSES SHOULD TRY
to prevent bedsores, you should be
watchful for any red or raw spots.
Pressure on an area impedes the flow
of blood, creating a tender spot that
can develop into an open wound if
not treated immediately. Be sure your
parent is being routinely repositioned
to alternate the pressure on vulnerable areas and alert the nurses to any

suspicious-looking marks. (See page 249 for more on bedsores.)

HOSPITAL-BORNE INFECTIONS

STUDIES HAVE FOUND THAT 5 TO 10
percent of patients develop infections
while in the hospital (called *nosocomial infections*). The combination of
germs and bacteria, on the one hand,
and patients who have weakened
immune systems, open wounds, and
tubes in their bodies, on the other, is
a volatile one.

Hand washing is the best weapon
against hospital infections. Doctors,
nurses, and staff are supposed to wash
before touching or examining a patient,
but they sometimes neglect to do it.
If you think this is the case, ask the
person handling your parent to please
wash his or her hands first and, preferably, to wear gloves.

Unfortunately, asking a health professional to wash his hands can be a
little uncomfortable. Be tactful, but ask
anyway, because this simple request
will reduce the risk of infection significantly. Most health-care providers
won't mind your asking. You should
wash your own hands frequently as
well when caring for your parent.

Urinary tract infections are one
of the most common nosocomial
infections. Older women, in particular,
are prone to them because menopause
leaves the urethra, the exit channel for
urine, susceptible to infection.

Your parent should drink plenty
of fluids and get to the bathroom at

least every two hours. Her genital area needs to be kept clean, and if she has a catheter, it should be changed regularly and checked often to make sure that it is draining smoothly.

If your parent (men get them too) has symptoms of a urinary tract infection—a persistent urge to urinate, burning during urination, and pain in the lower abdomen—alert the doctor or nurse. Urinary tract infections are treatable with medications, but they can lead to serious problems if ignored.

INADEQUATE PAIN RELIEF

PAIN WILL NOT ONLY MAKE YOUR PARent miserable, it will limit his ability to function and heal, and it will make him cranky and tired. Be sure your parent's pain receives ample attention.

Doctors almost universally undertreat pain, in all situations but especially at the end of life. With very few exceptions, your parent should receive as much pain medication as he needs to be comfortable.

If your parent is in considerable pain, talk to the doctor. If it turns out that the doctor has approved medications but the nurse is slow in bringing it, talk to the nurse or nurse supervisor about how to speed things up.

Some hospitals now allow patients to dispense their own pain medication by pushing a button on a pump that delivers a dose through a needle under the skin. This provides relief that goes beyond the medicine's physical properties. Studies show that people actually use less medication when it is

CONVALESCING: UP AND AT 'EM

When your parent is recuperating from illness or surgery, your instinct may say, "rest," while the doctor is saying, "move." Trust the doctor here.

In most cases, people need to get up and move about in order to get all the bodily systems functioning again (to avoid constipation, stroke, lung infections, and other complications), and they need to do simple tasks, like feeding themselves or combing their hair, to regain movement, coordination, and other abilities.

It may seem as if the nurses and therapists are being cruel if they are forcing your mother to move in ways that she doesn't want to move, or being lazy if they leave her to do certain things for herself, but often they are just practicing good medicine.

The process may be painful to watch, especially if your parent is struggling, complaining of pain, or spilling her food. But let her do it herself and encourage her to keep going. Restrain yourself from helping too much. It will allow her to recover faster and more fully.

at their disposal because they aren't worrying about getting the next dose and tensing up at the thought of the approaching pain. So ask the doctor about this.

Keep in mind, pain is much easier to fight when it is treated before it sets in rather than when it has become well established. This is yet another reason

After the operation, I tried to help my father get his teeth back in. I struggled for a time and they finally went in. Then I looked at him and thought, 'Pop, you look weird.' I called home to see if anyone knew a better way to get his teeth in. I tried that cushion stuff, but nothing made it better.

Finally I realized these weren't his teeth. They were someone else's! I went traipsing to the room he used to be in, and to the doctor's office, and even to the operating room, all over the hospital looking for the right teeth, but I never found them. It was really kind of funny because here I am looking around for a set of teeth and realizing that somebody else must be wearing Pop's teeth. Luckily, he thought it was funny, too, and we had a good laugh about it. He had another set at home, but he never did use them again. Once old people take their teeth out, they don't like to put them back in."

—JACQUI H.

to be sure your parent is getting ample relief, and getting it before pain becomes troublesome.

Often it is the patient, not the doctor, who is limiting pain medications. If your parent is doing this because she doesn't like the groggy or confused feeling caused by the medications, or she is afraid of falling while on these medications, talk to the doctor about switching to a lower dose or to some other drug that might not be so sedating.

If your parent is skipping pain medications because she feels that taking the drugs is a sign of weakness, she fears addiction, or she doesn't like to complain, talk to both the doctor and your parent. Your parent should be counseled on the benefits of pain management (comfort, sleep, more mobility, less anxiety) and the risks of not treating pain (discomfort, distress, insomnia, irritability, poor mobility, more illness). She should know that using pain medications does not say anything negative about her character and will not turn her into a drug addict.

If her pain and your concerns are not addressed adequately, ask the doctor if there is a palliative care or pain specialist in the hospital. Most large hospitals have such specialists. Pain relief, once a simple matter, has become so technical that most doctors don't know all they need to know about it.

STAFF OR DOCTOR NEGLECT

MOST DOCTORS ARE RESPONSIBLE and compassionate, but some are not,

BEYOND DRUGS

Pain is no simple matter. It stems from injury and illness, but it can also be rooted in fear, anxiety, and depression. And all these things become intertwined, making the original pain that much worse. Pain and illness lead to fear, which leads to anxiety, which leads to more pain, which leads to more anxiety or depression, which leads to more pain, which leads to more pain, and so on.

Be mindful of your parent's whole being and the sources of pain. Pain should be treated on many fronts. Medication is just one of those fronts. Relaxation exercises, peaceful music, anything that brings joy, reassurance, massage, visualization, biofeedback, and other nonmedical approaches can reduce pain significantly.

parent questions about her health and symptoms. And then he or she should listen to what she says. If your parent doesn't say much, take it upon yourself to give the doctor ample information.

Nurses and other staff may also give your parent short shrift. If your parent is left sitting on a bedpan, or if her lunch fails to materialize, chances are that the hospital unit is understaffed. If your questions to the unit supervisor or the hospital administrator don't improve the situation, talk to the hospital's patient representative.

Comfort on the Fifth Floor

Don't get so caught up in your role as advocate that you neglect the comfort and care that your parent needs now. Visit and recruit others to visit. Not only will visits from others cheer up your parent, but they will also ease some of the burden on you.

VISITS

VISITORS ARE THE BEST FIRST AID going. However, they should be polite and unobtrusive visitors. Visitors should always call first, as an unannounced visit, especially when someone is wearing a backless gown, can be awkward for everyone. They should also plan their trips so they come one at a time or in very small groups, and for only a brief interlude (less than thirty

and almost all are carrying heavy patient loads. While you need to respect the demands on his or her time, you should also make sure your parent's doctor is not spending dangerously little time with your parent. He or she should actually look up from the medical chart, and ask your

minutes is usually more than enough) as your parent will tire easily now.

Give visitors guidelines, if necessary, about how long to visit, what sort of visit your parent is up for (balloons and hearty cheer, or a quiet time for two), and whether to bring children or not.

At times, your parent may be too tired for visitors, but may not be willing to tell people for fear of hurting their feelings. It's your job to tell them, as tactfully as possible, to come another time. In fact, there may even be times when your parent doesn't want you to visit. Don't take it personally.

Some things to keep in mind when visiting:

◆ **Be prepared.** If your parent has had a sudden and severe illness or accident, you may be shocked by his appearance on your first visit. He may not only look different, but he may be confused, weak, or in pain, or he may be attached to a lot of machines. Brace yourself so you don't gasp in horror or burst into tears as you enter the room.

Understand that if your parent is in the intensive care unit, it doesn't mean that he is close to death, only that he is being watched closely. Elderly people are often put in ICUs after surgery, stroke, or accidents. Remain calm. Your parent needs your confidence and warmth.

◆ **Be yourself.** Hospitals and illness breed discomfort. *What do I say? Should I be cheery? Should I talk about what the doctor found or avoid mentioning her illness?* All of this is especially awkward if your parent is near, or seems to be near, death.

Relax. Your embarrassment will only make your parent ill at ease—and she is already ill enough. Be yourself. It's okay to ask about her ailments, her pain, and her feelings, if that's something you want to know about. In fact, she may welcome such hon-

"WHY DON'T YOU EVER COME SEE ME?"

If your parent suffers from dementia and doesn't remember that you have visited every day for the past week, or doesn't seem to know who you are while you are there, keep in mind that your visits are crucial nevertheless. They are comforting, even if he doesn't remember them. And, more important, they allow you to make sure that your parent is being well cared for (vitally important now because of his confusion). Your visits also show the staff that you are concerned about his condition and the quality of his care, and will act if that quality is inadequate. In other words, don't visit less just because your parent doesn't remember that you came.

esty and an opportunity to talk about her situation.

Take the cue from her when it's time to move to other topics. Often, hearing about day-to-day things, the weather, the grandchildren, is a welcome escape from constant talk and thoughts about illness.

◆ **Arrange for some privacy.** Interruptions are a way of life in hospitals. Someone comes in with medication, then it's time for a blood sample, and just as you and your parent start talking, her temperature must be taken.

If your parent shares a room, pull the curtain around his bed. If his condition allows it, get him into a wheelchair and move the conversation into a lounge. Otherwise, ask the nurse if you can have some uninterrupted time and put a note on the door.

◆ **Silence is golden.** If your parent can't speak or if she is too confused or tired for conversation, you might read to her or tell her a story and let her lie peacefully. Or just sit quietly with her. You can read a book to yourself, or do some work. Your presence alone is powerful and will relieve her fear and ease her loneliness.

◆ **Get physical.** Don't let tubes, monitors, or injury deter you from touching, stroking, and holding, especially if you've had that sort of relationship with your parent in the past (although this isn't a bad time to offer a hug or kiss even if you haven't done much of that before). Human contact

> *Quite often we'll see a family come, six or seven of them at one time. They all cram into the person's room and chat with each other, and the grandchildren run around, and there are a lot of gifts and food and flowers. It's all very hectic, and very exciting.*
>
> *And then they all leave. And no one comes to visit for two weeks. That's very sad."*
>
> LORRAINE N., R.N.

is potent medicine. Hug him, hold his hand, stroke his cheek, caress his arm—whatever body parts are available. If there are a lot of machines in the way, ask the nurse if there isn't some way to make physical contact easier. However you can do it, touch. It says more than any words can say, and it's healing.

◆ **Pamper her.** Do something to make your parent feel special and pampered—wash or comb her hair, massage her feet, or paint her nails. (Ask the nurse first if it's anything too physical or if it involves food.) You might bring in some favorite feast or simply jazz up the hospital tray with a red napkin and a few flowers. Give her a bright bed jacket or new slippers.

While you're making life more livable, replace the water in flower arrangements, read letters aloud, and then write letters for her.

◆ **Respect the rules.** Enforcing visiting hours allows patients—not just your parent but roommates and those who are down the hall—to get some rest. Stay within the rules whenever possible. If the only time you can visit is after hours, or if your parent is extremely ill and needs someone nearby all the time, the staff will usually adjust the rules.

(If your parent is in an intensive care unit, the rules will be stricter and need to be obeyed.)

◆ **Don't forget the children.** In most cases, a child is a welcome visitor, adding vitality and sparkle to a dreary hospital day, singing songs, asking funny questions, stroking Grandpa with tiny fingers. Children also tend to see beyond the ugliness of illness and don't notice the things that adults find worrisome (they may be more absorbed by an IV bag than by Grandpa's paralysis).

Your instinct may be to protect children from seeing Grandma ill, but children learn from seeing life and death, and all that falls between. However, if Grandma doesn't seem pleased at the prospect of a child's visit, or if your child is afraid or hesitant, don't press the matter.

GIFTS

FLOWERS ARE ALWAYS NICE, BUT a framed photo, child's art project, small pine-scented cushion, and cheerful cards are great gifts. The smallest thing can mean a lot when one is facing the four walls of a hospital room. You don't have to spend a lot of money. In fact,

some of the best gifts are a story, a special poem, or prayer. Anything at all that is made by a grandchild is wonderful—a child's drawing brings color and life into an impersonal hospital room.

If your parent is relatively alert, his hospital stay will seem awfully dull. Look for gifts that will entertain her—games, books, magazines, puzzles, playing cards, materials for a hobby, knitting supplies, music (an inexpensive radio), books on tape, and a tape player.

If your parent is going to be in the hospital for some time and you are able to spend a little more money, buy a robe, new slippers, a pouch that attaches to a walker or wheelchair, or a soft, downy pillow (but put it in a case that is anything but white so it doesn't get thrown in with the hospital supplies).

If your parent has a laptop computer, she can watch DVDs or play games without disturbing a roommate. Some hospitals have Internet access, or your parent might be able to plug a laptop into a telephone jack, which would allow for e-mails. Scan family photos and send them to her.

If your parent is confused, bring pictures, photo albums, and familiar items from home that will make the room seem more familiar and help to orient her.

MEALS

ALTHOUGH SOME HOSPITALS ARE sprucing up their menus, hospital food is still notoriously tasteless. It's also served at odd times and sometimes

REST FOR THE WEARY

Sometimes a parent's hospital stay is anything but a break from your caregiving role. As advocate you might be micro-managing your parent's care—which can be a rigorous test of your endurance. Deeply worried about your parent, you return to the hospital every free moment you have. Then, when you finally drag your weary body home, you're deluged by messages from family and friends. There isn't a minute when you aren't living and breathing your parent's hospital experience.

Protect yourself. Make one phone call and ask a sibling or relative to relay information to others in the inner circle. When others are visiting your parent, get away, even if only for a walk outside or a cup of tea in a nearby cafe. Ask one of the nurses if there is a lounge or an empty room where you can lie down. Take a day off and go out with a friend and talk about something—anything—else.

It's vital to take care of yourself now. Your parent will need your strength when he returns home.

---

left to grow cold in front of a patient who can't lift a fork or remove a piece of plastic wrap.

Your parent's diet isn't simply a matter of comfort; the rate of malnutrition among the hospitalized elderly is estimated to be as high as 50 percent. A poor diet will make your parent's recovery more difficult. So, whenever possible, visit during mealtimes so you can check on your parent's eating habits and, if necessary, help him eat.

Bring him an occasional home-cooked meal or favorite takeout food, as long as it's within his diet. (Ask the nurse what he's allowed to have.)

If you can't be there, ask other visitors to come at mealtime, or ask the hospital's patient advocate about volunteers who might help your parent dine. Simply having company may encourage your parent to eat more.

Although hospitals don't advertise it, many offer an array of foods and special meals—kosher, vegetarian, low-salt, and even sandwiches. You can order special meals, as long as they are within your parent's diet, and you can also ask that meals be brought at different times if that would help your parent to eat more. (They might not do it, but it's worth asking.)

RELIGION AND COUNSELING

WHETHER OR NOT YOUR PARENT WAS religious before her hospital stay, she

> ❝ *When my mother was in the hospital after her stroke, she turned to me and said, 'Pizza.'*
>
> *I said, 'What?!'*
>
> *And she said, 'I really want some pizza. And a chocolate milkshake. It's all I can think about.'*
>
> *My mother is not a pizza-eater. She usually eats like a bird. So I drove around town looking for pizza and a chocolate shake. She didn't eat much of it, but she ate enough. I guess it was just a craving. Her body was crying out for something caloric and filling, and I was glad to see her eat something with such gusto.*"
>
> —Fran M.

may have some spiritual thoughts now. She may want to talk with you or a member of the clergy. Someone from her church or synagogue should be willing to visit her. Otherwise, hospital clergy will gladly stop by a patient's room.

Hospitals also have counselors, social workers, or psychologists who will talk with your parent about particular issues—fears about dying, family relationships, a diagnosis of cancer, as well as practical matters like housing, finances, and community services.

DIGNITY

Ask the staff to address your parent by whatever title she is used to—Mrs. Asher, Professor Madison, or, if she prefers, a nickname. If her real name is Elizabeth but everyone always calls her Lizzie, then remind staff of her name, ask to have it written into her chart, or put a note on the wall next to her bed.

ROOMMATES AND ROOMS

If a roommate's habits or his visitors are keeping your parent awake, talk to the roommate or a nurse about setting up a schedule of "quiet time." Or get your parent some earplugs or a small cassette player with earphones to muffle any loud snoring or chatter. If the roommate is obnoxious, see if you can't leave a curtain drawn permanently between the two beds. If all else fails, request a room change. It involves a lot of paperwork and hassle, but sometimes it is necessary.

Problems and Disputes

If you are facing a dire problem and need immediate results—the nurse is violent, the doctor reeks of alcohol, your parent's Do Not Resuscitate order is being violated, for example—go straight to the hospital's administrator. (If you casually mention that you are talking with a lawyer about the problem, even if you aren't, you will get more attention. Hospitals do not like lawsuits.)

If you or your parent has a less severe problem with a doctor, nurse, or other staff member, talk with that person directly, if possible. Be specific about your concern and cite an example of the problem. Many problems are due to a lack of communication—the nurse didn't know that your parent is allergic to lactose because it hadn't been entered in her chart, or you didn't realize that the doctor had ordered her painkillers stopped.

If the problem isn't resolved, go up a step on the ladder to the head nurse on the unit or floor, for example, or the hospital's director of nursing. If it's a medical issue, go to the medical director of the hospital, or if it's a financial issue, to the financial administrator or the insurance company, Medicare, or Medicaid.

You can also use these channels:

◆ **Patient advocates.** Most hospitals hire patient representatives, or patient advocates, who serve as a link between patients and the hospital system. Their job is to represent the patient, making sure that questions are answered and that any problems are resolved. Your parent or you can ask a patient advocate to help with practically anything—disputes with staff, lost hearing aids, billing questions, faulty plumbing, late lunch trays, roommate problems, or inadequate insurance coverage. Of course, some patient advocates are more helpful than others, but the good ones are godsends.

Patient advocates should be listed in the hospital brochure or directory, or their phone number may be posted on the hospital room wall. If you don't see it, ask the nurse.

◆ **Hospital committees.** If a dispute is over a medical decision—you and the doctor disagree about when to withhold treatment or you believe your parent has received the wrong treatment—many hospitals have medical or ethics committees that review such dilemmas. Ask the hospital's patient advocate or, if there is no advocate, a nurse or administrator, how to appeal a medical decision.

◆ **Quality Improvement Organizations.** If you believe that your parent has received inadequate care or unnecessary treatment in the hospital, if she is refused admission, if she is being discharged too soon, or if you believe Medicare coverage is being denied unfairly, contact the state Quality Improvement Organization (or QIO, often referred to as a PRO, or Peer Review Organization).

A QIO is a group of physicians and other health-care professionals who are contracted by the federal government to ensure that Medicare patients receive proper care from hospitals, doctors, nursing homes, and home health-care agencies. To reach the QIO in your parent's state, contact Medicare (800-MEDICARE or www.medicare.gov) or the American Health Quality Association (www.ahqa.org). Or, you can ask the hospital discharge planner, the local Social Security office, or the area agency on aging.

A NOTE ON BILLS

If at all possible, keep a list of what was provided each day. Even a partial record will help when it comes time to decode a hospital bill.

And by the way, be forewarned that everything and anything costs—a lot—in a hospital. That relaxing bath? $30. A special meal? $15. A Tylenol? $7. When asking for a little extra, find out just how much "extra" is going to cost.

Hospitals are required to give your parent a pamphlet about Medicare, patient's rights, and the QIO (or PRO) appeals process. For a list of the Hospital Patient's Bill of Rights, see page 643. Often the hospital's patient advocate or discharge planner will contact the QIO on your parent's behalf and get the ball rolling. Otherwise, contact the QIO yourself and ask for instructions on how to appeal a decision or file a complaint.

◆ **State boards and agencies.** While they may not be that helpful, it is important to notify the appropriate state licensing board if your complaint involves the skills or conduct of a nurse, doctor, or other licensed professional. And if the state has a separate agency that oversees

"medical quality assurance," contact that as well.

When You Are Far Away

Absence can make the heart grow fonder, but in this case, the heart usually grows more anxious, and understandably so. If you can't be there to act as your parent's advocate, find a relative or friend who can. Or, if you can afford it, hire a geriatric care manager, health aide, or companion to monitor your parent's care while in the hospital.

When you are far away, collect information early—who to call if there's trouble, names of doctors and their phone numbers, numbers for insurance carriers. Talk with the hospital discharge planner early about when and how your parent will be discharged so you can make all necessary arrangements.

Call the head nurse on your parent's floor and explain your dilemma. Find out if there is a primary nurse overseeing your parent's care with whom you can speak on some regular basis. Ask if there is a time when you can call, perhaps each morning, when the nurse might have a moment to talk to you about your parent's progress and care.

Check in with the doctor, too, as regularly as possible. Be sure he or she knows your parent's symptoms and concerns, ask as many questions as you need to, and be sure the doctor can reach you at any time of the day or night if there is a change in your parent's health (thank goodness for cell phones).

One family member should be designated to speak with nurses and doctors, and then that person should relay information to other family and loved ones. More than one spokesperson is difficult for care providers and can lead to misunderstandings and miscommunication.

Make sure your parent has company as often as possible, not only to monitor her care, but also because it can get lonely on the fifth floor. Ask others who are nearby if they might drop by occasionally. (Most people don't mind doing this once or twice, even though it may feel to you like an imposition.) If you don't know anyone well enough, call a local church, synagogue, or other community organization to ask about volunteers.

When you can't be there, call and write. Send your parent a big, colorful card, a photo of yourself or the grandchildren, an audiocassette (and inexpensive tape player) of you and others talking about what you are doing with your day and how much you all miss him (or a videotape if the hospital has VCRs). Mundane, day-to-day things—what happened at the bus stop, what the kids did in school, what the dog brought home—may seem trivial, but for someone alone in the hospital, these are wonderful stories that temporarily bring him home and help him forget his pain.

Leaving the Hospital

Before your parent is discharged, be sure that she has written information about medications, dosages, potential side effects, meals, exercise, precautions, symptoms to watch for, and foods to avoid.

The hospital discharge planner is responsible for planning your parent's return home—ordering medical equipment, setting up home care, or arranging institutional care. The planner, who usually knows a fair amount about local home-care agencies and senior residences, can be very helpful, but be aware that his or her primary job is to get patients out with speed. Take sufficient time to study the options and make a careful choice, if at all possible.

While hospitals have gotten better about not discharging patients quite so early, people are still discharged in pretty miserable states. (Of course, most are eager to depart.) If you do not believe that your parent is ready for discharge, or if you simply need to buy an extra day or two while you make housing arrangements, talk with the doctor, the nurse, the hospital social worker, or the patient advocate.

There may be valid reasons why your parent shouldn't leave yet. The social worker, doctor, or you may be able to convince Medicare or another insurance carrier that your parent needs coverage for a longer hospital stay. Or you can usually squeeze an extra day out of Medicare by appealing the discharge decision.

When your parent entered the hospital, she should have been given a pamphlet on Medicare rights regarding discharge and appeals. If not, ask for it. Quite often, the discharge planner or the hospital's patient representative (ombudsman) will help with appeals.

You'll need to contact the state Quality Improvement Organization, which monitors health care financed by Medicare. You must ask for the review before noon on the first working day after the hospital has given you what's known as a "Notice of Non-Coverage." The appeal process usually takes at least twenty-four hours and can take up to three days. (If you appeal on Friday, for example, it's likely that little will happen before Monday.) During the appeal process, you don't have to pay for the hospital stay. So even if the QIO rejects the appeal, your parent will get a little extra time in the hospital.

Of course, your parent can stay in the hospital without coverage (although it's not a great idea because of the risks inherent in hospitals), but she will have to pay for it herself. And the cost at this point is not the Medicare rate, but full retail price.

Hospital Bills

Hospitals have perfected chaos when it comes to billing. They use so many codes, abbreviations, and notations that it is almost impossible for a human being to figure out what a bill actually covers. And your parent will not receive just one bill, but a seemingly endless series of bills—from the hospital, the surgeon, the anesthesiologist, the radiologist, the physical therapist, the laboratory—all of which may come from different billing offices. Then there are the insurance companies, and Medicare and Medigap agents, and claim forms to wrangle with. What does your parent's insurance cover? What does your parent really owe? Which bills are redundant?

If you are handling your parent's finances and trying to sort out his medical bills, be patient. Even doctors and health policy experts have trouble deciphering and confirming their own hospital bills.

Whatever you do, don't assume that health-care providers are honest and hospital billing departments know what they are doing. The U.S. General Accounting Office has found that nearly all hospital bills include overcharges. According to a survey by *Consumer Reports,* people are frequently charged for medications, lab work, tests, and procedures that were not given or performed; charged for more time in the operating room than actually took place; and charged for the day they were discharged even though hospitals are not supposed to do that. They are also charged for more expensive services and procedures than the ones they received.

First of all, save everything for your records. If a bill is confusing or some expense is questionable, call the hospital's billing department and ask for an itemized bill, including explanations of any notations. They should do this free of charge.

Scan the itemized bill for duplications, charges for services that your parent never received, or unauthorized tests or procedures. If anything seems out of place, ask for an explanation. If the explanation is not adequate, refuse to pay that portion of the bill.

If you need help, each state has a State Health Insurance Counseling and Assistance Program, or SHIP.

Counselors assist people on Medicare with all sorts of insurance questions, including help with billing. State SHIP numbers are listed in Appendix C, page 635. There are also private companies (which you can find on the Internet) that will sift through hospital bills, keeping some percent of what they recover.

For questions and concerns about Medicare coverage, contact Medicare (800-MEDICARE or www.medicare.gov). For questions about Medicaid coverage, contact the state medical assistance office, listed in Appendix D, page 639.

Chapter Fifteen

PAYING THE WAY

Financial Planning • Benefits and Discounts
• Homes as Collateral • Tax Tips
• Using Your Own Funds • Financial and Legal Counsel
• Frauds and Scams

....

CERTAINLY, LIFE IS A LOT EASIER IF YOUR PARENT IS financially set, but no one is free from financial headaches. If you are not concerned about your parent's day-to-day survival, you may be worried about his future security or a dwindling inheritance. If you are not dealing with a parent who is unwilling to spend a dime, you may be trying to contain one who doesn't realize how little money she has. On top of it all, there are siblings who may bicker about how finances are handled and what is being spent, saved, or given away.

Finances are a private and often touchy subject, but you need to talk and plan. Be sure that your parent can cover her expenses, both now and for the future; that she isn't hiding financial problems from you; that she is getting all the benefits to which she may be entitled; that she has adequate (but not too much) insurance and is not spending more than she should on taxes; and finally, that she is not losing money to financial scams. Simplify her finances and take steps so that you can take over, now or in the future.

This chapter lays out the financial groundwork. The next chapter looks specifically at paying for health and home care, which will be by far the biggest expense. And Chapter Seventeen looks at legal issues, many of which concern your parent's finances. Whatever financial problems your parent may face, the best solutions require advance planning, so don't delay.

Talking about Money

Whether your parent is financially proficient or financially challenged, you need to talk. At the very least you need to find out where relevant documents are kept and how you will assume power, if need be.

Tread gently. Money is a private matter, deeply connected to personal success, independence, control, and dignity. Your mother may be reluctant to divulge her financial situation. Your father may not want your advice. You walk a thin line between respecting such wishes and ensuring your parent's financial security.

Consider the issue from your parent's perspective. Not only did he grow up in an era when money wasn't discussed, but much of his identity may be invested in his role as a provider. He may feel that talking about his finances with you will strip him of that role.

Furthermore, your parent's view of saving and spending may be quite different from yours. If he lived

TAKING THE FINANCIAL REINS

If he hasn't done so already, your parent should sign a durable power of attorney giving someone the legal authority to handle his finances and property. He can ensure that the power does not go into effect until he is sick or deemed incompetent, if he is afraid of relinquishing control too early.

Your parent can also name you or someone else as a joint owner of a bank account, enabling you to sign checks, if necessary. And he can appoint someone as a joint renter for any safe deposit box.

As for Medicare and Social Security, your parent can authorize you to be her representative, or you can apply directly (if she is not able to do so). Contact the local Social Security office or the Social Security Administration (800-772-1213 or www.ssa.gov).

> " *I have a joint checking account with my mother, but I still pay for a number of things out of my own pocket. She examines the statements carefully and would have a fit if she knew what some things cost. I've hired extra help and paid for a few minor repairs on the house. I also paid some of her lawyer bills because otherwise she would never have hired a lawyer. Anytime I do this, I keep receipts so I can show my brother what I've spent. He's not apt to challenge things like that, but you can never be sure how people are going to react.*"
>
> —RHODA B.

through the Depression, watched prices rise astronomically throughout his lifetime, and now faces an unknown future on a fixed income, he may be fiercely protective of every penny. He may not be willing to spend now in order to save later, to hire a lawyer, to buy adequate insurance, or to pay for necessary home health care.

When things get really tough, your parent may not want you to know just how bad things are. She may be deciding between groceries and medications because she simply can't afford to pay for both. She may be turning off the lights and turning down the heat, putting herself in a dangerous situation.

Or perhaps your parent has enough money but simply doesn't want you to know how she's mismanaged it, or how much she has spent on lottery tickets. She might be afraid of losing her control over her finances once she opens that door. There are all sorts of reasons a parent might be unwilling to divulge financial information.

But you need to talk. If the topic is sensitive, you can bring it up in terms of your own financial planning and even turn it into an advice-seeking question that your parent might respond to more comfortably. *Dad, I've been putting money away, but I'm not sure how much I'll need. Did you save when you were my age? Do you feel you have enough now?* Or you might talk about the financial hardships of a relative or acquaintance, then lead into questions about whether your parent feels financially secure. You can also mention that you read something about elderly people becoming dependent and not getting adequate care because they didn't plan.

Or simply come out with it. Ask your parent if she has a financial plan, if she has ample insurance, if she has enough money to pay for long-term care, and if she knows about available benefits. Then listen to her thoughts—her view of what the problems are, her priorities, and her plans—before offering your own opinions.

As you talk about various options and solutions, let your parent make her own choices whenever possible. It's not easy, especially when you feel you know what's best, but remember, it's not just her money that is at stake, but her pride.

WHOSE MONEY IS IT?

You may find that, as much as you want the best for your parent, you are also eyeing her assets with some thought to yourself. How much is there? How much might be passed along? How can your parent's money be protected? To some extent, these are healthy thoughts—conscientious, not greedy. Your parent should protect whatever she can. Certainly, it is better that her money goes to her heirs than to the government.

But be very careful not to overstep the boundaries of helpful financial planning. This money belongs to your parent, not to you. It should be used, first and foremost, for her comfort and care, even if that means spending every last dime on private nurses and special medical equipment.

If your parent's money is disappearing because of decisions that you believe to be foolish, and there is nothing you can do to change her ways, resign yourself to the situation and accept the fact that you will not inherit anything. You will save yourself from aggravation now and from disappointment when everything is gone.

If your parent resists, go slowly, if possible. Discuss basic financial tools and options without prying into the specifics of his situation right away. Then, with time, move further into the conversation.

You might also recommend a professional. People are often more comfortable talking with someone outside of the family. Give your parent the name of a good financial planner or lawyer.

If that doesn't work, consider the gravity of the situation. If your parent is facing a serious and immediate problem, spell out the consequences. Tell him calmly and clearly that if he doesn't get a loan, he will have to move out of his house, or that if he doesn't

pay his health aides enough, he will be left to manage on his own. If you still come up against a brick wall, you need to decide how far to go on your own. Contact the area agency on aging, which often has counselors who are well versed in dealing both with parents and with various benefits programs and special services to protect elderly people from eviction, starvation, or danger.

If the issue isn't dire, you might have to back off on certain issues. Your parent should still plan, but he might not spend his money in the way you think he should. He might fall down the stairs because he's too cheap to install a ramp, or the government may get your inheritance, but there may be little you can do but live with his decision (and make sure there are sturdy handrails along those stairs). This is, after all, his money and his life.

If you believe your parent is making irrational decisions because of true incompetence (as opposed to foolishness), you will have to step in more forcefully. Talk to his doctor. Find out if depression, dementia, alcohol abuse, or another problem is getting in the way of rational thinking. If he has dementia and is unwilling to hand over the financial control, you may need to obtain guardianship over him. (See page 396 for more information on this.)

Financial Planning

Regardless of the size of your parent's estate, she should do some financial planning (or someone should, if she can't). Advance planning is the best way to avoid a financial crisis, at any income level.

A financial plan can be formal and extensive or simple and to the point. You can do a rough plan yourself or hire a professional to put one together.

Basically, financial planning means reviewing one's worth, income, budget, and future needs, and then creating a plan that will increase income, decrease spending, and protect assets, as necessary. It also means developing a strategy to pay for future expenses and care. If your parent has a relatively large estate, she will need to review her investments and insurance, and think about protecting her assets from taxes. Someone with a smaller estate might be looking into low-income benefits and studying Medicaid eligibility.

The Budget Planner on pages 328 and 329 will help you get started. But someone who knows about state laws and services and is savvy to financial issues will be of enormous help. You can hire a financial professional or lawyer, or ask your area agency on aging about free or inexpensive guidance.

A comprehensive financial plan shouldn't take an inordinate amount of time, and it will be time well spent. The following guidelines will help your parent (and you) get started. Collect information you will need, including tax records, bank statements, and financial reports.

If you are involved, restrain any urge to take over completely, unless your parent wants you to or needs you to. Respect her privacy, autonomy, and right to make her own choices.

ASSESS THE CURRENT SITUATION

MAKE A LIST OF ALL YOUR PARENT'S assets (savings, investments, real estate, etc.) and then calculate her debts (mortgages, loans, outstanding bills). This will give you her "net worth" and an overall framework to consider as you review her finances.

Once you have done this, add up all sources of income (pensions, Social Security, etc.). Then figure out her monthly expenses (mortgage, rent, utilities, etc.). Reviewing past entries in a checkbook may reveal some of her regular expenses.

If she is spending more than she is taking in each month, how is that gap being covered? Is your parent building up debts on a credit card? (Put an end to this right away. For help, contact the National Foundation for Credit Counseling at 800-388-2227 or www.nfcc.org.) Is she going through her savings? How long can she continue this way? Are there expenses that can be trimmed or eliminated? Are there other sources of income she might tap into (a home that can be used as collateral against a loan, a life insurance policy that can be cashed in, properties or other assets that can be sold)? Are there programs and services for senior citizens, particularly those living on a low income, that she might use?

Look at her insurance policies. Does she have enough coverage? Is the coverage redundant? Be sure that policies have not lapsed, or that he is not still paying for an old policy that is no longer necessary.

Study any investments or savings. Are they invested conservatively enough so that she'll have money for the future? Does she need a new broker or financial adviser?

ANTICIPATE THE FUTURE

WHAT DO YOU ANTICIPATE YOUR PARENT's income and expenses to be in one, three, five years? How will they change?

"My parents have done nothing to prepare for their old age. They have simply spent whatever money they had without thinking of the future. They never listened to us when we told them to save. Now they are running out of money. Neither one of them is healthy, and they are both growing helpless. I'm sure one of them, and probably both of them, will need nursing care at some point soon. And they won't be able to afford it.

My brothers and I are wondering who's going to pay for this. I probably have the most money of the three of us, but I also have four children. I can't afford to pay for nursing care, nor do I think I should. I feel for them and I want to help, but I'm also angry at them for dumping this responsibility on us."

—DIANE P.

The big question here is, what sort of care might your parent need? If he needs home care, nursing-home care, or some other long-term care, how might he pay for it? He can expect to spend anywhere from $20,000 to more than $100,000 a year on long-term care. If he has any long-term care insurance, how much of his care will it truly cover? (See Chapter Sixteen on paying for health care.)

Are there tax credits or deductions, or any free or low-cost services

BUDGET PLANNER: A STARTING POINT

Assets	
House and other real estate	
Cars, boats, and other property	
Valuables (jewels, antiques, collectibles)	
Checking accounts	
Savings accounts	
Stocks, bonds, mutual funds	
Annuities	
Trusts	
Life insurance	
Loans receivable	
Equity in a business	
Other	
Debts	
Mortgages	
Outstanding loans and debts	
Outstanding bills	
Credit cards	
Other	
Income	
Salary or wages	
Business income	
Pensions, IRAs, Keogh	
Social Security	
Dividends	
Interest (from investments, savings)	
Rental income	
SSI, food stamps, or other entitlements	
Other	

Current Expenses	
Mortgage or rent	
Taxes (property and income—federal, state, and local)	
Utilities (heat, AC, water, phone, Internet, electricity)	
Food (groceries and dining out)	
Travel (car payments, gas and upkeep, buses, taxis)	
Vacation travel (planes, hotels, etc.)	
Clothing	
Medications	
Other medical (vision and hearing aids, dental)	
Insurance premiums (homeowners, health, car, disability, flood, life, long-term care)	
Home and yard maintenance	
Housekeeping	
Home care (companions, aides, etc.)	
Interest payments (credit cards, outstanding loans)	
Hobbies and pastimes (subscriptions, club dues, classes, gym memberships, equipment)	
Pet care	
Entertainment	
Gifts	
Donations	
Other	
Possible Future Expenses	
Home renovations (to make it more accessible)	
Assisted living devices (automatic door openers, stair lift, various utensils, hearing and vision aids, etc.)	
Home health care	
Assisted-living and/or nursing home	
Increased medical bills	

PREPAID FUNERALS

If your parent is tempted by ads suggesting that she prepay for her funeral, assuage her concerns and convince her otherwise. Prepaying is generally not a good idea. So many things can go wrong. (The funeral home goes out of business, your parent moves, the funeral home later insists that the money won't cover all the expenses, etc.) And, really, what's the point?

If she's worried about this and it makes everyone feel better, she can simply put money into a "payable on death" account. She needs to put the account under her name and then "POD" followed by your name or the name of another sibling. Any bank can set it up for her easily. The money will be solely hers and then, upon her death, it is immediately available to the other person named on the account, in this case, for funeral expenses.

that he might be eligible for now or in the future?

How will inflation affect expenses, and what might a downturn in the market do to investments?

While looking at the future, your parent needs to consider ways to protect his assets. If they are substantial, he can protect some of them from estate and inheritance taxes, or if he is not all that far from Medicaid eligibility, he may be able to protect some of his money.

If both your parents are alive and you are helping them with their finances, explore how each of them would fare financially if the other became ill or died. Determine how each spouse's income and expenses would change and how they might protect themselves now.

YOUR PARENT'S PRIORITIES

As you and your parent create a financial plan, talk about your parent's goals and priorities. What does he need money for, and what is most important to him? Does he want to enjoy these years as much as possible, or is he committed to setting aside money for his children? Is he adamant that he pay all his bills without going on public assistance or borrowing? Encourage your parent to consider these issues so that he can arrange his assets to meet his goals.

DEVELOP (AND FOLLOW) A PLAN

Once you have a picture of your parent's financial strengths and weaknesses, come up with a plan to meet her needs. This may include changing her spending habits, buying a new insurance policy, renting out a room in her house, setting up a trust, selling some assets, or revising her investments to include more bonds and fewer stocks.

Be sure your parent follows the course that's been laid out. It does no good to spend hours figuring out ways to save money if the cost-cutting measures are ignored. Give your parent encouragement and support while she tries to alter fixed habits. And keep after her, because waiting is a dangerous game.

Review the plan in six months or a year, or any time there is a change in your parent's circumstances—illness, disability, injury, divorce, or financial windfall.

Make It Easy

With all that you have to do, and all that your parent may not be able to do, now is the time to simplify.

◆ Consolidate her accounts and, if possible, get them all within one financial institution so there is one statement and, hopefully, one person overseeing them.

◆ Consider selling any real estate beyond her own home, so that she is not playing landlord or worrying about other properties.

◆ Bills can be paid automatically, giving her, or you, one less thing to think about. It will protect her so that her utilities are not shut off, her insurance policies don't lapse, and her credit

is not jeopardized. (If your parent doesn't want her bills paid automatically, and you are concerned that she may forget to pay them, ask the creditor to notify you or another family member if bills become overdue.)

◆ Income, such as Social Security and pension checks, can be deposited automatically so that checks don't pile up or get thrown out accidentally.

◆ While direct deposit and automatic bill paying should take care of most day-to-day financial chores, you

HOLDING ON TO THE PURSE STRINGS

While it is tempting to throw your hands up in the air and assign the whole financial mess to a professional, finances are too important a matter to relinquish completely to someone else. Financial and legal advisers should be used for just that—advising. Your parent, you, or another family member should oversee everything a professional does. (If you don't understand something, keep asking until you do.) Generally, your parent should not give a financial planner, lawyer, or other professional the legal authority to make financial decisions on her behalf without her (or your) approval.

can also hire a money manager if you or your parent needs more help. A manager will pay bills, make deposits, balance checkbooks, organize tax records, deal with creditors, and handle medical bills and insurance claims. Hand over such duties with caution, however. Know who you are dealing with and keep an eye on things. You can find a money manager through the American Association of Daily Money Managers (301-593-5462 or www.aadmm.com). They generally charge between $25 and $60 an hour, depending upon the area.

◆ AARP, in conjunction with several states and financial institutions, has volunteers who help low-income elderly people budget their money, pay bills, make deposits, and keep track of finances. To learn more, contact AARP at 888-687-2277, or visit AARP's Web site for its money management program, www.aarpmmp.org).

Benefits and Discounts

Find out right away what services, discounts, and programs your parent might be eligible for. Way too often, people spend, worry, struggle, do without, and borrow from family when, in fact, help is available. So look into this before your parent spends more than she needs to or you dig into your own pockets.

Of course, there's Medicare and Medicaid (both discussed in the next chapter) and various programs that help people sort through health-care coverage and insurance questions. And there's Social Security, which provides income to all workers after they retire. But there are other, less well-known benefits that your parent should tap into.

Start by going online to www.benefitscheckup.org and fill out the questionnaire. This will give you a list of programs and benefits to which your parent is entitled. BenefitsCheckUp is run by the National Council on the Aging. Also try the government's site, www.govbenefits.org. These are fairly inclusive. Nevertheless, you should still contact the area agency on aging (page 628), which may know about other state and local programs.

Even if your parent is financially secure, there are programs that will lower her monthly bills or provide services and consulting at a discount, such as legal and insurance counseling, prescription drugs, home maintenance and repairs, health-care savings programs, and more.

You'll need to provide information about her income, assets, and monthly payments, but you can guesstimate these and then get the specifics when you want to apply for a particular program or service.

HELP FOR PEOPLE WITH LOW INCOMES

IF YOUR PARENT'S INCOME IS VERY limited and her assets negligible, she may qualify for a host of federal, state, and community programs. Again, www.benefitscheckup.org is a good place to start, as well as the area agency on aging.

DISCOUNTS AND SPECIAL SERVICES

The elderly are big business, and everyone is getting into the act. Shops and professionals of all types now offer special services and discounts to elderly customers. Some popular marketing programs aimed at seniors include:

◆ Grocery stores: free deliveries, senior discount days

◆ Veterinarians and other pet services: house calls, discounts, and pet-walking services

◆ Pharmacies: free deliveries and discounts

◆ Hair stylists and manicurists: house calls and discounts

◆ Phone and utility companies: discounts and other services, including amplified phones, large-button phone pads, and large-print bills. Also, call several providers to be sure your parent is getting the best deal based on her calling habits. Find out about one-rate calling and other plans.

◆ Local power and gas companies or energy agencies help people pay to insulate and otherwise "weatherize" their homes and lower utility bills. Some have special programs to help elderly and low-income customers with heat and power bills.

◆ Health clinics, hospitals, and public health departments: free health screenings and shots, and some discounted services

◆ Dentists and hygienists: discounts and services for the homebound

◆ Restaurants: discounts on certain nights or times (early-bird specials)

The government's Web site, www.gov benefits.gov, also lists benefits.

Supplemental Security Income

Elderly people (or blind or disabled people) on very limited incomes and with few assets are eligible for monthly payments of several hundred dollars a month from the federal program Supplemental Security Income or SSI. (This is not the same as Social Security.)

Income limits vary from state to state. A person's assets (usually excluding their home, clothing, furnishings, a car, and a small burial fund) cannot exceed $2,000 for an individual or $3,000 for a couple.

To learn more about SSI or apply for it, contact the local Social

Security office or the Social Security Administration (800-772-1213 or www.ssa.gov). Your parent will need her Social Security number, birth certificate or other proof of age, proof of where she lives (property tax bill, lease agreement, etc.), bank book, and/or payroll stubs.

Food Stamps

Many people don't realize that the government will help low-income elderly people with their grocery bills. Or maybe they realize it, but don't realize that they are eligible. For whatever reason, far more elderly people are eligible for food stamps than actually use them. It is certainly worth investigating whether your parent meets the standards.

To get food stamps, an elderly person must have only minimal assets (about $3,000, not including things like a house and a car, but this figure changes from year to year) and meet a somewhat complicated monthly income limit. The food stamps program looks at "net" income, which is your parent's income minus a deduction—most medical expenses, and some portion of household expenses (rent, mortgage, taxes, utilities). Anyone receiving SSI benefits, regardless of assets, is eligible for food stamps.

You don't actually get stamps. You use a card, called an Electronic Benefits Transfer (EBT) card, which looks much like a credit card. It is replenished automatically each month. The average benefit is under $100 per person per month.

For information, contact the local food stamp office or the national office

of the Food Stamp Program (800-221-5689 or www.fns.usda.gov/fsp).

Energy Assistance Programs

The government's Low Income Home Energy Assistance Program (which has the unmanageable acronym of LIHEAP) helps pay energy bills so your parent can stay warm in the winter and cool in the summer, which is critical for an elderly person. The elderly are very susceptible to both overheating and hypothermia. LIHEAP programs are federally funded but run locally, so eligibility and benefits vary. Some LIHEAPs also offer weatherization and energy-related home repairs.

To learn more, contact the National Energy Assistance Referral Project (which has the more manageable acronym, NEAR). NEAR can be reached at 866-674-6327 or you can find the local LIHEAP office at www.acf.dhhs.gov/programs/liheap. To apply, your parent will need recent copies of utility bills, recent proof of her income (including Social Security, payroll, pensions, disability, etc.), proof of address, and her Social Security number.

Phone Bills

All local telephone companies are required to take part in a program called Link-Up America, in which phone companies help cover the cost of installing a new phone service, and Lifeline Assistance, which helps cover the cost of monthly phone bills. These services are available to anyone eligible for Medicaid, Supplemental

Security Income, food stamps, or energy assistance programs.

Link-Up covers half the cost of installation of one phone line and allows you to delay the rest of the payment for a year with no interest. Lifeline provides a monthly discount, which, with matching state funds, may be between $10 and $15 a month.

For information, call your parent's local telephone company or department of human or social services.

Getting Cash Out of a Home

If your parent is cash poor but owns a home, or simply would like more liquidity, he can use his home to get cash. He can take in renters, or he can share his home with someone who can care for him and do some chores and home maintenance.

Or, your parent can borrow money by using his home as collateral. He can simply refinance his house, get a second mortgage, or get an equity line of credit and pay it back in installments with interest. He can also get what's known as a reverse mortgage, which, at his stage of life, may be the best choice.

Beware: Borrowing is a complex business and a bad deal can get your parent into serious trouble. He should consult a lawyer to make sure that any arrangement is a safe one. And he should be sure that a loan will actually cover his financial needs, now and in the future, because once he

has used the equity in his home—and some of these loans have high interest rates—he may have little else to offer as collateral.

Your parent also needs to consider how any mortgage will affect his income and taxes, as well as his eligibility for programs like Medicaid and SSI. For example, he might be able to go on Medicaid and keep his house, without any need to draw cash from it. (In fact, drawing cash from his house might make him incligible.)

REVERSE MORTGAGES

A REVERSE MORTGAGE CAN PROVIDE your parent with a lump of cash to renovate his house, a constant flow of cash to pay ongoing bills, a line of credit to cover unpredictable expenses, or some combination of these things. But unlike home equity lines of credit, which require that the debt be repaid in monthly installments, these loans do not have to be repaid until the home is sold, or your parent moves or dies.

Because of this, there are no income qualifications and no monthly payments on the loan. Furthermore, closing costs and fees can usually be financed within the mortgage. All your parent pays is his usual taxes, insurance, and the cost of any maintenance or repairs.

Typically, the loan is most expensive in the early years of the mortgage, meaning that a person loses the most value in his house right away. In other words, this isn't a great financial tool for the short term; it is a better deal the longer your parent stays in his home.

The full amount of the loan—principal, interest, fees and other charges—is owed as soon as your parent dies or moves away. Your parent cannot, however, owe more than the value of his house.

Reverse mortgages are widely available, from both private and public agencies. Again, be cautious. Know what you are buying. The various types include:

◆ **Federally insured loans.** These plans, known as Home Equity Conversion Mortgages (HECM), are the most popular and the most widely available reverse mortgages. They are provided by private lending institutions, but backed by the federal government. This guarantees that your parent will be allowed to stay in her home for as long as she likes, and that the lender cannot claim any other assets if the house depreciates. Also, payments to your parent are guaranteed in case the lender defaults on them—a reassuring advantage.

HECMS are usually less expensive and provide larger cash advances than other similar loans offered by the private sector.

To receive an HECM loan, your parent must be sixty-two or older; the house must be her primary residence and it must be at least a year old; and she must meet with a counselor from an agency that is approved by the U.S. Department of Housing and Urban Development (HUD). Her house can contain no more than four housing units and she must, obviously, occupy at least one of them. Condominiums,

townhouses, and "manufactured homes" must meet certain HUD guidelines. Finally, she cannot already have a large mortgage on her home.

For more information, contact HUD at 202-708-1112, or go to www.hud.gov on the Internet and click on "Information for Senior Citizens." You can also get the name of a local HUD-approved counseling agency and a list of local approved lenders by calling the Housing Counseling Clearinghouse at 800-569-4287.

◆ **Privately backed reverse mortgages.** Loans that are not insured by the Federal Housing Administration (FHA), but rather privately owned and backed, are referred to as "proprietary" reverse mortgages. These are generally more expensive, but useful if your home is worth quite a lot and doesn't meet HUD limits.

While the loan amount may appear to be larger than one your parent can get from an HECM, be sure you are accurate in your comparisons. Look at all costs and changes in the loan over time. Some credit lines grow with time, some do not. Sometimes the lender will want, in addition to the amount owed, a percent of the appreciation in the value of the home. Be sure you know what you are getting into and compare the options.

◆ **"Uninsured loans."** These loans are not insured by the FHA and have fixed terms, meaning that the loan must be paid back on a predetermined date, usually within a few years. Such loans are useful if your parent needs money for a specific period of time and expects to sell his home before or at the end of the term. However, fixed-term loans are available only in a few states, and sometimes only in certain areas of a state.

HOME-REPAIR LOANS

HOME-REPAIR LOANS, WHICH ARE typically offered by government housing agencies or nonprofit organizations, are terrific if you can find one. They provide a onetime lump sum for home repairs (fixing a roof, repairing plumbing, weather-stripping, insulating) or renovations that make a house accessible for people with disabilities (installing ramps, grab bars, a lift, or lower cabinets). Home-repair loans cannot be used for cosmetic work or additions judged to be unnecessary.

What makes these loans so great is that they are usually offered without interest or at a very low interest rate, and with no or low fees and closing costs. Sometimes, if a person lives in his home for a certain length of time, the loan is forgiven, meaning that your parent owes nothing. And the cherry on top of all of this is that the construction might increase the value of the home so much that it covers the loan or even leaves a profit. These loans, however, are usually available only to people with moderate or low incomes.

Home-repair loans (sometimes referred to as "deferred-payment loans" or DPLs) are often set up as a reverse mortgage so that nothing is paid on the loan until your parent dies or sells her house.

To find out about such loans, call the area agency on aging or the local housing department.

PROPERTY TAX DEFERRAL LOANS

IN MANY STATES, ELDERLY PEOPLE WHO meet certain income limits can defer paying property taxes. Again, the amount owed, plus any interest, is paid off when a person sells his house, moves, or dies. For more information, call the area agency on aging or the local tax collector.

SALE-LEASEBACK PLANS

UNLIKE OTHER PLANS, WHICH ARE offered by government agencies or

---

FOR MORE HELP

AARP
888-687-2277 or
www.aarp.org/revmort

AARP has an abundance of information on reverse mortgages, including a loan calculator.

The National Center for Home Equity Conversion
651-222-6775 or
www.reverse.org

This Web site operates in conjunction with the AARP site, offering more detailed information, help comparing loans, and guidance in finding a loan.

private lenders, sale-leaseback deals are usually made between individuals—sometimes between family members. Your parent sells his home to another person, but remains in it indefinitely as a tenant with a guaranteed lifelong lease. While your parent gets cash and no longer bears the burdens of home ownership, he also relinquishes some control over his home.

Tax Tips

◆ Many older people are not required to file federal tax returns, so make sure of your parent's tax status before doing unnecessary work.

◆ People over sixty-five are entitled to a tax credit and a higher standard deduction.

◆ Even if your parent does not need to file a federal tax return, call the local tax office about state tax laws. Individual states offer various tax-relief programs and tax credits for seniors.

◆ Elderly people are not required to pay taxes on most public assistance, such as mortgage assistance, home improvements paid for by the state to reduce home energy costs, nutrition programs, and veterans benefits. They may be required to pay taxes on part of their Social Security income, however.

◆ You can claim your parent as a dependent under the following circumstances: No one else claims him as a dependent; your parent's gross tax-able income is less than a few thousand dollars (the exact amount changes from year to year); and you pay for more than half of his care and living expenses for the year. (If your parent does not live with you, then you have to pay half the cost of keeping up his home for that year.)

◆ Your parent can deduct medical expenses that exceed 7.5 percent of his adjusted gross income (if he doesn't take the standard deduction and instead itemizes his deductions). This includes all medical and hospital care not reimbursed by insurance, dental care, health insurance premiums and co-payments (including a portion of premiums paid for long-term care insurance), prescription drugs, nursing services, medical aids (eyeglasses and hearing aids), medical supplies, and transportation to medical appointments. The entire cost of nursing-home care (including room and board) is deductible as long as the stay is medically necessary.

Your parent can also treat as a medical expense the cost of any home improvements that have been made because of a disability or medical condition, such as installing railings or widening hallways and doorways to accommodate a wheelchair. If the change increases the value of the house (say your parent installs central air conditioning because of his asthma), then he can deduct the amount spent minus the amount the property increases in value (which has to be determined by an appraiser).

> *After my father died, I had to file his tax return. My father was incredibly orderly. But I have never seen such a disorganized mess as his tax information, including masses of past tax forms and receipts. I hired an accountant to help me, and we sorted through papers for months.*
>
> *Dad always hated the IRS and taxes. He died on April 15, which has become a little joke in our family—maybe, lying in that hospital bed, he started thinking about his taxes and the IRS and it was just too much for him to bear. Taxes. It should be on his death certificate as cause of death."*
>
> —Gloria C.

◆ If you are paying your parent's medical bills, you can add them to your deductions if you provided more than half of his total living expenses in that year (whether or not you claim him as a dependent on your tax return). Again, you can only deduct medical expenses if they exceed 7.5 percent of your adjusted gross income.

◆ If several siblings are sharing the costs of parentcare, you can file a "multiple support agreement" and then each deduct the medical expenses that you pay for.

◆ Tax credits are available for certain home services, adult day care, and supervision. If, for example, you hire someone (and pay their Social Security contributions) to care for your parent while you work, you can take a credit of up to 30 percent of the cost of the care.

◆ Your parent may not have to report the sale of his home (his primary residence) on his tax return unless the gain was more than $250,000 ($500,000 if he is married and filing a joint return).

◆ Taxes can be filed and paid online. (The software even checks the math.)

For answers to tax questions, go online to www.irs.gov. Or call your local IRS office or the IRS tax information number, 800-829-1040.

FREE TAX HELP

IF YOUR PARENT DOESN'T HAVE AN ACCOUNTANT doing her taxes, she can get free help and advice. Tax Counseling for the Elderly is a program funded by the Internal Revenue Service that offers free tax help to older people. The counselors (who are volunteers) are trained in issues pertinent to the elderly, such as Social Security benefits, tax credits, and rebates. The volunteers set up shop each year in early February in public libraries, senior centers, and banks (some will make house calls).

To speak with a volunteer, contact a local senior center or IRS office, the federal IRS office at 800-829-1040 or www.irs.gov, or AARP at 888-687-2277 or www.aarp.org. As part of the IRS program, AARP sponsors volunteer tax counselors through its program, Tax-Aide.

Dipping into Your Own Funds

The costs associated with your parent's care can sneak up on you slowly—you're buying your mother groceries occasionally, paying to have a ramp installed, buying her a warmer coat, and, of course, there are all those trips back and forth. Or, it can come at you suddenly. Your mother needs an aide to take care of her and she has no way to pay for it. How do you regulate the smaller expenses, and do you ever pay the larger ones?

It's a tough question, and there is no right answer. It's an individual and very personal decision. What you decide to do will depend upon your

> *My mother-in-law lives on her Social Security payments, which come to less than $900 a month. She managed on it, sort of, but now she needs help at home and she can't afford it. My husband thinks we should pay for it, but his income and mine together barely cover our expenses, with the kids and all. I'm so angry. I feel like we shouldn't have to do this, but if we don't, I can't imagine what will happen."*
>
> —KATHY P.

own financial security, your parent's financial insecurity, your relationship with your parent, and your personal views. Do not compare yourself with others. Do not feel either righteous or immoral for the decision you make. It is perfectly reasonable not to want to use up your child's college fund or your own retirement savings to pay your parent's bills. And you should think very seriously before taking on debt or getting yourself into financial straits to cover your parent's bills.

Before you do anything, learn about benefits, services, and programs that might help your parent. Quite often, families with meager resources pay a parent's way without realizing that they might have tapped into public or private programs.

Learn about Medicare, Medicaid, PACE programs, VA benefits, benefits for government employees and their families, and work-related benefits that might extend to others in the family. Find out about adult day care, transportation, meals-on-wheels, legal aid, and other community services that are provided free or on a sliding scale. And consider reverse mortgages and other, more creative, solutions to her financial problems.

Before spending your own money, look carefully at your own financial resources. What do you need to live, to retire, to care for your children? What can you afford to spend? Are you willing to spend it?

If you decide to spend your own money and you have siblings who are willing to share the burden, create a fund to which all of you contribute. Then appoint someone to keep track of all expenses from the fund.

Or, if you are the only family member willing or able to help, you can treat any expenses as a business deal. For example, you could give your mother a loan that will be paid off, with interest, at her death. Or you might buy her house and let her remain in it until she moves or dies, which would provide her with more spending money. Write up a contract that clearly defines the terms of the arrangement, and have it signed by both parties.

If you find yourself paying for a little of this and a little of that, and it's beginning to add up, keep a record of what you spend. You might work things out so that you are able to deduct some of these expenses from your taxes, declaring your parent as a dependent. Also, you might work things out so that you are reimbursed from your parent's estate after her death. But alert your siblings to the expenses you are paying and make sure they agree to any reimbursement plan. Then send them regular financial reports and keep meticulous records, including all receipts, bills, and cancelled checks.

You are not betraying any assumptions of goodwill by being businesslike about these matters. Even the closest family relationships can be torn apart by financial issues. There will be less division and contention if everything is decided in advance and then handled in a businesslike manner.

Professional Help

Friends, colleagues, doctors, and social workers are all eager to offer financial and legal advice and share their own experiences. Be wary. Even people who are trained in these matters have a hard time keeping up with the fine print and the ever-changing rules. And each individual's situation is different.

Seek the advice of reputable and experienced professionals. While it is expensive, the savings and protection provided are worth the price.

Be careful also about taking a broad spectrum of financial guidance from one person. You don't want investment advice from an insurance broker or insurance advice from a tax adviser. Most people with a reasonable estate need an accountant, an estate attorney, and an investment adviser.

WHO ARE ALL THESE PEOPLE?

◆ **Financial planner** is a generic term for anyone offering financial advice. If your parent wants a financial plan, find someone who specializes in this work, and preferably an independent adviser who offers impartial advice—that is, someone who is not being paid commissions to sell products, l ike investments or insurance. The National Association of Personal Financial Advisors (800-366-2732 or www.napfa.org) represents financial planners who work on a fee-only basis.

Most financial planners come with a variety of letters after their names showing that they have taken courses and passed the exams and require-ments of a particular organization. Most are either Certified Financial Planners (CFP) or Chartered Financial Consultants (ChFC).

◆ **Accountants** primarily handle taxes and auditing. Most are Certified Public Accountants (CPAs), which means they have passed an exam and are licensed by the state. Those who are not actually CPAs may have been in the business before licensing laws went into effect. Some accountants have additional training in financial planning and so carry the title Personal Financial Specialist (PFS).

◆ **Lawyers** come in all stripes, but two are most apt to deal with the elderly. Estate attorneys generally stick to estates, wills, trusts, and the like. Elderlaw attorneys help with Medicaid and other public benefits, probate, guardianship, estate planning, and long-term care planning.

◆ **Brokers, investors, and money managers** buy and sell stocks, bonds, and other investment tools. Be care-ful that someone isn't pushing your parent to buy things (or buy and sell things) just to make a commission. For information about brokers, firms, and any disciplinary action against them, or to file a complaint, contact the National Association of Securities Dealers (800-289-9999 or www.

nasd.com) or the U.S. Securities and Exchange Commission (800-732-0330 or www.sec.gov).

HIRING A PROFESSIONAL

Get recommendations, preferably from other professionals—lawyers, financial planners, professors at law or business schools, business acquain-tances, accountants. Or consult library directories (for example, the *Martindale-Hubbell Law Directory*). For national organizations that provide referrals to various financial and legal experts, see Appendix A, pages 607 and 618.

Once you have the names of three or four people who sound promising, make an appointment to meet them. Some issues to discuss and questions to ask:

◆ **Training and credentials.** What degrees, certification, or special train-ing do you have? (Several organiza-tions test and certify financial planners.)

◆ **Experience and expertise.** What is your specialty—estate plan-ning, investing, taxes, insurance, health care? How long have you been prac-ticing? (With few exceptions, it should be at least three or four years, prefer-ably more.) What percentage of your clients are elderly, or the families of elderly people?

◆ **Services provided.** What, exactly, will you do for my parent and/or family? Outline what you want done and be sure you are getting at least that. If more than that is being offered, is it something your parent wants to pay for? Are these services personalized? That is, does a financial planner simply put your parent's financial information into a computer and then hand you a printout, or does he or she consider the specifics of your parent's situation and her priorities? Likewise, does a lawyer fill in the blanks on generic forms or tailor advice and legal documents to meet individual needs?

◆ **Cost.** How do you charge—an hourly fee, a flat fee? What is your estimate of the total cost? What happens if the cost exceeds this estimate? (The professional should get written permission before exceeding the estimate.) Are bills itemized? Is an advance payment required? How often do you bill?

Fees are almost always negotiable, so once you find someone you like, compare prices and ask if he or she can bring the price down. Then get a written agreement concerning bills, payments, penalties, and services provided.

◆ **Commissions.** Are you getting commissions for any services you provide? If so, consider whether this person will be acting in the best interests of your parent or simply working to sell a policy, an investment, or another financial or legal tool.

◆ **The time frame.** What needs to be accomplished, and how long do you estimate it will take? When will the plan or the portfolio be updated, and how much will this cost?

◆ **Other helpers.** Who else in the office will work on this matter? If it's an assistant or associate, will his fees be lower, and how much supervision will he receive?

◆ **References.** Get the names of two or three clients, preferably people in a similar situation, and then call and find out how long they have used this professional and how helpful, open, and knowledgeable they have found him or her to be.

◆ **Compatibility.** As you talk, get a sense of the person's character and

TOO MANY COOKS

If your parent or family is dealing with more than one professional—an estate lawyer, accountant, and investment adviser, for example—be sure they are able and willing to work together. In the best of circumstances, such professionals should work as a team, meeting every year or two to review a plan. Otherwise, a financial planner may be dedicating certain assets for future use while a lawyer is protecting them in an untouchable trust, and an insurance agent advises your parent to use the money to buy a new policy. Your parent, or you, should talk with each person involved and choose one to oversee everything, though none should have the right to make important decisions without your parent's approval.

personality. Do you like him or her? Do you share a basic approach or philosophy? Do you sense that this person will be honest and direct? Does he or she answer questions so that you and your parent can understand the situation clearly? Can this person assure you that he or she will return phone calls within one business day?

◆ **Handling disputes.** Find out, in advance, how a professional generally settles disputes. What happens, for example, if you disagree with a bill or feel that the service was inadequate?

Fraud, Scams, and Scoundrels

Financial fears, loneliness, and boredom make the elderly popular prey for sweepstakes, contests, investment fraud, and other rackets and rip-offs.

Nationally, consumers lose billions of dollars each year to telemarketing scams alone. That doesn't include unscrupulous insurance and mortgage agents, identity theft, e-mail scams, and other forms of deception.

Even if your parent has never bought into this nonsense before, he may be more susceptible now. Be alert to clues: His bank account is suddenly overdrawn, he has fifteen new magazine subscriptions, his wallet is packed with new credit cards, the mail is full of sweepstakes letters, etc.

Even if there are no signs of trouble, discuss the following do's and don'ts with your parent:

◆ Trust your instincts. If something sounds too good to be true, it probably is.

◆ Beware of lures of friendship and entertainment. Living alone, with little to do, elderly people are often eager to sign up for memberships and contests that cost them dearly in the end.

◆ Don't be tempted by easy money and promising investments. Financial troubles—real or imagined—may lead your parent into all sorts of scams.

◆ Don't be pressured into buying anything. Be leery of any salesman who ignores your refusals or urges you to act immediately. Expressions like "only good for a limited time," "free," and "no-risk offer," are warnings.

◆ Never give a credit card number over the telephone unless you have initiated the purchase. And do not give out your Social Security number.

◆ Give donations only to established, reputable charities or to causes with which you're personally familiar. If a group piques your interest, ask the solicitor to send you more information.

◆ Consider joining the federal "Do Not Call" registry (www.donotcall.gov). After three months, most telemarketers are not allowed to call you. Ask telemarketers not to call you again, and if they do, contact the Federal Trade Commission (877-382-4357 or www.ftc.gov).

◆ If salespeople come to the door, do not let them in. Ask for identification and then let them give their pitch from outside (or just say, "No thank you," and close the door).

◆ Always get receipts, avoid dealing in cash, and never send cash in the mail.

◆ Steer clear of contests and sweepstakes. The odds of winning are ridiculously low, and you can get yourself in trouble. If you do enter, you do not have to buy anything, and that's the law.

◆ Be suspect if anyone who is repairing your house or car suddenly finds a number of things that need fixing. Get another opinion before having any additional work done.

◆ Never leave workers unattended in your home or give a stranger your house key.

◆ Rip up any preapproved credit card offers, which can be filled out by someone else. Similarly, be careful when discarding credit card receipts and statements, which hold all the information necessary for new charges.

◆ When using an ATM machine, do so in private, and always have an eye on your card. Thieves can actually install a device that reads your card's encoded data, and then enter your PIN to drain your bank account.

◆ All of this and more is true of the Internet. Don't be tempted by "irresistible" offers. Don't open "spam," or unsolicited junk e-mail. Never open attachments on e-mails unless you know who it is from. Never give important information (address, credit

" Dad was always very careful about money, so it never occurred to us that there might be a problem or that this was something we should look into or even think about.

I guess we didn't want to see that there was a problem because, looking back, there were clues.

He has Alzheimer's, but we didn't know that then. He seemed okay. A little forgetful maybe, but nothing unusual. Now we realize it had already started to fog his judgment, and I think he was lonely and missing Mom. So, it turns out that he was buying into every sweepstakes and credit card offer and magazine subscription and scam that came his way. I don't know what he was thinking, but he went through thousands of dollars. He was really in trouble by the time we realized what was happening."

—PETER K.

card, Social Security number) over the Internet unless you initiated the deal and know exactly with whom you are dealing.

◆ For more information concerning fraud, call the local consumer protection agency, police department, area agency on aging, or local Better Business Bureau. The National Consumers League has a toll-free consumer protection line (800-876-7060) and a helpful Web site (www.fraud.org).

PAYING FOR HEALTH CARE

Medicare • Medigap • Medicaid • Long–Term Care Insurance

....

IF MEDICAL, NURSING, AND HOME-CARE BILLS ARE NOT POURING in now, the prospect that they soon will be lies ominously ahead. Premiums, deductibles, co-payments, excessive costs not covered by insurance, and the sky-high price of prescription drugs can quickly consume your parent's entire living allowance.

The biggest quandary, even for those with a comfortable savings and income, is how to cover the extraordinary cost of long-term care—nursing homes, assisted-living care, or help at home when a person simply can't care for himself. These costs can easily reach $50,000 to more than $100,000 a year. Medicare and most other insurance virtually never cover these costs.

Most people pay for long-term care out of their own pockets, using up every last dime they ever saved, and then they get onto Medicaid, the government's insurance program for low-income people.

If he hasn't done so already, your parent and/or you should evaluate his health insurance and consider ways that he might cover these bills. If his savings are meager, find out about early Medicaid eligibility.

Too little health insurance leaves him exposed to enormous financial risk, while too much means unnecessary payments for premiums and possible delays for reimbursement if plans overlap and insurance companies disagree on who should pay. Act now because your parent may become ineligible for certain types of insurance as he grows older, or for a life-care center once he is seriously ill or disabled.

Medicare

Medicare is federal health insurance for people over sixty-five and for certain disabled people under sixty-five. The program is run by the Centers for Medicare & Medicaid Services (CMS), previously known as the Health Care Financing Administration.

Anyone who receives Social Security benefits (or benefits from the Railroad Retirement Board) gets a Medicare card when they turn sixty-five. If your parent doesn't receive Social Security benefits (because she is still working, because neither she nor her husband paid Medicare taxes while working, or some other reason), she can still apply for Medicare. To do so, she should contact the local Social Security office or the Social Security Administration (800-722-1213 or www.ssa.gov).

Medicare offers choices. Your parent can opt for the Original Medicare Plan, or she can choose from a variety of other plans, called Medicare Advantage (formerly called Medicare + Choice). Those who choose a Medicare Advantage plan are still covered under Medicare and still get the coverage offered under the original plan. But in most cases, they get additional coverage for certain tests, exams, and medical services that are not included in the basic plan. However, they may not be able to choose any doctor they want; they may have to stay within a "network" of doctors and other health-care providers.

Which plan your parent chooses will depend upon what she is able or willing to spend up front, what her health needs are, what extra benefits she might need or want, which doctor she wants to see, and where various doctors are located.

For the most part, your parent can switch from one plan into another at any time. However, some plans limit the number of members they take, and they won't accept new members when they reach their maximum. (The rules are different for people with end-stage renal disease. Contact Medicare for more information on this.)

THE OPTIONS, IN BRIEF

Medicare: Federal health insurance for people over sixty-five. Medicare's basic coverage, called the "original plan," covers the bulk of medical and hospital care, but not long-term care.

Medicare Advantage: Offers the same or more coverage than the original plan, but with different premiums, deductibles, and co-payments. Insurers often limit care to a specific group of doctors, hospitals, and other providers.

Medigap: An additional policy meant to fill some of the gaps in Medicare's original plan.

Employee or retiree coverage: Sometimes a former employer or union provides health-care coverage beyond retirement.

Military benefits: Veterans and those with TRICARE coverage (expanded coverage for uniformed services retirees and their families) receive fairly ample coverage.

Prescription drug coverage: Medicare offers a plan for drug coverage. Other drug cards and discounts are available through states, charities, and businesses.

State programs: States help people with limited incomes pay their Medicare premiums, and sometimes the deductibles and co-payments as well.

Medicaid: Government health insurance for low-income people, which ends up paying for nearly half of all nursing-home care nationally.

Federally Qualified Health Centers (FQHC): Lower-cost health care at a community clinic.

Long-term care insurance: Private insurance that covers some of the cost of long-term care.

PACE: Programs of All-inclusive Care for the Elderly provide full medical and daily care for very frail elderly people living in the community. It is not widely available and is primarily for those who are eligible for Medicaid. (See page 159 for more information.)

Waiver programs: States can use Medicaid funds to offer a variety of programs and services that are not usually covered under Medicaid, and most of them do so. Some extend to people who are not yet eligible for Medicaid.

Continuing Care Retirement Communities (CCRC): Full care, from independence through nursing-home care, usually in deluxe settings, at a relatively steep price. (See page 423 for more information.)

To oversee your parent's Medicare coverage, contact the local Social Security office and ask for authorization to access her records and receive bills, checks, and other mail. If your parent is able, she can give you authorization to access her records by completing a form (Form SSA 1696-U4), which is available through the Social Security Administration. You can call (800-772-1213) or download it from the Internet (www.ssa.gov).

THE ORIGINAL MEDICARE PLAN

THE BASIC, "ORIGINAL MEDICARE Plan" is divided into two parts: Part A, hospital insurance; and Part B, medical insurance.

Part A covers most hospital bills, hospice care, and a very limited amount of nursing-home and home care. Most people do not have to pay anything to receive Part A, the hospital insurance, but your parent will be responsible for certain deductibles and co-payments once she needs care.

If for some reason your parent isn't enrolled in Part A, she should enroll right away; if she waits until she is hospitalized, she (or, most likely, you) will face a mountain of paperwork and bureaucratic delays at an already difficult time.

Part B, the medical insurance portion, covers most doctor's fees (but not annual checkups), medical equipment, diagnostic tests, outpatient care, and some mental health care and rehabilitative therapy.

Most people pay a monthly premium of about $70, which is taken directly out of their Social Security payments. (Starting in 2007, the premium will be linked to income, with higher rates for those making over $80,000 a year.)

An annual deductible of about $100 must be met before payments begin. After the deductible is covered, the enrollee pays a "coinsurance" or share of the cost of any covered service (about 20 percent) and Medicare pays the rest.

Part B is optional. If your parent receives Social Security payments, she is enrolled automatically. If, for some reason, your parent doesn't want Part

MEDICARE REQUIREMENTS

◆ Services must be provided by a Medicare-approved (certified) hospital, agency, institution, or company, except in emergencies.

◆ Services must be "medically necessary"—that is, ordered by a physician to diagnose or treat an acute or chronic illness.

◆ Services must be provided within the United States or, in some emergency situations, Canada or Mexico. (Some Medicare Advantage plans have different rules regarding travel.)

B (perhaps she is adequately covered by another policy), she needs to contact the local Social Security office and let them know. But there may be penalties if she changes her mind and signs up at a later date.

ACCEPTING ASSIGNMENT

MEDICARE TRIES TO KEEP COSTS UNDER control by determining in advance what it will pay for medical procedures and supplies. When a doctor, other health-care provider, or medical equipment supplier accepts this assigned fee as full payment for a given service—called "accepting assignment"—your parent pays only the deductible and any coinsurance (usually 20 percent).

More than 70 percent of doctors (excluding pediatricians and others who do not provide care for Medicare

---

HELP!

M edicare Part A and B, and now D? Medicare Select? Medicare Advantage? Medigap? Appeals? Notices and bills? How does anyone figure it all out? To ease the headaches and confusion, there are several sources of help.

◆ Medicare has a "Personal Plan Finder" (at www.medicare.gov, or, if you do not have Internet access, call 800-MEDICARE). Once your parent answers a few questions about her needs and preferences, the finder outlines plans available in her area that fit the bill, explaining what they cost and what they cover. It also provides some information about the quality of each plan.

◆ Each state has a State Health Insurance Counseling and Assistance Program (SHIP), in which counselors help people sort through the medley of insurance options, decode bills, and appeal Medicare decisions. (See Appendix C, page 635 for a list of SHIP programs by state.)

◆ The state insurance department can help if your parent is denied insurance coverage or believes that an insurer is committing fraud.

◆ For general questions about existing Medicare coverage, you can either call the SHIP or, for Part A, the "fiscal intermediary," which is a private company contracted by Medicare to pay Part A bills. For Part B, call the "Medicare carrier," which is the private company contracted by Medicare to pay, yes, the Part B bills.

beneficiaries) are "participating physicians," which means that they accept assignment on all Medicare claims.

If a doctor does not accept assignment—for example, if a doctor charges your parent $220 for a test when the approved Medicare fee is only $200—then your parent pays the usual 20 percent coinsurance on the Medicare amount *plus* the $20 difference between the doctor's fee and Medicare's approved fee. However, you may have to pay the bill in full and then get a partial reimbursement from Medicare.

There is a limit to how much doctors can charge. In most cases, doctors cannot add more than 15 percent to Medicare's approved fees. So if the approved fee for a service is $100, the most any doctor can charge is $115. (Of course, a doctor may charge any price he chooses for services that Medicare does not cover.)

If your parent is happy with his doctor, he may be willing to pay the extra charge. Otherwise, he can find a participating physician either by calling doctors' offices or by looking in the *Participating Physician Directory*, which can be found at www.medicare.gov or in public libraries, Social Security offices, and senior citizen centers. He can also call his Medicare carrier for a list.

MEDICARE ADVANTAGE

BEYOND THE ORIGINAL MEDICARE Plan described above, your parent may have other choices, depending upon where he lives. Private insurance companies contract with Medicare to pro-

DUAL COVERAGE

If your parent has coverage from more than one source, any group health plan, no-fault insurance, liability insurance, or worker's compensation must be billed first, before Medicare. If you are not sure where to send bills, contact the Coordination of Benefits Contractor at 800-999-1118.

vide coverage. They often offer broader coverage but limit which doctors, hospitals, and other health-care providers a person can see.

Your parent will still be in the Medicare program. He will still get the coverage included in Part A and Part B of the original plan.

The Medicare Advantage plans generally fall into one of these four categories:

◆ **Managed Care.** Under most managed-care plans, your parent can go only to doctors and other providers who are on the plan's list, or "network." Also, her primary-care doctor may have to make a referral in order for her to see a specialist. Be aware that doctors can leave the plan at any time. If your parent adores her current doctor, be sure he or she is in the network and is not thinking of leaving it.

Some managed-care plans offer an option called "point of service," which means that your parent can go

MEDICARE PART A: HOSPITAL INSURANCE*

	Covered (after an $875 deductible is paid)	Not Covered
Hospital stays	• The first sixty days of hospitalization; the next thirty days require a co-payment ($219 a day). This coverage begins anew with each "benefit period."** For days 91 to 150, the co-payment is quite high ($438 a day) and only sixty of these extra days will be covered in a lifetime.	• Co-payments and all costs beyond 150 days • Private-duty nurses • The extra cost of private rooms unless "medically necessary" • Television or telephone
Nursing-home care	• "Skilled care" (nurses, therapists) that follows a hospital stay of at least three days • The first twenty days in a benefit period are covered fully; a co-payment ($109.50 a day) is required for the next eighty days. • Medications, meals	• Co-payments and all costs beyond one hundred days in a benefit period • Custodial care (help with bathing, dressing, grooming, eating, etc.) • Any care that is not related to a hospital stay of three days or more • Extra charges for a private room
Home health care***	• Part-time or intermittent "skilled" care (nurses, therapists, and aides) when prescribed by a doctor for treatment or rehabilitation, and when the patient is homebound. Services must be provided by a "certified" home health care agency	• Custodial care (help with bathing, dressing, grooming, eating, etc.)
Hospice care	• All medical and nursing care, medical supplies, home care, and counseling • Short-term hospital or respite care • Drugs for pain and symptom relief • Some inpatient respite care	• A small co-payment for drugs (less than $5) • 5 percent of the cost of inpatient respite care
Inpatient psychiatric care	• 190 days, over a lifetime, in a free-standing psychiatric hospital (as opposed to inpatient care in a general hospital, which is covered like any other hospitalization)	• Any care in a psychiatric hospital that exceeds 190 days
Blood received as an inpatient	• All but the first three pints	• The first three pints in each calendar year

Dollar amounts are 2004 figures.
**A "benefit period" begins anew if someone does not use hospital or skilled nursing care for sixty days.*
***Covered under Part B if someone doesn't have Part A*

MEDICARE PART B: MEDICAL INSURANCE*

	Covered (at 80 percent, after a $100 deductible is paid each year)	**Not Covered** (20 percent of Medicare's approved fee)
Doctor's fees	• Most bills from doctors who "accept assignment"	• Charges in excess of "approved fees" • Most routine physical exams • Routine dental care, some chiropractic care and foot care
Outpatient hospital and mental health care	• Most medical services and supplies, including emergency-room visits, one-day surgery, and some rehabilitation • Outpatient mental health care	• 50 percent of the cost of outpatient mental health services
Therapy	• "Medically necessary" outpatient physical, occupational and speech therapy • No limit if therapy is provided by a hospital outpatient facility	
Diagnostic and laboratory services	• Blood and urine tests, X-rays, scans, EKGs, biopsies, some screening tests	
Medical equipment and supplies	• Durable equipment, including hospital beds, wheelchairs, oxygen supplies, walkers	• Eyeglasses, hearing aids, dentures
Ambulance service and emergency care	• Cost of ambulance transport (when medically necessary) • All emergency care	
Preventive care	• Mammograms, pap smears, and pelvic exam; pneumonia, hepatitis B, and flu shots; bone mass, colorectal, prostate, heart disease, and glaucoma screening; diabetes services	• Most other preventive care • While most of this is covered at 80 percent of the "approved amount," some care requires no coinsurance payment.
Drugs	• Coverage for a few (very few) prescription drugs	• Most prescription drugs
Blood received as an outpatient	• All but the first three pints	• The first three pints in each calendar year

* Prices as of 2004. Part B requires a monthly premium.

to doctors and hospitals not in the network, but he or she may have to pay deductibles and coinsurance to do so.

◆ **Preferred Provider Organization.** These work much like managed-care plans, except that people can see specialists without referrals from a primary doctor. In some cases, people can see any doctor or provider who accepts Medicare, but, again, they might have to pay extra if the provider is not within the plan's "network."

◆ **Private Fee-for-Service.** These plans operate much like the Original Medicare Plan, except that a private company, rather than Medicare, determines the "approved fees," premiums, deductibles, coinsurance, and co-payments. Your parent can go to any doctor or hospital that is approved by Medicare and accepts the plan's fees as payment.

◆ **Specialty Plan.** These are relatively new plans that provide normal Medicare coverage plus any extra care that is needed because of a specific disease or disorder (such as renal disease, congestive heart failure, or diabetes).

OTHER DRUG COVERAGE AND DISCOUNTS

Your parent may not need Medicare's drug plan. Some Medicare Advantage, Medigap, and other health insurance plans include drug coverage. Numerous public and private programs provide free or discounted prescription drugs to low-income people. And finally, many states, pharmaceutical companies, mail-order companies, and online drugstores have discounted drug programs with no eligibility requirements.

To learn more, you can go online, answer some basic questions, and see what discount plans and free prescriptions may be available to your parent. Try www.benefitscheckuprx.com, run by the National Council on the Aging, or www.medicare.gov, the government's site, which also has a similar search tool. Or you can call Medicare at 800-633-4227.

The Pharmaceutical Research and Manufacturers of America have a database of Patient Assistance Programs through which manufacturers provide free medications to eligible patients (www.helpingpatients.org).

For a list of reputable online drugstores (called Verified Internet Pharmacy Practice Sites, or VIPPS), some of which may offer discounts, go online to the National Association of Boards of Pharmacy (www.nabp.net).

For more ways to save on drugs, see page 222.

SAVINGS UNDER MEDICARE'S PRESCRIPTION DRUG COVERAGE

Annual cost of prescription drugs	Amount your parent pays	Amount saved
$1,000	$857.50	$142.50 or 14%
$2,000	$1,107.50	$892.50 or 45%
$3,000	$1,920	$1,080 or 36%
$4,000	$2,920	$1,080 or 27%
$5,000	$3,920	$1,080 or 22%
$6,000	$4,065	$1,935 or 32%
$8,000	$4,210	$3,790 or 47%
$10,000	$4,265	$5,735 or 57%

PRESCRIPTION DRUG COVERAGE UNDER MEDICARE

MEDICARE OFFERS A PRESCRIPTION drug plan, called Medicare Part D, which will be fully in place in 2006. In the meantime, your parent can buy (for about $30) a drug discount card that should help her save anywhere between 10 and 25 percent on prescription drugs.

As numerous companies offer the cards and each offers discounts on different drugs (and your parent can have only one Medicare drug card), your parent (or you) should make a list of the medications she takes and how much she pays for each, and then find out which cards offer the best discounts on her drugs. Medicare can help with this (800-MEDICARE or www. medicare.gov). If your parent is part of a Medicare Advantage plan, she might have no choice in discount cards; she might have to use the card offered by the plan. (Other drug discount cards are available and may give greater discounts on the drugs your parent uses; see the box on opposite page.)

People with low incomes (less than about $12,570 for a single person, or $16,870 for a couple in 2004, but the numbers change every year) may be able to get a $600 credit on their drug card.

Starting in 2006, there will be a number of Medicare prescription drug plans to choose from, but they will all follow a fairly complicated plan that goes something like this:

◆ A premium of about $35 a month

A NOTICE, NOT A BILL

Your parent will get a Medicare Summary Notice (MSN) each month. This is not a bill! Do not pay it. It is simply a summary of medical services received. Look it over to be sure it is accurate. If something is not right, call the number on the statement.

Your parent may also be able to get her MSNs online. To learn about this, go to www.medicare.gov.

♦ A deductible of $250 a year

♦ After the deductible is met, coverage of 75 percent of the bill, until the cost of drugs reaches $2,250 in a given year

♦ Beyond the $2,250 mark, there is no coverage until a person has spent $3,600 out of pocket (for a total of $5,100 in prescription drug bills)

♦ 95 percent coverage for drug costs beyond $5,100 (or $3,600 out of pocket)

Here's the math:

In any given year, your parent will pay $420 in premiums; plus the first $250 in bills; plus another $500 for the next $2,000 in drug bills.

At this point, the drug tally is $2,250, and your parent has paid only $1,170, for a savings of $1,080, or 48 percent. Now that's pretty good.

However, as her prescription drug tally rises, her savings drop rapidly, because the next $2,850 in drug costs is not covered at all.

Then it all begins to switch back again. When she has reached a total of $5,100 a year in prescription drugs (Medicare has paid $1,500, and she has paid $3,600 plus her premiums, or $4,020), Medicare begins to foot most of the bill and, as she spends more on drugs, her savings rise again.

Again, there is help for people on low incomes who have limited assets. Those who are eligible for Medicaid do not have to pay any premiums or deductibles and pay only $1 for generic prescription drugs and $3 for brand-name prescriptions. Others who have limited income and assets, but are not eligible for Medicaid, get varying degrees of help with drug costs.

For example, in 2006, a single person with an income of less than $13,000 a year and assets of less than $6,000 has to pay $2 for generic drugs and $5 for brand-name drugs, with no premiums or deductibles. A single person with an income of up to $14,400 a year and assets of up to $10,000 has to pay premiums on a sliding scale, a $50 deductible, and 15 percent of drug costs until out-of-pocket spending reaches $3,600, at which point generics are $2 and brand names are $5.

Note that your parent does not need to pay for Medicare's drug coverage if she has Medigap or other insurance that covers prescription drugs. In fact, she is not allowed to buy into Medicare's drug plan if she is already covered. She can, however, switch to a different Medigap plan that doesn't have drug coverage, and then buy into one of the prescription drug plans, if that works out to be a better deal for her.

APPEALING
A MEDICARE DECISION

DON'T THINK FOR A MINUTE THAT IT'S not worth challenging the bureaucracy of Medicare. It is. According to the Centers for Medicare & Medicaid Services, which manages Medicare, about 70 percent of all appeals are successful, at least to some extent.

If you disagree with a decision—if coverage has been refused, stopped, or is inadequate, or if there is some other problem—request a review of the claim. Tackling all that red tape may fill you with dread, but if your reasoning is sound, your chances of winning the case are quite good.

If your parent is under the Original Medicare Plan, ask the provider (doctor, hospital, home-care agency, etc.) to send in a claim. Then, when coverage is denied, follow the instructions on the back of the notice that comes back to you. It will say something like "Explanation of Medicare Benefits" and will tell you how to appeal a decision.

MEDICARE FOR LESS

If your parent has little in the way of income and assets, but is not eligible for Medicaid, he may be able to get under the Medicare umbrella at a discount—no premiums, and sometimes no deductibles or co-payments. States have various programs, called Medicare Savings Programs, to help cover these costs.

The rules are a bit different in every state, but broadly speaking, a person must have less than $5,000 in assets, and less than $1,500 in monthly income to be eligible. (The rates change every year and are higher for couples, so you should check on this.)

If there is any chance that your parent might qualify, apply. Many people who are eligible never apply and end up spending hundreds of dollars each year needlessly.

To learn more about such programs and to see if your parent is eligible, call the state medical assistance office (listed on page 639) or contact Medicare (800-633-4227 or www.medicare.gov).

Other Medicare plans must also tell your parent, in writing, how to appeal a decision. (If a medical decision threatens her health, demand fast action on the appeal. The plan must respond within seventy-two hours.) If the private plan does not decide in your parent's favor, the appeal is then sent on to an independent organization for review.

If your parent is in the hospital, she should be able to remain in the hospital, receiving care, while Medicare reviews any appeal.

For more information on filing appeals, contact the Medicare intermediary or carrier (the private insurance company contracted by the government to oversee Medicare and any claims) listed on her Medicare statement, or the State Health Insurance Counseling and Assistance Program (see page 635).

Medigap

Medigap is private health insurance—separate from Medicare and other federal programs—that fills some, but not all, of the holes in the basic, or original, Medicare plan. Typically, this supplemental insurance pays the cost of premiums, co-payments, deductibles, and any physician bills that exceed Medicare's approved charges. It does not cover much, if anything, outside of Medicare's realm, including long-term care.

Medigap insurance protects people from ongoing medical expenses, and it is a good idea for many. But it is not for everyone. For example, it is not for people who are enrolled in a Medicare Advantage plan or other managed-care or group health plan that provides ample coverage. (In fact, it may be illegal for a company to sell your parent a Medigap plan in these situations.)

Furthermore, anyone who is nearing the financial eligibility limits for Medicaid doesn't need a Medigap policy, and in most cases is it illegal for a company to sell Medigap to someone who is on Medicaid. (There are exceptions; Medicaid is run by states, and they all have their own arrangements.)

If your parent wants to fill some of the gaps in her basic Medicare plan, she also has the option of switching to a Medicare Advantage plan that offers more generous benefits.

Anyone who wants Medigap should buy it, ideally, within six months of enrolling in Medicare Part B. Of course, it may be way too late for that for your parent. But during this window of opportunity, your parent cannot be denied coverage because of existing medical problems.

After this six-month enrollment period is over, insurance companies may be allowed to increase the price of a policy, refuse to cover someone, or attach an array of conditions to a policy. Your parent is protected from these hikes, denials, and conditions if his current employer, group, or Medicare Advantage health coverage ends for some reason.

Your parent may switch from one Medigap policy to a different one, without penalty for preexisting illness or disability, as long as she has had her current policy for at least six months. The company can, however, delay any coverage, beyond what her original policy covered, for six months.

BASIC MEDIGAP BENEFITS

ALL MEDIGAP POLICIES COVER CERtain holes in Medicare. These include:

◆ Co-payments for hospitalization

◆ After Medicare's hospital benefits are used up, coverage for 365 additional days (over a lifetime)

◆ Co-payments required under Part B (20 percent of the Medicare-approved amount for doctor's services and 50 percent for mental health services)

◆ First three pints of blood each year (at which point Medicare picks up the tab)

TEN MEDIGAP PLANS

TO MAKE SHOPPING EASIER, MOST states limit Medigap to ten standard plans. They range from plan A, the core plan, which covers only the basic benefits described above and is available in all states, through plan J, the most comprehensive and expensive plan. By law, these plans cannot vary from company to company or state to state. And to further simplify life, the language and format used in the policies are also standardized.

But—yes, there is always a "but"—some states do not offer all of the

> " *The hospital was going to discharge my mother because Medicare allowed only so many hospital days for her procedure, and then they wouldn't pay anymore. But I knew she wasn't well enough to be discharged, so I told the discharge planner that I was leaving her there and contesting the decision.*
>
> *It was a battle, but in the end Medicare paid the additional hospital bill, which was about $5,000. It was definitely worth the trouble. You can't let these guys get the best of you. You have to fight for what's right."*
>
> —LUCILLE L.

plans, and a few states (Massachusetts, Minnesota, and Wisconsin) have their own version of these plans. So while these are meant to help you comparison shop, your mother in Minnesota may not be able to buy the same plan that Aunt Marjorie bought in Illinois.

Also, any of the standardized plans can be sold as "Medicare SELECT" policies, which work like managed-care plans. Clients are required to use a designated group of doctors, clinics, and hospitals, but they usually pay less for the plan. Finally, insurers are allowed to add benefits to a standard plan, thus making it, well, no longer standard.

The bottom line is, despite all these efforts at standardization, you or your

VETERANS AND MILITARY RETIREES

Veterans have a host of health benefits and coverage. For information, contact the Department of Veterans Affairs (800-827-1000 or www.va.gov).

Those retired from uniformed services can get expanded medical coverage called TRICARE. For information on this, call 888-363-2273 or go online to www.tricareonline.com.

parent should read any policy carefully to understand exactly what is covered and what, if any, exclusions or restrictions exist. Ask the company for a clearly worded summary, which insurance companies are required to provide. By and large, your parent will be comparing apples with apples, so she should be able to decide with relative ease which type of plan she wants, and then to shop around for the best price and service, and the most stable and reliable company.

MEDIGAP SHOPPING TIPS

WHILE THE TEN STANDARD POLICIES are the same, the prices for them can vary widely, so shop around. Figure out how much your parent spends on health care each year (premiums, deductibles, co-payments, excess charges, prescription drugs, etc.), how a policy might affect these costs, and what her future health care might entail.

Other shopping tips:

◆ **Don't buy more policies than needed.** Duplicate coverage is expensive and unnecessary. It's also widely prohibited.

◆ **Be careful when replacing an existing policy.** Your parent must be given credit for the time spent under the old policy in determining if any restrictions on preexisting conditions apply under a new policy. While he must verify that he plans to terminate the old policy, he shouldn't cancel until he is all set with a new policy.

◆ **Don't be pressured.** Take time to pick the best policy. Your parent shouldn't be forced or frightened into buying a policy, or into switching from one policy to another. (Pressuring prospective buyers is against the law.)

◆ **Know the company you're dealing with.** Check with the state insurance department to make sure a company or agent is licensed. And beware of any claims that a policy is sponsored by a state agency, or that an insurance agent is working for the government. Neither is true.

◆ **Check the right to renew.** States require that Medigap policies be guaranteed renewable. This means that a company cannot refuse to renew a policy unless a person fails to pay the premiums or has lied about his health on the application. Beware of older policies that let a company cancel policies on an individual basis.

THE TEN STANDARD MEDIGAP PLANS
(EXCEPT IN MASSACHUSETTS, MINNESOTA, OR WISCONSIN)

	Plan A	Plan B	Plan C	Plan D	Plan E	Plan F	Plan G	Plan H	Plan I	Plan J
Basic Medigap benefits*	✓	✓	✓	✓	✓	✓	✓	✓	✓	✓
Part A deductible ($876 in 2004)		✓	✓	✓	✓	✓	✓	✓	✓	✓
Nursing care co-payment**			✓	✓	✓	✓	✓	✓	✓	✓
Emergency care in foreign countries (80% after $260 deductible)			✓	✓	✓	✓	✓	✓	✓	✓
Part B deductible			✓			✓				✓
Part B doctor fees in excess of "approved fees"					✓		✓ only 80%		✓	✓
Personal care at home***			✓				✓		✓	✓
Prescription drugs ($250 deductible; 50% co-insurance)								✓ up to $1,250	✓ up to $1,250	✓ up to $3,000
Preventive medicine					✓					✓

* See description on page 359
** Co-payments through day one hundred; no coverage after one hundred days in a benefit period
*** Only when a person is receiving skilled home care covered by Medicare, and then for an additional eight weeks after skilled care is no longer needed, up to $1,600 a year

◆ **Check for preexisting-condition exclusions.** Don't be misled by the phrase "no medical examination required." If your parent has had a health problem recently, the insurer might not cover treatments related to that problem until the policy has been in effect for six months.

◆ **Decide on a date when it will become effective.** Your parent may need her coverage to begin when some other policy ends, or on some other date. That should not present any problems. Get an agreement in writing.

◆ **Complete the application carefully.** Do not believe an insurance agent who says that the medical history on an application is not important. If you or your parent leaves out any of the medical information requested, coverage could be refused for a period of time for any medical condition that you neglected to mention. The company could also cancel the policy.

◆ **Use the "free-look" provision.** Insurance companies must provide at least thirty days to review a Medigap policy. If your parent changes his mind during this time, he can cancel the policy and get a full refund of any premiums paid.

◆ **Don't pay cash.** Use a check, money order, or bank draft payable to the insurance company, not to the agent. Be sure to get a receipt that includes the insurance company's name, address, and telephone number.

Medicaid

Unless your parent is very comfortable financially, learn about Medicaid (sometimes referred to as "medical assistance" or Title 19), the government health insurance program for low-income people. It may seem that he's well off and would never need it, but long-term care is so expensive that many people who don't expect to go on Medicaid end up there.

Learn the rules (or, better yet, confer with a lawyer) early, so your parent doesn't scrape the bottom of his savings account needlessly. The fact is, he may qualify for Medicaid before he thinks he will.

Jumping on this early is also important because your parent may be able to protect some of his assets before going on Medicaid. (When people use up their money to become eligible for Medicaid, it is called "spending down.")

Unlike Medicare, which is fully regulated by the federal government, Medicaid is a joint program of both federal and state governments. The federal government sets guidelines, and then states set up their own rules and programs within these broad guidelines. As a result, states have various rules and programs, no two quite the same.

Many states have special programs specifically for the elderly, allowing them to get coverage under less stringent financial rules, especially if they need long-term care.

Elderly people who qualify for Medicaid are called "dual eligible," meaning that they are eligible to receive both Medicare (because of their age) and Medicaid (because of their finances). Anything covered by Medicare is paid for by that program first. Medicaid picks up where Medicare leaves off.

Medicaid covers the bulk of a person's health-care costs, including nursing-home care and some "skilled" care at home, but there is a price to pay. Some doctors and nursing homes won't take patients on Medicaid, or will accept only a limited number because the reimbursement rates are relatively low. As a result, Medicaid patients sometimes get health care in clinics where they wait and wait, and then receive mediocre care. Or, unable to find a place in one of the best nursing homes, they settle for substandard care.

Despite these liabilities, Medicaid is a vital and welcome safety net. Get your parent to talk with a state Medicaid counselor or to meet with a lawyer who specializes in Medicaid planning, because the rules are complicated. (A state counselor, by the way, cannot advise someone on how to protect assets.)

For information about Medicaid and nursing homes, see page 430.

WHAT'S COVERED

MEDICAID RULES VARY FROM STATE to state, but coverage must include:

♦ Inpatient and outpatient hospital services

NOTE FOR MEDICAID RECIPIENTS

Once on Medicaid, don't sit back and assume your parent is properly covered. To get the coverage and care that your parent deserves, you might have to fight the system. Any time you or your parent feels that Medicaid has refused to cover necessary or adequate services, contact the state medical assistance office (see page 639).

♦ Physician services

♦ Periodic diagnostic tests and screenings

♦ Laboratory and X-ray services

♦ Rural health clinic services

♦ Nursing-home care

♦ Home health care for people deemed eligible for nursing-home care

♦ Medical transportation

Beyond this list of "musts," many state Medicaid programs also cover:

♦ Prescription drugs

♦ Prosthetic devices

♦ Eye care and eyeglasses

♦ Transportation

♦ Rehabilitation and physical therapy

Our father told us years ago not to pay for expensive caretaking if he began to suffer from severe dementia the way his father did. He protected his assets so he would be eligible early for Medicaid. It all happened the way he'd imagined. I'm grateful he had such foresight."

—FRED S.

♦ Less intensive home care and community-based services

♦ A full array of health care and social services for people living in the community but eligible for nursing-home care

♦ Dental care

♦ Case management

Medicaid usually covers the entire cost of an eligible patient's health care, although some states charge a small deductible or co-payment for certain services to people in certain financial brackets.

WHO'S ELIGIBLE

BROADLY SPEAKING, IN ORDER TO qualify for Medicaid, a single person is permitted to own no more than a home, personal belongings, a car, some small amount of savings (perhaps $2,000, plus some money set aside for burial and funeral expenses), and can have only a meager income (a few

hundred dollars a month or less in most states). Income includes any payments your parent receives from a job, Social Security, a pension or other retirement fund, and interest from savings and investments.

Because a person who remains at home continues to need financial support when a spouse enters a nursing home, the rules for couples are more generous. Generally, the healthier spouse can keep, in addition to a home, car, and personal belongings, half of the couple's assets, but usually no more than $95,000 and certainly no less than $19,000 (in 2004). Spouses can also keep their own income and sometimes a portion of their partner's income, depending upon the healthier spouse's needs and the state's limits. (In some states, spouses can keep up to the maximum, regardless of whether it represents half of their assets.)

These standards vary, depending upon the individual's disability and medical needs, what other public assistance he receives, his life insurance, and other issues that a state deems important. (If your parent is eligible for Supplemental Security Income (SSI), he is automatically eligible for Medicaid.)

Beyond broad federal guidelines, each state has its own unique and bewildering set of rules and exceptions. As mentioned, many states have special programs to help people who do not quite meet these financial requirements. Some states also have created innovative programs to help people stay in their homes and receive home and community care, rather than going to a nursing home.

Here's an example of why it's important to know the rules: In some states the spouse who remains in the community is allowed to keep whatever assets are necessary to produce enough income to pay her regular bills. A person who receives $300 a month in Social Security but has $200,000 in the bank earning 3 percent (or $500 a month) might be allowed to keep the entire bank account so that she has enough income to live on. Most people are not aware of this provision and thus would wait until the $200,000 was virtually depleted before applying for Medicaid. In other states, a spouse can refuse to contribute to nursing-home bills and can keep all of her own income.

While Medicaid is generally limited to U.S. citizens, there are exceptions, and "emergency Medicaid" is available to anyone, regardless of citizenry.

To find out if your parent is eligible, go to www.benefitscheckup. org, www.govbenefits.gov, or www. cms.hhs.gov (click on "Medicaid" and then "Medicaid Information for Consumers"). You can also call the local medical assistance office (listed on page 639).

HOW TO APPLY FOR MEDICAID

THE AREA AGENCY ON AGING OR, IF your parent is in a hospital or nursing home, the facility's patient advocate can tell you how to apply. In most states you need to contact the local depart-

> " *When the lawyer talked to me about putting Dad's house in my name, I thought it was a great idea. Then I got home and I began to feel it was wrong. Dad believed in paying his own way. That was important to him. I didn't think he would want me to do this.*
>
> *The more I thought about it, the more confused I felt. I know he wanted us to have his house, but I also know he wouldn't want to be on welfare or have us do anything dishonest. Here I was, choosing between these two horrible things, and he couldn't express his opinion because he was too sick.*
>
> *In the end, I didn't put the house in my name. I just felt it was wrong. We still have it now, but the lawyer tells me that the government will come after it eventually."*
>
> —ANNE P.

ment of social services or the human resources administration. (See page 639 for a list of state contact numbers.)

Your parent has to have proof of his identity and citizenship (birth certificate or passport), proof of address (lease, cancelled rent checks, utility bills), proof of income (letter from Social Security, pay stubs, retirement benefits), proof of assets (bank statements, bank books, and other financial statements), proof of living expenses (rent, utility bills, etc.) as well as medical bills.

PROTECTING ASSETS TO QUALIFY FOR MEDICAID

....

YOUR PARENT SAVED DILIGENTLY SO he could pass something on to his children. Maybe he wanted his parent's home or a piece of land to stay in the family. But faced with the prospect of hospital and nursing-home bills, his savings and perhaps even the house or the land are in jeopardy.

Your parent may be able to protect some of his assets and still become eligible for Medicaid, but to do so he has to plan well in advance. The sooner he acts, the more he will be able to protect.

Of course, the notion of protecting one's money or property and then going on Medicaid raises troubling moral and legal questions. Medicaid and other public programs are meant for those who are truly needy. What your parent saves, taxpayers pay. Over the long run, such actions destroy the system for those who need it. Furthermore, your parent's money is for his own living expenses, not your inheritance. Going on public assistance is demeaning, and it often means inadequate care.

On the other hand, one can argue, as many do, that affluent people do all sorts of financial wrangling to protect their estates from taxes, so why shouldn't people with smaller estates protect themselves from nursing-home bills? Your family has to be guided by its own moral and political code on this matter.

For the time being, in most states, your parent can protect his assets by giving them outright to others or by putting them in an irrevocable trust, one that your parent cannot touch or benefit from. But this has to be done very early in the game.

For the most part, when a person applies for Medicaid, officials examine his financial records for the past thirty-six months to see what, if any, gifts or transfers have been made. Anyone who has given a substantial gift or otherwise transferred assets during this "look-back period" may not qualify for Medicaid until some time in the future. Usually the person must wait the number of months it would take for him to spend on nursing-home care the amount that was given away or transferred. However, attorneys have found ingenious ways to get around even this.

Let's say your parent finds that he needs nursing-home care, so he immediately gives you and your siblings his savings of $180,000. If the average cost of nursing-home care in his area is $9,000 a month, then he would not be eligible to receive Medicaid for twenty months, the length of time it would take for him to spend the entire $180,000 on his nursing-home care. Of course, he no longer has that money, so all he's got is trouble and he hasn't saved a dime.

One way people get around this rule is to give away half of their money—keeping just enough to pay for care during those months that they aren't covered. So instead of giving away the whole kit and caboodle, your parent now gives away (or puts into an irrevocable trust for his heirs), only

PAYING FOR LONG-TERM CARE WITH LIFE INSURANCE

If your parent needs more care than he can afford, under certain circumstances he may be able to collect life insurance money to pay his bills. Many insurance companies now offer an arrangement known as "living benefits" (or "advanced benefits" or "accelerated benefits"), in which policyholders collect benefits early—rather than passing them on to dependents or heirs—in order to pay for a nursing home, home care, and other such expenses.

The specifics of each plan vary, though most require that the policyholder be expected to live for less than a year. Some life insurance companies pay only a fraction of the total benefit, while others pay almost all of it. Some pay the benefit in one large check, while others provide monthly payments. Some offer living benefits only on new policies, while others will add riders to existing ones.

Living benefits should not be confused with "viatical settlements," which means selling an insurance policy to a company or individual for a fraction of its value—often just 50 to 80 percent, depending upon life expectancy. The company takes over the life insurance policy, becoming the beneficiary; pays the remaining premiums; and collects when the original owner dies. These arrangements are often more flexible than living benefits, but they pay less and may affect taxes and other benefits. They are also subject to abuse.

Before your parent cashes in his life insurance, he, and preferably a lawyer or accountant, should study any agreement carefully. Consider the reasons for cashing in, look at other options, find out if the income will be taxed, and see if this will affect his eligibility for Medicaid and other entitlements.

---

half of his savings, or $90,000. He now has to pay for his own nursing home care for ten months, using up the $90,000 he has kept. But he has protected the other $90,000.

Also, while a person can keep a home and certain personal belongings, states claim anything remaining in the estate after the person dies to recoup what has been spent on their care. Depending upon the state's rules, your parent may be able to protect his home by putting the deed in someone else's name. Even if your parent lives in the house during his lifetime, it would then be out of reach of state officials and other creditors. But again, officials will look back thirty-six months, so he needs to act well in advance.

If your parent chooses to give away his assets and go on Medicaid, he shouldn't be overly zealous about it; he needs money to live on. And he would be well advised to keep enough money so that he can apply to a good nursing home as a self-paying resident.

Also, keep in mind that the opportunities to protect assets are becoming narrower and may eventually disappear; what is permitted today may not be permitted tomorrow.

Long-Term Care Insurance

The missing piece in Medicare and other health insurance plans is coverage for long-term care, and as we've noted, it's a very large piece indeed. Nursing-home care averages more than $60,000 a year nationally, but it costs well over $100,000 a year in many areas. Home care is usually less, but not always. (Some math: At $15 an hour, round-the-clock care would cost more than $130,000 a year.)

If that doesn't send you home crying, consider this: These prices don't include drugs, medical supplies, doctor's fees, or special services that might be needed. And, nursing-home costs are expected to rise 5 percent a year.

Because these policies are relatively new, it's unlikely your parent has long-term care insurance. And if she is already quite old or ill, she will not be eligible for it. These policies are usually not a viable option after age eighty or if a person has already been diagnosed with a debilitating illness.

If your parent is eligible, and has substantial assets to protect, long-term care insurance is worth investigating. Or, if you're looking at fifty or sixty, it is worth considering for yourself. However, don't jump too fast. These plans are not for everyone.

Prices vary, depending upon the type of plan and the age and health of the buyer. A sixty-year-old person in good health can expect to pay about $3,000 a year for a policy, but premiums can reach more than $8,000 a year for an older person.

Be aware that insurance companies have, by and large, grossly miscalculated the costs of these policies and are imposing steep rate hikes. Customers are also finding that companies are resistant to actually paying out benefits when the time comes.

WHO NEEDS IT?

THIS IS A GAMBLE, AS IS THE CASE with most insurance. If someone ends up needing years of supervision and care, then the insurance was a good buy; if they die suddenly, never using any sort of personal or nursing care, then it was a bust. And remember, no policy covers all the costs; there will still be bills to pay, even with coverage.

As your parent (or you) consider such insurance, beware of pushy salespeople and scare tactics. The costs are high and the fear is great, but don't buy in a panic. Many people shouldn't bother with these policies. Agents get enormous commissions (often 50 percent of the first year's premium and another 10 percent for every year after that), so they have plenty of incentive. Think long and hard about whether this is a worthwhile investment.

Long-term care insurance helps protect assets and preserve inheritance for heirs. However, it's not cheap, it doesn't cover the full cost of care, and some people never need such care.

So, who should consider buying a policy?

◆ **Those with ample assets.** The primary reason to buy long-term care insurance is to protect one's assets from the excessive costs of long-term care. Certainly your parent should not buy a policy if he would be eligible for Medicaid within, say, twelve to eighteen months of entering a nursing home. Nursing-home costs vary widely, so look at costs in the area. As a rough guideline, your parent should have at least $100,000 in assets (not including his house and personal belongings) before considering a long-term care insurance policy.

◆ **Those with ample income.** Can your parent afford to pay $300 to $600 a month in premiums without affecting her lifestyle? Some experts suggest that long-term care insurance should not cost more than 5 percent of a person's total income, and that seems to be a pretty good guideline.

> ## FOR VETERANS ONLY
>
> I f your parent is a veteran, he may be eligible for free or low-cost medical and nursing-home care, and he may not need much in the way of supplementary health insurance. Call the local Veterans Affairs Office for more information on services and coverage, or contact the U.S. Department of Veterans Affairs at 800 827 1000 or www.va.gov.

Also, will your parent be able to continue to pay these premiums if they rise or her income dips? Keep in mind, if your parent fails to pay premiums, her policy will be cancelled; she shouldn't start this if she isn't sure that she can continue it.

◆ **Those whose assets and income are not overly ample.** People with a large income or, say, more than a million dollars in savings generally don't need such insurance because they will be able to pay for their care out of pocket. They might still want it, however, in order to protect assets for heirs and perhaps for a little peace of mind.

◆ **Those who are likely to need long-term care.** No one has a crystal ball, but you can make an educated guess.

After age sixty-five, the odds of entering a nursing home at some point

" *I'm looking at long-term care insurance for myself, because it's too late for my parents. But when I think about the expense I wonder if it's really worth it. I'm only fifty-three—too young to think about nursing homes. But then, that's what always happens with these things. You don't think about them until you really need them, and then it's too late.*"

—NELLY O.

in life are about 40 percent. The average length of stay is 2.5 years. But 45 percent of nursing-home stays are three months or less and the majority are less than one year. What tips the scales is that 10 percent are five years or more. Another 30 percent of people end up needing assisted-living care or substantial help at home.

So what does all this tell you? That there is a very good chance that your parent will need nursing-home, assisted-living, or home care at some point, but perhaps not for more than a year or two.

Now you can fine-tune those odds by considering your parent's health and family history. If he has a family history of sudden and fatal heart attacks, then he is less likely to need extended care than, say, a person who has a family history of Alzheimer's disease. Is your parent a smoker? Does he exercise? How's your mother's bone density? All of these things play a role in how much care a person might one day need.

Finally, is there a lot of family support, a wealth of local volunteers, and inexpensive services on which your parent can rely, or does he live in a community with little in the way of social services? If your mother lives near your sister, who is a retired nurse with time on her hands, she is less apt to need nursing-home care than a person who lives alone, far from family support.

◆ **Those who have no plans to enter a continuing care retirement community.** CCRCs, as they are called, charge hefty admission and monthly fees, but they provide almost all care that is necessary, from assisted-living to nursing-home care. Having long-term care insurance would be redundant.

SELECTING A LONG-TERM CARE POLICY

COMPARE SEVERAL POLICIES TO FIND the one that best suits your parent's needs (or, if you're considering insurance for yourself, your needs). See page 587 for further information about long-term care insurance for yourself. The state insurance department can tell you which companies sell long-term care insurance locally. You might also look into the possibility of adding a rider onto a current health insurance policy. Several companies provide free quotes by mail or over the Internet. (Any Web search for "long-term care insurance" will turn them up.)

It's not easy to compare policies. They vary in so many ways—when they kick in, what they cover, how benefits are paid, etc. Ask to see an "outline of coverage" detailing a policy's benefits, costs, restrictions, and limitations.

When reviewing policies, be sure that any special features are worth the price paid in higher premiums. Any extras will add substantially to the cost. Your parent shouldn't simply decide what she wants and get a price. She should compare basic packages with more extensive policies, see what each item adds to the price of the policy, and then determine if it makes sense to pay the higher amount.

A growing number of employers now offer long-term care insurance to employees, retirees, and sometimes employee's parents as well. Usually this means discounted premiums (they are often paid with pretax dollars, to boot). The federal government offers long-term care insurance options to most federal and U.S. Postal Service employees, active and retired members of the uniformed services, and their spouses and adult children (employees can also get insurance to cover their parents, parents-in-law, and stepparents). For more information about the federal program, go to www.ltcfeds.com or call 800-582-3337.

But even if your employer offers such an option, look at other plans and compare. Just because a company has a group plan doesn't mean it's the best option for your parent (or you).

MEDICAID PARTNERSHIP

A few states have established innovative partnerships between Medicaid and the insurance industry to help people get the care they need and protect their assets. Generally, the programs allow people who buy long-term care insurance to get Medicaid coverage when their insurance runs out, and still protect all or some of their assets (within certain income limits). Call the state insurance department to find out if such programs exist in your parent's state.

Some features to look for:

◆ **A solid company.** Find a well-known, stable company with a good reputation. Buying from a strong company is essential because the field is relatively young, and companies have little history upon which to base their underwriting assumptions. A strong company will be better able to absorb errors.

Check the company's rating with Standard & Poor's (www.standardand poors.com), A.M. Best (www.ambest. com), or Moody's (www.moodys.com). Look for one that falls into the top two categories on financial strength.

Ask the company how long it's been selling long-term care insurance.

A company that's been at this for some time (perhaps ten years or more), will have more experience, and rates will be more stable.

It's also worth calling the state insurance department, which may have information about any complaints against particular insurance companies.

Be leery if a salesperson tells you that the state guarantees coverage if the company defaults. The premiums may be higher for such policies, and if the company fails, the coverage offered by the state won't be as generous as the terms of your parent's original policy.

◆ **Tax qualified.** Most policies are qualified, but it's worth checking. "Tax qualified" means that a policy conforms with the 1996 Health Insurance Portability and Accountability Act, or HIPAA. What it really means is that the benefits can't be taxed. Also, a policy must be qualified if someone wants to deduct the premiums as "medical expenses" from their taxes. (Such expenses must be greater than 7.5 percent of a person's adjusted gross income.)

◆ **Comprehensive coverage.** "Facility-only" policies cover only one type of care, usually nursing-home care. Most policies, however, offer "comprehensive" coverage. These policies should cover care in a nursing home or assisted-living facility, as well as care at home, adult day care, hospice care, and respite care. For most people, it makes more sense to buy a comprehensive policy, which gives them more options and broader coverage.

◆ **Early eligibility.** When does a policy consider someone eligible for benefits? That is, what are the "benefit triggers?" Most policies kick in when someone cannot handle two or more "activities of daily living," or ADLs. These include bathing, dressing, eating, getting from a bed to a chair, toileting, and continence. A good policy should also cover dementia or any other cognitive impairment that requires supervision. Some will cover care deemed "medically necessary," as well, such as care for someone with congestive heart failure.

◆ **A reasonable deductible period.** Most policies include a waiting period (called a "deductible" or "elimination" period), which means that the policy doesn't kick in until a person has paid for care themselves for a certain number of days. The longer the waiting period, the cheaper the policy.

Any waiting period of less than twenty days will make a policy quite expensive. On the other hand, a waiting period of more than one hundred days reduces the chance significantly that a person will ever put the policy to use. Usually thirty or forty days is reasonable.

◆ **Adequate reimbursement.** Most policies pay a fixed amount for each day of long-term care, and you pay the rest. Benefit rates usually run somewhere between $50 and $300 a day. Of course, the higher the daily coverage, the higher the premium.

Home care is usually covered at about 50 or 60 percent of the rate of nursing-home or assisted-living care. So a policy that pays $100 a day for nursing-home care might pay only $50 a day for home care.

To determine how much daily coverage your parent needs, calculate how much he can afford to spend on long-term care (or is willing to pay). That is, how much is left over after he has paid his regular bills (including his new insurance premiums). Now find out the average per-day cost of nursing-home care in his area. From there, it's a matter of subtraction. If nursing-home care costs $160 a day, and he has $70 a day in discretionary income, then he needs a policy that offers at least $90 a day in coverage. (Take into account that nursing-home rates will climb, while his income may not. Also, daily rates do not include some expenses, such as drugs and supplies, so the actual daily cost will be higher.)

◆ **A reasonable time line.** Very few long-term care policies offer unlimited, lifetime coverage, and those that do are extremely expensive. Most will pay a set daily amount for a set number of years—the more years, the higher the premium.

If you want to play the odds, remember the average nursing-home stay is about two-and-a-half years, but the majority are less than one year. That doesn't include time that a person might have home care before entering a nursing home, however. A four-year policy is usually ample, covering enough care without raising premiums prohibitively.

> ❝ *"My sisters think that my father should be in a nursing home because it would be cheaper, and they say he doesn't know or care where he is anymore. I think he should stay in his home with private nurses because I believe he does know the difference.*
>
> *It's true, we're spending a tremendous amount of money for his care. All of his money is disappearing. I know what they're feeling because I'd planned on having some inheritance, too. But I think we have to make his life as comfortable as possible. I don't want the inheritance if it comes at such a price."*
>
> —KATHERINE S.

Some policies offer coverage based on "benefit periods." A policy might, for example, cover a year of nursing-home care (at the chosen daily rate), and then, as long as there's a break of at least ninety days in between, it will cover another year. Other policies have lifetime limits—a given number of days or a specific dollar amount that will be covered over a person's lifetime.

Check the coverage for nursing-home, assisted-living, and home care, as some policies provide different benefits for each type of care.

◆ **Flexibility.** The market is changing. New options may be offered in the future. A good policy will have provisions to allow coverage of new types of care, or will be willing to update a policy for a nominal fee.

◆ **Inflation protection.** If someone buys $80-a-day coverage today, but doesn't need it for fifteen years, the price of nursing-home care may have gone up so much that his policy won't even cover meals. For most people, a policy should allow for at least 5 percent inflation, compounded annually.

This sort of protection is particularly important for relatively young people (in their fifties and sixties). Inflation protection that is not compounded may be fine for someone who is seventy-five or older.

◆ **Fixed premiums.** Once a policy is purchased and the terms agreed upon, a company is not permitted to raise premiums unless it does so for all its policyholders or for a certain group of policyholders. It cannot raise the premiums on an individual policy.

Be certain about this before signing, and find out about recent premium hikes. Otherwise your parent may find that just when he most needs this coverage, he can no longer afford to keep it.

◆ **Waivers.** A policy should include a waiver that frees your parent from paying premiums while he is receiving long-term care. Check for any restrictions on this, such as the number of days of care or the type of care that must be received before premiums are waived.

◆ **Coverage for dementia.** Almost all policies cover Alzheimer's and other "organic diseases of the brain" (as opposed to mental illness, alcoholism, and drug addiction, which most policies do not cover). But check to be sure.

◆ **Guarantee of renewal and protection from cancellation.** Virtually all long-term care policies are guaranteed renewable, but check because this is imperative. A company should not be allowed to cancel a policy unless the premiums are not paid or someone lied on his application.

◆ **Return clause.** You can usually return a policy within thirty days of buying it and get your money back.

◆ **Nonforfeiture protection.** This provision can add 20 to 50 percent (or even more) to the price of a policy, but it is important for buyers who are relatively young (under seventy). Nonforfeiture guarantees that the buyer will receive some value from the policy if he decides he doesn't want it anymore. The value—either some money back or partial long-term care coverage—is based on the premiums paid prior to cancellation. The longer the policy is held, the more value it accumulates.

For those who don't buy nonforfeiture protection, some companies offer "contingent nonforfeiture benefits," which is a definite plus. These kick in if premiums rise more than a certain amount. Say someone buys coverage at age sixty-five, and five years later the premiums go up 40 percent. He could opt to stick with his old premium rate and either reduce the amount that will be covered per day, or shorten the benefit period.

◆ **Marital discounts.** Some plans offer discounts of 5 to 15 percent if both halves of a couple buy policies. Other plans allow couples to "split benefits," in which case they buy two policies, but if one person dies, the other gets the total coverage remaining. In other words, if each person buys a policy covering three years of nursing-home care, and one dies without ever needing such care, the surviving spouse now has six years of coverage.

◆ **Few restrictions and exclusions.** Once you know what a policy covers, consider what it doesn't cover. Most don't cover self-inflicted injuries, alcoholism, drug addiction, or mental illness.

Some policies won't cover any illness that existed at the time the policy was purchased, or they deny coverage for a certain amount of time. In this case, the restriction should last for no more than six months.

Also, beware of restrictive clauses in a policy, like "usual and customary costs," "prevailing costs," or "appropriate costs." What does this mean? How will it limit coverage?

Most policies no longer do this, but be sure that there are no restrictions requiring hospitalization or skilled nursing care before receiving home care or some other less intensive care.

Ask how a plan deems someone eligible for benefits. Do they send someone to do an assessment, must a doctor certify that care is needed, or is there some other method?

Chapter Seventeen

LEGAL ISSUES

Wills • Power of Attorney • Advance Directives
• Trusts • Reducing Estate Taxes • Probate
• Competency and Guardianship • Legal Help

....

Y OUR PARENT HAS $5,000, OR MAYBE $5 MILLION, ALONG with a home and some personal property. Either way, legal issues arise. What if your father becomes incapacitated? Someone has to have the legal authority to pay his bills and make housing and health-care decisions for him. Your mother might want to avoid expensive probate proceedings or protect her money from estate taxes.

Whatever the specifics, your parent should do a little estate planning. If that conjures up images of *The Great Gatsby,* wide rolling lawns, pillared porches, and polo fields, don't be put off. In a legal context, an estate is simply a person's property and possessions, however grand or modest. Estate planning ensures that your parent's affairs will be taken care of, that he will be cared for properly, that his savings and other assets are protected, and, when he dies, that his "estate" is distributed according to his wishes.

Whatever else he does, or doesn't do, your parent should have an up-to-date will, power of attorney, and advance directives. These documents don't cost much (if his estate is simple, you can get them for free), and they will guard your family against costly legal proceedings and bitter arguments.

This chapter describes these essential documents along with other basic legal tools. Obviously, the information here is meant to serve only as a broad guideline; your family should work with a lawyer who is knowledgeable about the laws in your parent's state and experienced in issues concerning the elderly.

Wills

Lawyers will tell you that pretty much everyone of legal age should have a will. Of course, they have a vested interest in getting people to execute wills, but in this regard, they are absolutely right. Anyone with children or assets—a house, a savings account—should have a will.

Most lawyers will draft a simple will for a few hundred dollars. For a larger estate, or when there are more complicated issues, drafting a will could cost $2,000 or $3,000. But it's money well spent.

A properly drafted will ensures that your parent's belongings will be divided according to her wishes. It can prevent, or at least diminish, family squabbles and reduce the time and cost of probate. And in some cases it can reduce taxes.

If your parent dies without a will, the court will decide how his property is to be distributed, and appoint someone to oversee the closing of the estate—someone who may charge a fee that can be as much as 5 percent of the value of the estate. When your parent dies you will have a lot on your mind; a clearly drafted will can make this period easier for everyone.

If both your parents are alive, they should each have a will, as a joint will can complicate matters. If your parent already has a will, be sure it is up to date. A will should be reviewed every couple of years, and whenever there is a significant change in your parent's assets, his family (a death, a divorce), or his beneficiaries, or if he moves to another state.

Typically, a will explains how a person's finances, property, and other belongings are to be doled out after the person dies. Most wills include a general bequest, giving all assets to a spouse, or dividing them among the children. Some dictate that assets are to be put in a trust for children or grandchildren or some other person, either to reduce taxes or to hold money for a disabled relative or young child. A will might include specific instructions, assigning certain items to individuals (a ring, a medal, a painting), or describing burial wishes. A will also names an executor (or executrix, if it's a woman), who will pay taxes, bills, and other debts out of the estate, and be sure that money and other assets are distributed in accord with the will's instructions.

Of course, once a will is written, your parent's assets must be set up so that the instructions in his will can be

GENERIC LEGAL FORMS

Many of the forms that your parent needs—a will, power of attorney, advance directives, and even the papers to set up a trust—can be found at stationery or legal supply stores, public libraries, the county recorder's office, and on the Internet. Some computer software and Web sites have interactive programs, which allow your parent to answer questions and set parameters to create a document that meets her particular needs. But is this a safe bet?

In some cases, these forms are fine. Generic advance directives, for example, are commonly used and widely accepted. Just be sure they are specific to your parent's state and include any special instructions she might have.

A computer-generated will may be sufficient as long as your parent's estate is small and uncomplicated, and a power of attorney, as long as it's written precisely, should work (you can get forms from individual banks, etc., as well).

While generic is better than nothing, it is usually worth the money to have a lawyer draft these documents, even if your parent has a modest estate. If the language in a generic document is loose, or if a small detail, like the date, is missing or wrong, the entire form may be declared invalid. Some states will declare a will invalid if it is not precise enough. And banks and other financial institutions may not honor a generic power of attorney, especially if anything at all is amiss.

Because generic forms are not customized, they may not accomplish what your parent hopes they will. Lack of clarity can lead to family arguments and even lawsuits over their terms, language, and even the validity of the document.

carried out. A will is of little use if, say, his assets are held jointly or held in a trust, and therefore do not fall under the jurisdiction of a will.

Legally, a will affects only that part of the estate that goes through probate. Anything that is jointly owned, in a trust, or passed directly to a beneficiary (such as life insurance proceeds) does not go through probate and so is not bound by the terms of a will.

Be sure you know where your parent keeps the original copy of his will, codicils (amendments) to the will, and any letter of instruction that accompanies the will. If he doesn't already have a safe spot for it, suggest that he keep it in a lawyer's office, in a strongbox, or with a state registry service. A safe deposit box in your parent's name is not a good place to store a will because the court may seal the box at the time of death.

LETTER OF INSTRUCTION

YOUR PARENT'S WILL EXPLAINS IN broad legal terms how his estate is to be passed on, but does anyone know what is to be done with his beloved cat, Pester? Or who should get the family's photo albums? Or which of his colleagues should receive the books, files, and computer equipment from his office?

Beyond the scope of a will, there are often a number of practical matters that need attention. Get your parent to write (or dictate, if he can no longer write) a letter of instruction, which is an informal, nonbinding document that explains any personal matters not mentioned in the will. The more comprehensive it is, the better, especially if your family is prone to disagreements or your parent has failed to talk with the family about these issues in advance. A letter of instruction might include:

◆ Wishes about how personal property that is not mentioned in the will, such as furniture, diaries, jewelry, military medals, photo albums, or letters, are to be divided.

◆ Instructions on what to do with business files, equipment, and computer software, including a computer password.

◆ Funeral and burial instructions.

◆ Names and addresses of lawyers, doctors, brokers, accountants, and other advisers. The location of important financial and legal documents.

◆ An inventory and possibly an appraisal of personal belongings.

◆ Explanations or instructions regarding investments, income tax returns, outstanding debts, credit card accounts, other properties, mortgages, renters, insurance policies, and death benefits.

◆ Special instructions on how to operate or maintain a house or other property. For example, a list of regular maintenance people, such as the plumber, handyman, electrician, veterinarian, or auto mechanic.

◆ Personal wishes, such as thoughts on how beneficiaries are to use their inheritances, or how children should divide personal belongings if they can't come to an agreement.

◆ Any special messages to an individual or last comments to the family (although personal thoughts to an individual might be better conveyed in a private letter).

> " *I had my mother-in-law write down all her specific bequests on a sheet of paper and sign it, right across the whole thing, and then I tucked that in with her will. It wasn't terribly official looking, but it worked in her case. Everyone honored her wishes.*"
>
> —NELLY O.

Power of Attorney

More important than a will is a power of attorney. This doesn't give anyone the power of a lawyer. It is a simple document by which one person (the "principal") authorizes another person (the "agent" or "attorney-in-fact") to take care of business and personal affairs—to sign checks, sign contracts (to, say, admit someone to a nursing home), and buy and sell properties, for example.

> *My mother-in-law's will was so poorly written and rewritten that we couldn't make any sense out of it. We asked her lawyer about certain sentences, and even he didn't seem exactly sure what it meant. I mean, that's scary. He wrote the darn thing. I don't know how he let this happen. It seems that she wanted certain things to go to certain people, but anytime she was upset with one of us, she'd call him up and tell him to change it. In the end, there was one painting that was actually given to two of us. We don't even live in the same state. How could a lawyer let that happen? Looking back, I'm sure we should have sued him or reported him or something. It was a mess."*
>
> —Peg G.

A power of attorney won't strip your parent of her own legal powers. She can still make decisions, vote, and control her own legal and financial affairs. It simply names a deputy who can handle some or all of these matters in case your parent is unable to handle them herself, or if she simply wants someone else to take on certain tasks for her.

It is a critical document that she, you, and anyone else over the age of eighteen should have, absolutely. It is easy to do, costs virtually nothing, and will save your family from grave financial and emotional hardship. If your parent were to become ill or confused and she could not fully understand the legal ramifications of the document, then she would no longer be permitted to sign one. Without it, your family will have to petition the court to have someone named as her legal guardian, a lengthy and humiliating process that can cost thousands of dollars. So do this right away.

Your parent needs to execute a document known as a *durable* power of attorney, which will remain in effect when she needs it most—when she is incapacitated. A regular power of attorney is useful if your parent wants to give someone short-lived legal authority, such as paying her bills while she is on vacation. But if she becomes incapacitated, this power will be revoked. A durable power of attorney remains valid until she dies.

Power-of-attorney documents should be written to suit the specific needs of your parent and the laws of her state. Typically, the form includes the name of the person granting the power; the name of the person who will serve as attorney-in-fact; the name of a backup person to serve if the first person can't; a list of the duties and powers being granted; an explanation of when, for how long, and under what circumstances the power is valid; and the signatures and seals required by the state.

If your parent has assets in more than one state, she needs a durable power of attorney for each state. Your parent, the attorney-in-fact, and any backup person should all have copies of the document. The original should be filed with a county recorder's office, with your parent's attorney, or in an office file to which you both have access.

To be sure that nothing goes wrong, she should also get a power of attorney form from individual financial institutions. Banks and brokerage firms are uncomfortable about handing over money and accounts to someone not named on the account, and rightfully so. To ease any doubt, most have their own versions of these documents on hand, and they give them out for free.

DEFINING THE POWER

MAKE SURE YOUR PARENT'S WISHES are very clear on the form. Some states limit the powers of an attorney-in-fact unless specific provisions are written in, such as the authority to give money to others, to deal with the IRS, and to transfer assets into or out of a

> " *I told my mother how important it was for her to sign a durable power of attorney, and she said no. And that was it. No more discussion. She has always been controlling, but now that she is sick she is clinging more desperately to that control. She can't handle the idea that anyone else would ever manage her money or anything else in her life.*
>
> *I didn't push it. It's her choice. I was upset for a while because I think she is making a mistake, one that may mean more work for me. But I realize that there's nothing I can do about it. And honestly, I don't want her doing something that makes her uncomfortable.*"
>
> —DIANE P.

trust. Your parent has to expressly write in such powers.

Your parent can give his attorney-in-fact broad powers, including the authority to handle all financial, business, real estate, and legal matters, as well as all personal matters, such as housing decisions. Or he can turn over limited power, such as the authority only to sign checks from a single account. He can also decide when the power goes into effect (say, when he becomes incapacitated) by signing a "springing" power of attorney, which "springs" into effect at a predetermined time in the future.

In general, a straightforward, broad power of attorney is best. First of all, who's to say when your parent is incapacitated? Perhaps the document states that a particular doctor, or maybe even two doctors, have to make this declaration, but what if a doctor is out of town, or if the two doctors disagree? One might think your parent is completely incompetent, while another feels that she is still able to make certain decisions for herself. Even if they agree, a bank might question this, wanting more proof of incapacity or incompetence.

Also, if your parent turns over only limited powers to, say, one bank account, what happens if you need broader power? What if you need to deal with his taxes, or sign a contract, or gain access to another account? You'll end up in court doing just what everyone wanted to avoid.

If your parent trusts someone enough to give them this power, he should trust them to know when to

A LEGAL LEXICON

A **decedent** is a person who has died.

A **personal representative** is the general name for anyone overseeing the estate of a decedent—paying taxes and bills, and then distributing property according to the terms of the will.

An **executor** or **executrix** is a title used in many states for a personal representative who is named in a will to manage an estate.

An **administrator** or **administratrix**

is named by the court to manage the estate when no will exists, no executor is named in the will, or the executor named cannot serve.

A **fiduciary** is anyone acting on behalf of others. In the case of wills, an executor is acting as a fiduciary. In the case of trusts, the trustee who manages the trust is a fiduciary.

Probate is the court proceeding in which it is determined that a will is genuine and an executor is given

the power to handle the distribution of an estate.

A **grantor** is a person who establishes a trust.

A **beneficiary** is a person who is designated to receive funds, property, or other assets from an estate, trust, or insurance policy.

A **trustee** is a person who manages the trust for the beneficiaries.

An **attorney-in-fact** is a person who has the legal power to act on behalf of another person.

use it and how to use it. A wide berth will cover all angles and ensure that you don't have to go to court.

If your parent is uneasy about giving someone such power, he can sign a broad durable power of attorney and simply give the original to a third party, a lawyer, or other trusted professional or friend, who determines when to pass it on to the attorney-in-fact. Or he can keep it in his own files and simply alert the person named in the document that it exists, where it is, and when it should be used. Your parent must notify this person of the document's existence, however, or it will be of no use.

CHOOSING AN ATTORNEY-IN-FACT

YOUR PARENT SHOULD THINK VERY carefully about whom to designate as her attorney-in-fact because this is a powerful tool. Having access to another person's money can be tempting when one's own finances are in trouble. The person should be someone whom she trusts completely, someone with whom others in the family feel comfortable, and preferably someone who lives nearby and can meet easily with lawyers, accountants, bankers, or others. Be sure she has a second person assigned as a backup, in case the first person named is away or unavailable.

An attorney-in-fact has a legal obligation to deal with your parent's finances and affairs responsibly. If others feel this is not happening, they can go to court to have the attorney-in-fact changed.

YOU, TOO

This is a good time to get your own affairs in order. Do you have a will, a durable power of attorney, a living will, and a health-care proxy? Have you thought about ways of protecting your estate from taxes and the future costs of long-term care? Do it now. Everything here applies to you as well. See Chapter Twenty-Seven for more on planning for your own old age.

Advance Directives

A straight power of attorney covers pretty much everything, with one exception: decisions regarding health care. This is why your parent needs two other documents. Both of them are easy to get and absolutely vital.

When a person is too confused to make medical decisions or too ill to communicate his preferences, doctors usually confer directly with family members and rely on them to make decisions. Some states allow this by law; others permit it by practice. But all too often, family members disagree with each other or with the doctor, or they simply don't know what the patient would have wanted in a given situation.

These decisions become particularly onerous and vexing at the end of life.

Oh, you say, you know what your parent wants. She doesn't want to be hooked up to machines, her death dragged out. You don't need to worry about this. But are you sure? Do you know, with certainty, what your parent would want in a given situation? Do you understand the kinds of choices that arise at the end of life? Are you sure no one in the family will suddenly have doubts? And are you prepared to carry out your parent's wishes? Could you say no to a procedure that might, just possibly, keep her alive?

Most people think they are prepared, and then they are sadly, very sadly, surprised to find that they weren't. It turns out that they had no inkling of what was involved, and weren't exactly sure what their parent would have wanted.

Death pulls us up short. The medical decisions we, as loved ones, must make are agonizing. Without written documents and good long discussions, you could easily find yourself at the bedside of your parent, paralyzed by grief and stymied by ignorance. The decisions are too big, the pain too acute, the loss too large.

TAKING THE REINS—EVER SO GENTLY

If you are taking over some or all of your parent's finances, do so gently and with great respect for the power entrusted to you. Not only do you need to be responsible with his money, but you also need to be sensitive to his feelings. Personal financial control is a source of independence and pride; turning it over to someone else hurts.

Whenever you take over a new task, do so with your parent's consent or only when you determine that he is truly unable or unwilling to handle it himself. Proceed slowly, keeping him in charge to whatever extent possible. You might start by getting his Social Security, pension, and other income deposited directly into his bank account (contact the Social Security office, bank manager, or other agency representatives about this). Likewise, find out about having certain fixed bills, like mortgages, insurance premiums, and utilities, paid automatically from his account. This way, you are simply making life easier for him, freeing him from a task; you are not taking over.

Let your parent retain whatever financial powers he still can. If he can't handle the important bills, he might continue to write checks for his weekly groceries, donations, gifts, and other expenses.

As a result, most people die after a bout of intensive and extraordinary medical treatment, treatment that is agonizingly painful and that distances them from the very people they most need at their side. Death is not a peaceful passage spent at home with ample pain relief, a time of final good-byes and tender touches. It is, instead, a trauma, played out in a hospital and controlled by a vast medical and technological system.

To avoid court battles, family battles, and, most of all, a horrendous death dragged out by extensive and brutal treatments, several things need to happen. And they need to happen now, before your parent is too sick or confused to discuss her wishes.

Do the work. Be prepared.

STEP ONE: SIGN

"ADVANCE DIRECTIVES" INCLUDE A living will and a health care proxy. A living will outlines your parent's wishes regarding life-sustaining medical care. A health-care proxy, or power of attorney for health care, allows her to name someone to make treatment decisions in her stead.

These two papers protect her, to some degree, from getting unwanted treatment (or from being refused treatment that she might want). They also give your family some guidance when making health-care decisions, and they reduce the likelihood of sibling fights and court battles.

Although most people have heard of advance directives and even think that they are a good idea, only a small fraction of the population has actually executed them. People put it off or assume that advance directives are not really necessary. But these forms are not for the rare occurrence, the freak incidence. At least one study suggests that more than 70 percent of deaths in hospitals occur after a decision is made to forgo life-sustaining treatment, and in most of those cases, it is not the patient, but the family who makes the decision. In addition, family members routinely make many other treatment decisions that do not have to do with end-of-life care.

Advance directives must be signed while your parent is competent, so don't wait. Everyone over the age of eighteen should have them. They are easy to get. Easy to fill out. Easy to file. And they are free. So there are no excuses.

You can get state-specific advance directives from a lawyer, the public library, or Last Acts Partnership (800 989-9455 or www.lastactspartner ship.org). If your parent spends time in more than one state, then he needs advance directives for each state.

He should keep the originals in a safe place—an office file or strongbox, but not a safe deposit box—and inform the rest of the family of its location. Copies should be given to family members, agents, doctors, lawyers, and others involved in your parent's care. He might also put information about the documents (where they are, and the name and phone number of his health-care agent) on a card, with other vital medical information, in his wallet.

STEP TWO: TALK
....

DON'T STOP WITH A SIGNATURE. THIS is only the beginning. A living will and a power of attorney for health care should serve as a springboard for ongoing discussions about your parent's thoughts on her future medical care, so that when you have to step in, you have a good understanding of what she would want.

Simply saying that she doesn't want to be hooked up to a lot of machines is too broad a statement

---

ADVANCE DIRECTIVES

A living will states a person's wishes in the event that she is close to death and unable to make decisions about her medical care. Typically, it requests that the person be allowed to die free of pain and free of aggressive medical treatment when the end is in sight and there is no reasonable chance for recovery. Usually the terms are broad, but your parent can list specific treatments that are either wanted or not wanted in given situations. For example, a person may state that he does not want to be put on a respirator or receive artificial nutrition, but does want to receive antibiotics.

Although it is not commonly done, a living will can also be used to express a person's desire to be kept alive with aggressive medical intervention.

While a living will provides assurance that your parent's wishes will be upheld, it has limitations. For example, in some states the documents are valid only when a patient is "terminally ill," which does not include situations in which a patient is in a coma or suffering from a debilitating but not terminal illness. Furthermore, some states exclude artificial nutrition and hydration unless they are explicitly written into the document.

Be certain you know the laws in your parent's state. And urge your parent to sign a health-care proxy in addition to a living will.

A health-care proxy (or power of attorney for health care) form covers a wider range of situations than a living will, and rather than asking a person to make decisions in advance about unimaginable situations, it allows him to appoint someone he trusts to make medical decisions on his behalf. Of the two, this is the more important document to have. It should include a list of specific instructions and the powers that are granted. (Some states, for example, require that the power to stop artificial nutrition and hydration be written in separately.)

applied to a vast number of possibilities, all of which are inconceivable to a relatively healthy person. You need to know more about her views, her wishes, and her fears.

You can get into this discussion by asking your parent if she has advance directives (you should have them too, and can tell her that you have, or are drafting, your own), and then finding out who her health-care proxy is. This is the person she needs to talk with at length, but others need to know what she has said.

Here are some of the issues that should be covered, but these are just openers. Take this conversation as far as you can, and bring it up more than once, covering new turf each time. You might be surprised where it goes.

◆ Is she afraid of dying? What does she fear, dread, or worry about? (Being a burden? Being alone? Being in pain?)

◆ What can you and she do to ease those fears (learn about pain control, talk about hospice care, etc.)?

◆ What are her religious beliefs about life and death, and how does that affect her feelings about death and dying?

◆ What are her overall feelings about receiving life-sustaining medical treatment—ventilators, surgery, or even something as simple as antibiotics—when she is terminally ill or severely incapacitated? Would she want to try a treatment for a brief time to see if it got her through a crisis, or does she want to stop all efforts at prolonging life and focus instead on comfort care?

◆ What illness, disability, or treatment would be unacceptable to her?

◆ Which is more important to your parent, to be free of pain or to be mentally alert? (You may have to make decisions about the quantity of pain medication she receives.)

◆ What are your parent's feelings about receiving artificial hydration and nutrition? (See page 547.)

◆ What might she find comforting at the end of life? When she has been sick in the past, what was comforting (physical touch, music, readings from a religious text, etc.)?

◆ What are her feelings about hospice programs, which focus on keeping people comfortable instead of battling death?

◆ If you face a wrenching decision about odds and possibilities—a treatment holds a 20 percent chance of giving her another six months of life—what would she want you to consider at such a moment?

◆ If a friend or relative is hospitalized or has died recently, talk about the illness, the treatment, and the outcome. How does your parent feel about the decisions that were made? How does she think the situation should have been handled, and why?

◆ Does your parent trust her doctor's judgment about treatments? Has she expressed her philosophy and

> " *My father had a bout in the hospital last year when things didn't look good for him, and after that I got much firmer. When he got out of the hospital, I said, 'Listen, Dad, there are several things that we have to face head-on, and one of them is a living will.'*
>
> *My brother had said that we had to be delicate, but I said, 'I don't think we're going to have to be careful. I think we're going to find him ready for this.'*
>
> *And he was. Ready, and even relieved to talk about it.*"
>
> —ELEANOR R.

feelings about medical intervention and end-of-life care to her doctor? Does he (or she) understand her wishes, and is he prepared to abide by them?

STEP THREE: PREPARE

SHE'S SIGNED THE PAPERS AND you've had the talks, but are you truly ready? Do you understand what's involved? If your parent were in the emergency room struggling for air, could you refuse a respirator? When the doctor asks whether to go ahead with a blood transfusion or relatively simple surgery, even though it might only give her two more months of pain and suffering, could you say no?

Think about the reality of this. It's unimaginable, of course, especially if your parent is not facing death and has no life-threatening disease, but do what you can to prepare yourself.

If your parent has a particular illness, speak with her doctors about her prognosis, what choices are likely to arise, and how you might handle them. You might have to push the doctor to have such honest conversations, but keep at it.

Talk with your parent about the options, if possible. Then, think not only about what you won't do, but what you will do. How will you provide comfort and care at the end? How will you say good-bye?

For more on protecting your parent from a dreadful death and understanding the issues that often arise at the end of life, see Chapter Twenty-Four. It may seem morbid, and perhaps it feels a bit like you are tempting fate, but learning about death doesn't make it happen. It only relieves fears and makes it a gentler passage. Learn about it now, talk, and prepare, before a crisis strikes.

Trusts

Don't be put off by the language. A trust is merely a way of holding money, property, or other assets. Rather than having a bank account in your parent's name, for example, the account is held in the name of a trust (for example, the John Parker Trust Fund).

Trusts are not just for the rich. Yes, they are commonly used to protect large estates from taxes, but they have other important uses as well, such as:

◆ **To avoid guardianship proceedings.** A trust can be set up to give you or someone else control of your parent's assets. In this way, a trust is like a glorified power of attorney, giving someone access to property, financial accounts, and any other assets held in the trust.

A trust, in this instance, allows your parent to dictate, in advance, exactly how certain assets are to be managed, and to monitor the actions of a trustee for a while. As he loses his ability to manage these matters, the trustee steps in and gradually takes over.

In most cases, a power of attorney is fine. The advantage of a trust is that it will not be questioned, while a power of attorney might be. People generally establish a trust when an estate is large or complex, involving, perhaps, a business, several real estate holdings, numerous accounts, or a sizeable art collection. But even when a trust exists, your parent should still assign power of attorney because it is nearly impossible to put all assets into a trust, and there may be issues and decisions that are outside the terms of a trust.

◆ **To avoid probate.** Probate, the legal proceedings in which a person's will is settled, can be time-consuming and expensive. The contents of a trust, however, are not subject to the terms of a will, and therefore do not pass through probate. (They are still subject to taxes, though.)

Setting up a trust costs money, too, so this may or may not be a financial savings. (Setting up a trust may cost a few thousand dollars, while probate can cost between 2 and 7 percent of the value of the estate.) Establishing a trust to avoid probate is useful in states that have onerous probate proceedings; when something about an estate would make probate particularly complicated; or when a person has property in several states, requiring multiple probate proceedings. But, to avoid probate completely, absolutely everything must be in the trust.

◆ **To hold money until a certain time or for a specific use.** Trusts are often established to hold money until an heir reaches maturity, or to care for an heir who is disabled and needs someone else to oversee his funds. If, say, you have a brother who is mentally retarded, your parent might put money into a trust that is to be used for his care and needs. Or your parent may hold money in a trust for a grandchild, and then dictate that he can have the money when he reaches a certain age, graduates from college, or reaches some other benchmark.

◆ **To provide for a spouse or sibling.** Money can be put in a trust with explicit instructions that the interest or some portion of the principal can be used by a spouse, sibling, or other person during that person's lifetime. Then the trust dictates who the remaining money goes to once that first beneficiary dies. For example, your parent might want his wife to have access to an account, but then have the money go to his children, and not to her children from a previous marriage.

◆ **To simplify life.** When relatives will be hard to locate, a trust is easier. Before a will is read, all potential heirs must be notified, even if they are not mentioned in the will. If assets are in a trust, long-lost family members don't need to be notified.

◆ **To reduce the risk and cost of disputes.** While a trust can be fought, it's a bit more difficult than fighting a will. First of all, all potential heirs must be notified of probate proceedings for a will, and anyone can show up and dispute its terms. This battle prolongs the hearings, which are paid for out of the estate. If there is a trust, potential heirs do not need to be notified and, if someone wants to make a stink, they have to initiate court proceedings themselves.

◆ **And yes, to reduce taxes on large estates.** There are a number of ways trusts are used to shrink an estate and reduce any federal and state estate taxes. These are described later, in the section "Reducing Estate Taxes."

THREE BASIC TYPES

TRUSTS FALL INTO TWO BROAD categories: *testamentary trusts,* which are set up after a person dies, under the terms of a will; and *living trusts,* which are established while a person is still alive. Living trusts are either "revocable," which means that the person who set it up maintains control over it and can change it at any point, or "irrevocable," which means that the person has no power to revoke or alter the trust in any way. Your parent, the "grantor," appoints a "trustee" to manage the trust—often a family member or a professional. The "beneficiaries" are the folks who get money or assets from the trust.

A trustee has a legal responsibility (known as a "fiduciary duty") to manage the trust carefully and in the best interests of the beneficiaries. If the beneficiaries question the actions of the trustee, they can challenge him or her in court.

◆ **Testamentary trusts.** A testamentary trust is described in a will and created after the grantor's death. Such a trust is often set up to hold assets for a specific purpose, such as a child's education or the care of a disabled relative, or until a specific time, say, when an heir matures. They are also commonly used to reduce estates taxes.

◆ **Revocable living trusts.** A revocable living trust is set up during the grantor's lifetime and can be changed or canceled at any time by the grantor (in this case, your parent). The grantor usually acts as the primary trustee, retaining full control of the assets. A secondary or successor trustee (you, some other person, or a bank or other financial institution) steps in when the primary trustee becomes incompetent, relinquishes control for some other reason, or dies. This person now manages and distributes the assets according to the terms of the trust.

Such trusts are used to avoid guardianship proceedings, to reduce the cost and time of probate (or, when done correctly, to eliminate probate completely), to protect a person's privacy (because assets do not pass through probate), and to hold assets until heirs mature.

◆ **Irrevocable living trusts.** Setting up an irrevocable trust, which can be neither changed nor destroyed, is a serious step that requires a good deal of thought.

Irrevocable trusts are sometimes used to reduce estate taxes. As long as your parent is not a beneficiary of the trust and has no control over it, then she is no longer considered the owner of the assets, and they are not considered as part of the estate. The trust would still be subject to gift taxes and capital gains taxes, but these are generally less than estate taxes.

Irrevocable trusts are used to shelter life insurance policies so the proceeds are not included in the estate, or to keep assets that are expected to appreciate significantly out of an estate. A house can also be put into an irrevocable trust, allowing your parent to take his house out of his taxable estate. (For more information, see page 393.)

CHOOSING A TRUSTEE

A TRUSTEE, LIKE AN ATTORNEY-IN-fact, should be a family member who is respected and trusted by the beneficiaries of the trust and is at least somewhat savvy or capable financially. Or, it might be a professional trust manager or financial adviser. A relative can be appointed in conjunction with a professional, which makes a good mix—the heart and soul of a family member combined with the business instincts and neutrality of an outsider. (For an irrevocable trust to be excluded from an estate, the professional must be able to outvote a spouse.)

Reducing Estate Taxes

Your parent should consider more extensive legal wrangling to dodge hefty estate taxes if he has assets worth more than, say, $1 million, although this number is changing.

You may not think your parent's assets are anywhere near this, but if he has a house, life insurance, a retirement plan, and some savings, you might be surprised, particularly if the house is in a desirable area and his 401(k) has been quietly growing. Older people are often worth more than they realize, as they may rely exclusively on their incomes for living expenses and not be aware of what has accumulated in their bank accounts or how a piece of property has grown in value.

Why $1 million? Because that is the point at which federal estate taxes used to kick in, and it is a number that is scheduled to come back and haunt us in a few years. The federal

> " *I was the executor of my mother-in-law's estate, and it was an eye-opener, seeing how much money is paid out in taxes unless you do something to protect yourself. It's shocking. More than half of her estate went to Uncle Sam.*
>
> *Having been through all that, my husband and I have made sure that our affairs are in order. We each have a will and a durable power of attorney, and we have started to give our money to our children each year.*
>
> *We learned the hard way, and we don't want them to have to go through what we did.*"
>
> —NELLY O.

tax exemption (the amount that is not subject to taxes) is rising gradually and will hit $3.5 million in 2009. The tax is set to be repealed completely in 2010. Then, in a frightening zap of a political wand, on January 1, 2011, the tax is resurrected and the exemption slides back down to $1 million (making some wonder if there won't be a nationwide unplugging of life support on New Year's Eve).

With all this uncertainty in the air, it's best to cover all bases. The rules could change at any time, which is why people who may think they are free and clear should still do some planning. You simply never know. Furthermore, there are state estate taxes to consider, and avoid.

Here are a few of the most common ways in which people shrink their estates to minimize taxes:

◆ **Gifts.** If your parent wants to shrink a large estate, or if he is simply generous, he can give up to $11,000 per year to any number of individuals without paying gift taxes. If both your parents are alive, they can each give this gift to an individual, boosting the total gift to $22,000 per person per year, tax-free. If both parents give to children and their spouses, they are now giving away $44,000 per couple per year. It certainly starts to add up.

Your parents can make tax-free gifts in excess of $11,000 to an individual if the additional money is paid, on behalf of this other person, directly to an institution for medical care or education. That is, your parent can put $11,000 into an account for a grandchild and then send a check to a college to pay her tuition, and not owe gift taxes (or, later, inheritance taxes) on any of it.

◆ **Bypass, or credit shelter, trust.** This type of trust, also referred to as a family or AB trust, is one of the most often-used and effective ways of avoiding estate taxes. It actually doubles a family's tax exemption, potentially saving them hundreds of thousands of dollars.

Here's how it works:

Normally, when a person dies, all his assets go to his spouse, tax-free. Then, when that spouse dies, all the assets go to the children or other heirs. Anything over the amount of the current tax exemption will be heavily taxed. For the sake of illustration, let's say the tax exemption is $1 million and that anything over that amount is taxed at 45 percent. In this case, the family is exempt from taxes on $1 million, saving them $450,000.

But this family could do better, much better. In fact, they could have saved themselves twice that amount. The trick is to be sure that both parents pass on the maximum amount allowed tax-free. There are two ways to do this. One is to give the money outright to the next generation, either during one's lifetime or through the terms of a will. But this should be done only when an estate is quite large and the surviving spouse will still have plenty of money left. The other way is to put money into a bypass trust.

When the first parent dies, his will states that up to $1 million (or whatever the current tax exemption might be) is to be put into a bypass trust for his children, but that the money can be used by the surviving spouse during her lifetime. He has effectively given the money to his children (tax-free), but given his spouse access to it. Then, when the second spouse dies, the children receive the trust from the first parent, and then another $1 million tax-free (or the current exemption amount) from the second parent. By doing this, the couple has saved, in this illustration, $900,000.

As an added bonus, even if the money in the trust grows, it is still free from estate taxes (although not free from capital gains taxes).

In order to do this, wills must include provisions for the trust, and each spouse must have assets in his or her own name that can be put into a trust. Anything that is jointly owned goes automatically to the surviving spouse and cannot be put into a trust.

♦ **Irrevocable life insurance trust.** Putting a life insurance policy into a trust is one of the most painless ways of shrinking an estate. Ordinarily, the benefits of a life insurance policy are included in the taxable estate of the

A LIVING TRUST IS NOT A WILL

Some people call living trusts "substitute wills" because a trust dictates how assets will be distributed, just as a will does. However, it is virtually impossible to put all assets into a trust; some part of an estate is usually left out. Therefore, regardless of any trusts that are established, your parent should still have a will, as well.

And while a living trust mimics a power of attorney, it should not replace a power of attorney. Your parent should still sign a durable power of attorney, giving someone the authority to manage assets that are not in the trust, sign contracts, and handle other legal and personal affairs.

owner. By putting a life insurance policy into an irrevocable trust, your parent removes it from his taxable estate. This means that he can no longer borrow against it or change beneficiaries. But it saves on taxes, the proceeds can be used by the next generation to pay any estate taxes, and it provides them with quick cash, which is useful when most of the value of an estate is in real estate or a business.

(Note: Once the trust is set up, the premiums will be a gift to beneficiaries. Also, if an existing policy is transferred into a trust and your parent dies within three years, the benefit will be included in his estate.)

◆ **QPRT trust.** A Qualified Personal Residence Trust (referred to as a "Q-pert") allows a person to give his house to his children, thereby removing it from his taxable estate, but he can remain in it during his lifetime. This is particularly beneficial if the value of the house is expected to appreciate significantly. Then by all means,

get it out of the estate. But this requires some serious advance planning.

The advantage of this is that the IRS values the house at far less than its true value because your parent will continue to live in it for a certain number of years, and you and your siblings won't take possession of it right away. So a house that is worth $500,000 might be valued at, say, $300,000.

The problem is that the trust must set some time frame, say five years, at which point the house is turned over to the children. If your parent dies before the five years are up, then the trust is void and the full market value of the house at the time of death is included in the value of the estate. If, on the other hand, your parent outlives the trust period, then he must either move out of the house or pay fair market rent to his children. This is fine if you have friendly family relations. In fact, by paying rent, he further reduces his estate. However, if the kids are feeling nasty, Dad could, in theory, end up living on the streets.

◆ **Charitable remainder trust.** Of course, anyone can shrink an estate by giving money to charities, either during one's life or after death. This is particularly useful when an asset has appreciated significantly because you don't pay any tax on the gain, and you get a tax deduction on the gift. But then, of course, the money has been given away.

Another option is to put an asset into what's known as a charitable remainder trust, which removes the

HOLD BACK

Don't let your parents be overly zealous about giving money away to reduce estate taxes. They shouldn't give away so much that they jeopardize their own financial security. And they certainly shouldn't give away items that they still use and enjoy.

asset from the estate and creates a tax deduction, while also providing income for your parent during his life.

Let's say your father bought a stock ten years ago for $5,000. That stock is now worth $50,000. If he puts the stock into a charitable trust, the trust can sell the stock tax-free, and then, depending upon the terms of the trust, it would pay your parent some percent of the value of the principal (say 6 percent of $50,000, or $3,000 a year). This way, he removes the stock from his estate, doesn't pay capital gains taxes, gets a deduction for the charitable gift, gets annual income, and feels good about giving to charity. The trust can be set up to give to one charity or any number of charities. However, this is only useful if your parent wants to give money to a charity; it's not really a money-saving tool.

OWNERSHIP

OWNERSHIP SHOULD BE A SIMPLE matter; something belongs to one person or it belongs to another. But by law, an item can belong to one person, to another, or to two or more people in a variety of ways. The way in which a person owns a house, a stock, an account, or other assets affects how vulnerable the property is to creditors, how it is passed on, and, most important, how it is taxed.

◆ **Sole ownership.** Sole ownership is fairly straightforward, but even here there are gray areas. For example, if your parent puts her house into

your name, but remains in the house as a tenant, some states, along with the IRS, might still consider the house part of her estate. Likewise, if an item is in your parent's house, it is usually still considered hers. That is, in most states your parent can't write notes on the back of valuable objects ("This painting belongs to Jane," "This silver belongs to Ann") and assume that the objects are no longer part of her estate.

◆ **Joint ownership with right of survivorship.** Married couples typically own a house and other assets as joint owners with right of survivorship. The primary advantage of this type of ownership, from a legal point of view, is that the property passes directly to the other person without going through probate.

Your parent might own something jointly with someone other than a spouse. For example, he might have a joint checking account with you so that you can pay his bills for him.

The big concern of any joint ownership agreement is whether one owner trusts the other. When a bank account is owned jointly, all owners can draw on the account (even empty the account) without the approval of the others. The joint assets are also vulnerable to all owners' creditors.

◆ **Tenants in common.** As tenants in common, the parties own property jointly, but there is no right of survivorship. Each person owns a share that is passed on directly to his heirs. For example, if your father owns a business equally with two partners.

When he dies, his third would be passed on to his heirs, not to the other business owners.

If your parents' estate is worth more than the amount exempt from federal estate taxes, each should maintain assets in his or her own names so each can pass on the maximum amount tax-free. Because a house is usually the most valuable asset and cannot be split and put into each name, like a bank account or stock portfolio, your parents might want to own it as tenants in common.

Probate

Probate, the legal process of determining the validity of a will, notifying potential heirs, and authorizing an executor to manage an estate, has a nasty reputation, much of which is deserved. It often involves enormous amounts of paperwork and thousands of dollars in legal fees. The process usually lasts at least six to twelve months, but it can go even longer.

As for the cost, probate itself isn't that expensive. The court might charge a couple hundred dollars. The bills start coming in when the lawyers get involved, and lawyers are often necessary. A lawyer will fill out paperwork (which must be done precisely), notify family members, and get permission to pay bills or sell a house, for example, during this time. Appraisers and accountants might also be involved, adding their bills to the total.

The cost and time involved depends largely upon state law, but also upon the whims of the presiding judge, the complexity of the estate, the clarity of the will, the efficiency of the executor, and whether the will is contested. If property is owned in more than one state, each state will conduct its own probate proceeding, adding to the time and cost.

But probate, or estate administration, as it is sometimes called, isn't always so onerous, and sometimes it is far easier and cheaper than anyone expects. In many states, it's relatively easy and inexpensive. Small estates, or those that contain only a small amount of probate property, may qualify for a streamlined version of probate, called small estate administration or summary administration. In this case, the transfer of assets is handled through an affidavit, or court order, that takes no longer than a few months to complete.

While experienced local attorneys can usually expedite probate proceedings, it is possible, in some states and some situations, to do it yourself. A probate clerk can guide you through the process.

A Question of Competency

Your father's confusion has you wondering. Is he still able to pay his bills? Your mother's dementia has gotten so bad that she doesn't know a coffee maker from a blender. Should she be making decisions about where she lives? Your parent has to decide whether to have chemotherapy, but he just nods his head in agreement any-time the doctor makes a suggestion. Is he really making an informed decision?

These are not easy questions because there is no clear line between competence and incompetence, no simple test to determine your parent's ability to make decisions and handle her own affairs.

Competency is defined as the ability to receive and understand information, evaluate choices, make a decision that is consistent with a set of personal values and goals, and communicate that decision to others. Certainly, just because your parent makes decisions that you consider foolish—he refuses a simple medical treatment or gives his money to a questionable cause—does not mean that he is incompetent.

Competency is not an all-or-nothing matter. Your parent may be quite competent in one area and not in another. Someone who cannot handle his own financial affairs may be perfectly able to make decisions about where he wants to live, for example. Or a person may be competent at one moment, during a phase of lucidity or when strong painkillers wear off, and incompetent at another.

If you have concerns about your parent's competency and are not sure whether you should step in and act on his behalf, get his doctor or a geriatric care manager to guide you. If someone has been assigned durable power of attorney, that person can step in right

> *My mother-in-law died almost a year ago, and I am still in contact with the lawyer almost weekly. I thought her financial situation was simple, but it turns out she made a number of gifts years ago and never paid any gift taxes. And she has property in a couple of states. It's a nightmare. I think she named me as her executor so she could torture me even after she was gone."*
>
> —SUSAN V.

away. If not, you may have to go to court to have your parent declared incompetent and be named her legal guardian. People often need guardianship to gain access to an ill parent's funds so they can pay bills; to have a severely confused parent admitted to a nursing home against her will; or to handle a business or sell a house.

SECURING A COURT MANDATE

GOING TO COURT IS, OBVIOUSLY, A grave step and therefore always a last resort. If your parent is declared incompetent by the court, he will be stripped of some or all of his legal rights—the right to make decisions about his medical care or living arrangements, to handle his own finances, to write checks or buy or sell property, to vote, to marry or divorce, to drive, and to enter into contracts. It is a potentially time-consuming and expensive process that can be draining for everyone involved, especially if your parent puts up a fight. But sometimes going to court is unavoidable and truly in the best interest of your parent.

States have different rules regarding guardianship, all of them, understandably, stringent. In most cases, you must retain a lawyer who files a petition with the court. A hearing date is set, and an attorney is assigned to represent your parent, who is now referred to as "the proposed ward" (a troubling expression, but remember it's only a legal term). A judge, or in some cases a panel or jury, interviews

THE GRIEF OF GUARDIANSHIP

Your father, who represented strength and vitality, who guided you through much of your life, is now unable to make basic decisions for himself. It's painful to see a parent become powerless and vulnerable, and even more painful to have to go to court to have him declared unfit. When it's over, you may feel uncomfortable in the position of chief decision maker.

◆ Be gentle with yourself. A lot is being asked of you right now. You are doing the right thing, and yet at times it can feel very wrong. Take time off, if possible, to handle this new workload and to give yourself a chance to grieve.

◆ Move slowly, keeping your parent informed and in control, as much as possible and for as long as possible. When you make decisions, explain to him what is happening and why, even if you think he cannot understand you.

◆ Remember, this may be harder on you than on your parent. He may be relieved to let go of his duties and concerns, or he may be unaware of what is happening.

◆ If your parent has dementia and becomes angry with you for taking over, remember that his anger is, in part, due to the disease. Try not to take it personally. Remind yourself daily why you are doing this and how important it is that you take on this responsibility.

◆ During this time, everyone will have an opinion about what you are doing. The only "right" decision is the one that you believe is right. Trust your instincts.

family members, doctors, and others involved in your parent's life to determine if he is truly unfit to handle his own affairs and to what extent. In most states, your parent does not have to be present at the hearing, but if he wants to fight the judgment, he may go to court.

If the court declares your parent incompetent, someone will be named to take over all or some of his decisions, duties, and legal rights. This surrogate decision maker, also called a guardian or a conservator, is usually a family member, but it can be an outsider, a group, an agency, or an institution. (The court will go outside the family if no family member is able to assume this role or act in the best interest of "the ward.") Guardians can be granted total or limited authority. For example, you may be given the authority to handle your parent's personal affairs, while a bank trustee is assigned to oversee his finances.

In most states, a guardian must report back to the court at specific intervals or whenever a major decision is made, to show that he or she is acting responsibly.

Legal Help

Most people get referrals to lawyers from family, friends, and respected professionals, or from established organizations. You can get information and referrals from the state bar association or from the American Bar Association (312-988-5000 or www. abanet.org). You can also get information about local lawyers from the state agency that licenses them, often called the legal, or bar, examining agency. The American Bar Association has a state-by-state list of them.

The National Academy of Elder Law Attorneys (520-881-4005 or www. naela.com) gives referrals from its list of members. Elder law attorneys, as the name implies, specialize in the needs of elderly. They deal with issues such as long-term care, Medicaid planning (protecting assets prior to getting Medicaid), nursing-home rights, Medicare, and estate planning. While any lawyer can call himself an elder law attorney, a few are actually certified (very few, as such certification is relatively new). For the name of a certified attorney, visit the Web site of the National Elder Law Foundation (www.nelf.org).

Beyond word of mouth and bar association referrals, the Internet offers a number of ways to find a lawyer. So many, in fact, it's a bit intimidating. Numerous sites have online directories of lawyers. Such lists from bar associations or other respected organizations are totally legitimate, but beyond that, be wary.

Some Web sites match clients, based on their needs, with lawyers who fit the bill. The Web site might either charge a fee directly, get a fee from the lawyer, or make money by selling forms and information on the Web site.

Other Web services ask clients to explain their situation, and then lawyers bid for the job. Be extremely careful about doing this or, better yet, don't do it at all. First, posting your legal problems on the Internet raises certain confidentiality questions. Second, what sort of lawyers get business by bidding on the Web? Who are you dealing with? Is this person actually a licensed lawyer?

> *After my mother died, my father's dementia got much worse. He started doing bizarre things, and a couple of times he became violent. Eventually I had to establish a guardianship for him, and I can tell you, doing it was horrendous. My father has always been very proud and independent. He would never accept help from anyone. He fought the guardianship, and the court proceedings dragged on for almost five months. During all of that time he argued with me, screamed at me, and once he even threatened to kill me.*
>
> *All the way through it I kept telling myself, over and over: 'This is for him. This is my gift to him. I am doing this for him.' Some days I believed it, some days I didn't. Some days it felt as though I was punishing him. He certainly saw it that way. But I know now that it was the right thing to do."*
>
> —RONA S.

Is he or she licensed in your state? (Many laws vary by state.)

A few lawyers actually conduct business over the Internet. Best to avoid this. But if you go for it, use extreme caution, and consider the above questions.

The process of hiring a lawyer and questions to ask are described on page 342.

FREE AND LOW-COST LEGAL HELP

◆ Under the Older Americans Act, every area on aging must offer some sort of free legal help to people over sixty. While these services are available to all seniors, most states gear such programs to people who are living on lower incomes, giving legal advice primarily about public benefits.

◆ Legal aid societies throughout the country also offer free or low-cost help to low-income seniors. These are sometimes referred to as LSC services, because federal funds are funneled into the programs through an organization called Legal Services Corporation. But some societies are not federally funded and not associated with LSC.

These services are usually listed in the telephone book under "legal aid," or you can do a search on the Internet for "legal aid" and the name of the state. Be careful, however, that these are true legal aid societies and that services are free. LSC also has a listing of its federally funded programs on its Web site (www.lsc.gov).

◆ Many bar associations (membership groups for lawyers) offer "pro bono," or free, legal services or reduced fees for clients living on low incomes. The state bar association will know of these, or you can contact the American Bar Association (312-988-5000 or www.abanet.org).

◆ In some states, people over sixty, regardless of their finances, can call legal hotlines for legal advice. To find one, go to www.aoa.gov, click on "Elders and Families," "Elder Rights & Resources," and then "Legal Assistance." Again, be wary of hotlines that are not sponsored by the state or by a bar association, as someone may be trying to dupe you.

◆ Many unions, organizations, and employers offer low-cost or free legal services, such as the AFL-CIO, NEA, UAW, and AARP.

LEGAL HELP ON THE WEB

The Internet is loaded with all sorts of free legal advice. Be careful. Use only those sites set up by large, well-respected organizations. Some good sites were set up by SmartMoney magazine (www.smartmoney.com), and CNN and Money magazine (www.money cnn.com), although there are others.

Avoid Web sites not associated with established organizations or approach with a large dose of caution. You can get bad legal advice, or be hoodwinked.

Chapter Eighteen

HOME AWAY FROM HOME

Is It Time to Move? • Sharing Your Home with Your Parent • Senior Apartments, Group Homes, Assisted Living, and Other Options

HOME CERTAINLY IS WHERE THE HEART IS, AND IT IS generally the best place for your parent to be, but at some point it may not be feasible or desirable for your parent to stay in his own home. He might not want to care for such a large house anymore. He may be isolated and lonely living alone. His confusion or medical needs may be too extensive for independent living. His finances may necessitate a move.

Whatever the reasons, when your parent can no longer stay in his own home, it's a major turning point for everyone involved. For your parent, it may mean leaving a cherished place of his past, and losing his independence and privacy. It may also represent a final move, a last stop, which can be very sad and demoralizing.

For you, it's a time of doubt, worry, and, once again, guilt. *Is this the best place for Dad? Will he be all right? Are we doing the right thing?* You may find yourself sparring with siblings, and even with your parent if he sees you as the force behind a move he doesn't want to make. And if he's moving in with you, well then, you have a whole other set of concerns and worries.

A move might come slowly after years of caregiving, renovations, home care, deliberations, and waiting lists. Or, your parent might be lying in a hospital bed while you run frantically about trying to find a nursing home because he suddenly is unable to live on his own. However this move happens, once the dust settles, a new living arrangement can, over time, provide friendship and stimulation, as well as the care your parent needs.

Where should he live? Fortunately, your home or a nursing home are not the only alternatives. There is an expanding array of options, ranging from shared housing and assisted-living homes to full-service life-care centers. As soon as possible, talk with your parent about his needs and preferences, think about what his future might be, and learn what's out there. Planning ahead and becoming familiar with the options will help both of you navigate this difficult terrain and make the best choice.

Launching the Discussion

If you aren't facing a crisis already, don't wait until one arises to consider housing, because then you will be left with few choices and little time. As hard as it may be to discuss these issues in advance, you need to find out what your parent wants. What is most important to her—privacy, companionship, activities, a garden, proximity to family? What will her finances allow? If she were to need constant supervision or more complex medical care, where would she want to be? How important is it to her (and you) that she not move a second time?

Unfortunately, most people have more trouble talking about changing homes than about living wills, perhaps because they find it easier to imagine a time when they will be disconnected from a respirator than a time when they will be disconnected from their homes. But urge your parent to talk about this as soon as possible.

Remember, your parent's home, no matter how modest or messy, means the world to her. It is where she built her life, raised a family, and welcomed her friends. It holds her memories and her past. It is molded to fit her needs—or was before illness or disability changed them. More than perhaps anything else, her home represents her independence and her privacy. Leaving it, especially to go to a place that is earmarked for the elderly, may be devastating or unthinkable for her.

BEFORE MAKING A MOVE

Before you pack her bags, be sure that your parent can't stay in her own home, if that's what she'd like to do. Think about ways to renovate and rearrange her home to make it more accessible and to make daily life more manageable. Talk with someone from the area agency on aging (page 628) about community services and home care. And study some of the financial options that might free up some cash or reduce her costs, if finances are a deciding factor. Some communities are making great strides in allowing elderly people to stay in their homes by improving community services, helping with home renovations, and providing some financial support through Medicaid and other programs.

If your parent skirts this subject, delays a decision, and, in general, clutches defiantly at the status quo—frustrating you to no end—she may have valid reasons. What you perceive as stubbornness may be a perfectly normal desire to stay in her own home, and a deep-rooted fear of what lies ahead.

Keep in mind, you will be in her shoes before you know it. Be sympathetic to these feelings and get her to share her grief about this move and her fears about the future.

Is It Time to Move?

It may be possible to renovate your parent's house and hire home aides, but is that affordable or practical? How long will it last? Is it best for your parent or manageable for you? If there's time, your parent should weigh all the reasons for moving and for staying, visit a few residences, and then let the idea sit for a month or two before making a decision. While her personal wishes are the top priority, there are other issues to consider:

◆ **Her safety.** Your parent may need more medical care and supervision than visiting nurses and aides can reasonably provide at home. If her confusion or disability makes living at home dangerous, then staying where she is may not be an option. Your family needs to weigh the risks along with her right to decide.

◆ **Your limits.** Your ability to help your parent will play a major role in determining when it's time for him to move. You and other family members may not have the time or the stamina to tend to his needs, juggle schedules, coordinate, and oversee home-care services and fill in when workers cancel. Accept your own limits and recognize that they are important.

◆ **Costs.** Paying property taxes or a mortgage, keeping up with home maintenance, and hiring aides and nurses may all be too much for your parent's purse. If finances are the only problem, look into homeowner loans that are not paid off until a person dies, sells the house, or moves (see page 335). Ask someone at the area agency on aging about programs that help older homeowners stay in their homes, save on property taxes and utility bills, and get affordable help. Also, consider innovative options, like taking in renters or adding an apartment to your parent's house to help defray costs.

Assisted-living or nursing-home care may very well cost more than staying at home. It all depends upon your parent's needs, how much family help is available, and whether she is eligible for assistance (or might soon be eligible for Medicaid). Calculate your parent's current expenses, the costs at home (rent or mortgage, taxes, utilities, maintenance, food, home-care workers, etc.). Learn the costs of other housing (but be sure to get a complete picture; a base rate at an assisted-living residence, for example, is not all-inclusive).

◆ **Location.** If your mother lives in the boondocks and cannot drive because of poor eyesight, she might need to move closer to public transportation. If winters in Maine are too hard on your father's ailing heart, he may want to head south or find a housing situation that doesn't require scraping windshields, shoveling snow, or plodding through drifts.

◆ **Loneliness.** Loneliness is no small issue. Your parent may love his home, but it may be a little too hollow and quiet these days, especially if a spouse has recently died, or a beloved neighbor has moved, or your parent is unable to get out to see friends. Companions and community visitors may fill the void for a time, but he may yearn for more reliable and meaningful friendships. He might have someone move in with him, or he might move into an apartment building or a group living situation. Or he might simply move into town so he is closer to friends and shops. More communal living, however, will offer company and activities.

> *My mother made the decision herself, without discussing it with anyone. She moved out of New York and into an elderly housing complex near me. I was upset because, you know, this is a thing that you dread. I thought she would be miserable. But she seemed happy there, and looking back, I remembered that she had talked about going into an old-age home once with my father before he died. She said, 'Wouldn't it be nice to be in a place where they do everything for us?'*
>
> —BARBARA F.

◆ **Her future.** A diagnosis of Parkinson's, Alzheimer's, or another debilitating disease means it's time to prepare for a future when your parent may not be able to live at home. It's often better to move while she can still make her own decisions and can adjust more easily to the change. Once something like dementia is entrenched, a move can be catastrophic.

PROMISES MADE . . .

Even though you may believe that you will never put your parent in a nursing home, you simply don't know what the future holds, either for your parent or for you. Your parent may become so ill or so perilously unaware that you cannot continue to manage her care. Your own life may change in such a way that you cannot give your parent the attention that you assumed you could. Given such possibilities, don't put yourself in the position of having to break a promise; don't make it in the first place.

If your parent asks you to promise that you will never put her in a nursing home, tell her that you will do whatever you can to avoid it, and that you will never abandon her.

Should Mom Move Closer?

When your mother needs to move, you may be tempted to lure her to your own neighborhood. That way, you could spend more time with her; keep an eye on her; help her with shopping, cooking, and other chores; and arrange local services for her. She could see more of her grandchildren, and you would save a lot of time and money on travel. Certainly being near family is a top consideration.

But think about this very carefully. If your parent has been living in the same community for several decades, what will she lose by moving? Are you uprooting her from dear friends, a longtime doctor, a beloved congregation and clergy, paths she knows, and people she trusts?

Think about the pros and cons of moving her away, perhaps far away, from her home. Do you want her to move because it will truly make her life better, or because it will allow you to sleep at night? What will she do in this new place, without her old friends and familiar haunts? Once she is nearby (or living with you), will you really be able to do all that you say you will?

On the other hand, if your parent is so frail that she couldn't get to her old stomping grounds even if they were down the block, and her old friends have moved on or passed away, then moving closer to you or other relatives makes sense. And if she is going to move into an institution—a nursing home or assisted-living home—then being near those who can visit is critical.

Before suggesting this move, be sure it is really the best thing for her, because once she moves, having her return home or move somewhere else will be difficult and disruptive.

Should Dad Move In?

Now here's a biggie. When a parent can't live alone any longer, you may have an instinctive response to take him in.

It's a generous thought, certainly, but it's not always the best option, and sometimes it can be an enormous mistake. Having your parent move in with you is a serious commitment, so think it over carefully before extending the invitation. It entails a lot of work—more than most people realize—and it can be emotionally draining as well.

When in doubt, test the waters for a time. Ask your parent to live with you for a few months or even a few weeks, being clear about the trial nature of the arrangement, and see how it goes.

If you decide against family living, that's okay. A lot of people couldn't live compatibly with a parent at this time of life. Nothing is wrong with deciding against doing so. It is simply honest.

On the other hand, if you think it will work, and you've had a successful trial run, and your parent thinks it's a

> *Dad wasn't all that frail, but he was lonely. He would come up with a hundred reasons to ask one of us to come over. A lightbulb was out or a gutter was full or he couldn't get the television to work. There was always something, and I was always running over there or worrying about him and feeling bad that I wasn't with him. I turned to my sister one day and said, 'This has got to stop.'*
>
> *I have three kids at home and a job and I couldn't keep doing it. I couldn't handle the work and I couldn't handle the worry. That's when we started looking into other housing possibilities."*
>
> —Skip R.

great idea, go for it. Living together like this works for many families, and it can be a wonderful arrangement for an aging, frail parent. Just know what you are in for.

Some things to consider as you ponder the possibility of long-term togetherness:

◆ **Can you get along?** It's not worth trying this if your blood pressure rises at the mere thought of it. Think about your relationship with your parent. What was your most recent visit like? Did you enjoy a pleasant afternoon together, or did you watch the clock until you could leave? Is your parent capable of respecting your

“ *My mother moved in with us at age ninety-five. I bought a reclining chair for our guestroom and a television set and flowers, and I bought her a beautiful nightgown and robe so that she looked lovely all the time. She started to accept herself again and her spirits came back.*

It was very draining, though, because I was getting up during the night to change my mother's colostomy bag. And from the very beginning my husband and I missed our privacy.

I was glad to see Mother so happy, but I couldn't keep it up, so I brainstormed with my sisters, and we decided to split up the care. Now Mother goes to one sister's in May and June and to another sister's in July and August. The moving around is a little tough on Mother, but other than that it works pretty well.”

—MARGARET F.

privacy, your lifestyle, and your authority in your own home? Can he respect your relationship with your spouse or other mate? Can you respect his privacy, lifestyle, and decisions? While you might develop a closer relationship, it's also likely that old problems and annoyances will be more pronounced when you are under one roof.

◆ **What about the rest of the family?** How do your spouse and children (or roommates) feel about having your mother move in? Do others in the house get along with her? Call a family meeting or talk with each person individually and listen to his or her views.

◆ **Do you have the space?** This seems like an obvious question, but it's one that many people fail to consider fully. Communal living is far more successful in larger homes or those with a separate apartment or a bedroom that's set off from the rest of the house. Tight quarters will exacerbate everyday problems and strip everyone of their privacy.

If you have the space, are you willing to give it up? How will it change your life to lose a study or a guestroom, or to move two children into the same room? If you are adamant about this move, you may want to consider renovating the basement, building an attached apartment, or buying a prefab unit for the backyard.

◆ **Is your house equipped for this?** Ample space won't do any good if the extra room is upstairs and your father can't climb stairs (although you can buy conveyors to get him up and down the stairs). Take a good look at your house in light of your parent's needs and disabilities. Are the hallways, doorways, and at least one bathroom wide enough for his wheelchair? Can you make needed changes, such as installing handrails, ramps, or whatever else might be necessary?

◆ **How much care does your parent need now?** Consider his daily needs—meal preparation, transportation, help getting showered, dressed, and to the toilet. Can you meet his needs? Are there adequate community services? Can you afford home care? Will you be able to coordinate and oversee workers? Are you willing to have strangers in your house?

What about entertainment? Will he be sitting in the living room every day with nothing to do, waiting for you to play a game or chat with him?

◆ **How much care will he need in the future?** Perhaps you can give him what he needs today, but what about up the road? If he's just been diagnosed with dementia or has Parkinson's disease, what sort of care will he need in the future, and will you be able to provide that? If not, it still might make sense to have him move in with you, at least for a while. But moves are traumatic, and you don't want to have him move in with you only to have him move out six months later.

◆ **Do your lifestyles meld?** Do you sleep late, but your parent gets up with the sun? Does your teenager listen to loud music in the afternoon when your parent likes to nap? Will you have to make meat-and-potato meals even though everyone else in the family is a vegetarian? Is your parent a chain-smoker, but your spouse is sensitive to smoke? Does she have three cats and you have allergies? If your lifestyles clash, is there any way of living together in peace?

◆ **Are there friends and family nearby?** Do others live nearby who might be able to help or even take your parent in occasionally so you can have a break? Are they willing to get involved? Extra hands will certainly make living together easier.

Or will all these relatives, whom you're not all that fond of, be congregating at your house regularly?

If none of her friends or family live in your community, will your parent be dependent upon you for all her daily needs?

◆ **Can your community meet her needs?** Will your parent be moving from an urban area that has a plethora of senior services into a town that has very little to offer? Are there volunteers, companions, adult day-care services,

CLOSE, BUT NOT TOO CLOSE

If you want proximity but not total immersion, accessory apartments and ECHO housing (described on page 414) allow you and your parent each to retain your privacy and your own space, but spend time together as well. If your house can be easily renovated to add a separate apartment, such arrangements are also less expensive than most other housing options.

My father has always been a big drinker and sometimes he likes to smoke a cigar after dinner. That was fine in his own home. But Mary and I don't like it.

When we invited him to move here, I told him right away that the drinking and smoking would have to stop, or at least be cut back. I was amazed at how well he took it. I'm not sure I've ever stood up to him like that. I think it caught him off guard. But he listened and, so far, he's respected our wishes."

—BEN W.

home-care agencies, and other programs that will be of assistance?

If your parent loves gardening, moving her into a tenth-floor apartment might not be a good idea. If she loves art and music, shopping, and restaurants, she might be miserable in your country home.

◆ **What are the costs?** There are all sorts of costs to this arrangement, both fiscal and otherwise. Certainly you'll have less privacy (maybe none). You'll have less time for your spouse and children and friends. You'll have less sleep and exercise and downtime. You'll have more worry and anxiety and stress.

Financially, if you have to renovate a basement or add a wing or make a bathroom wheelchair accessible, what will that cost? If you have

to cut back on work hours, what will that do to the family budget? If you have to hire a companion or other help, who will pay for that?

Sort through some of these costs. What are you willing to give up? What can you afford to pay? What will this really cost you in the end?

If your parent is financially solvent, she should pay for her own care and any needed renovations, and contribute to general household expenses. Your siblings might also help share the cost of her care. Families make all sorts of financial arrangements to compensate the person who has taken on this task. If your parent is eligible for Medicaid, it may cover some of her expenses.

◆ **What are the advantages?** This can be a wonderful arrangement for your parent because she does not have to be alone; she does not have to maintain a property; she does not have to be in an institution; she can be with her family; and she will have supervision and care, as well as a trustworthy person overseeing any hired care.

You also stand to gain by caring for your parent during these last years of her life. While the task is exhausting and consuming, and will certainly take you away from other things (job, kids, friends, hobbies, vacations, sleep), it is a gift you will be glad you gave. Your children will also benefit from time spent with their grandparent.

There may also be tangible advantages to this arrangement. If your parent is still in relatively good health, she may be able to help around the house, do some shopping, or stay with the children when you're out.

◆ **Are siblings supportive?** This will be a whole lot easier if other family members think it's a great idea and are willing to support you in any way they can. One sibling who thinks Mom should have gone elsewhere, or is angry about this arrangement for any reason, can make life miserable. It's not a reason to forgo this plan, but certainly an issue to keep in mind. This is a big job, and it is nice to have siblings on your side, offering you support by phone, days of respite, help with daily tasks, or any other assistance.

RULES FOR
LIVING TOGETHER

WHEN A GROWN CHILD LIVES WITH an elderly parent, whether by choice or by default, there can be warmth and humor, and wonderful memories for the future. But the stage is also set for trouble. You are giving up space not just to any boarder, but to a boarder who needs your help and care and supervision on a regular basis. More problematic, this is a boarder whose opinions matter to you, who may be able to electrify you with a simple comment.

For your parent, he is not only becoming dependent, but he is becoming dependent upon his child, a person who has depended on him and looked up to him. He may feel embarrassed by this living situation and his own inabilities. He may feel that he is a burden and may connect you to his loss of independence. As a result, his gratitude may be mixed with resentment. So as you try to do things for him, he may be fighting to retain his autonomy. He may criticize you and yell at you. And if he does, you are surely going to yell back at times.

Even if you and your parent are best of friends and get along perfectly, under these circumstances that relationship will be tested.

Anticipating bad feelings and understanding the reasons for any antagonism, should ease them—a bit. Having clear house rules can help. Many families don't need them, but if you have any doubt, write down rules or at least establish some routines right away. Work out the guidelines with your parent, spouse, and children, if possible.

◆ **Remember your limits.** Your parent took care of you, so why can't you take care of her? Well, because she's not your child. Remember, you cannot ever repay what your parent has done for you. You need to accept the limits to what you can do for your parent, and make room for your own needs as well as hers.

◆ **Identify the head of the household.** Your parent used to rule the roost, but it is your turn now. If this might be a problem, make your roles clear from the start. Let your parent know that you will listen to his views, but that you and your spouse run this household and that you cast the tie-breaking vote on any disagreements.

If you have children, you may need to assert your role as the parent. Your

« I spent the better part of an afternoon trying to convince my mother that I was her daughter, not a servant, and when I went to bed that night I thought, 'We have to make another arrangement.' And that was it. I'd put up with this for too long. I'd had it.

The next morning I started making phone calls, and we found her an assisted living home within a few weeks."

—Jane D.

parent should not usurp your job or undermine your authority. You and your spouse are the ones who decide how your children will be raised, and your parent has to follow your lead.

◆ **Set down rules, assign tasks.** If you are concerned about a specific issue—noise levels, smoking, telephone bills—or worried that you will end up serving as butler, cook, and bottle-washer, make a list of rules and tasks on day one, so there are no questions or misunderstandings. Give your parent certain chores to do, even if they are menial. He might make the morning juice, set the table, or weed the garden. He'll be happier if he feels useful and knows what is expected of him, and you will feel less resentful.

◆ **Protect everyone's privacy.** Devise a way to give everyone in the household a bit of privacy. Be sure your parent has a space where he can shut the door and be alone without being disturbed. And, of course, you need a similar space. If you plan on going out for dinners or away on vacations without your parent, make that clear from the start. Clarity will not only preserve some of your privacy, it will also allow your parent to enjoy your time together without worrying that he is intruding.

◆ **Choose your battles.** When things don't work out, consider what you can live with and what is genuinely unbearable. Everyone will have to make compromises now. Decide which battles are worth fighting, and try to solve others. If your parent is on the telephone too much, get another line. If she falls asleep with the television on each night, buy yourself some earplugs or program the TV to turn off at a certain time.

◆ **Establish a forum for complaints.** Problems should be aired before frustrations reach a breaking point. Talk about this in advance. How will each of you approach conflicts and problems? Perhaps you can have a family dinner once a month in which the living situation is reviewed and disagreements are discussed.

◆ **Give it time.** The beginning may be turbulent, but in a few months you should all settle into a routine. Don't pack your parent's bags before you've allowed ample time for adjustment.

◆ **Know when to quit.** Once you've given this arrangement a reasonable chance, listen to your instincts. Any number of issues can bring family togetherness to a painful, grinding halt. There may be no single moment, no simple reason, just a realization that this living arrangement is not working. You can try to ignore it, and it may last a few more months, but eventually you will have to speak up and make a change.

If this arrangement is damaging your marriage and ruining your career, or simply making you pull your hair out, see what can be done to solve the problem. Talk with a family counselor, if necessary.

Then, when you've done what you can, act. Don't wait until you are physically sick or screaming at your parent. Start looking into alternatives. Talk with your parent about the move and begin preparing for it. The transition will be smoother for everyone if it is done before you're at your wit's end.

Housing Options

Fortunately, the range of housing options available to the elderly is growing rapidly. Traditional nursing homes now represent only one end of the spectrum, and they are a last resort. In the widening middle ground between home and nursing home are a variety of living arrangements. To find out about specific housing options in your parent's community, call the area agency on aging and the long-term care ombudsman (page 628).

ACCESSORY APARTMENTS

ALSO CALLED IN-LAW APARTMENTS, accessory dwellings, mother-daughter homes, and granny apartments, these are separate apartments within or attached to a home or over a garage. An accessory apartment usually consists of a bedroom, bathroom, sitting area or small living room, and kitchenette, often with a separate entrance. They can be created by renovating a basement or garage, or by attaching a wing to a house.

Accessory apartments often work well for parents who want to live near their children, but each party wants a little space and privacy. They also can be used for people who are not related. Your parent could move into an accessory apartment attached to someone else's house, allowing her to stay in her community in a smaller and less expensive dwelling, where she has a close "neighbor" who might provide a little oversight and help.

Or, if your parent wants to stay in her own home, but it's too big for her, or the expenses are too high, she might create an accessory apartment, live in either the apartment or the house, and rent the other section to a tenant.

Some owners make special arrangements, such as keeping the rent low in exchange for help with chores or other assistance. (Be sure your parent understands that taking in renters requires some work on her part and that there can be problems if, say, a renter fails to pay the rent.)

Before building an accessory apartment, you may need to:

◆ Call the local zoning board or building department. Accessory apartments are not allowed in some communities zoned for single-family residences, and if they are permitted, certain restrictions and regulations may apply. If you are told that accessory apartments are not allowed, ask about getting a variance or a special-use permit.

◆ Call the local housing authority and area agency on aging. Some communities offer low-interest construction loans, tax deductions, and other financial assistance to help people build accessory apartments for the elderly.

◆ Consider the finances. Get an estimate on what it will cost to create a separate apartment. Adding a few small kitchen appliances to an existing studio or guest suite might not be all that expensive, but building a bathroom, kitchenette, and separate entrance onto a second floor might be prohibitive. Also, property taxes might be higher because of the addition. If your parent takes in renters, the rent will change his income level, which may affect his eligibility for Medicaid or Supplementary Security Income.

◆ Talk with a real estate agent if you need someone to find renters and draw up lease agreements. (You can find generic lease agreements in most stationery stores.)

> *Twenty years ago my husband was transferred. My mother was all alone, so we told her to sell her house and come live with us.*
>
> *She is pretty easy to live with, except that she complains a lot. As the kids got older, the complaining got worse. It caused a lot of conflict. 'You should do this with the kids. You shouldn't do that.' You know, that sort of thing. I said, 'I'm the mother here. You're not their mother.' But it didn't work. So we sold our house and bought one with an in-law apartment. I see her in the afternoon, drop off her meals, and drive her around, but we also have our own, separate lives. It's much better this way."*
>
> —LUCILLE L.

ECHO HOUSING

ELDER COTTAGE HOUSING OPPORTUNITY (ECHO) homes are modular homes that are temporarily placed on the property of a single-family house, usually in the backyard. They are about the size of a large garage, and include a bedroom, bathroom, living area, kitchen, and eating area. They are designed specifically for older people and so are single level, wheelchair accessible, energy efficient, and well lighted.

An ECHO home does not have to look like Mom drove up in a mobile home, although some do. Most can be designed to match an existing house, with the same windows, siding, roofing, and roof pitch, or they can be adapted to look like a guest house on the property.

The area agency on aging or housing department should be able to give you information about local manufacturers of ECHO homes. A typical ECHO home is about 500 square feet and costs about $25,000. Most can be removed when they are no longer needed.

Check with the local zoning board to see if ECHO homes are allowed in the neighborhood. And find out whether local regulations require a minimum of yard space; what the requirements for access and parking are; whether utility hookups are possible; and how such a structure will affect the property taxes.

SHARED HOUSING

SHARED HOUSING HAS BECOME POPular among the elderly in recent years, and understandably so. It saves money, provides companionship, and allows residents to keep their autonomy, a precious asset. These arrangements may also include meals, housekeeping, and other services.

By definition, shared housing is a situation in which two or more unrelated people live together as a family. The specific arrangements, however, vary from house to house and apartment to apartment. Your parent can move into someone else's house and pay rent and/or a share of the household expenses. Or he might find a per-

---

WANTED: HOUSEMATES

Some communities have services that link people with potential roommates or find group housing for them. Most provide this service free, although some charge a fee. To find out if such a program exists in your parent's community, and to get more information about shared housing (including a list of interview questions for prospective roommates and a model lease agreement), contact the National Shared Housing Resource Center (www.nationalsharedhousing.org).

---

son to move in with him who will do chores in lieu of rent. Sometimes friends get together, find a house, and share tasks and expenses. Several friends living together can, for example, hire a full-time housekeeper or aide and get the care they need without paying an arm and a leg for it.

Group homes are sometimes set up by an outside person or agency for people who can live independently but need some help with activities of daily living. These are also called "board and care homes."

Your parent needs to think about whether this is a plan that will work for her. Is she good at sharing and getting along with others? If she is sharing a

HOUSING OPTIONS AT A GLANCE

Type	Description	Costs
Accessory Apartments	An apartment within or attached to a house, or an outbuilding on the property of a single-family house.	Renovations for an accessory apartment vary, as will any rent, if applicable.
ECHO Housing	Modular homes placed temporarily on the property of a family home.	$25,000 and up for about 500-square-foot building.
Shared and Congregate Housing	Anything from a roommate situation between friends to group housing arranged by an outside agency.	Varies widely, depending upon housing costs in the area. Anywhere from $200 to $1,000 a month.
Senior Apartments	Apartments for independent, elderly residents. Often set up by charitable organizations with government monies for people with low incomes.	Subsidized apartments accept only low-income residents. Others range anywhere from $300 to $1,500 a month.
Assisted Living	Facilities that provide a range of services for elderly people who need some supervision and help getting through the day. A good midway point between home and nursing home.	Anywhere from $600 to $4,000 a month. Costs may be higher, depending upon the area and services needed.
Foster Homes	A family takes in an elderly person and provides meals, housekeeping, laundry, and some other services.	Varies widely, depending upon the area—from $300 to $3,000 a month.(SSI will cover some of the cost.)
Continuing Care Retirement Communities	Large complexes that offer the full spectrum of care, from apartments to assisted-living units to nursing-home care.	Usually, one hefty entrance fee, plus monthly rents of $1,500 and up.

Advantages	Disadvantages
Offers proximity while preserving privacy, if your parent moves in with you. Or your parent can take in renters who pay rent or help out.	These are not allowed in some towns. They can be expensive to build.
Independence and proximity to family, without full immersion.	Not allowed in some neighborhoods.
Companionship, shared expenses, and, in some cases, services such as meals, transportation, and housekeeping.	Less privacy than independent living Older people who have lived alone for years may have no interest in group living.
Privacy and independence, without home maintenance. Most offer meals, housekeeping, laundry, and transportation, as well as recreational and social activities.	Typically there are long waiting lists for subsidized apartments, and they are sometimes poorly maintained.
Help and support—meals, housekeeping, supervision, activities, and custodial care—while maintaining independence and privacy.	May not be appropriate for someone who needs, or will soon need, extensive care.
With the right family, loving care, emotional, and physical support.	With the wrong family, a disaster.
Peace of mind that all future care is covered and no more moves are necessary. Activities, independence, and a mix of residents.	The high cost makes this an option only for middle- and upper-income people. Residents usually must sign up while they are still relatively healthy, so it requires advance planning.

house with a friend, is this someone with whom she has spent a lot of time, and is she sure that they can get along?

If she is finding a roommate through the want ads or a roommate-matching program, she needs to decide what she wants in a housemate. When your parent (or you) interviews potential roommates, ask about pets, smoking, noise levels, visitors, laundry, sleep habits, and arrangements for shared meals and chores, as well as checking personal and financial references.

Once a match is made, prepare a detailed list of the house rules and each person's responsibilities. If a roommate has agreed to help around the house instead of paying rent, be specific about the chores and how often they need to be done. Be clear about how rent, utilities, groceries, repairs, and other bills will be paid—how the costs will be split and when payments are due. Housemates should also agree in advance how bills and responsibilities will be handled if one person becomes ill.

Be aware that two or three people sharing a house usually goes unnoticed, but once four or more unrelated people share the same residence, local zoning officials may be alerted. Depending on local ordinances, the situation may be considered "group or multifamily housing," which may be prohibited. So check the local zoning codes.

CONGREGATE HOUSING

ALTHOUGH IN SOME AREAS THE TERMS *congregate* and *shared* housing are used interchangeably, congregate housing is typically a more formal arrangement, includes more people, and offers services such as meals, housekeeping, recreation, and transportation. Residents may have bedrooms within a large house or a multifamily home, or they may have separate apartments within a building, often supervised by a house manager. All or most meals are shared in a central dining room, and residents sometimes share a living area.

Congregate housing can be better than a less formal arrangement for people who need more care and services. But it can also cost considerably more.

Many communities are leery of congregate housing because of the challenges it has posed to local zoning ordinances, but resistance is fading, some. Government, nonprofit, for-profit, religious, and community groups have all gotten into the act, building, organizing and sponsoring such homes. The local housing department, senior center, or area agency on aging should be able to give you information about any congregate housing opportunities in your parent's neighborhood.

SENIOR APARTMENTS

SOME APARTMENT BUILDINGS specialize in the needs of the elderly. Not only are all of the tenants older, but the buildings are also constructed for seniors—no stairs, ample pathways for wheelchairs, sturdy and stable furniture, good lighting, tight security. From small buildings with a few units to massive high-rises, these apartments are usually situated near shops or public transportation, and they often provide meals, activities, and other services.

Many senior apartments are government subsidized, through the U.S. Department of Housing and Urban Development's Section 202 program. However, these often have waiting lists of up to four years, and they are available only to people with low incomes.

If your parent is frail and contemplating a move into a senior apartment, find out exactly what services are provided, including whether there are emergency provisions—an emergency call button in the bedroom and round-the-clock staff who can respond to emergencies. Also, find out in advance if your parent would have to move should he become ill or immobile. Some senior apartments evict residents who become infirm, even if they can afford to hire personal health aides or companions.

FOSTER HOMES

SOME FAMILIES WILL TAKE IN AN older person for a fee (anywhere from $500 to $3,000 a month). Most elderly people who live in foster homes have some physical and/or mental limitations and need help with daily tasks. The foster family cooks meals, does laundry, provides transportation, and generally helps the person through the day.

Foster care can be great if the foster family embraces and nurtures your parent. You may feel considerable

COMMUNAL? SCHAMMUNAL!

Group living arrangements like home-sharing and congregate housing are not for everyone. They are economical and provide companionship, stimulation, and sometimes other support. However, if your father has been a loner all his life, he's not likely to adapt well to communal living.

Is your parent ready to share a living space, or does he need a good deal of privacy? Can he get along with others and enjoy their company, or does he find most people to be a nuisance? Can he compromise, adjust his schedule and habits, and be sensitive to other people's needs? If he doubts his capacity to be flexible in these areas, he may want to have a trial run before signing any long-term lease agreements.

relief, and you may even develop your own close relationship with the foster family.

However, foster care can also elicit unexpected reactions. You may worry about whether a foster family is treating your parent well, whether they are neglecting or even abusing him (so far, few such problems have been

> *One day when she called and sounded particularly low I said, 'Oh Mum, I think I really missed the boat. I should have helped get you into a retirement home where you could have been with other people, because you love people so much.'*
>
> *I made it sound like a compliment. And I left it so that if she was interested, she could bring the subject up later, as though it were her own idea, not something that I was pushing on her. It takes some time for this sort of thing to settle in her mind. She needs to mull it over, without any pressure from me. If I had suggested straight out that she move, she would have gotten all indignant and resistant."*
>
> —KATHY L.

reported). You may also be visited in the late hours of the night by your old companion, Guilt, who tells you that strangers are doing what you should be doing. Or you may grow jealous of the relationship that is developing between your parent and his foster family. *Mom wants to spend the holidays with them instead of us. I can't believe it.*

In the clear light of morning, the fact that your parent has found a good home should outweigh such anxieties and concerns. Your best assurance is to visit frequently and establish a rapport with the foster family, letting them know how much you value and respect your parent, and how much you appreciate all that they are doing.

States have their own rules on foster care, specifying how many adults can live in one foster home, regulating costs, and defining eligibility requirements to become a foster family. The area agency on aging should know about any adult foster-care programs in your parent's state. Usually the older person or his family shoulders the cost, although some states are now allowing partial Medicaid and SSI coverage for foster care.

ASSISTED LIVING

THESE RESIDENCES ARE CALLED BY dozens of names, including personal-care homes, sheltered care, adult homes, and residential care. Whatever they are called, they are ideal for people who need a little help getting through the day but don't require the intensive supervision and medical services of a nursing home. Residents may need help with bathing, dressing, eating, and other personal tasks. Many use walkers or wheelchairs. About a third, overall, are incontinent.

Because residents generally have quite a bit of privacy, are (ideally) encouraged to do as much as possible on their own, and are surrounded by others who are still fairly independent, they tend to remain healthier and more active than people who enter nursing homes prematurely.

Furthermore, assisted living is, on average, about two-thirds the cost of nursing-home care.

Assisted-living facilities range from large houses with a few rooms to tall buildings with more than 200 units. Most range from 25 to 125 units. Smaller facilities, often called "board and care homes," usually offer fewer services and less medical care, and are only loosely monitored, if at all.

In some residences, people share bedrooms; in others, they have private apartments. Whatever the size and style, most offer round-the-clock, on-call help, two or three meals a day, transportation, recreation, and exercise programs, housekeeping and laundry services, social services, and help with bathing, dressing, toileting, and other personal tasks.

The Search

Find a home that is near family and friends who can visit. Ideally, it should be near shops or offer transportation services, and have gardens and other outdoor areas where residents can stroll.

The services offered can vary enormously, so find out exactly what is provided. Get a detailed list. All meals or just some? Full laundry services or only sheets and towels? Housekeeping in your parent's room or only in the common areas? Is there custodial care (bathing, dressing, grooming, toileting) available around the clock or just during certain hours? Is there any nursing care at all?

The more services that are offered, the more expensive this will be. But

A QUALITY CHECK

When you research housing options, ask the local area agency on aging or the long-term care ombudsman about licensing or any "quality assurance" program within the state. Also, check with the Department of Consumer Affairs or the Better Business Bureau to see if any complaints have been filed against a particular residence. Most important, talk with people who reside in the facilities you are considering. Ask what they like and don't like about it.

some services, particularly custodial and nursing care, also mean that as your parent grows more frail, she can get what she needs and may not have to move to another facility to receive a higher level of care.

Find a residence that fosters independence, offers plenty of stimulating activities, gets residents outdoors and doing things, encourages people to remain independent, and provides some privacy.

Visit a facility both on a formal tour and then again during off-hours, such as in the evening or on a weekend, when staffing levels may be lower. Go during a meal and see how the food is. Talk to residents, talk to staff, watch how they interact, and get a feel for the place.

Does the residence seem clean, well-kept, and secure? Are some residents at a comparable level of functioning as your parent? Are they active and interesting? Do they like to do some of the things that your parent likes to do? Are they encouraged to care for themselves and remain as independent as possible? Do they get along well with the staff?

If people share rooms, how are roommates matched? What happens if your parent does not get along with her roommate?

Find out the staff-to-patient ratio and whether there is a high rate of staff turnover (which suggests something is wrong).

Be sure a facility can meet the particular needs of your parent. Many assisted-living residences accept people with dementia, incontinence, or other problems that require a good deal of attention. What sort of training does the staff have to deal with dementia? What sorts of provisions does the residence make for people with dementia (are they separated from other residents? How is the space physically arranged?) How does the staff handle wandering, repetition, agitation, abusive behavior, odd eating hours and habits?

For a list of other issues to consider, see Appendix F, page 646.

The Cost

Assisted living can cost anywhere from $1,500 to $5,000 a month, with the national average falling somewhere around $2,500 ($30,000 a year). But

HOW LONG WILL THIS LAST?

Find out what happens as your parent needs more care. If she needs help now getting meals, vacuuming, and doing her laundry, what happens when she needs help with toileting and dressing? Will a home health aide help her? How long can she stay in this facility? Who decides when she must leave, and how do they decide that? How much warning will you receive? Do they help in finding a nursing home or other living situation for her? What happens if she is hospitalized and then in rehab for a period of time? Does she lose her space at the facility?

this is a base price and does not include various services. Be sure you know exactly what is included in the price and what is extra. You don't want to have your mother move in, only to find out that telephone, television, linen service, and meals are all extras. Sometimes help with particular tasks, say bathing or dressing, is charged hourly ($20 to $25 per hour). Also, find out how much the rates might increase each year. Is there some cap on rate increases?

Medicare and most private insurance do not cover the costs; however, if your parent has long-term care insurance, it should pay for room and board and perhaps a little more.

Some states have arrangements to provide some coverage under Medicaid, and some residences offer financial assistance.

For more information and a list of assisted-living residences where your parent lives, contact the long-term care ombudsman in your parent's area (see page 628), the Assisted Living Federation of America (703-691-8100 or www.alfa.org) and/or the National Center for Assisted Living (202-842-4444 or www.ncal.org).

CONTINUING CARE RETIREMENT COMMUNITIES

Continuing care retirement communities (CCRCs), also known as life-care centers, are the *prix fixe* meal on the menu of housing options. They offer it all—from independent living to nursing-home care—usually for one fairly hefty fixed price.

Most such communities accept only people who can get around and live independently. Once a resident has been admitted, however, he receives whatever care is necessary for the duration of his life.

The centers usually include apartments for those who are living independently and offer a variety of activities, such as golf, swimming, tennis, a gym, lectures, movies, and trips. They also have an assisted-living complex, which provides care and services for people who need help with daily tasks like bathing, dressing, and eating. Then there is a nursing-home wing or unit for residents who are very frail or ill. Consequently, there is a mix of residents, many of them healthy and active, so the atmosphere is often less dreary than in a nursing home.

While they are expensive, these communities can offer companionship, care, and enormous peace of mind. Your parent doesn't have to worry about if or when he will need nursing-home care, where he will go, and how he will pay for it. Everything he will ever need is paid for (depending upon the type of contract signed), and he will never need to move again (except within the facility).

Entrance fees vary greatly, ranging anywhere from $20,000 to more

> "About three years ago, my parents moved into a life-care center in the neighboring town. My sisters and I were shocked. They were healthy and active. It seemed as if they were giving up.
>
> Now I am grateful. They love being there. They don't have the responsibility of caring for a house, and they do what they want to do. It's not gloomy or depressing. In fact, it's nice—much more like a country club than an old folks' home. Best of all, we don't worry about the future. It's all taken care of. It's really a blessing."
>
> —Elizabeth J.

CONTINUING CARE INFORMATION

The Continuing Care Accreditation Commission (202-783-7286 or www.ccaconline.org) inspects and accredits these communities. The Commission can send your parent a list of accredited CCRCs in her area that meet certain criteria with regard to finances, medical care, resident life, and management. There is also a list on its Web site. Keep in mind that accreditation is a helpful, but far from perfect, yardstick. Application is voluntary, and the CCRCs pay a fee to be evaluated. Those that are not accredited may still have high standards.

The American Association of Homes and Services for the Aging (202-783-2242 or www.aahsa.org/public/ccrc.htm) has quite a bit of information on CCRCs and how to look for one. It also puts out a Consumers' Directory of Continuing Care Retirement Communities, which contains information about hundreds of these communities. The most recent directory can be found in some public libraries.

than $400,000. Sometimes the entrance fee is actually the cost of a house or apartment. In some cases, part or all of the entrance fee (or cost of the residence) is returned to the resident's estate when the resident either dies or moves. There are also monthly fees, ranging from $500 to more than $4,000.

CCRCs offer various and usually pretty complicated financial contracts, making it difficult to compare apples with apples. Generally, residents are asked to choose from among three types of arrangements:

◆ Extended, or all-inclusive, contracts cover everything. The entry fee and monthly fees cover all health care that is needed, including unlimited nursing care, without an increase in those fees while the person is receiving that care. This usually involves higher monthly fees, but everything is paid for.

◆ Modified contracts cover only a limited number of days of nursing care each year. After that, the resident pays a fee that is usually about 80 percent of the full rate.

◆ Fee-for-service contracts provide residents with independent-living and assisted-living services, but require that they pay the full cost of any nursing care needed. In this case, monthly fees are lower.

Because this is a long-term commitment and an enormous financial investment, your parent should do a lot of research and have a lawyer experienced in such matters examine the contract. He (or you) should check the financial stability of the residence, the refund policy, Medicare and Medicaid certification, any costs not included in the monthly fees, health insurance requirements, possible increases in fees, and the availability of nursing-home beds. Also, find out how decisions are made to move residents from one level of care to the next.

Keep in mind that if your parent is moving into a life-care center, long-term care insurance may be redundant.

Tour a CCRC as you would any other facility. Go on an official tour and then return unannounced. Have a meal, talk to residents and staff, watch people interact, visit an activity, see if anyone is using the weight room or pool and what kind of supervision they have, ask about staff to patient ratio in the nursing home, etc. See Appendix F, page 646, for a list of questions to ask when choosing any long-term care facility.

A Good Nursing Home

The Decision • Who Pays? • The Search
• What to Look for in a Nursing Home
• Getting In

Y OU HOPED IT WOULD NEVER HAPPEN. MAYBE YOU EVEN promised yourself or your parent it would never happen. But at some point—often after great effort to avoid it and agonizing days of sadness and guilt—it becomes clear that the time has come. You need to move your parent into a nursing home.

It is a devastating decision to make. But if your parent has an illness or ailment that demands an enormous amount of care and attention, and staying in her home simply isn't an option any longer, a nursing home can provide a level of medical care, supervision, companionship, and activity that she cannot possibly receive at home. About 40 percent of people over the age of sixty-five will spend at least some time in a nursing home during their lives. And while there are plenty of horror stories, many of them get very good care.

While a move to a nursing home should relieve some of the daily demands and pressures on you, your job is far from over. Your involvement, and the involvement of other family members and friends, is vital to the success of this move. Your parent needs someone to monitor her care and to act on her behalf. She needs someone who will talk with staff members regularly, and speak up when things aren't right. And, of course, she needs your support, your love, and your warm touch, now more than ever.

Sorrow may be unavoidable, but try to shake off any guilt you may be feeling. You are doing your best, you will continue to do your best, and that's all that you can do.

Learn about local nursing homes early. Don't wait until there's a crisis. Even if you think that you would never let your parent move into a nursing home, know the options, just in case.

The Decision

The mere thought of a nursing home may conjure up images of muttering old people warehoused in stench and isolation, of abusive orderlies, indifferent nurses, and helpless patients strapped to chairs.

It happens, absolutely, but it happens less than it used to. Public lobbying, consumer advocacy, litigation, and federal reforms have all forced nursing homes to rethink their mission and responsibilities. As a result, many have hired more staff, improved staff training, cut back on the use of physical restraints and sedative medications, eased rigid schedules, renovated rooms, and developed a range of activities to keep residents engaged and stimulated.

Inspections routinely discover negligent and even abusive situations, but there are more and more examples of success—nursing homes where residents make friends, become involved, and receive good medical and personal care. If you do some legwork and get your parent into the best nursing home you can find, then visit her regularly and advocate on her behalf, her move to a nursing home may very well be a good one.

Nursing homes are invaluable if your parent needs more medical care or supervision than is practical or possible at home; when family members cannot handle the physical and emotional demands of caring for an acutely infirm person at home; and when living in any other type of residence is not an option because of the severity of your parent's disabilities or behaviors.

Despite the problems inherent in nursing homes, care at home is not always better. Sometimes the caregiver cannot possibly provide the level of care that is needed. Sometimes even family members can be neglectful or abusive. And sometimes the care required is so intensive that the caregiver actually ends up sick and needing care.

Most nursing homes offer basic medical care and round-the-clock nursing supervision in addition to meals, laundry services, personal care, counseling, recreation, social services, rehabilitative programs, and pharmacy and laboratory services. Some also offer "subacute medical care"—special wings or floors that provide hospital-level care.

While they are typically needed for long-term care, nursing homes are also used for brief periods—a few days, a couple of weeks—while a person recuperates from an injury or illness, or to give a family a break from the rigors of home care. Homes are usually privately owned, publicly supported, or run by a nonprofit religious or civic group.

Who Pays?

What shocks most families is not just the exorbitant cost of nursing home care, but the fact that Medicare and private insurance pays for almost none of it.

The average cost of nursing home care nationally is more than $60,000 a year, but that does not include therapy, rehabilitation, medications, doctor's fees, and other services, all of which bring the price tag significantly higher.

And that's only an average. In many parts of the country, the rates are far higher. For example, in Alaska the average cost of nursing home care is around $170,000 a year.

The bottom line: Your parent's stay at a nursing home can easily surpass $100,000 a year.

Private long-term care insurance will pick up some of the tab, but most people don't have such insurance. As a result, the vast majority of people pay out-of-pocket until their pockets are empty, at which point they apply for Medicaid.

All of this comes as a great surprise to people who thought that they had a sufficient nest egg and then suddenly find that it is completely gone. Even a fairly hefty savings can be depleted quickly.

Before your parent drains her savings account and sells her house to pay for nursing-home care, learn about Medicaid eligibility in her state and ways that your family might protect at least some assets. Also, if there is any chance that your parent will go on Medicaid, be sure a nursing home can guarantee her a bed once she switches payment sources.

Medicare

Medicare does not pay for what's known as "custodial" care, which is help with the tasks of daily life—bathing, dressing, eating, toileting, etc. And this is just the sort of care most frail, elderly people who are entering a nursing home need. It pays only for nursing care that is "medically necessary," and even that care is covered for only a few months, only partially, and only in very specific situations. (See page 347 for more on Medicare.) Here it is, in a nutshell:

Medicare will pay for "skilled" nursing care in a Medicare-certified nursing home (meaning that it meets certain federal standards). "Skilled" care, by definition, is authorized by a

FOR MORE HELP

For information about paying for long-term care, contact Medicare (800-MEDICARE or www.medicare.gov). The State Health Insurance Counseling and Assistance Program (page 635) and the long-term care ombudsman can also answer questions and guide you (page 628). The state medical assistance office (page 639) can tell you about Medicaid rules in your parent's state.

If your parent is a military veteran, call the local veterans' affairs office to find out if he is eligible for free or low-cost nursing-home care. (Medicare, Medicaid, and long-term care insurance are all discussed further in Chapter Sixteen.)

> *I know my limitations as a person. I knew what I could do for her and what I couldn't. My mother lived with us for almost five years, and at the beginning we were able to manage. But she became too sick, too demanding. Moving her into a nursing home was the only choice. It was time. I don't have any guilt about it."*
>
> —NANCY S.

doctor and requires the oversight of nurses and/or rehabilitation therapists. That is, it is medical care—changing bandages, giving intravenous medications, providing physical therapy, etc. Furthermore, this "skilled" care must be necessary within thirty days of a hospital stay that lasts at least three full days, and it must be directly related to that hospitalization.

If your parent meets all of these requirements, Medicare will pay for twenty days in the nursing home, and then pay only a portion of the tab for the next eighty days. After that, you're on your own. Many supplemental insurance policies will cover the extra cost between days twenty-one and one hundred, but that's it.

Medicaid

Medicaid, health insurance for low income people, is run by both the federal and state governments, which means that the rules vary from state to state. However, it does cover most nursing home bills. In fact, Medicaid covers nearly half of all nursing home care in this country, so most nursing homes accept Medicaid patients. However, they favor self-paying and Medicare patients, and many limit the number of Medicaid patients they will take. For example, a nursing home with 200 beds might have only 20 beds earmarked for Medicaid patients.

If there is any chance your parent will end up on Medicaid, be sure that any facility you consider accepts Medicaid, and can guarantee that your parent will be able to stay at the residence if she switches from Medicare or private pay to Medicaid.

Things get a little tricky here. If a nursing home is fully certified to take Medicare and Medicaid, it cannot legally discharge your parent for switching to Medicaid, even if no Medicaid beds are available. But many nursing homes have just one wing or unit that is certified. In this case, a home can evict a patient who is newly on Medicaid on the grounds that no Medicaid beds are available. However—and nothing is simple on the nursing home front (only nuclear power plants have more regulations)—states have their own rules regarding Medicaid, and some states require that nursing homes guarantee a bed if a resident goes on Medicaid. Some nursing homes have their own similar policies internally. The bottom line: Know the policies and get something in writing before your parent enters any nursing home.

As for what sort of care your parent will receive, it is a myth that anyone on Medicaid will end up in a dreadful nursing home. It's true that in most areas the plushest nursing homes do not accept people on Medicaid. And it's also true that some homes have units designated for Medicaid patients that are not as nice or as well staffed as the rest of the residence. Nevertheless, there are some very good, attractive, and well-managed nursing homes that accept Medicaid patients.

Remember, an expensive nursing home is not a guarantee that your parent will get loving, devoted care, just as a run-down exterior doesn't always mean shabby care. Appearance is an important clue to what kind of service is provided, but the quality of care comes from the people who work in the facility. The philosophy of the administrators and the devotion of the staff is what matters most.

To get your parent into one of the better nursing homes, get his name on waiting lists early. Sometimes it helps if he sets aside enough money so that he can apply as a self-paying resident. If your parent can cover even six months of nursing-home care, he may have a better chance of being accepted by the home of his choice.

> " *I refused to put my mother in a nursing home. I wouldn't have it. My sister and brothers kept telling me that we had to do it, that she was too difficult to manage, but I wouldn't listen. I cut back my hours at work and used up pretty much all of her savings to pay for aides and nurses at home. I stuck to my resolve.*
>
> *Then a friend of mine told me that I had created a home for my mother that was worse than any nursing home. And she was right. My mother didn't do anything or see anyone. She never got out or had any stimulation. And, in the meantime, I was ruining my own life.*
>
> *I finally gave in, but I was mortified any time I had to tell people where she lived. The staff at the nursing home was reassuring and I gradually felt better, but it took time. I regret being so stubborn, but I was only doing what I thought she would want.*"
>
> —ALEX B.

Checking the Cost

When comparing nursing-home prices, use caution. Any daily or monthly price quoted is apt to be only a base rate. Find out exactly what is covered in that rate, and what is not. Every extra service will be added on to the base price. Often, medications, doctor visits, wheelchairs, walkers, and other such services are extra. In some homes, doing laundry, monitoring catheters, and preventing bedsores are considered extras. A survey by *Consumer Reports* found that nursing homes sometimes charge up to $1,000 a month for such extras.

Also, know that one home's "enriched care" may not be the same as another home's "enhanced care." (The Health Care Financing Administration

KEEP YOUR PARENT AT THE HELM (EVEN IF YOU'RE CHARTING THE COURSE)

No matter what your parent's physical and mental limitations—even if she isn't fully aware of what is happening around her—try to keep her involved in all stages of this decision, talking about the options, touring homes if she can, choosing one, and signing up. Keeping her involved and informed should make the transition easier.

If your parent can't tour nursing homes, collect brochures, menus, and activity schedules for her; take photos or, better yet, a video; and describe what you saw and the people you met.

While reviewing the options, keep in mind what makes her happy and what would be best for her. A common mistake adult children make when helping a parent relocate is selecting a place that is convenient for them but far from people who might visit. Or they pick a place that is attractive and pleasant to visit, but not so great to live in. A beautifully renovated building may wow you, but your parent may feel more at home in a smaller, less fancy facility with a warm and caring staff.

---

has identified forty-four different names for the various levels of care provided by nursing homes.) Ask what is provided and visit the home, to be sure you are comparing apples with apples.

The Search

Ideally, to find a good nursing home you need time to tour a number of facilities, revisit one or two that look promising, and ask a lot of questions. But quite often, time is not on your side and the search is hurried, or even frantic.

If your parent is in the hospital, the discharge planner can lead the way.

Discharge planners should know quite a bit about local nursing homes, and they often have relationships with administrators, so they may be able to expedite your parent's admission. They also know something about your parent's medical situation, so they can advise you on which homes are best suited for her. Sometimes nursing-home administrators give priority to a hospital patient whose care will be covered, at least in the beginning, by Medicare.

Be aware, however, that a discharge planner's main objective is to get your parent out of the hospital, so she may pressure your family to make a hasty decision. A hospital may also have a tie to a particular facility, biasing the planner's recommendations. (But if you ask, they should tell you about any links they have.)

Whenever possible, look at residences yourself, check out nursing homes that the planner may not have suggested, and use your own judgment—or your parent's judgment—as you inspect and review the options.

This decision is too important to hurry if you don't absolutely have to. If your parent is about to be discharged from the hospital and you need a little extra time, you can usually get a reprieve of a day or two by appealing your parent's discharge.

Take any extra time you can because moving is very disruptive at this point. If you "try out" a nursing home with the thought of moving your parent to a better one later, you will throw her life into chaos twice, create more work for yourself, and possibly hurt her chances of getting into another residence, as her placement may seem less urgent.

Start your search by putting together a list of nursing homes. Look in an area that is near relatives or friends who will visit frequently, as visitors are crucial to the success of this move.

Talk with friends and acquaintances, ask your parent's doctor, and call the state or local long-term care ombudsman (page 628). Each state has an ombudsman, and some communities have a local ombudsman, who acts as an advocate for nursing-home residents and their families.

They help people find good residences and help resolve problems within a facility. These ombudsmen visit nursing homes routinely, so they know a great deal about what each offers and the quality of care available.

Be aware, however, that while ombudsmen can be an excellent source of information, they are government employees and don't like to make waves. An ombudsman may not come right out and say that a nursing home is dreadful; he or she may try to redirect you more subtly. *Why would you select Serene Acres? I think you should look at Barton's Landing. Are you sure Cedar Hollow is right for your parent?* Listen carefully for those cues.

Many communities have citizen advocacy groups, which keep tabs on nursing homes, and guide and support residents and their families. They can be very helpful to those searching for a good residence. (To find an advocacy group, see page 654.)

Medicare has a program called Nursing Home Compare, which lists and compares all certified nursing homes in a particular region. Of course, this means that some perfectly good nursing homes, those that are not certified, will not be included in this list.

Also, call geriatric care managers, local senior centers, the area agency on aging, and members of the clergy, who visit people in nursing homes and may have some recommendations.

As you gather your initial list, don't pass over nursing homes sponsored by religious organizations even

NURSING HOME COMPARE

Medicare's Nursing Home Compare program, available at www.medicare.gov or 800-MEDICARE, is a good starting point for your search. It will tell you the names of nursing homes in the area, along with basic information about the home, staffing levels, certain quality measures, and any problems cited in recent inspections.

While this information is useful, it is only a starting point. Talk to the long-term care ombudsman, and visit nursing homes yourself to see what is really going on.

Here's what Nursing Home Compare describes:

◆ **Quality measures.** Medicare tries to give a picture of the actual health status and care of the residents, and then compares that information with both statewide and national averages.

Looking at long-term residents, it examines the percentage who have lost some function since they were last tested (they are less able to feed themselves, move about, go to the bathroom alone, etc.), who are physically restrained in some way (arm bands, vests, body straps, etc.), and who have pressure sores, pain, or infections (signs of inadequate care). For short-term residents, it examines delirium, pain, and improvement in mobility. With the exception of mobility, these are all negatives, which means that low percentages are better.

◆ **Inspection results.** Certified nursing homes are inspected by state agencies. Nursing Home Compare ranks each deficiency according to its severity and how many residents were affected. Clearly, failing to file a medical report correctly is less serious than failing to prevent bedsores. So look beyond the number of deficiencies to see what the problem actually is. Then, when you tour the home, ask what is being done to remedy the situation.

◆ **Nursing staff.** This is one of the most important factors, in terms of your parent's care. Medicare calculates the number of nursing hours worked each day, on average, and divides that by the number of residents. Keep in mind that nursing assistants, as well as administrative nurses, are included in this number. Nursing assistants are the ones who really spend time with the residents. For more information, ask nursing-home administrators directly.

if your parent is not affiliated with that religion. While your parent should be in a place where she feels comfortable and won't be isolated because of her religious beliefs, a good home, no matter who runs it, is certainly worth considering.

WHAT TO LOOK FOR

AS YOU INITIALLY CONSIDER YOUR LIST, location will be a primary factor. Do you move your parent closer to you or another sibling who can keep an eye on things, or do you find a residence near your parent's current home and friends? Generally, it's best to choose the former, a place you and other family members can easily visit. It is imperative that someone checks on your parent as often as possible.

During this initial review, you'll also have to consider cost, bed availability, and whether a residence can meet the particular needs of your parent.

For anyone in a rural area, the choices may be slim. But if you live in a metropolitan area, there may be several options. Narrow down your list and then begin your on-site research. Visit several nursing homes so you have something to compare.

Visit any residences of interest more than once, and go at different times of day. Go on a formal tour, then return during the evening or on weekends when staffing levels tend to be lower.

Talk with residents and staff, and don't be afraid to ask questions. If you don't understand something or if a situation seems amiss, ask. This will tell you far more about the home than you will learn in any guided tour.

When you go on a formal tour, go beyond the public rooms—the lounges, library, gym, dining room, game room, etc. Ask to look at several bedrooms and bathrooms, the kitchen, the infirmary, and the dementia wing or any other special unit. Meet the director or manager of the residence, the heads of nursing and admissions, and staff members in charge of various aspects of residential life—the social worker, activity director, nutritionist, medical director.

Appendix F, page 646, provides a detailed list of issues to consider and questions to ask when searching for a nursing home. Here are some general issues to consider:

♦ **Certification and licensing.** As we've noted, to receive Medicare or Medicaid payments, a nursing home must be certified by the federal government. Certification means that the home meets certain standards, has passed an inspection by the state survey agency, and is monitored routinely. Some states have further regulations and requirements.

It's generally best to find a nursing home that is fully certified, so it comes under federal rules and policies, and so, if your parent needs Medicaid at some point, she cannot be discharged solely because of finances.

♦ **Gut instincts.** Your first instinct is often a pretty good one. You need to look further, of course, but don't forget that first reaction. What turned you off? What surprised you? What

" I visited two homes with wonderful reputations and found that while the grounds and buildings were beautiful, the staff were nasty to the residents and clearly unhappy in their work. Four others I visited were better—but I still wasn't satisfied. I kept calling friends and friends of friends, trying to get more leads. Then a friend's mother mentioned a place that she said had been a wonderful nursing home years ago, but now was in a bad neighborhood.

I went out to see it anyway— the neighborhood was poor, but not dangerous—and while it didn't compare aesthetically with the other places I'd seen, it was immaculately clean and the staff was actually cheerful. They seemed truly fond of the residents, and never seemed to be exasperated, even when patients were difficult.

My mother was very weak and confused, but she seemed content there and I felt good about it."

—SARA B.

did you like? Don't be blinded by fancy interior decorating or lush gardens, however. Walk the corridors and observe how the residents are cared for, because that's what really matters.

♦ **Well scrubbed and maintained.** That first waft is a good indicator of cleanliness. A facility shouldn't smell musty or rancid, but it also shouldn't be filled with perfumes or heavy ammonia. Does it appear clean and well maintained, not just in the lobby and public rooms, but elsewhere as well? Are the buildings and furnishings in good repair, or is there plaster cracking off the walls?

♦ **Safe.** Is there ample security? Are the pathways cleared to prevent falls, or are there ladders and drop cloths in the hallways? Are there grab bars and ramps? And what about the neighborhood? Is it relatively safe?

♦ **Staffing levels.** The National Citizens' Coalition for Nursing Home Reform recommends that nursing homes have at least one "direct care" staff member for every five residents during the day. (These are registered nurses, licensed practical nurses, or certified nursing assistants who directly care for patients, as opposed to those in administrative roles.) The ratio in the evening should be at least one to ten, and at night, one to fifteen. These should be higher in special wings, such as a dementia unit, or at mealtimes if numerous residents need assistance eating.

Nearly 90 percent of nursing homes fail to meet these criteria. But the residence that you are considering should not fail by much.

Nursing homes are required to post current staffing levels (not those assigned, but those who actually showed up for work) in a clearly visible place near the entrance of the home.

◆ **The hominess factor.** Would this be a comfortable place to live? Are the lounges cozy and the rooms adequate? Can your parent bring furniture and other items from home? Do the rooms look individualized, or are they all exactly the same? Is there privacy as well as a sense of community? Are there gardens or grounds where residents are free to roam? Can your parent have a pet?

◆ **A caring staff.** Is the staff pleasant and helpful, or do they seem overworked and on edge? Do they seem to have warm relationships with the residents? Do they treat residents with respect? Are they generally cheerful? Is there a high rate of turnover (which suggests trouble)?

◆ **The folks that live there.** The single most important part of your tour will be the residents themselves. Do they look well cared for and content? Are they groomed and neat? Are they alert, or do they look sedated? Are they restrained physically in beds, chairs, or wheelchairs? Are they engaged in interesting activities, watching television, or sitting alone in their rooms? Do they have friendships within the facility? Talk with them and their family members out of earshot of staff so they can be candid. Are they happy with the care they are receiving? Do they like the staff? What are their biggest complaints?

◆ **What's in a day?** Is independence encouraged and stimulation provided? Do residents get fresh air and exercise? Is there a range of activities? How many people actually participate in a given activity? Is there a workout room or pool?

◆ **Is a bed available?** If not, how long will your parent have to wait? If you and your parent like a particular home, and a bed is not available, talk with the discharge planner at the hospital or director of admissions at the nursing home about short-term possibilities. Could she be cared for at home until a bed is available? Could she stay in another nursing home until a bed becomes available in the desired facility?

◆ **Medical care.** Are nurses available around-the-clock? Are there doctors on staff? Is the facility close to a

A FRIENDLY TAG-ALONG

If you are touring without your parent or a sibling, ask a friend to come with you, preferably someone who has been through this experience. It's not easy looking at nursing homes and imagining your parent living in one of them, and it's physically tiring to do so much walking and interviewing. A friend can help you think more clearly and less emotionally, and give you the moral support you need on such a difficult trip.

hospital? Does the home have an arrangement with the hospital to deal with emergencies? Are residents unnecessarily restrained, either physically or with medications?

◆ **The chow.** When you go on your tour, arrange to have a meal so you can sample the daily fare. Does it look appetizing? Does it taste good? Is it nutritious? Does the daily menu

SPECIAL CARE FOR DEMENTIA

If a nursing home claims to have special programs and services for people with dementia, find out exactly what that means. An "Alzheimer's wing" may be a few rooms with a locked door, or it may be a carefully designed unit with a highly trained staff. The only way to know what's really offered is to see for yourself.

A program doesn't have to be solely for people with dementia; many of the best facilities mingle residents. A good unit should be quiet and calm, but also provide physical and mental stimulation. Residents should be encouraged to do simple exercises, engage in easy and entertaining projects, and receive lots of encouragement to do all that they can for themselves.

The floor plan should allow them to find their way around easily and to wander safely. The staff-to-patient ratio should be high, with at least one staff person to every three or four patients during the day. Schedules should be flexible to meet the diverse needs of residents,

including those who are awake during the night or want to eat at odd hours.

The number of patients on sedatives or other psychotropic (mind-altering) medications should be low, and the use of physical restraints, such as straps or body vests, should be virtually nonexistent.

Once in a residence, be sure your parent receives a thorough assessment and that any plan of care takes into account her special needs and unusual quirks——what she can and cannot do, what she enjoys and what makes her anxious, what she eats, what medications she's on, what gives her comfort, and the best way for the staff to help her.

Stay abreast of whether the staff is actually following the plan and whether changes are necessary. People with dementia can change quickly, going from critical and jumpy to calm and withdrawn in a matter of months. (See Chapters Twenty-Two and Twenty-Three for more on caring for someone with dementia.)

offer several alternatives, and does it change often? Can the kitchen accommodate any special dietary needs of your parent (kosher, vegetarian, etc)?

◆ **The head honchos.** While you certainly need to discuss finances, services, and eligibility with administrators, get a feel for the philosophy of the institution, as well. An administration that is genuinely concerned about residents will see to it that your parent gets good, continuous care.

◆ **Resident and/or family council.** Is there an active council? How often do they meet? What kinds of issues do they discuss? How receptive is the home to suggestions and criticisms? If possible, attend a meeting of the resident or family council.

◆ **Rules for room changes and discharge.** You don't want your parent moved from room to room or, for heaven's sake, evicted. Find out under what circumstances the nursing home would move your parent to a new room or refuse to keep her at the home. For example, what happens if she's hospitalized? Does she lose her room? Find out if your parent might be moved to another section of the nursing home once he is on Medicaid. While this isn't as horrible as being discharged or transferred, it is disruptive for an older person to switch rooms, especially if he has made friends on a certain floor or wing. Furthermore, some nursing homes put all Medicaid patients onto a floor or unit that is not renovated, more

crowded, less well staffed, and otherwise grubbier.

Under what circumstances would they discharge or transfer a resident? When was the last time they did so, and what were the reasons?

◆ **Special needs.** What sort of care is offered to residents with dementia? Incontinence? Trouble bathing or eating? Insomnia? Can residents get a snack at night? Are they helped to the toilet immediately? Are there people on hand who will help them eat?

◆ **Culture and religion.** Is the home sensitive to the ethnic and cultural norms of your parent? Are there other residents in the home that follow your parent's religion or are ethnically similar? Do they serve appropriate foods and have places where your parent can worship? Are there plenty of people who speak the same language as your parent?

◆ **Hospice care.** If hospice care is of interest to your parent and you, ask if the nursing home has any arrangement with a nearby hospice or dedicated beds for hospice care.

ASK FOR THE INSPECTION REPORT

ALTHOUGH MEDICARE'S NURSING Home Compare lists some of the deficiencies in a residence's inspection report, it's best to look at the full report yourself. Nursing homes that receive Medicare or Medicaid funding are examined once every 15 months by inspectors from a state survey agency.

Getting my father into a good nursing home was like getting someone with very poor grades into college. He was on Medicaid because we'd spent all of my parents' money during my mother's illness. He had advanced dementia, and he had become angry and disruptive. A social worker said that nursing homes in the area would not consider taking such a patient and suggested that we get him admitted to a hospital and let the hospital staff pull some strings.

We represented my father as being cooperative and agreeable, as he had been before the dementia set in, and finally found a nursing home that we liked that was willing to admit him. We whizzed through the application process because we were afraid they would refuse him once they understood how difficult he could be. They took him, thank goodness, but it was quite an experience."

—Sara B.

Their reports reveal any violations, from the temperature of the tap water to cases of outright physical abuse.

Your request may ruffle some feathers, as many nursing homes would rather keep these reports private, but don't be intimidated. Inspection reports —also known as surveys—must, by law, be made available to the public. If the nursing home makes this difficult, ask the state long-term care ombudsman (page 628) or the state office that licenses nursing homes for a copy of the report.

When you review the inspection report don't seek perfection because it doesn't exist. Instead, look for repeated violations and the kinds of violations that directly affect a patient's well-being, such as failure to follow a "plan of care" or overuse of restraints.

Ask about any violations that concern you. The way the staff answers your questions—whether they are direct and apologetic, or indifferent— will tell you a great deal about how they regard their mission.

Getting In

Finding a good nursing home is only half the battle. The second half is getting your parent accepted. In some places, where there are more beds than patients, getting in isn't a problem. But in many areas, popular nursing homes will have plenty of candidates vying for admission, and administrators pick and choose freely when accepting residents. The person with the most money or the best Medicare coverage or the fewest problems will be given priority.

When you meet with an administrator, be discreet in what you say about your parent's angry outbursts or demanding personality. Focus on the side of her that is calm and easygoing. And while you shouldn't hesitate to ask questions, be tactful. A family perceived as unreasonably demanding may be turned away in favor of one who understands the pressures of nursing-home work.

You can't hide your parent's financial problems because the nursing home will look through his records. Homes prefer residents who qualify for Medicare coverage and self-paying residents. The longer someone can foot the bills privately, the better. If your parent is on Medicaid, he may have fewer choices and may face lengthy waiting lists.

If he has trouble being admitted, talk to the long-term care ombudsman, a local citizens' coalition, and, if possible, a savvy eldercare attorney.

Build a rapport with the nursing home's administration, and if your parent is put on a waiting list, call often and be persistent about making sure that he gets the first bed available.

Admission

The admissions process can be lengthy and exhausting, and it requires that you submit a variety of your parent's personal, medical, financial, and legal records. The nursing home's admissions or financial officer will tell you what is needed.

A nursing home might ask for a large deposit before admission. Find out what this covers and whether it will be refunded if your parent leaves early. Get any agreement in writing. If your parent's care is to be covered by Medicare or Medicaid, the home cannot require a deposit in advance.

Any nursing-home contract should include detailed information about costs, payment schedules, services to be provided, penalties for failure to pay, the facility's refund policy and bed-holding policy should your parent be hospitalized or temporarily absent for some other reason, the discharge policy, the rules of the house, and the responsibilities and rights of residents.

Read the contract carefully or have an experienced lawyer read it. Ask the nursing home's director or the state's long-term care ombudsman to clarify any provision that concerns you or your parent. Beware of clauses in the contract that free an institution from liability for injury or lost possessions.

MAKING THE MOVE WORK

*Moving Day • A Plan of Care
• Your Role as Visitor and Advocate
• Long–Distance Caregiving • When Trouble Brews*

Y OU'VE FOUND A NURSING HOME FOR YOUR PARENT, OR perhaps an assisted-living residence, but your job is far from over. Just because your parent is moving into a place that offers supervision, it doesn't mean that you have relinquished responsibility for her care.

A week or two of nursing-home care may mean a break for you, but when your parent moves in for an extended stay, you need to stay on top of things. Nursing homes are not safe havens. Unfortunately, residents are neglected and sometimes even abused.

It is up to you and others in the family to help your parent make the initial adjustment, which can be very rocky, and then be sure that she gets adequate care for the duration of her stay. Your involvement will help keep her spirits up. But most important, it allows you to develop relationships with staff members who care for her, and to be sure that she is being cared for properly.

While this chapter is geared toward those who have a parent moving into a nursing home, much of this advice and information is relevant to any institutional housing situation.

Moving Day

Moving day can be wrenching for everyone. You may feel anxious, sad, guilt-ridden, and uncertain. Your parent may be nervous, depressed, angry, or frightened. Put your own worries aside for the moment so you can empathize with her and reassure her.

Know that anger, depression, and even some hostility are normal responses. This is a big move. It's scary. It feels final. She is leaving a lot behind and facing a great unknown at a very fragile time of life. Let her express these things. Listen to her calmly and acknowledge what she's saying. Let her know that you love her and that you will not desert her. Her reaction is part of a process of letting go and moving on.

Whatever you do, don't suddenly make a change of plan at the eleventh hour. *I can't do this. I'll figure something else out.* You've given this move a lot of thought. You've both come this far. Now give it a chance.

If you have some time before the move, that is, if she is not going unexpectedly from the hospital into a nursing home, there are ways to make the transition easier:

♦ In the weeks before the move, bring your parent to visit her new home, several times, if possible. Even if she's been there before, she will now see it through the eyes of a future resident, which will give her a different perspective. Introduce her to other residents and staff and tell them when she will be arriving so they can greet her.

♦ Ask friends and family to offer encouragement and support. They might tour the home themselves and talk with her about some of the things they saw that they liked.

♦ Hold a party for your parent a few days before the move. (Have it around her hospital bed, if necessary.) Guests should bring gifts for her new life—framed photos, silk flowers, a bathrobe, slippers, a scarf, scents and powders, a calendar with lots of visits already written in, some potpourri, a bed quilt, soft new sheets, a featherbed, a child's drawing for the wall.

♦ Before packing the car, find out exactly what your parent is permitted to bring, and what is not allowed, so you don't arrive only to be sent home with half of her belongings. Leave valuables behind unless they are absolutely necessary (things get lost and stolen in any institution), but include objects of comfort, such as a special chair, a favorite afghan, or family photos. Clearly label all of your parent's clothes and belongings, down to each book and bathroom kit.

♦ Get others to lend a hand. They might help you arrange your parent's room and then stay and have a meal with her. Or someone might stay home with your children so you aren't hurried while getting your mother adjusted.

♦ If a group of people helps with this move, be sure to space your departures so that your parent doesn't have to deal with one enormous goodbye. Later that day, the group might meet back at your house to give you some support and comfort at the end of what is bound to be an emotionally draining time.

◆ If your parent has fixed habits and routines, ask the staff if they can be accommodated. After years of doing something a certain way—having a cup of coffee first thing in the morning, staying up every evening to watch *The Late Show*—it's hard to change the pattern. Being able to maintain old routines and habits will make this move easier. Likewise, if your parent gets certain magazine subscriptions or likes certain newspapers, see if they can be delivered. Or if there are special foods she enjoys, perhaps that too can be arranged.

A Plan of Care

Once your parent is admitted, a nursing home must conduct a full assessment of his physical, functional, social, mental, and emotional condition. Staff will examine his overall health, hearing and vision, and his ability to perform "activities of daily living" (bathing, toileting, grooming, eating, walking), as well as his ability to communicate, understand, and remember. They should take note of his past, lifestyle, habits, hobbies, and relationships.

This assessment must be done within fourteen days of a resident's admission, or seven days after the admission of someone whose care is covered by Medicare. (Since Medicare only covers short-term, very intensive nursing care, these residents are usually in more serious shape than others.)

The staff then has a week to put together a "plan of care" that outlines your parent's medical treatments; describes the therapy and nursing care he will receive; recommends activities he should or shouldn't do; and specifies his diet, exercise regime, and daily schedule. The plan should be devised in a way that keeps your parent as active and independent as possible. It should be drafted by an interdisciplinary team that includes nurses, dietitians, social workers, rehabilitation and occupational therapists, members from the activities staff, and any others who play a role in your parent's daily care.

You, other family members, and, if possible, your parent, should all be integrally involved in designing the plan of care. Ask (insist if necessary) that the conference take place when family members can attend. Ask in advance how much time has been scheduled for it—it might last up to an hour, even longer. Be sure ample time is set aside so it isn't hurried.

If your parent can't speak for herself, be sure the staff understands her schedule, what gives her pleasure, what upsets her, what calms her down, what times and tasks are most confusing for her, and anything else that might help them create a plan. You should have a voice in her daily schedule, activities, and services.

Get a written copy of the plan, and be sure it is specific and reflects your concerns. When you visit, check to see that the plan is being followed.

A plan of care must be updated every three months, or any time there is a change in your parent's physical or mental health.

Your Role as a Visitor

Visiting can be stressful and time-consuming, but remember, even if a visit is brief, your parent complains the whole time, or she forgets that you came, your presence is invaluable. It lets her know that you care and that she is not alone, and it helps you keep tabs on how she is doing and any trouble there might be.

Visit as often as you can manage. And when you do visit, make it count. Take note of your parent's well-being, consult with staff members about how she is faring, and offer her lots of reassurance. A few visiting tips:

◆ While nurses and aides can be helpful in letting you know when your parent needs a visit, don't routinely schedule your trips via the staff. By dropping in unexpectedly now and then, you will be better able to monitor her care.

◆ Nursing homes often have posted visiting hours, but these do not apply to immediate family. The nursing home might want you to think that they do, but by law, relatives can visit whenever

> *I was prepared to be uncomfortable, to hate this place. But I was surprised. It was attractive, and, more than that, many of the people living there were much healthier than I expected. One older gentleman even flirted with my mother in the elevator. I think we both liked the home more than we expected, and that came as a great relief."*
>
> —FRAN M.

the resident wants them to. You might have to go someplace where you won't bother other residents or keep your parent's roommate awake. But visiting at off times lets you see what is happening when staffing is lean. Be respectful of any particular reasons for limiting visiting hours, but know your rights.

◆ Plan your visits around your parent's schedule. For example, don't interrupt her nap time or her favorite class.

◆ Visits can be short; in fact, short is often better. Your parent may tire easily. Thirty minutes may be an ample visit.

◆ If your visits are tense or uncomfortable, do something new. Play a game of cards, take your parent to lunch, help her write letters, take her for a drive, or read her mail, a newspaper, or a book aloud to her. If your parent has dementia, tour the home together (it will always be fairly new to her), or look through a photo album with her. Get your parent to reminisce about her youth or your youth. You will learn about who she was, and she gets to recall wonderful times in her life. You can also diffuse tension by talking to other residents. That will help your parent make friends and allow her to show you off as well.

◆ Pamper her. If you are used to having a hand in your parent's physical care, don't hesitate to continue in that role. Fix her hair, help her put on makeup, rub her back, give her a manicure or a foot massage. Looking good makes people feel better.

◆ Hugs are potent medicine, and nursing-home residents are woefully lacking in warm physical contact. Unless your parent is uncomfortable with touch, go ahead and be close.

◆ While your parent will enjoy hearing about what's happening at home, don't feel that someone always has to be talking. Sometimes just sitting with her, being in the room, is reassuring. Bring some knitting or a book or work and sit quietly with her.

◆ If your parent has trouble eating, visit during mealtimes and ask others to do the same. You can help her eat and, if you are eating too, she might eat more than she would otherwise. You'll know that at least one meal a day is getting in.

◆ Bring the children, unless your parent or a child specifically asks you not to. Children radiate joy, spirit, and energy—which is appreciated by most elderly people.

◆ If you have a cold or the flu or some other contagious illness, postpone your visit until you are better. Nursing-home residents are very susceptible to germs.

◆ Don't say you will visit at a certain time unless you are sure you can do so. If your parent is mentally alert, visits can trigger a lot of excitement, and a canceled visit can be a huge letdown. If you have to cancel, let her know as soon as possible, and reschedule. You might let the staff know of your parent's disappointment.

◆ Keep your parent up-to-date on what is happening with friends and family. News from the home front is gold. Photos and home videos are wonderful. Keep her posted on any local gossip or town events. And don't hide bad news, as tempting as that may be. It's best to be open and let your parent grieve when a friend or relative dies, and to react to other unhappy news.

◆ Take a few minutes during a visit to review your parent's wardrobe. Does she need new clothing or shoes? Ask an aide who regularly cares for her if there is something that might make your parent more comfortable, such as sneakers, slippers, a new robe, or elastic-waisted pants.

◆ Use your visits to establish a rapport with the staff. Get to know them and let them know how much you appreciate their efforts.

WHEN COMMUNICATION FAILS

When your parent cannot communicate, or perhaps can't even look up at you, visits can become particularly awkward. She is sitting hunched over in her wheelchair, staring blankly. You are trying vainly to make conversation, to find something to say. If you're busy with other things and squeezing this into a tight schedule, you may wonder why you bother.

Of course you know that your visits are more critical than ever now that she can't speak for herself. But there is more to it than that. Even if she seems oblivious, your parent is probably more aware of these visits than you think she is. She may not know it is you, but she will sense the presence of someone kind and familiar. She will hear your voice, smell your familiar scent, and feel your hand stroking hers. Your visits are probably very reassuring and calming, even though it may not seem so at times.

Come prepared with stories to tell—about your day, what's happening with friends and family members, changes in her town, the past—or bring a book or magazine article to read aloud. If she likes physical touch, gently stroke her hands and the back of her neck, brush her hair, or put lotion on her. You might also bring some favorite music.

Speak slowly, explaining what you are doing, so you don't startle her. Touch her, but also let her touch things, your hands, your face, or perhaps a cat or new scarf. And if possible, get her outdoors to smell the fresh air and feel the sunshine.

Don't worry. She knows.

Your Role as an Advocate

When you visit or call, take time to build a rapport with those staff members who care for your parent regularly. Support them in their work, thank them for caring for your parent, and talk to them about who she was, her daily routines, her likes and dislikes, and any tips that might make their job easier.

Then speak up when you have concerns. If your father's roommate keeps him up at night; if you notice a change in his moods, sleep habits, or weight; if he can't or won't eat the food from the dining room; speak up. Talk to the staff members and try to come up with solutions that work for

A CAREFUL EYE ON DEMENTIA

A failing memory or sedated mind is a cruel foe. Your parent may not remember that you visited and insist that you never come to see him. Or his agitation may make him yell at you when you arrive and scream that you should leave. Do not be dissuaded. You have to be his friend and advocate now.

Be aware of mood shifts and changes in behavior that might signal trouble. Look out for sores and bruises, weight loss, poor hygiene and grooming, and other signs of poor care or even abuse.

When you visit, tell the staff about your parent, who he was, and what he once enjoyed. Put photos up of your parent in his younger days. Remind them about his needs, quirks, and preferences. What is the best way to calm him? What schedule works best for him? What triggers anger and agitation? What does he enjoy?

As for his forgetting your visits, you might mark a large calendar with your name written in large, bright red letters on the days that you will visit. Ask the staff to remind him that you are coming before your arrival. (If your parent is very forgetful, put a photo of yourself in his room, and the staff can show him who you are.) Then send notes between visits reminding him of what took place during your last visit and when you will visit next.

If none of this helps, don't push your parent to remember something that he can't. What difference does it make, really, if he knows when he last saw you? Live in the present with him. And definitely ignore any urge to visit less. Your advocacy is critical, and your presence is still reassuring to him.

your parent, but don't overburden the staff. If you aren't sure of his rights and yours, see "A Nursing-Home Resident's Bill of Rights," page 652.

Obviously, you need to be alert to any signs of possible abuse or neglect: bruises or wounds, bedsores, soiled bedsheets, incontinence, poor hygiene, weight loss, excessive fear, diminished self-esteem. (See pages 453–457 for information on these and other similar issues.)

Beyond that, be sure your parent is safe. Be alert if he is at risk of falling. Stay abreast of those ailments that are often overlooked or not adequately treated by nursing-home staff, such as vision and hearing problems, bedsores, incontinence, nutrition, insomnia, pain, and overmedication.

Be particularly aware of depression, as it is very common in nursing-home residents and often ignored. Feeling morose and lethargic, losing weight, and lacking sleep are not normal parts of aging. They require attention and treatment.

If you can't be there in person, ask the staff about these issues, and ask to be notified if your parent falls, becomes ill, or requires a change in treatment or medications. She should not be overly sedated, another common problem in nursing homes.

Even if your parent is very frail, immobile, and suffering from dementia, she should get fresh air, proper nutrition, and some exercise. Talk to the activities director about options. She should not be alone, staring at a television screen, all day.

If your mother used to have a particular interest, say, in gardening, talk with the activities director about how she might become engaged in some relevant task. If your father's days are meaningless, ask if he can visit people in the infirmary, read to residents who can't see, help in the gift shop, or deliver flowers or mail to others. It's amazing how a little giving can lift the spirits.

Also, be sure that your parent is treated with respect and that he has some privacy, as these are vital to self-esteem, yet so often lacking in communal living situations. If your mother is uncomfortable about having strangers help her dress or bathe, see if the job might be limited to one or two regular attendants. They might drape towels in such a way that she retains her dignity.

TWO GOLDEN RULES

◆ Strike a balance between advocating assertively and supporting those who care for your parent, from supervisors to the cleaning crew. Certainly you should expect, and demand, reasonable care, and you should be outspoken when care is lacking. But keep in mind, many people working in nursing homes have almost no training, receive little more than minimum wage, and have far more work than they can handle. Staff will usually show your parent the same kindness, understanding, and respect that you show them.

Develop a rapport with those who care for your parent. Ask them about their own families and lives, and let them know that you are sympathetic to the pressures they face.

> " *There were a couple of very bad months at first. I spoke to the social worker at the home, and she asked me if I could hire a part-time aide to help my father adjust. Because he was on Medicaid, this wasn't really aboveboard—he would have been cut off if they knew we were paying for private care—but we did it anyway. And it succeeded beyond our expectations. The place became a home for him. He joked with the aides and nurses, and they treated him with affection.*"
>
> —Lillian R.

When someone makes a special effort or is especially kind, be sure to thank him or her. If you want to go a step further, give the person a gift and send a letter of praise to a supervisor. Ask a floor supervisor or the family council if tips are allowed. If not, the family council might pool contributions for a staff gift or party.

When you have a concern, work together with the staff to find solutions or resolve problems. Staff members can often make adjustments once they are made aware of a problem, but they will do so more readily, and care about your parent and your family more genuinely, if you show them respect. Have patience and a sense of humor about any minor mishaps.

It's difficult letting go of a parent's care. It's hard not to constantly correct and criticize those who now care for your parent because, of course, they are not doing it as you would. But you aren't taking care of your parent day in and day out. And they are. Try not to take out your grief and pain on an overworked aide or orderly.

◆ Choose one person from your family to act as a spokesperson. You don't want a phone call from your brother to jeopardize an understanding you have carefully developed with an aide, or a visit from your sister to discontinue a special menu you have worked out with the dietitian. Talk among yourselves and agree upon a plan. Then have one spokesperson. This is easier for nurses and aides, and it reduces the possibility of mix-ups.

Long-Distance Caregiving

If you cannot visit your parent, find someone who can. Talk with relatives and friends, and find out about local volunteer visitors. A social worker from the nursing home, the state long-term care ombudsman, or a local consumer advocacy group should be able to tell you about volunteers and groups that visit the facility. If you cannot find volunteers, consider hiring someone to visit regularly and keep tabs on your parent's care. This is expensive, but if you can afford it, it's a worthwhile investment.

Ask a nurse supervisor how to best stay in touch with the staff and when you should call to get regular updates on your parent's care and condition.

Create a relationship with one or two nurses or aides who see your parent regularly. Find someone whom you trust and who is sympathetic to your situation.

Also, contact the nursing home's family/resident council, which represents the needs and concerns of residents and their families. It will keep you abreast of what's happening in the home and make others aware of your parent's situation.

Use the telephone. Lots of calls, even short ones, can fend off the loneliness your parent may be feeling now. Send her a video of you and others in the family. If she has trouble seeing, send a letter dictated into a tape machine. Talk about your day, your kids, your life, time spent with her in the past and other memories. If she has access to the Internet and can use it, e-mail notes and photos of yourself and grandchildren regularly.

Send pictures drawn by grandchildren. Send care packages of special foods or small gifts. Send jokes or cartoons you read, short articles you enjoyed, recipes you just made—anything so that there is a constant flow of mail and communication.

When you can't be there, be sure any special instructions are very, very clear. You'll want to do this in any case, but when you are not around, it is especially important to do whatever you can to avoid mix-ups. If your father is lactose intolerant, place a clearly visible note over his bed reminding the staff of this fact. Talk to staff personally about any issues or concerns. Ask what is being done to avoid problems.

You might even post a note asking the staff to be kind to your parent, reminding them that, while his body is failing and mind is fading, your love for him is still strong, and let them know that you appreciate their hard work and compassion. Post photos of your parent when she was younger, as well, and perhaps even some information about who she was and what she used to do.

Sometimes families who are far away or busy at work want to install webcams—also known, in this case, as "granny cams"—in their parents' rooms. This way a view of your parent's room is always available to you, either by videotape or on the Internet. Be aware, however, that nursing homes have their own

> " *When my mother stopped recognizing me, I stopped visiting her as much, not because I thought she didn't know the difference, but because it was so hard for me. To have her turn and look blankly at me, to have her ask, 'Who is this woman in my room?' was very painful. I used to shout at her, 'Mom, it's Nancy!' and then be depressed for days after the visit.*
>
> *I still don't go quite as often as I used to, but I've learned something that helps. When I visit, we look through this old album together. It is filled with pictures of her and her brothers when they were little. We look at the same pictures every time. She doesn't have any idea who I am, but she knows who they are, and I see how it comforts her to tell me about them. For that one hour, she is a child again, living in a brown house in Richmond, Indiana, with a great big slide and two fun-loving brothers. And for that hour, I think she is happy.*"
>
> —NANCY S.

policies on this. Generally, you cannot install a granny cam without the full permission of any roommates. You must also consider your parent's right to privacy—is this something she agrees to, or would agree to if she was competent?

Also, consider the practical value of a granny cam: Your parent is not always going to be within the camera's view, and it might create some animosity between you and the staff.

Use your own best judgment and, if possible, discuss it with your parent, any roommate, and the staff.

When Trouble Brews

When you notice a problem in your parent's care, bring it to the attention of the staff as soon as possible. First, talk with the person directly involved—the orderly who has repeatedly left your parent sitting unattended, the housekeeper who fails to change his wet sheets, the aide who should be helping your parent get to the toilet.

When raising a problem with a member of the staff, be patient and understanding of the demands on her time. Try to be helpful rather than reproachful at this stage. The worker may not even know that the problem existed. Be specific about your concerns. Explain what you've noticed, when the problem occurred, and why it is a concern. Then listen to the staff member's thoughts on why this is happening and what might be done to resolve the matter. Offer possible solutions yourself, if you have some ideas.

If the problem is not resolved, talk to an immediate supervisor, again, being as specific as you can. If you still hit a roadblock, move on up the ladder, from the aide to the nursing supervisor or medical director to the administrator, until you get results.

Be calm and respectful when you deal with each person, but remain firm in your resolve. Being rude, critical, or otherwise difficult might adversely affect your parent's care, but reasonable complaints that are thoughtfully registered should not. In fact, once the staff realizes that you are not turning your back on things, your parent may receive more attention.

Throughout this process, document everything. Keep notes on what happened and when, whom you spoke with, when you spoke with them, and what their responses were. Keep track of the time and date. Follow up phone calls with letters, and request a written response. This assures that any agreement is clear, and it gives you backing in case the problem is repeated or becomes more serious.

If there is no resolution from the staff and administration, look into the facility's grievance procedure and file a formal complaint. By law, all nursing homes are required to have such a procedure.

Talk also with members of any resident or family council. Some are more helpful than others, but they should be alerted to complaints or problems. Most will at least advise you on how to proceed; some may step in on your parent's behalf.

OUTSIDE HELP

IF THE PROBLEM IS NOT RESOLVED from within the nursing home, or if a problem is dire, go outside for help:

◆ Long-term care ombudsmen have both the authority and the experience to work with a nursing home to resolve problems. They are required by law to investigate all complaints and can refer serious ones to other agencies. Some states permit ombudsmen to file lawsuits on behalf of residents.

If you want to keep your complaint confidential, an ombudsman can still investigate the matter and find out if other residents are having similar problems. The ombudsman can also explain laws and your rights and can advise you on how to proceed with a particular problem. (See page 628 for the numbers of state ombudsmen offices.)

◆ The state survey agency, which licenses and certifies nursing homes and conducts regular inspections, must, by federal law, investigate any dire situation (one in which a resident is in immediate danger) within two working days. (Contact the long-term care ombudsman to find the state survey agency.)

Unfortunately, less pressing complaints might not be investigated until the next time the residence is inspected, which could be months away. If the problem is recurring or affecting a number of residents, be persistent. Get other families to join you in the effort. There is power in numbers.

◆ If you believe the nursing home is exploiting your parent financially, notify his bank and ask that his account be monitored.

◆ Contact a local nursing-home residents' advocacy group. These groups monitor nursing-home care within certain areas or states. They often assist families who are facing conflicts or worried about inadequate or dangerous care. (See Appendix H, page 654, for a state-by-state list). The National Citizens' Coalition for Nursing Home Reform (202-332-2275 or www.ncc nhr.org) has a lot of good information about resident's rights and laws on their Web site.

◆ The long-term care ombudsman can direct you to other state offices you need to notify (the Medicaid office, a senior advocacy agency, the attorney general's office) and should also be able to refer you to available legal services if necessary.

◆ Consider other local agencies that might be helpful in your particular situation, such as the health department, adult protective services, the medical assistance office (for Medicaid patients), the attorney general's office, or legal services.

NEGLECT, ABUSE, AND EXPLOITATION

PHYSICAL AND EMOTIONAL ABUSE and neglect, financial exploitation, and theft occur with shocking frequency, especially when residents are too sick or confused to fend for themselves, and families are not able to visit regularly or at all. Be alert to signs of trouble and act immediately. Don't ignore subtle warning signs; if something doesn't seem right to you, follow up on it.

Again (again and yet again), visit often or have others check in. Drop in unexpectedly. Ask about any unusual marks or bruises. (If your parent has fallen or otherwise been injured, you should have been notified immediately.) Be sure that his possessions and bank accounts are safe. If your parent has dementia, note changes in his behavior—accusations, fear, agitation, outbursts—and try to ascertain whether there might be a valid reason for his distrust and anxiety.

Obviously, any sort of hitting, shoving, pinching, slapping, or other such attacks are abusive, but a person doesn't have to touch your parent to be abusive. Saying things that make

RESTRAINING RESTRAINTS

Nursing homes have been ordered by Congress to cut back on the use of restraints—both physical and chemical means of controlling patients —but some facilities have been more successful than others at curtailing this practice. Know what to look for and how to keep your parent as free from restraint as possible.

Physical restraints include everything from full body vests to straps that tie a person's arms down and innocuous-looking wheelchair trays that basically prevent a person from getting up. Chemical restraints include tranquilizers, antianxiety drugs, antidepressants, sedatives, and hypnotics.

Any restraint is dehumanizing and potentially dangerous. The drugs can cause side effects—from confusion, agitation, and insomnia to hypertension and change in appetite. Physical restraints can lead to anxiety, depression, bedsores, constipation, poor circulation, incontinence, and loss of appetite. They can also choke or severely injure a person who, in a state of panic, tries to escape, or who simply tries to get up in the middle of the night.

Indeed, restraining a person is often more dangerous than leaving him be. And oddly enough, research also shows that people who are restrained often require more time, not less, from nurses, when compared to similar residents who are not restrained.

With a little ingenuity, risks can be reduced so falls don't happen or, when they do, they are not harmful. They can be prevented through exercise (which improves balance and strength, and relieves agitation and insomnia), the use of supportive shoes, lower beds and chairs, better lighting, clear pathways, handrails, and walkers.

him feel threatened, demeaned, or afraid also constitute abuse.

Isolating a person, ignoring his physical or emotional needs, or failing to keep him safe, clean, fed, and toileted all constitute neglect. It is neglectful to repeatedly ignore a resident's call bell, to fail to reposition her to avoid bedsores, to fail to help her eat and drink, or to leave her to walk unassisted when she needs help. However, unlike abuse, neglect may not be intentional. Staff might not have time to help or know how to help. Sometimes the problem can be remedied simply by talking to staff members.

Abuse, on the other hand, requires immediate and aggressive action. If there

A wedge of foam tucked into a chair can prevent a person from sliding out, and sensors can be attached to a bed to alert the staff when a confused person is trying to get up. Also, wheelchairs and canes should be tailored to the individual size and needs of the resident.

Residents of nursing homes generally do better in terms of falls, as well as agitation, when they are allowed to operate on their own schedules, have friends and companionship, be involved in activities they enjoy, get outdoors regularly, exercise, have ample opportunities to use the toilet, and have a safe environment. Talk with the staff about creative solutions to any seemingly dangerous behaviors and the true risks involved.

Anytime your parent is restrained, find out why. Restraints can be used only under a doctor's order. Mind-altering medications are more difficult to monitor because there can be many reasons for prescribing various medications. If your parent is unusually groggy or inattentive, find out what drugs she is being given and why. If a drug is necessary to treat an ailment, perhaps she can take a lower dose or be treated with a nonsedative or short-acting alternative.

When falls or other problems cannot be avoided without restraints, weigh the risks and benefits of the situation. While your instinct may be to protect her at all costs, remember that it is usually better to risk a minor fall than to have your parent restrained and risk more serious injuries and complications.

If your parent is threatening the safety of others, talk with the doctor, social worker, or nurses about other solutions. There may be reasons why he is combative and ways to make him feel less threatened.

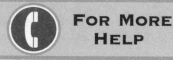

FOR MORE HELP

Long Term Care Ombudsman Resource Center
202-332-2275
www.ltcombudsman.org
To find your state ombudsman agency, see page 628.

AARP
888-687-2277
www.aarp.org
For brochures on finding a nursing home and protecting your parents' rights once they are in one.

National Citizens' Coalition for Nursing Home Reform
202-332-2275
www.nccnhr.org
For information about residents' rights and the laws governing nursing homes, as well as information about particular issues. The NCCNHR Web site is particularly helpful.

is any question at all of danger, get your parent out of the situation right away or ask that the person or people responsible be removed from your parent's care immediately. Document any problems in writing and be specific about when, where, and what happened and who was involved. Alert the staff supervisor, the director of the home, and the doctor. Contact the local ombudsman,

the local adult protective services agency, the nursing-home licensing agency, and the citizens' advocacy group.

UNWANTED ROOM CHANGES AND DISCHARGES

COULD YOUR FATHER SUDDENLY BE evicted or transferred out of his nursing home? It shouldn't happen, but it does, all too often.

Nursing homes can legally discharge or transfer residents who, after reasonable notice, fail to pay their bills. They can also discharge residents who go on Medicaid if the home is not fully certified and has no specially earmarked "Medicaid beds" available. (However, if the home is fully certified, it cannot evict residents who are waiting for Medicaid eligibility, regardless of beds.)

Nursing homes can also discharge residents or transfer them to another facility if the resident no longer needs nursing-home care, if the nursing home closes, if the facility cannot provide adequate care for some reason, or if the resident presents a danger to himself or others.

These last two reasons really should not be an issue, as nursing homes, by nature, provide complex care and should be able to adjust that care and implement plans to meet the needs of almost any resident and head off any violent behavior.

Unfortunately, nursing homes occasionally use these reasons to get rid of residents who are difficult, who have families who are seen as difficult, or who are switching from self-payment to

Medicaid, which means less income for the nursing home.

Before notifying a family and resident of any plans for discharge, the nursing home must make some real effort to meet the needs of the resident or alleviate any troubling behavior through a plan of care. If, after this effort has been made, a resident is to be transferred to another nursing home or simply discharged, the nursing home must give thirty days' notice. It must explain, in writing, why the resident is being transferred, where the resident will be moved to, and when the move will occur.

This written notification must also include information about how a resident or family can appeal the decision. States have different rules about discharge and transfer, and the rules are also different if, say, your parent is on Medicaid. Contact the long-term care ombudsman if you are concerned about a discharge or transfer plan.

Sometimes, a resident who has been living in a facility, perhaps for several years, and paying privately for that care, goes on Medicaid and is suddenly transferred to another unit or wing of the residence. Such a move, as we've already noted, is very disruptive for an elderly person distancing him from friends he has made and a familiar environment. Worst of all, it may be a move into a wing with inferior care. This is legal, but you can still fight it. Talk with administrators and contact the long-term care ombudsman and any local advocacy group.

Is This Move Working?

Your mother's belongings are in place, her room is relatively comfortable, the staff is nice, and you have both settled into a new routine. But she seems unhappy. Her health has deteriorated. She is more confused than before, and she complains endlessly. Was this the best thing to do?

Give it time. Elderly people usually need at least six months, and often longer, to adjust to a new environment, a new routine, and new relationships. There are often setbacks early on, but your parent probably will adapt with time.

If your parent's complaints are vague, help him to be specific. Is there something he needs or wants, or does

> *One of the aides, whom my mother loved, had heard a rumor that I had complained about her. I hadn't, but it took over a year to break down this barrier. I said to one of the home's social workers, 'Look, if she wants to be angry with me, fine. I can take it. I just don't want her to be angry with my mother.' I tried very hard to mend the fences because I knew that much of the quality of my mother's care depended on what they thought of me."*
>
> —Barbara F.

> " *At first my father didn't want to stay, and he kept trying to leave. The staff was kind and understanding about it, but we were really afraid that they would decide that he couldn't stay. He was angry and demanding a lot of the time, he was notoriously picky about what he ate, and he complained about everything. The staff told me not to worry, that he would adjust, but I couldn't believe it. I was sure he would wear them out, and then what would we do? I also felt like a monster for leaving him there because he seemed so miserable.*
>
> *About two months after his move, I went to see him and arrived to find him all smiling and happy. I have never been so grateful to anyone in my life as I was to the nurses who were so patient and good to him. They never suggested medicating him to make him less rambunctious, or made me feel that he was in any way a burden. It's odd. You love these people, these strangers, who care so tenderly for your parent, who do what you wish you could do. They become your friends, and you want to do good things for them."*
>
> —BRENDA S.

he simply need to air his fears and worries? Once you've discussed his complaints and addressed any real problems, ask your parent to think of three things he likes about this new home. Redirecting his attention to the positive aspects of this move will take his mind off the less desirable factors, at least temporarily.

If you believe that your parent's care is good, keep these realities in mind:

◆ Nursing-home residents sometimes complain bitterly and appear depressed when visitors are around and then, as soon as the guests are gone, they return to activities, friends, and a more pleasant mood. If there is a staff member who has a good rapport with your parent, ask how your parent's mood changes with your visits. If your father simply needs to complain and you are an easy target, let him. Just be aware that you are getting all the bad news and none of the good, and take his complaints with a grain of salt.

◆ If your mother appears worse each time you visit, it may not be that her condition is rapidly deteriorating, but simply that you are more aware of her decline. When you see someone every day, you are less apt to notice subtle changes in health or mental abilities. When you visit only once every couple of weeks, the changes become more apparent.

◆ Adult children often project their own emotions onto parents they have placed in nursing homes. Who is really unhappy, your parent or you? You may not like seeing her in a nursing home, but she may be doing just fine.

NURSING-HOME REFORM

Take a hundred or so very sick, elderly people, place them out of public view, provide little funding and hire too few workers, most of them with no training and low wages, and you have a recipe for disaster. Abuse, neglect, dangerous living conditions, and generally woeful care are serious and common problems in nursing homes.

The 1987 Nursing Home Reform Act attempted to rectify this and it helped, but not as much as people had hoped. More than ten years later, federal studies found that more than a quarter of nursing homes had serious violations—deficiencies that led to injuries or put residents in immediate danger of serious harm. More than 40 percent had violations that created a risk for less serious harm. Nursing homes were found to be understaffed, complaints often went uninvestigated, and enforcement was weak.

New efforts, particularly the 1998 Nursing Home Initiative, have increased the number of investigators and imposed financial penalties for serious violations, among other things.

The effort to improve nursing-home care nationally will continue, but it's an enormous challenge, largely because nursing homes don't have enough funding and, perhaps more important, because the vast majority of people in nursing homes today have no family or friends monitoring their care. Nursing homes are largely out of view of society.

We can all help by getting involved in local nursing homes— volunteering, visiting, bringing in school groups, organizing excursions, etc. Perhaps a garden club would volunteer to plant annuals or hang flowerpots; some friends might make a special dinner for a small group of residents; the Boy Scouts might visit and bring homemade gifts; a singing group might put on a show.

Nursing homes should be a part of the community rather than apart from the community. By shunning older people and leaving them behind closed doors, we not only invite disaster, we lose an invaluable element of our society.

Chapter Twenty-One

THE AGING BRAIN

What Is Normal? • Getting Tested
• Alzheimer's Disease • Multi-Infarct Dementia
• Treatments

A PILE OF UNOPENED BILLS SITS ON YOUR MOTHER'S DESK, which is odd because she's always been extremely organized and punctual about paying her bills. Now that you think about it, you've noticed a number of unusual things about your mother recently. She missed two lunch dates with you. There was that silly incident over the dog that enraged her. And last week she called and asked you to come over right away, but when you got there she couldn't remember what was so urgent. In fact, she couldn't even remember calling you.

A cold wave passes through you. *Could it be . . . ?*

When elderly people become forgetful or confused, the possibility of Alzheimer's disease looms ominously, and for good reason. Alzheimer's is a cruel disease, and caring for someone with dementia is overwhelmingly painful and difficult. But don't assume that your parent's waning awareness or inability to concentrate is because of irreversible brain disease. Mild forgetfulness and confusion may be benign side effects of old age and mental inactivity, or they may be symptoms of depression or some other treatable disorder.

Before you panic, urge your parent to see a doctor who is well versed in such matters, and find out exactly what is wrong and what can be done about it. Because even if the symptoms are due to Alzheimer's disease, there are things that can be done about it, new drugs that are available, and much planning to attend to now.

What Is Normal?

The human brain, a chunk of jelly weighing about three pounds, is made up of a hundred billion nerve cells, all interconnected to form an elaborate communication web. But just as skin sags and bellies protrude, this fabulous control center reflects its age. However, lots of people remain sharp, imaginative, and productive well past 100. Most people are affected only mildly, in inconsequential ways. They may need an extra few minutes to remember a person's name or what it is they came into the kitchen to get; they may have some trouble balancing a checkbook or following a long story. But a little forgetfulness is nothing to worry about. Up to half of people over sixty-five say they have more trouble remembering things than they used to. (In fact, plenty of people over forty say exactly the same thing.) Given ample time, healthy people in their seventies and eighties can do just as well as young people on memory tests.

After eighty, almost everyone experiences some decline in their memory, as well as in mathematical, verbal, and spatial skills (although verbal skills seem to weather the storm pretty well in general). This is what doctors call "minimum cognitive impairment" (or "age-related memory loss" or "benign senescent forgetfulness").

While changes in the brain may be largely to blame, other factors certainly play a role in forgetfulness. Sometimes brains shift into low gear simply because they are inactive. If a vibrant, brilliant man loses his job and has little to do all day but stare at a television, his mental engine is bound to slip into idle.

Unfortunately, about 40 percent of people with minimum cognitive impairment go on to develop Alzheimer's within about three years. But that means that 60 percent do not.

Keep an eye on what's happening with your parent, and be sure her doctor knows of your concerns. A number of things can cause or exacerbate confusion and memory loss, including poor vision and hearing, hormonal changes, medications (including many over-the-counter drugs), illness, high blood pressure, vitamin deficiencies, dehydration, alcohol, depression, stress, and anxiety. All of these issues should be addressed when there is any concern about her mental mastery.

Be patient with your parent. Help her cope with her absentmindedness with notes, reminders, lists, and other memory tools. Encourage her to find some humor in her slipups. Assure her that mild forgetfulness is normal and nothing to be overly concerned about. In fact, excessive worrying about memory loss may only exacerbate the problem. Most important, urge your parent to use her mind more, not less.

Dementia

The word *dementia* comes from the Latin *de,* meaning without, and *mens,* which means mind. Dementia is not a specific illness, but rather a group of symptoms that have dozens of causes, in the same way a fever and chills may be caused by the flu, meningitis, malaria, or other illnesses. The symptoms of dementia include severe memory loss (especially short-term memory), confusion, disorientation, delusions, personality changes, and difficulty with language, math, and visual-spatial relationships (seeing and understanding three dimensions).

Dementia is not an inevitable part of aging, but the result of disease, infection, injury, or another ailment. Still, it is common in the elderly, especially in the very old. While the statistics vary, it's generally thought that about 10 percent of people over sixty-five and nearly half of those over eighty-five suffer from dementia.

About 60 percent of all cases of dementia are the result of Alzheimer's disease. About 30 percent are caused by small, often unnoticeable strokes, something called vascular or multi-infarct dementia. Quite often, however, Alzheimer's and vascular disease occur in combination, making it unclear exactly what is causing what.

The remaining 10 percent of dementia cases are due to other causes, such as long-term alcoholism, HIV infection, normal pressure hydrocephalus (in which spinal fluid builds up in the brain, causing memory loss, incontinence, and an unusual, shuffling gait), and Creutzfeldt-Jakob, Huntington's, Parkinson's, and Pick's disease. (If your parent has Parkinson's disease, don't assume that dementia is a future certainty. Most estimates suggest that less than half of these patients will develop dementia, and it tends to affect memory and the speed at which one thinks rather than language skills.)

Some causes of dementia—albeit very few—are, happily, reversible. These include vitamin deficiency, reactions to medications, thyroid disorder, dehydration, and, when diagnosed early, normal pressure hydrocephalus.

DEMENTIA OR OLD AGE?

In the early stages, it is difficult to distinguish between dementia and benign memory loss. (And, as we've noted, given enough time, benign loss may end up becoming dementia.) The symptoms of dementia can be

MENTAL HYGIENE

The adage "use it or lose it" seems to apply to the brain as well as the body. Studies suggest that elderly people who continue to read, work, travel, learn new skills, and pursue intellectual interests maintain a higher level of mental functioning than those who do not. In fact, those who exercise their minds may be able to slow, and in some cases actually reverse, the effects of time, recovering mental abilities they had ten or twenty years earlier. (See Chapter Five on ways to exercise the mind.)

Encourage your parent to use his mind more. If he is mobile, get him to attend continuing education classes, to travel, to volunteer, or to learn something brand new, like a language or computer skills. If he is less mobile, he might read (or listen to books on tape), play bridge or Scrabble, or do crossword puzzles.

Your parent needs to keep the rest of the package fit too, as there is convincing evidence that low blood pressure, low cholesterol, exercise, good nutrition, minimal or no alcohol use, and overall good health all contribute to a keener mind.

---

fairly innocuous at first, and most people compensate for minor mental slipups with reminders and notes, or they find excuses for their errors. *Oh, I'm sorry about our date. I was sure we said Tuesday.* Social skills are usually the last to go, so during short visits a person with early dementia may seem perfectly fine. He may chat about old times and remember who's who and what's happening. Families and friends, who don't want to believe that something might be wrong, are more than happy to dismiss a slightly disheveled appearance or a few memory lapses.

At some point, however, the problems become hard to ignore. The dementia begins to interfere with rela-tionships and the details of daily life, such as shopping, paying bills, or selecting clothing. Your parent might lose a particular skill—an avid crossword puzzle fan may have trouble filling in the blanks, or a lifetime golfer may fumble over selecting the proper clubs.

If you suspect dementia, think carefully about what your parent was like before. Are these problems new? All of us are far more aware of memory slips in older people than in younger ones. When Grandma loses her hat repeatedly an alarm goes off, but no one gives it a second thought when a teenager keeps losing his.

The primary symptom of dementia is short-term memory loss, which means that a person might remember

> " Mom would forget something on the stove, or forget what she just did, and I'd think, 'Well, she's getting older. Maybe I'm just looking for problems.' But finally I said, 'No, something is not right.'
>
> She would wear the same clothes over and over and not care if she took a shower or washed her hair or anything, which is really out of character because she used to be immaculate. She would say, 'No, I didn't wear this yesterday,' or 'I washed them,' when I knew she hadn't."
>
> —LINDA K.

the distant past vividly, but not remember recent events—what she had for breakfast, what she did yesterday, who she just spoke with on the phone, where she put her coat, what you told her last week or even an hour ago. A person might ask the same question over and over again.

Generally, a person's memory doesn't just slip, it disappears. That is, when you try to jog her memory— *Remember, I came over yesterday and we talked about going to Aunt Carol's today?*—it doesn't jog. (She might pretend she remembers, however.) A person doesn't simply forget what you said; she forgets speaking to you at all. She doesn't miss an appointment; she insists she never had one. She doesn't forget the name of the movie

she saw; she forgets that she went to a movie.

In the early stages, people may have trouble remembering the names of family and friends, or everyday objects. And they often have difficulty doing everyday tasks, such as paying bills, cleaning the kitchen, or shaving. As memories and abilities slowly slip away, people often, understandably, become anxious, agitated, frustrated, worried, and accusatory. *If I can't find my glasses, then somebody must have stolen them.* A change in environment and routine often compounds the confusion.

Getting Tested

If you suspect dementia, urge your parent to consult her doctor, and perhaps see a specialist or medical team for a diagnosis.

One pressing reason for getting tested early is that some cases of dementia are at least partially, if not fully, reversible. For example, depression can mimic the early phases of dementia, causing a disorder sometimes known as pseudodementia.

If your parent's illness cannot be cured, doctors can ease the symptoms and perhaps slow the progress of the disease, and take care of any medical problems that may be exacerbating the confusion, such as medications or depression.

In follow-up consultations, a social worker can counsel your family, teach you about lifestyle changes that will make everyone's life easier, and lead you to community programs that provide services and support to patients and their families.

A diagnosis will help your parent to understand what is happening to her. It should prompt her to attend to important business and perhaps do things that she has put off. And it allows your family to plan for the future while your parent can still be part of that planning. Learning the biological reasons for your parent's behavior should also give you all a little more patience, empathy, and tolerance.

MAKING
THE SUGGESTION

CONVINCING YOUR PARENT TO HAVE an evaluation is another matter, of course. It will be easier if she has noticed the problems and wants to know what is happening to her. But if your parent is like most people and denies that there are problems, insists that it's just old age, and resents any suggestion that something is wrong, then you have a challenge before you.

Wait for the right moment, when your parent is calm and at her most lucid. Discuss your concerns as delicately as possible, touching on some of the changes you have noticed, without criticizing or alarming her. Better yet, next time she has just forgotten something she shouldn't have, casually ask if she has noticed more of these slips than before, and if it bothers her. Ask what she thinks it might be and if she has mentioned it to her

doctor. Assure her that such memory lapses may be due to simple things, like medications or a vitamin deficiency, which can be fixed. Then urge her to see her doctor. And then be sure that she does.

If she resists, try the do-it-for-me approach: "It would really put my mind at ease if you were tested." Or call your parent's doctor and alert him or her to your concerns.

If you get nowhere, make an appointment for yourself to see her doctor, a geriatric social worker, or someone from the local Alzheimer's Association to discuss your parent's symptoms, issues that worry you, and how to proceed. Then, in a week or so, raise the issue again with your parent. Maybe now that she's had a little time to think about it, she will be more amenable to the idea. Or maybe she's forgotten that you ever mentioned it in the first place.

WHERE TO GET
AN EVALUATION

YOUR PARENT'S PRIMARY DOCTOR should be able to determine if there is evidence of dementia through a brief mental exam, and should also rule out or treat any reversible or contributing causes. Some will go on to do a full evaluation themselves; others will refer your parent to a specialist or group of specialists.

If the doctor dismisses the symptoms as part of old age or prescribes drugs for the symptoms without looking for the cause, consult another doctor. Look for a geriatric specialist or neurologist, or find out if there is a geriatric assessment center nearby. For a referral, call the local chapter of the Alzheimer's Association (800-272-3900 or www.alz.org), a large municipal hospital, or other medical professionals.

WHAT HAPPENS IN AN EVALUATION

ALZHEIMER'S CAN BE DIAGNOSED WITH certainty only by studying the brain during an autopsy. But doctors can rule out other possibilities and make

SYMPTOMS OF DEMENTIA

The symptoms of dementia represent a change from how a person used to be. They are persistent and grow steadily worse.

◆ **Memory loss:** Information, dates, events, and conversations, especially recent ones, are forgotten, frequently and often permanently.

◆ **Confusion:** Simple, everyday tasks, like cleaning the kitchen or paying the bills, may be difficult to perform.

◆ **Language difficulty:** Words are forgotten, misused, or garbled. Instead of saying "car keys," a person might say, "the thing you use to start up the car."

◆ **Disorientation:** A person gets lost or disoriented, even in familiar places.

◆ **Poor grooming:** Personal hygiene is neglected, and clothing may be

soiled or inappropriate for the event or the weather.

◆ **Poor judgment:** A person makes unsafe or unusual decisions.

◆ **Mood swings:** A person can easily become upset, agitated, or angry (especially when confronted with her memory loss). She may also have periods of unfounded euphoria.

◆ **Personality changes:** People are "not themselves." They might become uncharacteristically aggressive, or unpleasant personality traits may be amplified. Depression, social withdrawal, and anxiety are common, especially as the disease progresses.

◆ **Math difficulty:** Counting or balancing a checkbook is a challenge.

◆ **Repetition:** A person says or does the same thing over and over.

a diagnosis by process of elimination. This may seem like a crude technique, but it is a surprisingly good one, with an accuracy rate of about 95 percent. They also should look for factors that might be contributing to any confusion.

Doctors take different approaches in an evaluation. Some immediately order tests and set up appointments with specialists, while others focus on the family's recollections, complaints, and immediate needs in the beginning (a preferable approach).

In general, a thorough evaluation takes at least two or three hours and may include some or all of the following:

◆ **A patient history**. This is a critical first step. The doctor will talk to your parent, as well as to you and other family members, about your parent's health, past medical problems, medications used now and in the past (including over-the-counter medications), memory problems, any difficulty he might have in carrying out daily tasks, changes in behavior, and other such matters.

◆ **Examination of mood and mental state.** The doctor will take note of your parent's appearance and speech and ask about his moods and any psychiatric problems he might have, such as hallucinations, obsessions, depression, anxiety, or phobias. Several easy tests can assess the presence of depression, with questions about life, moods, hopefulness, etc.

In a preliminary evaluation, most doctors will conduct what is known as a Mini-Mental State Examination (MMSE). This fifteen-minute test assesses your parent's ability to perform simple tasks, recall new information, think abstractly, calculate, and communicate. He might be asked, for example, to count backward by sevens, say the date and location of where he is, follow a simple instruction (hold this piece of paper in your right hand, fold it, and put it on that table), recall information given moments ago, and perhaps draw some familiar object like a clock or a shape. Incorrect answers do not mean that a person has dementia, and doctors take into account the patient's education, age, degree of nervousness in the presence of an examiner, and previous abilities in judging the results.

During these questions, your parent may be frightened or embarrassed if she has trouble answering them. If you are present, don't give clues or advice, but do offer some quiet reassurance and comfort.

If your parent does poorly on this test, the doctor will try to determine when the problems began and how they have progressed over time, and may order a neurological exam and laboratory tests.

◆ **Laboratory tests.** Blood and urine samples will be examined for the presence of a variety of disorders that cause or contribute to confusion, such as infections, anemia, kidney and liver disease, thyroid abnormalities, heavy metal or drug poisoning, vitamin B-12 deficiency, syphilis, and AIDS.

" *My parents were married for fifty years, and about five years ago my mother started to be really horrible toward my father. She went through these wild ups and downs when she would yell at him r become terribly depressed and not want to go out or do anything. I think she finally exhausted him, because he died two years ago.*

We all blamed her, and for a time I would have as little as possible to do with her. I was so angry with her for being so cruel to Daddy. Then, last year, she became so depressed while visiting my brother in Florida that he took her to the hospital. They said she had been having mini-strokes.

Oh boy, did I feel badly. I mean, she didn't know what she had been doing. She couldn't control her rage or depression or paranoia. I'm just glad that I know now so that I can take care of her and stop resenting her so much. She really has no idea what she is doing."

— MARGE W.

◆ **Neurological exam.** Looking for physical signs of illness or injury, a doctor will test your parent's reflexes, sensory and motor function, gait, and coordination.

◆ **Psychiatric exam.** If depression, paranoia, anxiety, or other psychiatric problem is evident in preliminary test-ing, a doctor may suggest that your parent see a psychiatrist for a more thorough psychiatric exam and treatment.

◆ **Scans and spinal tap.** Imaging technology (CT, MRI, and other scans) is used to take pictures of the brain to detect damage from seizures, strokes, blood clots, tumors, bleeding, or a buildup of spinal fluid. While most doctors will order some sort of scan of the brain, some will not, as it is not always necessary.

A spinal tap, in which the doctor inserts a slender, hollow needle into the spine and draws a small sample of fluid, is usually used only if the doctor suspects an infection or disease of the nervous system. Current research suggests that spinal fluid might be used in the future to diagnose Alzheimer's.

Alzheimer's Disease

While dozens of diseases cause dementia, by far the most common cause is Alzheimer's disease, affecting more than four million people in this country.

In Alzheimer's disease, brain cells degenerate and the brain becomes littered with telltale debris, known as plaques and tangles. Amyloid plaques are clumps of an abnormal protein surrounded by dead or damaged tissue. Neurofibrillary tangles are twisted bundles of fibers that build up within brain cells. What causes this destruction is unknown. In fact, scientists are not even sure if Alzheimer's is a single disease with a single cause, or a number of related diseases caused by a variety of factors. In other words, different paths may lead to the same type of brain damage and symptoms.

Growing old is clearly the greatest risk factor for Alzheimer's disease. After age sixty-five, the rate of disease doubles with every five years of age.

Genetics also plays a role, which means that anyone with a parent or sibling with the disease is at greater risk. However, if your parent has Alzheimer's, don't become overly alarmed about your own future health. The genetic link is not an overwhelming one. The disease may require that you inherit a faulty gene from both parents. Or you may inherit only a propensity for the illness, and some second assault, such as an injury or exposure to a particular environmental toxin, may be necessary for the disease to develop.

There is also mounting evidence that high blood pressure, high cholesterol, and elevated levels of homocysteine (an amino acid associated with heart disease) increase the risk of getting Alzheimer's. (And taking cholesterol-lowering drugs appears to lower the risk.)

Beyond these causes, researchers are looking at a number of other possible causes for Alzheimer's, including toxins in the environment, the role of the immune system, prior brain injury, viruses, or simply worn-out brain cells that run amok.

> " When the doctor told me it was probably Alzheimer's, I just kept saying, 'It's got to be something else. It can't be right.' Here was a woman who was such an active person. She raised eight of us by herself. She was completely independent. I just couldn't believe that her mind could be affected like that.
>
> I was very frightened. You read and hear so much about people with Alzheimer's. My first thought was, she's going to become like a baby, like a vegetable.
>
> So far, I've been managing. It's a challenge, that's for sure. We have good days and bad days, but somehow we got through them all."
>
> —LINDA K.

Multi-Infarct Dementia

Thirty to 40 percent of all cases of dementia are thought to be wholly or partially caused by a series of strokes so small they can occur unnoticed. Blood flow is blocked to some part of the brain, usually because of a clog, clot, or rupture, leaving behind a pocket of damaged or dead tissue. With each successive stroke, the brain loses more and more of its ability to function.

THE STAGES OF ALZHEIMER'S DISEASE

Although people with Alzheimer's react uniquely to the illness and follow an unpredictable course, experts have tracked a few of the more common symptoms of the illness. The stages described below are only a rough outline of what may occur over the course of a person's illness, which typically lasts five to twelve years.

Stage I: *A person with the disease is usually still alert and social, and may be very much enjoying life, although she may know that something is not quite right. Frustrated by the forgetfulness and afraid of what is happening, some people become anxious and/or depressed, which only exacerbates the memory loss and confusion.*

Short-term memory fades. A person has trouble remembering recent events, learning new things, retaining information, and concentrating.

Speech is slightly impaired. A person confuses one word for another, can't remember the right word or a name.

Hygiene is not what it once was. Clothing may be soiled or disheveled, and bathing and grooming forgotten.

Judgment is hindered, and thinking abstractly is difficult.

Emotional responses are erratic and exaggerated. A person may become easily upset, anxious, angry, or depressed, often in response to the changes taking place.

Daily tasks, such as tying a shoe, balancing a checkbook, or putting dishes in the dishwasher, can be challenging and may take longer to do.

A person at this stage might get disoriented in familiar places and on often-used roads.

Stage II: *The signs are obvious. A person may exhibit bizarre behavior, such as getting lost on the way to the bathroom in his own house, stockpiling food, or becoming outraged for no apparent reason.*

Short-term memory is largely gone. A person is unable to learn new information or skills, and may forget the names and identities of friends and family. He may also have trouble dealing with new or unexpected situations.

Coordination is poor, creating a risk for falls and accidents.

Confusion and poor coordination combine to make daily tasks difficult. At this stage, a person often requires some assistance with bathing, eating, and dressing.

Complex tasks that require any decision making or a series of steps are overwhelming.

Disorientation is pronounced. A person might not be able to find the bathroom in his own home.

People may wander away at this stage, especially if they are in an unfamiliar place.

Agitation and pacing are common.

Moods are even more exaggerated. A person may be uncooperative, hostile, or aggressive, although some people become serene and peaceful. (They may be less frustrated by the illness because they don't remember what they used to be able to do.)

Many people become paranoid and have hallucinations and/or delusions.

People often have trouble controlling impulses at this point, so they might be rude or vulgar. They might undress in public or make sexual comments or advances.

Language and speech troubles worsen.

Ability to add, subtract, or do other calculations is virtually lost. (The checkbook may be overdrawn or bills left unpaid.)

Sleep cycles fall out of sync, so a person may sleep at odd hours.

Stories or actions are repeated monotonously.

Stage III: *At this point, people are totally dependent and require constant care.*

Confusion is acute. All short-term memory, and most or all long-term memory, is gone.

Communication skills, as well as the ability to walk, are also usually gone by this point.

People are incontinent.

People often lose a good deal of weight.

Physical rigidity and seizures may occur.

Hallucinations (seeing or hearing things that don't exist), delusions (irrational or unfounded beliefs), and paranoia (in particular, a belief that others are trying to kill the person or that a spouse is cheating) are all common.

Eventually, people are unable to speak, get out of bed, or feed themselves. They become susceptible to malnutrition, infections, dehydration, pneumonia, and other illness. The cause of death is usually due to infections (of the lungs, skin, or urinary tract).

People with multi-infarct dementia (also referred to as vascular dementia or chronic cerebrovascular lesions) are often at risk of having strokes because of diabetes, high blood pressure, or other cardiovascular disease. Doctors can spot the disease with a scan of the brain.

While the symptoms are similar to those described for Alzheimer's, multi-infarct dementia often affects physical abilities before it affects the mind. A person might become weak, lose some vision, or become incontinent before he becomes forgetful or confused. Symptoms typically appear suddenly and grow worse in spurts, more like walking down stairs as opposed to the slow slide that occurs in Alzheimer's disease.

If diagnosed early, the progression of multi-infarct dementia can often be slowed by lowering the risk of stroke. This is done by giving medications that treat high blood pressure, high cholesterol, or vascular disease; improving circulation through diet and exercise; and improving the management of diabetes.

Dealing with the Diagnosis

Under normal conditions, doctors meet privately with patients to discuss a diagnosis, and then let the patients decide how much, if anything, they want to tell their families. But dementia derails everything in life, including the doctor-patient relationship. Quite often doctors confer with the entire family, which is helpful because every family member is affected by this illness. But this should be done only with your parent's consent. And, as tempting as it might be, the doctor should never discuss the diagnosis only with the family, bypassing your parent completely.

No matter how confused your parent is, and no matter how painful the news may be to her, she should be told her diagnosis. When it comes to an individual's health, honesty is always the best policy. All of us have a fundamental right to know what is happening to us, regardless of the severity. Knowledge about our own health allows us to retain some control over our lives, to plan for the future, and to understand the present.

People with dementia often take the news far more calmly than their families expect. Of course it is upsetting, terribly upsetting, but they already know something is wrong, even if they haven't readily admitted it. They have been worried and have had their suspicions and fears about what is happening. A diagnosis lets them know why their world is so askew. It also gives them the opportunity to begin to deal, both practically and emotionally, for what is to come.

If you think that for some reason your parent doesn't want to know, then ask. *The doctor wants us to come in and discuss the results of your tests. Do you want to come? Do you want us to come with you?*

BREAKING THE NEWS

WHEN YOU OR THE DOCTOR TALKS with your parent about a diagnosis of dementia, try to understand what she may be experiencing. In addition to obvious feelings of devastation, she is, most likely, afraid of losing dignity and respect, and of becoming a burden to the family, among other things. Listen, share her concerns, offer warmth and support, and reassure her that she will not be alone. Tell her that you all, as a family, are going to get through this together. Without dismissing her fears, focus on all she can still do and on the good times she and her family can still have together.

Of course, you will have your own turbulent emotions to contend with as well. You may have suspected Alzheimer's and now realize you were totally unprepared for the truth. You may feel shock, horror, anger, grief, and helplessness. You may feel even more sorry for yourself than for your parent and deeply afraid of the work that lies ahead. You may secretly hope that the disease runs its course quickly. You are surely going to experience some grief over what you have already lost and what you are going to lose.

These are all normal reactions. Don't be ashamed of them. You have a great deal to comprehend and to come to terms with. Be kind to yourself. Take time to digest all this. Spend time with family and friends, or carve out some time to be alone. Let the grief and tears come. And then know that there is a lot of good support out there for you, as well.

NOW WHAT?

THE DOCTOR OR A MEMBER OF HIS or her staff should talk with your family about the future and set you up with a social worker who can provide referrals and counseling. If you ask for this assistance and none is offered, do some research on your own, because a diagnosis by itself is of little use. You need help. Whether your parent has Alzheimer's disease or vascular

---

FORGIVE YOURSELF

If you have been snapping impatiently at your father or criticizing him for being disruptive, forgetful, or rude, you may feel guilty once you realize that his behavior is due to an illness. Forgive yourself. You reacted perfectly normally under the circumstances and have nothing to feel guilty about. In fact, even now that you know the diagnosis, you are sure to have plenty of angry outbursts in the future. It would be almost impossible not to, given the nature of this disease. Give your parent as much love as you can, forget about what happened yesterday, and focus your energy on today.

ON THE LOOKOUT FOR COMPLICATING FACTORS

If your parent has dementia, be aware of other problems that can exacerbate the symptoms (or cause confusion on their own).

◆ **Depression.** Depression can mimic early Alzheimer's, or it can coincide with dementia, especially in the early stages. Frustrated and saddened by the symptoms of dementia, people often become depressed. But depression will only worsen forgetfulness, confusion, and other symptoms. Identifying and treating depression—and it is extremely treatable—can noticeably alleviate early confusion and memory loss.

◆ **Delirium.** While it typically comes on suddenly—in a matter of days or even hours—delirium is sometimes confused with dementia or may coexist with it. Be on the lookout for delirium because when someone with dementia becomes sick with some other ailment, and especially if he is moved to a hospital, he is apt to become delirious. Symptoms vary widely but often include disorientation, inattentiveness, and changes in personality. Delirium is reversible, but it must be treated immediately.

◆ **Medication.** Antidepressants, heart medications, anti-inflammatory drugs, sleeping pills, ulcer medications, insulin, and cold medications can all cause confusion, agitation, and other symptoms. Your parent's doctor should be aware of all drugs that he takes, including nonprescription ones.

---

dementia, call the Alzheimer's Association (800-272-3900 or www.alz.org), which has local chapters throughout the country that run invaluable support groups and provide referrals to local services, from housing and legal aid to financial and medical assistance. Call other local senior service organizations as well, if you need further guidance and information on specific topics.

PLANNING FOR THE FUTURE

BECAUSE YOUR PARENT IS GOING TO need extensive care, and at some point will be unable to make decisions for herself, your family needs to plan now for the future. If she has not already done so, your parent should name a durable power of attorney, have a will drafted, and sign and fully discuss advance directives (see Chapter

◆ **Alcohol**. While prolonged, heavy use of alcohol can cause permanent brain damage and dementia, even moderate drinking can worsen confusion, agitation, and depression. Urge your parent to stop, or at least cut way back.

◆ **Vision and hearing impairment**. Make sure that your parent gets his eyes and ears checked regularly, as poor hearing or blurred vision will make his world that much more confusing.

◆ **Vitamin B-12 deficiency**. Medications or age can impede a body's absorption of vitamin B-12, causing fatigue, depression, anxiety, memory loss, and other problems typical of dementia. The deficiency is treated with injections of the vitamin.

Seventeen). It's vital that she have a medical health-care proxy giving someone else the authority to make medical decisions on her behalf. Also, she, or you, should compile other important documents, such as tax returns and insurance information (all listed on page 12). Be sure that family members know where these items are kept (because she certainly won't remember).

Your family also needs to consider how future medical and living expenses will be paid, and you should all discuss, at some length, your parent's future care and living situation. You should learn about communtiy service. And while you may be loath even to contemplate it, most families deplete their financial, physical, and emotional resources and eventually have to look for some other housing situation. In most cases, that means a nursing home.

Even if you believe that you would never, ever put your parent in a nursing home, learn what's available, because you simply never know and it's best to be prepared. Start looking sooner rather than later, as many facilities are full and have waiting lists.

While a diagnosis like this forces one to think about the future, it can also magnify the true value of the present. Talk with your parent about her priorities. If your mother is still relatively lucid, find out if there is anything that she wants to do while she still can. Does she need to resolve an old conflict or visit a distant friend? Has she always wanted to take a trip to San Francisco? Try Thai food? Go back to a childhood home? Remember, while it may be hard to believe right now, life is not over, either for you or your parent.

Finally, while it's terrifying to consider, think about who would care for your parent if something were to happen to you or another primary caregiver. Choose a family member, close friend, or trusted adviser who can take over as surrogate. Or talk with her doctor, the local mental health office, or local adult protective services office.

Treating Dementia

The best medicine for your parent will come from you, not the pharmacist. Right now, more than anything else, your parent needs a safe and familiar environment, a simple and calm routine that can be adjusted to meet her changing needs, easy mental stimulation, a lot of reminders and cues, a good diet, exercise, social activities, and a hefty helping of love and patience.

Even troubling behavioral problems, such as irritability, agitation, and aggression, can often be improved with changes in your parent's environment, her routines, and your approach.

To give your parent what she needs now, you need to take care of yourself, learn about this disease, master some tricks for coping, find ways to deal with stress, and dig deep inside yourself to muster up the strength, courage, flexibility, and patience for all that lies ahead.

MEDICATIONS

THERE ARE NO MAGIC BULLETS FOR dementia. Scientists have not found a way to stop the illness or even markedly slow it. But some drugs do ease and even temporarily reverse symptoms in some patients. And while it's not all that useful to those in the throes of it now, current research is promising.

Multi-infarct dementia is treated with drugs that reduce the likelihood of further strokes, as well as with dietary changes and exercise. Several newer medications slow the progression of some symptoms of Alzheimer's, but only in some patients. They do not, however, stop or even slow the eventual course of the illness. Most of these drugs must be started in the early or middle stages of the disease.

In Alzheimer's disease, levels of acetylcholine, a chemical involved in thinking and memory, decline. Three drugs, donepezil (Aricept), rivastigmine (Exelon), and galantamine (Reminyl), stop or slow the breakdown of acetylcholine. When taken early in the course of the disease (by people with mild to moderate Alzheimer's), these drugs appear to improve memory and thinking in some patients. They also seem to ease symptoms, such as delusions and agitation. (It is difficult for scientists, and even families, to know exactly what the drugs are doing or not doing, or how a person might fare without them.) Medications do not, unfortunately, cure the disease. They are useful for a limited time, but eventually the disease runs its course.

A fourth drug, memantine (Namenda), works on a different chemical in the brain, glutamate, and is used for patients with moderate to severe Alzheimer's. Its effectiveness is still unclear. (Most physicians no longer prescribe tacrine, or Cognex because it does not act specifically in the brain, and so it is more toxic than the other drugs and can cause liver damage.) Scientists are looking at a number of other possibilities for treating Alzheimer's in the future, and several drugs look promising.

Beyond these drugs, which aim at treating the actual disease, there are several medications that alleviate specific symptoms, such as extreme anxiety, agitation, violence, depression, aggression, insomnia, delusions, and hallucinations.

Although they can be invaluable, these drugs should be used only when other approaches (discussed in the next chapter) have failed, because, for the most part, they simply sedate the patient and can increase confusion. They should also be used hand-in-hand with continuing efforts to change behaviors through changes in the environment.

For example, antipsychotic drugs, are useful in treating psychotic behaviors such as delusions, paranoia, and hallucinations. But when it comes to nonpsychotic behaviors, such as agitation and violence, they do little more than knock the person out. When

DRUGS COMMONLY USED TO TREAT MENTAL PROBLEMS

Problem	Drugs Commonly Used	Possible Side Effects
Depression (low mood, weight loss, irritability, social withdrawal)	Paxil, Zoloft, Remeron, Lexapro, Effexor, Prozac	Drowsiness, constipation, anxiety, dry mouth
Anxiety (agitation, restlessness, excessive fear or worry, combative behavior)	Ativan, Xanax, BuSpar, and Serax Antidepressants (Zoloft, Remeron, and Paxil) are sometimes used to treat depression, especially when it is mixed with anxiety. Some anti-epileptics, such as Valproate, Neurontin, and Lamictal, are used for agitation.	Drowsiness, loss of inhibition, agitation, anger, and increasing tolerance to the drug
Psychosis (hallucinations, delusions, paranoia) and nonpsychotic symptoms, such as aggression, violence, and hostility	Zyprexa, Haldol, Seroquel, and Risperdal	Drowsiness, rigidity, tremors, jerking, twitching, confusion, dry mouth, constipation, urinary retention

antipsychotics are stopped, the problem behavior actually often improves on its own.

Antipsychotic medications often cause tremors, jerks, and other involuntary motions (called "extrapyramidal symptoms"). These are then treated with other drugs that can ease the tremors but often increase confusion. And so, as can easily happen in medicine, one drug followed by the next begins to pull the patient into a downward cycle of more confusion and more sedation.

Despite all this, these drugs are often necessary—particularly when someone is violent, combative, or dangerous and cannot be controlled with other means. But try alternatives, and be keenly aware of what is happening with your parent's medications. Nursing-home patients, in particular,

FOR MORE HELP

Alzheimer's Association
800-272-3900
www.alz.org

Alzheimer's Disease Education and Referral Center
800-438-4380
www.alzheimers.org

National Institute of Neurological Disorders and Stroke
800-352-9424
www.ninds.nih.gov

are often given sedatives and antipsychotics when other nondrug approaches would be far more effective. (Also know that antipsychotics can cause a more extreme form of jerking and tremors, called tardive dyskinesia, which may not improve even after the medication is stopped.)

When you must resort to drugs, remember the rule "low and slow"—start with a very low dose and then slowly increase it as necessary. Once a drug has had the desired effect, ask the doctor when your parent might be weaned off it, to see if it is still needed. People with Alzheimer's change quickly—a jumping bean who needs something to calm her down can turn into a couch potato as the disease progresses, making a drug unnecessary and dangerous.

Be careful about mixing drugs. Drugs that act on the brain to reduce hallucinations or paranoia, for example, do not mix well with alcohol or a number of other drugs, including over-the-counter pills found in most household medicine cabinets. The combined effect on the brain may cause greater confusion, agitation, and disorientation.

Consult your parent's doctor before she takes any new medicine, even if it seems benign. Some drugs, such as over-the-counter sleeping pills, act by lowering levels of acetylcholine, the very chemical that is already in dire shortage in the brains of people with Alzheimer's disease. These will only worsen confusion and other symptoms.

ANTIOXIDANTS
AND OTHER POSSIBILITIES
....

SOME STUDIES SUGGEST THAT VITA-
min E might slow the progression of
Alzheimer's by defending the body
from molecules called "free radicals."
Free radicals, which are a byproduct
of normal cell function, damage healthy
cells and, according to some research,
contribute to Alzheimer's disease.
Vitamin E is a natural antioxidant and
defends the body against such attacks.
And vitamin E is often in short supply late in life.

Scientists are also examining
whether gingko, a tree extract, might
delay or prevent some symptoms of
dementia. They are studying estrogen,
to see if it might prevent development
of Alzheimer's in women who have a
family history of the illness. And they
are looking at whether inflammation
contributes to dementia, and if nonsteroidal anti-inflammatory drugs
(NSAIDs), such as aspirin or ibuprofen, might slow onset of the disease.
(Do not give your parent anti-inflammatory drugs without the doctor's
approval, as they should not be used
with the medications usually used to
treat Alzheimer's.)

Your parent should talk with her
doctor before taking any dietary supplements, herbal extracts, hormones,
or drugs.

If she is interested in being involved
in research, she might consider being
part of a clinical trial. To find out about
current studies and possible participa-
tion in them, contact the Alzheimer's
Disease Education and Referral Center
(800-438-4380 or www.alzheimers.org)
or the National Institute of Neurological
Disorders and Stroke (800-352-9424 or
www.ninds.nih.gov).

Chapter Twenty-Two

LIVING WITH DEMENTIA

*Deflating Stress • Forgetting Logic
• Finding Patience • Simplifying the World
• Using Diversions • And More*

....

IF MARRIAGE AND CHILDREN TEST A PERSON'S FLEXIBILITY AND patience, then caring for a person with dementia is the final exam. Rarely is one asked to give so much only to receive so much aggravation and anguish in return. Dementia doesn't just take away a person's ability to remember names, calculate numbers, or tell a good joke; it steals his personality, his endearing quirks, and his beloved memories. You are left to care for a hauntingly familiar stranger, someone whose physical features and occasional glances may be heartwarming, but whose behavior and personality, more and more, seem to belong to someone else—someone else whom you might not like in the least.

For you, as the child in this relationship, witnessing such a transformation is unnerving. Your parent, the person who had the wisdom of experience, the person who made vital decisions, the person who was once your sole caregiver, is increasingly dependent, incompetent, and childlike. Your father may throw tantrums, have trouble feeding himself, or forget his way home. Your mother may become slovenly and self-centered. She may become rude, critical, and tyrannical. And with all this, you will be called upon to care for her in ways you never imagined, sometimes against her wishes or without her understanding.

While you still love the person you knew, you may feel disdain, resentment, or even disgust toward the person she has become. At the same time, you are grieving the loss, one painful step at a time, of the person she used to be. It's a confusing and sharp stew of emotions that can wear a person down very quickly.

The cruelty and heartbreak of this disease can't be avoided. Nevertheless, you can alleviate some of the symptoms, learn tricks for coping with others, and get outside support, all of which will make this ride a little bit smoother for both of you.

Helping Yourself

Dementia calls for a stronger-than-usual arsenal of self-preservation measures. This illness takes such an enormous toll on family members that many families end up, bedraggled and beaten, at the door of the nearest nursing home.

So now more than ever, you have to take care of yourself. People caring for dementia patients are at extremely high risk of illness and depression. And you'll be no good to your parent if you're in a hospital bed. This is an enormous undertaking. Don't underrate what is happening to you.

Exercise, eat well (sure you know it, but now you really have to do it), join a support group, schedule breaks, get plenty of help, and find ways to relieve stress and anger. Review Chapter Three and try the suggestions outlined below.

Keep in mind, your own care and your parent's care are now inseparable. Not only do you need to preserve your energy, health, and sanity so you can provide care, but your parent's mental state is going to reflect yours. If you are on the verge of exploding or crying, he will feel it and become that much more anxious and unsettled himself. This, of course, will make you much more stressed. And so on. Life can easily swirl downward into a tailspin of mounting aggravation and agitation. If, on the other hand, you are rested, calm, and patient, your parent will be more calm and composed.

ACKNOWLEDGE THE SITUATION

EARLY IN THIS DISEASE, IT'S NATURAL to believe, on some level, that your parent will wake up one day and be the person she used to be. That kind of hopefulness gets people through the day. But it also leads to frustration and despair when, instead, your parent wakes up each day to be less of who she was.

If your parent has irreversible dementia, she will not get better. She will not be able to do things today that she couldn't do yesterday (except perhaps very briefly, with the help of new medications). She will probably be even less capable tomorrow. You cannot teach her new things or remind her of old things.

Acknowledging the situation and accepting these harsh realities is extraordinarily painful, but it is the only way to appreciate whatever you still have, reduce the frustration, find new ways to deal with her, and prepare for what lies ahead.

REMEMBER, IT IS A DISEASE

WITH DEMENTIA, THERE ARE NO physical signs of illness—no cast, no bandages, not even a temperature for you to check. Your mother looks the same as she always did, so it's natural

> " *Sometimes it's as if my mother were dead, the woman who raised me, the one that I used to go to for comfort. I don't have her anymore, and I miss her terribly.*"
> —FRANCINE R.

to expect her to be the same. But she is not. She cannot control her behavior. She is not repeating the same questions over and over to exasperate you. She is not fidgeting frantically to annoy you. She cannot force herself to remember the answers any more than someone with a broken leg can force himself to walk.

Because of severe damage to her brain, your mother has not only lost her memory of people and events, she also has lost her ability to interpret the world or express her needs. She paces frantically because her bladder is full and she doesn't remember what she is supposed to do about it. She yells at you because her belly hurts. She wanders because she feels lost. She thinks that the nurse who is wrapping her arm in a blood pressure cuff is trying to hurt her.

Your mother may seem as if she has reverted back to childhood, but she has not. A child can learn and take instructions. A child remembers that the stove was hot and burned him, so he doesn't touch it again. A child feels safe in your arms and knows that you are not trying to kill him with your embrace.

Your mother's world is not just fading, it is topsy-turvy, illogical, and at times very, very scary. She is lost, out of control, and unable to understand her own fear, much less the cause of her fear.

But it is not her; it is a disease. Her brain cells are being destroyed daily. If you could put a bandage on her head—say, a bathing cap painted with damaged cells and dead debris—perhaps you would approach her a bit differently.

Bathing caps aside, just keep this fact planted firmly in your mind, and repeat it daily: *This is a disease; she can't help it; she is not doing this, the disease is.* It should alleviate some of the frustration and help you to keep some perspective.

TAKE TIME TO GRIEVE

WHETHER YOU HAVE ALWAYS ADORED your parent, or battled with her daily, or resented her silently, you are losing her now, one small piece at a time. This is the longest, slowest good-bye ever said. And no matter what sort of relationship the two of you have, saying good-bye to a parent is painful.

You are desperately busy facing the challenge, trying to get through each minute, and anticipating the future, but take time to grieve, because that is largely what this is about. Grieving means allowing the pain and tears, it means recognizing a loss, and it means being kind to yourself.

BE ALERT TO DEPRESSION

DEPRESSION IS VERY COMMON among those caring for someone with dementia. Be alert to the signs in yourself and others caring for your parent. If you feel that you can't get out of bed in the morning, can't face the day, can't stop crying or yelling at people, can't eat or eat too much, can't sleep or can't wake up, can't stop feel-ing miserable and worthless, and question the reasons for being alive, get help immediately. Call your doctor, a therapist, or a psychiatrist.

DEFLATING STRESS AND FINDING PATIENCE

YOUR MISSION IS TO STAY CALM, always, in a situation that evokes every emotion but calm. As your parent pees on your couch or accuses you of trying to kill her, and you finally find your lost car keys in the freezer, you may be feeling anything but calm. But it is the only emotion that will get you through this.

You need to find ways to relieve the pressure, to think clearly, and to draw out that calm, patient caregiver that resides deep within you. Yoga, tai chi, deep breathing exercises, support groups, walking around the block a few times, and practicing relaxation techniques will help a lot. Of course, going into your room and yelling, punching pillows, swearing furiously, and falling into a puddle of tears has its benefits as well.

In addition to some long-term approaches, like a regular lunch date with a friend who's in the same situation, and a stint at the gym each morning, you need some emergency techniques that will bring you to that serene, superhuman place in a pinch.

When your parent pours a whole bottle of shampoo on your rug because she saw a dirt spot, or throws dinner in the garbage because she saw bugs crawling on it (they were black pepper

✔ A SAFETY CHECKLIST

☐ Turn the temperature on the water heater down to 120°F. and label all hot-water faucets clearly with large red letters. A person with dementia may not test the water temperature. If it's too hot, he may not realize immediately that he is being burned and may not react quickly enough to escape serious injury.

☐ Because people with dementia can easily get lost, get your parent an identification bracelet that says "memory loss" and an address and phone number. If he wanders (or even if he doesn't), alert local police and neighbors to the situation. Have a photo of him on hand and perhaps a piece of unwashed clothing (for police dogs). Better yet, sign your parent up with the Alzheimer's Association's Safe Return Program, a national program that helps locate people with Alzheimer's who get lost.

☐ If your parent wanders, put locks on doors leading outside. Place them high or low on the door where he won't easily find them. You can also place bells on doors so you know when your parent has exited.

☐ Post by every phone a clearly written list of emergency numbers (police, fire, poison control, doctor) and instructions for calling 911. You can also get phones with memory-dial buttons labeled with photos—a picture of you on one, a picture of a fire on another, a picture of a police officer on another, and so on.

☐ Install handrails and grab bars throughout the house, as dementia affects coordination and balance. Remove loose rugs and clutter on the floor. Check that chairs are sturdy and have strong armrests. Buy a cane or walker if necessary.

---

flakes), pause before responding. Just pause. Don't say anything. Look quietly at the situation and decide if it has truly ruined your life. Take a few deep breaths. Roll your neck from side to side several times. Repeat your mantra: "I am calm. I am calm. I am calm." Breathe deeply a few more times. And then calmly, ever so calmly, tell your mother that she's probably right. When she's not looking, pull the roast out of the garbage and rinse it off, or make some peanut butter sandwiches.

From time to time, give yourself a hug. (If you've never tried to hug yourself, go ahead, wrap your arms around yourself, and squeeze. You need a big one right about now.)

☐ Lock (or install childproof latches on) any cabinets that contain household cleaners, solvents, medicines, matches, lighters, liquor, knives, laundry detergents and bleach, scissors, or other dangerous items. Check for hazards outside the house as well, such as paints, clippers, saws, grills, and lighter fluid.

☐ Remove bedroom and bathroom door locks that are operated from the inside so he can't accidentally lock himself in. Hide a spare key outside your house in case your parent locks you out.

☐ Your parent should not smoke when unattended. He might forget a burning cigarette or drop a smoldering butt in the wrong place.

☐ If your parent has trouble operating the stove, remove the knobs or encase them so he can't leave the burner or the oven on. Or put the electric stove on a timer so it can be operated only between certain hours. Ask an electrician for other possibilities.

☐ Driving will have to stop fairly early on. See page 129 for how to deal with an elderly, incompetent driver. The good news about Alzheimer's is, if you tell him the car is not working and headed for the repair shop, he might not remember that you've been telling him the same story for weeks.

☐ Remove artificial fruit, food-shaped magnets, or anything else that might be confused for food. Sometimes even small items stored in the kitchen, such as tacks, erasers, corks, and paper clips, can be mistaken for food, so store them elsewhere.

☐ Place decals at eye level on any glass doors or large windows so your parent doesn't mistakenly try to walk through the glass.

PUT YOURSELF
IN HER SHOES

IMAGINE BEING GIVEN A COLOSSAL assignment, one that you simply cannot do. You are overwhelmed by the challenge and humiliated by your lack of ability. You know, on some level, it's not difficult. In fact, you think perhaps you've been able to do it in the past. But today it feels like scaling the Empire State Building. Making matters worse, someone is standing over you growing increasingly impatient and annoyed as you struggle and fail. The pressure and embarrassment make it harder for you to think, so you fumble even more.

66 *I have said things that I*
would never have dreamed
I could say to my mother. I yell
and scream at her. I've cursed her.
Sometimes I hate her. I was brought
up to know that you don't do those
kinds of things. But you get to a
point where you just don't know
what else to do. I'm usually a pretty
controlled person, but with this, you
don't have any control. Or I don't.

    I don't like these sides of myself.
I don't like what's happening to me.
Every day I pray for patience."

—MARTHA S.

For your parent, getting dressed or eating a meal that involves several foods and an assortment of utensils are formidable tasks. She can't remember what to do next or why she is doing this at all. If you criticize her, hurry her, or become annoyed, she will only become more anxious and confused, and less able to perform. But if you can lower your expectations, muster a good dose of patience and compassion, and give her ample time, she might actually be more successful with the task at hand. Or at least she might not get as angry about it.

FORGET LOGIC

OF COURSE BANANAS SHOULD NOT BE put in the oven and hair should not be combed with a toothbrush. But if you attempt to explain why to your parent, you will be wasting your breath. She is living in a world where everything is changing. Nothing is familiar and nothing makes sense. You can't reason with her, so stop trying. You are wasting your breath and raising your blood pressure needlessly. Instead, give her a hug and hand her the hairbrush.

VENT YOUR ANGER— SOMEPLACE ELSE

YOUR WORST ANGER MAY ERUPT DURing the early stages of the disease, when you are still fighting what is happening, trying to hold on to the person your parent was, and struggling unsuccessfully for a logical explanation. You go for a visit (or to another part of your house) and, before seeing your parent, you promise yourself that today you will be patient. But within minutes of walking in the door, you find yourself snapping, "Mother!! What have you done? How many times have I told you not to rip up the mail? Why do you do this to me?" Minutes later, you hate yourself for getting so irate, and you hate her, or this disease, for turning you into a shrew.

    Welcome to dementia. This disease distorts the personalities not only of patients, but of their caregivers as well. People who never used to swear suddenly know every curse in the book. People who were kind become crabby. People who love their parents dearly suddenly want them to disappear.

    The problem is that while dementia breeds anger, it also feeds off it.

Yelling at your parent or yanking his shirt off because you can't stand to wait while he fumbles with each button may trigger a wild, emotional tirade. If you can back off and cool down, things will go more smoothly, and you may actually get him dressed and fed faster.

When you can't cool off, vent your anger elsewhere. Make sure your parent is safe, and then leave the room. Yell out loud or punch a pillow. And always have a list of friends or support group members you can call when you need to release some steam.

When you do slip and lose your temper with your parent, which you are bound to do fairly frequently, forgive yourself. You acted naturally, and if there is anything positive about this disease, it's that your parent will forget that you ever even raised your voice.

FOCUS ON THE GOOD TIMES

EMBRACE ANY PASSING MOMENTS OF intimacy or apparent awareness. You may not get them toward the end, but early on there may be breaks in this storm when your parent returns to you. Suddenly, there is a moment of singing or dancing or hugging, or maybe your parent tells an old story or gives you a familiar look or thanks you for all you are doing. Savor it. Remember it. Make a note of it and pin it to your wall. This is a shot of strength and pleasure that you may not get again.

DON'T ASSUME SHE'S MISERABLE

EARLY ON, WHEN YOUR PARENT IS still aware of what her abilities used to be, she may be extremely upset about what she can no longer do. But as the disease progresses, she may become perfectly content in her mixed-up, timeless world. She may not know that life used to be different. No matter how involved she used to be, she may be happy just sitting, stroking a pet, watching the leaves blow in the breeze, or listening to a favorite song.

BEWARE OF ABUSE

When a parent has dementia, the stress can become overwhelming, and you may find yourself lashing out, shaking, pushing, or even striking your parent. If this happens, get away from him immediately. Drop whatever you are doing and walk away. Call a neighbor, a relative, or a friend to take over for you. You need support and you need a break, and you need it right now.

Call the local chapter of the Alzheimer's Association. Most chapters have help lines that can get you through the moment of crisis and help arrange emergency respite care.

It may seem sad to you, but this may be all she needs right now.

REMEMBER YOUR SENSE OF HUMOR

IF YOUR MOTHER THINKS YOU STOLE her stockings so that you could wear them over your head and rob her, it's sad, but it's also amusing. Help her look for her stockings and assure her that you are not going to rob her. Then, when you repeat the story to your sister, go ahead, pull the stockings over your head, and have a good laugh about it. *What was I going to steal, her dentures?*

You need to grieve, of course. You are losing your parent in a very painful way. Yet despite the gravity of the situation—and because of it—you have to give yourself permission to laugh.

GIVE YOURSELF *A LOT* OF CREDIT

IT MAY NOT FEEL AS IF YOU ARE doing a good job. In fact, most of the time it may feel quite the opposite. You may not give your parent the time or attention he needs. You may lash out at him. At times, you may wish that he would die. You would have to be a saint to do otherwise.

Give yourself a lot of credit. If it helps, write a list of all that you are doing for your parent and put it someplace where you will see it regularly. Then stand in front of the mirror and tell yourself that you are a good per-

> " *Sometimes, she says something—a little joke or a comment—that shows me she is still there. Buried under that disease, a piece of my mother still survives. It's that little piece that remains, the memories of who she was and those soft, familiar hands that keep me going."*
> —MARGE W.

son. You are. In fact, anyone caring for someone with dementia is an unsung hero.

Remember, if you are in a support group or know people who are in a similar situation, don't compare yourself to them. Their parents may have different symptoms of dementia, they may have a very different relationship with their parents, and their lives may hold entirely different pressures. Furthermore, they may treat their parents better when people are watching than when they are alone at home.

USE HELP AND RESPITE

TO PRESERVE YOUR SANITY AND health, get help early and take regular breaks. Before your parent is accustomed to a routine that includes only you, get her used to other caregivers—people in the family, companions, or a day-care program. The longer you wait to take a break, the harder it will be for her to accept change, a new place, or unfamiliar people.

Once you arrange for help or respite:

◆ Don't ask your parent if she wants to go to day care or if she wants to have a particular person care for her, because she'll say no. Gently tell her what is going to happen (and how wonderful it's going to be). Don't make it a choice.

◆ Whenever possible, ease into the arrangement gradually. If you are having a companion or aide come to the house, have the person come very briefly the first time, and then build up. Or, if you are taking your parent to day care, and your parent clings to you, stay with her for the first day or two. Then leave her for an hour, working up to half a day, and so on.

◆ Schedule the changing of the guard for a time of day when your parent tends to be calm. Don't have a new companion or aide come in the late afternoon if that is when your father is most anxious and confused.

◆ Provide detailed instructions about your parent's daily routines and habits, and suggest ways of dealing with outbursts, wandering, accusations, or other difficult behavior. If possible, have the aide watch you in action once or twice, so he or she can follow in the same path.

◆ Make it clear to your parent when you will return. (She may ask for you every five minutes.) Put a calendar or clock, depending upon how long you will be gone, on the wall, marking the day or indicating the time that you will return. The companion or aide can draw an X through each day or count down each hour as it passes.

◆ Keep a regular schedule. Your parent should go to day care at the same time each day, or have a home-care

> *I tried to leave my mother at a day-care program, and the next thing I knew she was running after me.*
>
> *I'd spent so much time finding a situation that would be right for her, and I was very upset that she refused to cooperate. Several months later I tried again, at a new place. But this time I got my mother there early, before anyone else. It was like starting somebody off in kindergarten. We began with one day a week until we had worked up to four days. It was all very gradual. When my mother got anxious, the staff put a sign up: 'Sally will be here to pick you up at four.'*
>
> *She came to love the place. That's the funny part. She looked forward to it. Of course, as soon as she got off the van, she couldn't tell me where she had been or what she had done. But while she was there she was happy, that's all I know. And that's all I cared about."*
>
> —SALLY T.

worker come to the house at the same time each day, if possible.

◆ If your parent says you are abandoning her, accuses the aide of stealing, refuses to go to day care, or locks a visiting nurse out, consider any underlying reasons she might have for behaving this way. Maybe she is afraid you are leaving her for good, or worried that this other person is going to hurt her. Help her overcome her fears (for example, leave a large picture of yourself and a note saying that you love her and will return soon).

◆ Be committed to this arrangement. Give yourself a month or so to put up with the fussing that may accompany it. Don't give in. The longer the new arrangement is sustained, the easier it will become for your parent to accept it.

◆ Leave a list of emergency phone numbers, including your number and any cell phone number, near the phone.

Helping Your Parent

Just as keeping your cool will help your parent remain calm, making life easier for her will make life more manageable for both of you. It's all terribly intertwined.

Keep your parent's environment simple and predictable. Lower your expectations. And learn what makes her anxious, what helps her to relax, what distracts her, and what reassures her.

SIMPLIFY HIS WORLD

THE SIMPLER YOUR PARENT'S WORLD is—his house, his tasks, his conversations, his visits—the better life will be for everyone. Your parent may not realize that the volume is too loud or the lighting too bright or the room too crowded. He just knows that he is unhappy, and so he becomes agitated or angry. It is up to you to keep his surroundings manageable.

Here are a few guidelines:

◆ Get rid of knickknacks, small rugs, mirrors, piles of papers, and clutter, especially in the room where your parent lives.

◆ Furniture should be simple, and placed so that it can be easily used. Pathways should be clear. Once you arrange the furniture, heaven forbid, don't rearrange it.

◆ Keep the noise down. You may not notice that the television is blaring, the dog's barking, and that several people are talking at once, but it may confound him.

◆ Use signs wherever you can— on the bathroom door, in bedrooms, on cabinets, and on bureau drawers ("socks," "shirts," "pants," etc.). If your parent can't figure out which item in the refrigerator he should eat, write LUNCH across his sandwich bag. Use symbols if written words don't work.

◆ Get phones with large push-buttons, which are easier to read and easier to use. Some have memory dial with pictures.

◆ Offer simple choices. Don't ask your parent what he wants for dinner. Say, "Do you want chicken or fish?" Or, better yet, just tell him what you're going to have for dinner.

◆ When giving instructions, eliminate unnecessary steps and offer instructions one at a time. Each should require only a single action. For example, instead of asking him to bathe,

walk through each step with him, one at a time: "Unbutton your shirt. Take the shirt off. Step into the shower." And so forth.

◆ Avoid change. Simply going to the doctor's office may trigger a frenzy of fear and frustration. Certainly a change in living situation, or even a room change within your house, can cause pandemonium. The more life can stay the same, the better. New people, new foods, new activities, new schedules are likely to throw him off. If your parent has to move into a

SOCIALIZING WITH YOUR PARENT

Social isolation is one of the more serious side effects of this job. If your parent lives with you, the problem can become dire. You must find ways to meet your need for change and companionship and your parent's need for an unchanging environment. Get out on your own regularly, but if you need to include your parent in your socializing:

◆ Keep gatherings small. One or two people may be manageable, but a large party will confuse your parent.

◆ Whenever possible, socialize around a regular daily activity. Invite people over for a meal during your parent's regular mealtime, or have friends join you on your parent's daily walk.

◆ Invite people to come to your house, rather than moving your parent to a new environment. This way she will be more settled and can choose to go to her room when she gets tired. (Don't urge her to be part of a gathering if she doesn't want to be.)

◆ If your parent has odd habits or troubling behaviors, warn guests in advance. Everyone will be more comfortable, and most people will understand and be supportive when they know what to expect.

nursing home or other facility, keep it as simple as possible (for example, move all furniture from his old room to his new room and make it look as similar as possible). And then, be prepared for a decline in his behavior and ability.

LOOK FOR THE MESSAGE

YOUR PARENT CAN NO LONGER UNDERstand the world around her or communicate her needs. Both the input and the output are muddled. And so, you need to try to see the world from her perspective and decipher her signals as best you can.

If your parent is agitated and anxious, maybe the radio is too loud. If your parent strikes at a visitor, maybe that person came at her unexpectedly

---

Over the years we tried to convince my father to use a cane when he became unsteady on his feet, but he always refused. He'd say he got around much better than any of us, or he'd get angry and change the subject. When his dementia got worse, he also became much frailer, and one day I took out the cane we'd gotten for him and tried to slip it into his hand. Before I could do it, he looked at me with a concerned expression on his face and said, 'Eric! I didn't know you used a cane!'"

—ERIC S.

---

and frightened her. If your parent is screaming obscenities or throwing things, maybe it's because her leg hurts, or she has an infection, or she has to go to the bathroom. She can't remember how to say, "I need to go to the bathroom," or "My leg hurts." She is simply reacting to her discomfort, or trying to get something to change.

Look for things that might be upsetting her. Why is she angry or agitated? Watch for patterns in her behavior. If she is more anxious at a certain time of day or in a certain place, perhaps there is something about that time or place that reminds her of something she should be doing, or something frightens her. Also, think about how she used to be and what she used to enjoy. If she has always loved the outdoors and doesn't get outside at all now, perhaps she is agitated because of that.

Your mother is not trying to annoy you. She is not suddenly expressing moods that were always hidden within her. She simply doesn't understand her surroundings and doesn't know how to get what she needs or remedy what she doesn't like.

REMAIN CALM

DID WE SAY THIS ALREADY? WELL, IT'S worth repeating. It will help you cope, and it will certainly help your parent get through life a little more easily, which will, in turn, help you again. Whatever happens, remain calm. Your anger and frustration and criticism will only send your parent into more turmoil and deeper confusion. If she's made a mistake (another one), remain calm. If she's agitated, remain calm. If she's criticizing you and embarrassing you in public, remain calm.

TREAT HER
WITH RESPECT

RESPECTING YOUR PARENT AND treating her as an adult can be challenging when dementia strikes. But even when you are cutting her food or helping her bathe or calming her down, remember that your parent is not a child and shouldn't be treated like one. She has lived a long life and has well-formed opinions, dreams, likes, and dislikes—even if she can't remember what they are. Help her maintain a sense of dignity. Address her with the same respect you always have.

Make sure that your tone of voice is not condescending. Don't scold your parent as if she were a child. She is not a child. Furthermore, she hasn't done anything bad; it's the disease that is making her behave this way. Refrain from talking about her as if she were not in the room or unable to comprehend your words. Protect her self-esteem and modesty and ask others who care for her to do the same.

LET HIM DO WHAT HE CAN

WHATEVER HIS LIMITATIONS, YOUR parent should be encouraged to do whatever he still can (without pushing him to do things that he can't do). Day-to-day, it may be easier to do things for him, and it may seem like

> " *I had everybody here for Easter a few weeks before my mother died. I thought, 'What did I get myself into?' because I couldn't give my attention to anything else. She needed all my time.*
>
> *But she really enjoyed herself. My niece is a psychologist and they were trying to trigger her memory, asking her lots of questions, mentioning composers and songs. She loved music.*
>
> *I asked her that night if she had enjoyed her company. And the way she smiled at me I know that it was a very, very successful day."*
>
> —SALLY T.

an act of kindness to let him just stay in his chair, but, early on, it is important for your parent to maintain as much independence and self-esteem as possible. And later, he will fare better if he keeps busy.

Think of tasks that he can manage on his own or with minimal help. Have him polish the silver, make the orange juice, get the mail, or water the flowers. Ask him to hand you ingredients while you cook dinner. It may seem demeaning to have your father cut out coupons or pot plants, but the task may be quite enjoyable to him— at least more enjoyable than sitting on the couch, staring at the walls.

Of course, letting your parent help may require more work from you and others (the laundry may need to be refolded, the spilled juice wiped up). But studies show that people with dementia who are encouraged to stay active, remain social, do hobbies, and otherwise have some sort of a life, are less depressed, less aggressive and agitated, and generally less dependent.

BUT DON'T EXPECT TOO MUCH

OF COURSE, YOUR PARENT CANNOT learn new things, remember old things, follow a list of instructions, or suddenly understand what it is that you are telling him. Don't give him tasks that are too difficult or urge him to get back into model building when he can't even tie his own shoes. Avoid the urge to repeat instructions that he doesn't get, teach him, or instruct him. A louder voice, repetition, confrontation, shame, anger, criticism, or force will not bring back old skills or memories.

STICK TO A ROUTINE

CREATE A SCHEDULE THAT WORKS FOR your parent, and then stick to it. If she is most lucid in the morning, schedule complex activities, like bathing, for that time. If she gets restless and fidgety in the middle of the day, create a calm environment at that time.

Likewise, plan your visits for the same time and the same day every week. Or if your parent goes to day care every weekday, then try to follow the same routine on the weekend by getting her up and dressed and then giving her some activity to do that is similar to what she does in day care. She won't remember the schedule, but she won't be surprised by it either.

SUPPORT FOR PATIENTS, TOO

There are hundreds of support groups for the families of people with Alzheimer's and other forms of dementia, but also there are support groups for the patients themselves. Patients, at least those in the early stages of the illness, are often relieved to talk about their fears, losses, aggravations, and other reactions, as well as how they and their families plan to cope in the future.

To find out if there is a patient support group near your parent, or to get some pointers on how to start one, call the local chapter of the Alzheimer's Association.

You might also consider some psychotherapy for your parent if she simply needs to talk to someone about her fears and angers or any unresolved relationships.

DIVERT HER ATTENTION

SOMETIMES FORGETFULNESS CAN BE used in your favor. When your parent is about to do something that you don't want her to do, divert her attention.

When your mother starts into a tantrum or begins to tell a repetitive story, don't tell her to stop or say, "You've already told me that." Quickly change the subject or suggest a new activity. Have her look at a photo album, sip a cup of tea, go for a walk, knit, listen to music, sing a song, play a tune on the piano, or flip through catalogs. Or engage her in a chore she enjoys.

If she gets riled up in the middle of a task that has to be finished, like getting dressed, divert her from her frustration. Pause for a moment and sing a familiar song or tell an old family story. It should calm her down, and when you return to the task, she may forget that this is something she didn't want to do. A short break may calm you as well.

IGNORE SOME THINGS

DON'T CORRECT YOUR PARENT ALL the time. In fact, do it as little as possible. It is demeaning and confusing for him (he probably won't understand what it is he is doing wrong), and it is exhausting for you. Instead, ignore some things—a lot of things— as long as they aren't dangerous or harmful. Does it really matter if your parent remembers the dog's name or if he talks about his late wife as though she were still alive? Who is it hurting

> " *I've learned that I have to think ahead and make it look like I really don't want my mother to do something, and then she'll do it.*
>
> *I came home Thursday afternoon to find her physically wrestling with Mildred, the aide who takes care of her while I'm at work. It was raining and Mildred wanted her to go inside, but she wouldn't do it. I suggested that Mildred tell Mom to sit outside, that she didn't want her to go in the house. Then Mom wanted to come inside. You learn to do whatever works.*"
>
> —CAROL G.

if he wears mismatched clothes or if he wants to eat cereal for dinner and turkey for breakfast? You have enough struggles in the day. Some battles just aren't worth fighting. Ignore his mistakes, don't correct him, and agree with him sometimes even when he's wrong. Join him in his world.

When you need to correct him, say something that will get him back on track without being critical. *You probably did take your medication, but let's check your pillbox just to be sure.*

Interestingly enough, over time, ignoring certain habits often helps to curtail them. If you can stay out of a struggle, maybe not even look up, your parent may stop doing something that you don't want him to do. This technique works best if you pick just one

> *When my mother was in the nursing home, I used to visit her at lunchtime and feed her. After she had eaten, I would hold her hand and talk about the past, and she would lie there and listen. She never really said anything, or at least anything that made sense.*
>
> *One time I was flipping through old photos and she reached out and touched my cheek and there was a warm and connected look in her eye when she stared up at me. She said, 'They're all gone, aren't they?' I said, 'Yes, they are. But I'm still here and Polly is still here.' And that was it. She was gone again. But I don't think I'll ever forget that moment."*
>
> —GLORIA C.

behavior to ignore and alert everyone else caring for your parent to the plan so they all ignore that behavior as well.

BEWARE THE WITCHING HOUR

IF YOU NOTICE THAT YOUR MOTHER is more confused and agitated in the early evening, schedule any complicated activities for an earlier part of the day, and keep the evening calm and soothing. People with dementia often suffer what is known as "sundowning." That is, as the sun goes down, disruptive behaviors become worse. Agitation, in particular, becomes heightened.

It's not clear why this happens, whether it is the change in lighting or simply that the day has been tiring and exhaustion is playing its part. Certainly children are less well behaved around five o'clock in the evening, and it's the time of day many adults reach for a cocktail, so this affect doesn't seem to be limited to dementia.

Sometimes turning the lights on in the afternoon, before the sun starts to set, can help. But for the most part, it is best simply to be aware of it, schedule life accordingly, and brace yourself.

GET HER TO EXERCISE

IT SOUNDS LIKE AN UNNECESSARY hardship for you. Why bother? Even if your parent is very confused, some fresh air and sunshine and a walk around the neighborhood, or even some modest stretching and lifting light hand weights, will help her get through the rest of the day. Studies show that when people have dementia, exercise reduces agitation, improves sleep habits, reduces falls, helps people perform daily tasks, alleviates depression, boosts mood and self-esteem, and, best of all, improves people's interactions with their caregivers. Even if your parent is very frail, there are still things she can do to exercise (see page 66).

BE AWARE OF DEPRESSION, DELIRIUM, AND OTHER SIGNS OF ILLNESS

IN ALL LIKELIHOOD, YOUR PARENT cannot tell you when her head aches,

IN NEED OF SUPERVISION

Your parent might be able to live alone for some time after receiving a diagnosis of dementia, but not for long. Whenever she is alone, be sure to follow all the safety tips given earlier. See if she can use the phone, or install a phone with memory dial and photos, and then see if she can actually operate it. Think whether she would be able to respond to an emergency, or whether she might wander off. Is there a neighbor close by who might be put on alert? Perhaps you can put a bell on the door so someone is alerted if she leaves.

If your parent becomes confused easily, has trouble using a telephone, would not know how to get help, might wander, or presents some other risk to herself or others, she needs supervision. If you can't be with her 24/7, and you probably can't, find out about adult day-care programs, companions, volunteers, or other ways she might be supervised during the day. (Webcams and security cameras allow you to watch your parent from afar, but this is rarely useful because you would have to have cameras in every room where she might wander, and you would have to keep one eye on the screen at all times. Plus, what would you do if something did happen to her?)

or if she has abdominal pain, or if it hurts when she urinates. You need to be on the lookout for medical problems and alert to behavioral changes that might signal trouble. If she moans, is suddenly angry, or resists using the toilet, for example, talk with her doctor.

As we've noted, people with dementia often become depressed, especially in the early stages of the disease. Depression is treatable. Beware of the signs of depression and alert your parent's doctor. Even if there are no overt signs, ask the doctor about this. If the doctor doesn't take your concerns seriously, then find another doctor who does. (See page 281 for more on depression.)

Delirium, the sudden onset of acute confusion and inattention, is common in elderly people, especially if they are suddenly moved to a new location or become sick. Again, know the symptoms and alert the doctor immediately, as delirium is a medical emergency. (See page 292 for more on delirium.)

PETS, IMAGERY, AND MUSIC AND ART THERAPY

STUDIES SHOW THAT A PET CAN CALM people when they're agitated, alleviate depression, and boost self-esteem. Your parent probably can't care for a pet now, but if someone else is around to do that, she might enjoy having a gentle companion to talk to, stroke, and hold. Find a pet that is gentle and a bit of a couch potato. You don't need two agitated souls in the house.

Music can also be soothing and relaxing. Sometimes soft "white" noise, such as the sound of ocean waves or other continuous sounds from nature, can decrease nervous chatter and calm a person with dementia. Music from her youth will transport her to better times. She might sing along or even dance a little (good exercise).

Simple art projects can be an outlet for frustrations, fears, and hopes. Good colored pencils or some paints and paper, a soft chunk of clay, or other art supplies might tap a creative side of her (and keep her busy and distracted for a little while).

Imagery can be very effective in calming an agitated soul, especially when someone has dementia. Talk slowly and gently to your parent, describing a place or time she loved. Walk her through it, describing, for example, a walk on the beach, or the smell of the pine trees and sound of water lapping up on the rocks of a lake. Help her to relax in this place, to languish in it.

REASSURANCE AND HUGS

WARMTH AND LOVE ARE POTENT medicine. When your father gets riled, discombobulated, frustrated, anxious, or depressed, stroke his hand or cheek. Tell him that you understand, that he's doing a good job, that you are there for him, that you won't abandon him. A gentle touch and a kind word will help both of you get through the next few minutes—and a few minutes of peace can be a saving grace at this time.

Chapter Twenty-Three

MANAGING DAY TO DAY

Bathing, Dressing, and Eating • Communication • Dealing with Agitation, Wandering, and Anger • Coping with Special Problems

....

WHEN YOUR PARENT HAS DEMENTIA, MANAGING DAY-to-day is an exhausting test of will. It requires imagination, ingenuity, perseverance, and, yes, an enormous dose of patience. Every day, and sometimes every minute, brings a new challenge. Your parent's left the stove on, or insists that camels are in her room, or worries that she'll be late for her wedding, or keeps putting her clothes in the oven instead of the washing machine. Beyond the pain and grief of this loss are the daily questions of how to cope, how to survive.

Unfortunately, there are no uniform rules or answers. What helps one person may not be of any use to another. You simply have to try different approaches and see what works. Of course, just when you find something that calms your mother's pacing, the disease will progress and she'll pick up a new but equally troubling habit. And you are left to find yet another trick, a new approach.

Chapter Six suggests general tips for managing every day when a parent is elderly, many of which may be helpful to you. This chapter focuses on issues and problems that are particular to dementia.

Good luck.

Tackling Specific Issues

It's been a long day already. Now the mail has disappeared, your mother is insisting that you are her sister Margaret (whom she never liked), she's refusing to eat dinner, and tonight, of all night's, is bath night. Surely she could skip her bath. Again. But food?

It's enough to make someone buy a large bottle of wine and a ticket to Borneo. But before you do, try some

---

DOOHICKEYS AND DOODADS

A vast array of gadgets exists to make life easier for people with dementia—reminders, alerts, motion detectors, easy-to-use phones, medication dispensers, battery switches for the car, stove-top fire fighters, automatic faucet controls, etc. See page 131 for some guidance on this. The Alzheimer's Store (800-752-3238 or www.alzstore.com) specializes in products and clothing for people with dementia. Even if you don't buy anything, some of these devices might give you ideas for things you can do yourself.

---

of these approaches and see if you can't protect your mail, and your sanity.

BATHING AND HYGIENE

WHEN THE SMALLEST TASKS BECOME Herculean battles, it's tempting to let things go. But your parent's hygiene affects not only her health (increasing the risk of infections), but also her self-esteem and the reactions of others who spend time with her.

Daily baths are not necessary; she only needs to bathe two or three times a week. Sponge baths are fine when proper bathing isn't possible. You can also split up the task. You might buy a basin for washing her hair, and do that on one day. Then, she can bathe on another day, so she is not trying to accomplish too much at one time.

Also, set up a schedule and routine that works for her, if you can make it work for you as well. If she's more lucid first thing in the morning, for example, that might be a good time for a bath or shower. If she always brushes her teeth before bathing, do that first. A routine and predictable order should help in getting these things done.

Beyond that:

◆ Give her, and yourself, plenty of time for demanding tasks like this. Schedule them when you aren't hurried.

◆ Take a moment beforehand to gather your patience.

◆ Plan it out in advance. Draw the bath, have towels nearby, open the

GENERAL RULES FOR PHYSICALLY ASSISTING SOMEONE WITH DEMENTIA

When you are lifting or moving your parent, helping to bathe or dress him, or assisting in some other way,

◆ Approach from the front, so as to not startle him. Make eye contact and try to keep it.

◆ Take it slow. Whatever else is going on, try not to hurry. It will inevitably add only more time to this task.

◆ Speak gently, letting him know what is going to happen before it happens.

◆ Reassure him that he is doing fine, that everything is going well.

◆ Keep instructions short and simple, taking one small step at a time.

◆ Support him along his larger muscles and bones. Rather than holding a hand, hold a shoulder. Rather than turning him over by pulling an arm and leg, pull the hip and thigh.

◆ Lift with your legs, not your back. Bend your knees and push up using your leg muscles, not your back.

◆ If you can't lift or maneuver your parent, don't. Call for help from a neighbor, friend or, if necessary, the police.

◆ You can buy a "transfer belt" at any medical supply store or on the Web, which helps in lifting people to a standing position, or consider buying chair lifts, straps for cars, and other devices aimed at lifting and maneuvering people.

---

shampoo bottle, warm up the bathroom, have clothes laid out in the order that they go on, etc.

◆ Create an easy environment. Install grab bars on bathroom walls and safety handles on the tub. If she has trouble standing, put a small, sturdy seat in the shower stall. If you help her wash her hair in the tub, buy a handheld attachment for the faucet.

◆ Speak calmly and soothingly, encouraging her all the way. Remind her that you are there, helping her, and that she's doing it just right.

◆ Give simple instructions. Work on one small task at a time, like, "Put some shampoo in your hand," instead of "wash your hair." Minimize conversation to just those instructions and comments that are necessary.

◆ Respect her modesty, as much as possible. Give her a towel to hold in front of herself, or stand behind the shower curtain while aiding her.

◆ Tell her that this is a treat, something wonderful and relaxing, a special prize, a day at the spa.

◆ When things get rough, try a new tactic. Switch bath time to a different time of day. See if a bath, rather than a shower, is easier. Buy no-slip bath shoes or a seat for the shower. Sometimes a handheld shower head is easier to maneuver and less anxiety-provoking.

◆ Depending on her personality and where she is in this disease, buy her something special—lavender bath soap or a soft new towel—and see if it doesn't pique her interest in bathing.

◆ Keep up with oral hygiene as well, even if it's tempting to let this task go. Again, your attitude will help. Remain calm and act as if this is a good thing the two of you are doing, not a horrible chore that you dread.

◆ An electric toothbrush is often easier, if your parent can handle the change, because it requires little hand or wrist movement. (Of course, it might just be another new gizmo complicating life; but it's worth a try.) At some point you might have to use disposable dental swabs.

◆ Be sure dentures are kept clean.

◆ Talk with your parent's dentist about other ways to keep up with oral hygiene.

GROOMING AND DRESSING

FIND SOME BALANCE BETWEEN WHAT'S easy and manageable (the same pair of sweatpants every day) and what looks appropriate and might boost your parent's self-esteem (a bright dress or stylish blouse). Most of the time, you'll want to lean toward the former. But where you draw this line depends upon who your parent was, who she is, and how far along this disease has progressed.

Again, take a deep breath and gather your patience. Allow plenty of time, plan ahead, and keep instructions very, *very* simple.

◆ Find simple-to-wear clothing, such as slip-on shoes or sneakers that close with Velcro or have elastic laces that never need tying; elastic-waisted pants or sweatpants; shirts that pull over the head or snap up the front; and tube socks, which don't have a front or back.

◆ Clearly label dresser drawers, and mark the front and back of clothing. For example, sew a tag into the back of your father's pants that says BACK.

◆ In the morning, lay out your parent's clothes in the order in which they go on.

◆ Minimize choices. Keep only a few outfits in the closet. If your parent wears ratty clothing or bizarre outfits, get rid of some things (unless that old flannel shirt is his favorite), and put away any clothing that is inappropriate for the weather.

◆ If your parent is prone to undressing at inappropriate times, get him clothes that are not easily shed. Consider one-piece suits, or shirts that zip or have Velcro up the back, or something that has buttons.

EATING

SOMETIMES PEOPLE WITH DEMENTIA fail to eat because shopping and cooking are too confusing. Sometimes people have trouble getting the food from the kitchen to the plate, or from the plate into their mouths. Some people think they have just eaten when they haven't, and other times they forget they've just eaten and they insist on having another meal. Some forget what to eat, and have a box of chocolates for lunch.

In addition, hunger patterns and sense of smell change as one ages. Medications can interfere with the absorption of certain nutrients, further alter appetite and sense of taste, and cause an upset stomach.

Keep tabs on whether your parent is eating, what she's eating, and how much she's eating; be aware of weight gain and loss; and adopt some strategies for making a decent diet possible. (See page 119 for other tips on making eating easier, and pages 73 and 658 for nutritional information.)

◆ Again, make it easy. When you're not around, be sure your parent has food that is ready to eat (sand-wiches, stews, soups) or link her up with a meal-delivery service. As her confusion gets worse, be sure food is on the table when she sits down (no waiting time) and that it is easy to eat (no long spaghetti to spin on a fork, shells to crack, meat to cut up, etc.). Cut food up in advance and place only a napkin and fork at her plate.

◆ When utensils present an obstacle, serve bite-size finger foods, such as chicken nuggets, cut-up fruits and vegetables, tiny egg rolls, stuffed mushrooms, and tea sandwiches. This sort of food is easy to manage, and if your parent likes to pace, he can take finger foods with him as he strolls.

◆ Use unbreakable dinnerware in case something is dropped, or thrown. Try cups with handles on both sides, cups with straws, utensils with thicker, weighted handles, and anything else that might help.

◆ If you are dealing with a constant eater, place a mark on the clock, showing what time the next meal will be served. Or simply keep some low-calorie snacks in the house—carrots, celery, cucumber, raisins, low-salt crackers, or butterless popcorn. Instead of arguing with your parent about whether he did or didn't just eat, give him a plate of healthful food.

◆ The snack approach is also helpful for a noneater. Instead of forcing your father to the dinner table, leave a plate of healthful, filling snacks in front of him at all times—fruit, yogurt and wheat germ shake, chunks

> *My mother will eat with each member of the family as they come and go. Sometimes on Sunday mornings, my daughter's boyfriend will get her coffee and an egg sandwich before he leaves, and she won't say anything to anyone about it. Then she'll eat breakfast again with my husband and me an hour later. It's not a big deal, I guess, but how much can one person eat?*
>
> *She got four boxes of candy for Mother's Day and ate all of them single-handedly. I keep imploring people, 'Please don't give her candy,' but they don't listen. Now I sometimes hide the candy or even throw it away. She doesn't remember it existed."*
>
> —CAROL G.

of cheese, crackers or vegetables with a hearty dip, peanut butter on crackers, or a rich diet-supplement drink.

◆ Keep distractions to a minimum during mealtime—soft music but no loud conversation and activity.

SLEEPING, OR LACK THEREOF

RESTLESSNESS, CONFUSION, AND A disrupted internal clock all make getting a good night's rest difficult. People can also have trouble separating dreams from reality, which further disrupts sleep. Studies show that some people with dementia not only have trouble getting to sleep, but they wake up at least twice every hour during the night.

If your parent is wandering the halls at 2 A.M., tossing and turning at 3 A.M., and hunting for the bathroom at 4 A.M., not only will she be tired, but so will you. Trouble sleeping, and its effect on the whole household, is one of the top reasons why people with dementia eventually end up in nursing homes.

Whatever the causes, sleep problems eventually subside in most cases. In the meantime, here are some sleeping tips specifically for people with dementia (other sleeping tips are listed on page 240):

◆ Make sure your parent gets outside in the fresh air and gets some exercise most every day.

◆ Ban caffeine and other stimulants.

◆ Since her internal clock is irregular or absent, your parent has to rely on external clocks. Schedule naps and bedtime and then stick to the schedule. Don't let her doze off at 7 P.M. or she'll want to start her day at 3 A.M. Try to keep her awake until other people in the household retire.

◆ Guide her to activities that are calming before bedtime, like listening to music or, if she can, reading. If undressing is a nightmare, help your parent get into her night clothes half an hour before bedtime so she can calm down from the effort and isn't flustered on retiring.

◆ Make sure your parent has gone to the bathroom before going to bed.

◆ Don't lay out clothing the night before. Your parent might wake up in the middle of the night and think it's time to get dressed.

◆ Make sure your parent feels safe in her bed. Keep familiar furnishings and photographs near her bed. Also be sure the room is at a comfortable temperature and that she has appropriate covers.

◆ Be sure there's a night-light or other dim lighting in your parent's bedroom and put night-lights in the hallway so she doesn't become disoriented on the way to the bathroom.

TELEPHONES AND MAIL

IF YOUR PARENT LIVES WITH YOU AND you aren't getting your bills or are wondering why there are never any messages on your answering machine, it is time to make some changes.

Get a post office box or put a latch on your mailbox that is a little difficult to undo. If you live in a suburban or rural area, you might be able to work out a plan with your mail carrier to leave the mail on a shelf in the garage or in the neighbor's box.

Ask the phone company for a call-forwarding service so your calls can follow you, keep the answering machine in a locked drawer (so your parent can't turn it off), or turn the ringer on the phone and the volume on the answering machine off.

MEDICAL ALERT

Remember, your parent may not be able to tell you when she's ill or in pain, so you or some other caregiver must be on the lookout. Sudden changes in behavior—increased confusion or agitation, unusual exhaustion or lack of appetite, or grimacing while eating, for example—may be signs of illness or medication problems. Be aware of such shifts in behavior, and when you note one, alert the doctor.

If your parent lives alone and is having trouble handling the mail, arrange with creditors to have her bills sent to your address, or arrange to have them paid automatically from a bank account.

MONEY

EVEN IF YOUR PARENT USED TO BE thrifty, you may find that he is suddenly spending money recklessly. Or if he can't count anymore, you may discover that he's giving the checkout person $20 for a bag of candy that costs 70¢ and walking away without any change.

If you have control over your parent's finances (and if you don't, you should start that process), let him carry

> **"** *Last week Mom raced me to the mailbox and I actually had to wrestle the mail away from her. She had it all stuffed under her sweatshirt, and I knew I would never see it again. Finally I put a bungee cord on the box. She can't figure out how to get it off. The mailman has a little trouble with it, too, but he's getting better at it."*
>
> —CAROL G.

some cash, but only as much as you are willing to let him lose. If he doesn't go to the store often, you might also leave him with his credit cards, or perhaps only the expired ones.

DRIVING

THE QUESTION OF WHEN TO GIVE UP the car keys is a sensitive subject with any older person (see page 127), but it can be explosive when a parent has dementia. When you express your concern, your parent may have no idea what you are talking about, despite several recent fender-benders. Or when you steer him away from the ignition, he may accuse you of holding him captive.

Talk with your parent about driving early in this disease, before he needs to quit. (Although, he should quit pretty early on because disorientation and confusion can easily lead to a serious accident.) If he is already a danger and needs to be stopped immediately, take action regardless of his response.

If possible, get rid of the car so there is no threat of his driving. If the car is needed, get an auto mechanic to show you how to remove the distributor cap so the car won't start. When you need to use the car, you can easily put the cap back on. There are also gadgets you can buy that will temporarily disable a car. Talk with a mechanic.

TIME AND ORIENTATION

TO HELP YOUR PARENT TRACK THE hours and days, keep clocks and calendars clearly in sight. When you go out, put colored tape on the clock where the hands will be when you return, with the words, "Janie will be home at this time."

Various timers are available that can help remind your mother when to take her medications, when to eat, when to use the toilet, etc.

Your parent may be aware of her lost ability to track time and, as a result, be constantly worried about doing things at the wrong time. She may get nervous that she is late for an appointment that isn't scheduled until next week. Or she may be concerned about wearing out a welcome and say it's time to go just minutes after she's arrived for a visit.

Try to understand her concerns. Imagine how confusing it would be if you had no idea what day it was or how much time was passing. If large

A PLACE IN THE PAST

Your parent may have trouble remembering not only the day and the hour, but also the decade. Many people with dementia become lost in the past, talking about people who are long dead or a job that they left many years ago. This can be extremely upsetting, not only because it is a stark reminder of just how confused your parent is, but also because you may want to talk about today when your parent can talk only about yesterday. You may want to tell your father that you love him, but he is lost in 1940, a time when you didn't even exist.

As hard as this is on you, keep in mind that the past may be a very comforting and safe place for your parent. It is a place he can remember and a time when he was fit and able. In any case, trying to bring him into the present may only disorient and upset him. So don't frustrate yourself or him by trying to pull him into your world. If he is happy in 1940, let him stay there.

When he says that he is going to visit Wayne, a friend who died ten years ago, don't try to convince him that Wayne is gone. Instead, try something like, "Wouldn't it be nice for you to see your friend Wayne? Tell me about how you met him, Dad."

---

clocks and notes don't help, reassure your parent, yes, repeatedly, that you or someone else will help her get to where she needs to go on time, and that you will keep track of when it's time to leave.

COMMUNICATION

OVER TIME, DEMENTIA SKEWS communication in a number of ways. People may have trouble with grammar or finding the right word. They may talk fluidly, but the words may have no meaning. They may be able to formulate and write words and sentences, but have difficulty pronouncing them. They might lose their train of thought, drifting off in mid-sentence. They may not be able to find the right word for an object and say instead, "that thing that you play music on." Or, they might jumble their words, so that *needle* becomes *beedle*, or *food* becomes *fide*.

Your parent may not only have trouble expressing herself, she may also have difficulty understanding what others say. She may be able to read a sign, but have no idea what it means. She may understand what you say in person, but not what you say over the phone. She may be able to repeat a message, but not interpret it, so she repeats your instructions but doesn't follow them.

> " *Eventually my mother couldn't express what she was feeling. I would say, 'What's wrong?' and she really didn't know. One time she said, 'I want to be free,' and I understood that she wanted to leave, to be free of the disease, to go back to some other part of her life. Later, it was about her mother. She wanted to go home and she wanted to go to her mother, who was waiting for her, she said. And that made me very sad because I figured she was preparing to die.*
>
> *I realized that she wasn't sad. In fact, I think she was quite ready to go. I was projecting my own sadness, my own sorrow, onto her.*"
>
> —MARY W.

When communication fades:

◆ Have your parent's hearing checked, and be sure she has no dental problems that might be hindering her speech.

◆ When you talk with your parent, find a quiet place and do it at a time when you won't be interrupted or distracted.

◆ Use simple words and sentences. Speak slowly and deliberately. Use a calm, but amply loud voice. A deep voice is better than a high-pitched tone, which can be more difficult to under-stand and may suggest that you are upset.

◆ Supplement your words with nonverbal cues. Point to things. Use photographs, pantomime, and touch.

◆ If you are giving your parent instructions, don't assume she under-stands what you are saying, even if she assures you that she does. Double-check by asking her to repeat the instructions and explain what they mean. (Of course, if the instructions pertain to something in the future, she may not remember them, even if she understands them.)

◆ Listen carefully when your parent speaks. Give her your complete attention. Be patient, look directly at her, and try not to interrupt. If she hesitates, forgetting her thought, give her time to try to finish.

◆ When communicating becomes more difficult for her, listen for words that are repeated or seem meaning-ful, and respond to those. As you look for meaning in her words, be aware that common themes people with dementia try to express are loneliness and fear, concern about family, and a desire to be well again.

◆ Let your parent talk even if she is making no sense. She thinks she's making sense, and the sound of her voice and feeling that someone is lis-tening may be calming and reassur-ing for her.

◆ Correcting her mistakes will only increase her frustration and confusion. Encourage your parent and, even if you don't understand what she's saying, praise her for her efforts.

◆ Late in the disease, your parent may lose all ability to communicate. It's hard to know which of the many losses of dementia is the most difficult or the most painful, but when the lines of communication fall silent, you may feel shut out completely. Your parent, no longer able to relay his needs, his pain, his fears, or his wishes, becomes isolated. Caring for him becomes even more challenging and very lonely.

Monitor your parent's comfort and health carefully now because he can no longer explain when something is amiss. Watch your parent's body language carefully. Facial expressions, like a smile, a grimace, or a frown, or body movements, like a clenched fist or a turn of the head, can be revealing.

When he can't talk to you, keep talking to him. He may still understand what you are saying, and your presence and the sound of your voice will bring him comfort. Do not talk about him to others as if he were not in the room.

INCONTINENCE

WHEN YOUR PARENT BECOMES incontinent, it may not be caused by a problem in her urinary tract, but by a disruption in the brain's messages. Or, she might not be able to get her clothes off fast enough, or she might not remember how she's supposed to respond to this urgent feeling. In any case, some of the more common incontinence remedies may not be effective. Talk to her doctor to rule out urinary tract infections, medication problems, and problems with the pelvic muscles. Some of the tips on pages 264–267 should help. Also:

◆ Make sure the bathroom is clearly marked with large letters or a picture on the door. Better yet, leave the door open and the light on at all times.

◆ Clear a path to the toilet.

◆ Use clothing that is as manageable as possible.

◆ Remind your parent to use the bathroom or set a timer for established intervals. Monitor her habits and schedule bathroom visits accordingly. Have her go just before she normally does, say, every two hours or so, even if she insists she doesn't need to.

◆ Once you help your parent to the bathroom, you may have trouble getting him to actually use the toilet. If possible, leave the room to give him privacy or at least look the other way. Encourage his urination by turning on the tap water. Remind him gently why he is there and what he needs to do. Then give him all the time he needs to empty bladder and bowels.

◆ Draw attention to the toilet by using bright lights and/or hanging a brightly colored fabric behind it.

◆ If your parent confuses other objects, such as buckets, wastebaskets, and flower pots, for toilets, put lids on them, move them out of your parent's path, get them out of the bathroom, or label them.

◆ Look for cues that your parent has to go to the bathroom. He might play with his fly, suddenly become fidgety, or look toward the bathroom without actually getting up and going. If he has speech trouble, he may say, "I have to key." Or he may revert to childish words, such as *doo-doo* or *poopie*. Listen for any such hints that he needs to go to the toilet.

◆ Try not to be angry with your parent when there is an accident. He cannot help it. Set up his house or living area with plastic liners and other protection. If this doesn't suffice, he may need to use diapers or a catheter, but only as a last resort. Talk with his doctor.

Coping with Behavior Problems

No matter what your parent is doing that is making your life miserable, it will change. Maybe not tomorrow, but in a matter of weeks or months. A person who is hitting people and having tantrums often becomes calmer and quieter with time. A person who is always poised on the edge of danger, turning the gas burner on high and hiding scissors

under the couch cushions, will eventually lose interest in such things. A lot of patience, a list of strategies, and the knowledge that this too shall pass will help you cope.

When a particular behavior is causing trouble, keep a record for several days or weeks. Write down what time the trouble began and when it stopped, anything that might have happened to set off the behavior, and what approach was taken to resolve the problem (distraction, reassurance, medications, etc.). You might begin to see a pattern and find ways to head off trouble before it starts.

As noted, it can also help, in some situations, if everyone involved agrees to ignore the behavior. If what your parent is doing isn't dangerous, this approach is certainly worth a try.

LOSING, HIDING, AND HOARDING THINGS

If your parent is hoarding food, money, or other items, and her actions are not harmful, let her do it. People with dementia sometimes hoard things because they are afraid that they will have to care for themselves in the future, that they will be abandoned, that people are stealing from them, or that people are trying to harm them. It may give your parent some peace of mind to squirrel things away.

If you can, help. Provide a tin for food, or a safe hiding place for money. You will be less apt to find moldy cookies and spoiled cheese in drawers and closets.

A "LOSING" STRATEGY

Losing and hiding things is par for the course with dementia. Be prepared.

◆ Keep two sets of anything that's important—eyeglasses, keys, dentures, hearing aids.

◆ Attach small items to large key chains so they can be found more easily.

◆ Get in the habit of checking wastebaskets before emptying them.

◆ Keep important things in the same place, always. The house keys hang next to the door, the dentures go in the glass by the sink, etc.

◆ Attach house keys or glasses to a string that hangs around your parent's neck.

◆ Check all pockets carefully before clothing is laundered or dry-cleaned.

◆ Limit hiding places by locking cabinets and closets.

◆ Keep a neat and orderly house if at all possible, so there are fewer places to lose items.

◆ You can buy gadgets that allow you to connect a pager to items that are frequently lost—TV remote controls, cell phones, house keys, etc.

Also, keep an eye out for new hiding places and check them occasionally, without letting your parent know that you're on to them.

AGITATION

YOUR PARENT PICKS UP A MAGAZINE. Puts it down. Goes into the bathroom. Comes back. Sits down. Stands up. Walks into the kitchen. Comes back into the living room. Rocks in her chair. Asks you what she should do. Goes into the kitchen again. Comes back. Asks you what she should do.

Sedatives start to look awfully tempting about now. While they are sometimes necessary, they are not the best solution. First, try some of the tips offered already in this chapter, and, as always, remember your mantra: Stay calm.

◆ Make sure your parent isn't consuming any caffeine or drugs that contain stimulants.

◆ Encourage your parent to exercise daily so she'll use up some of the nervous energy. If she wants to pace, let her pace. Or get someone to go for

> **"** *For somebody whose mind is deteriorating, she does really well. She's fast. She'll snatch things off the table and put them in her pockets faster than you can see her.*
>
> *I made hot-cross buns for Easter, and by the end of the meal her pockets were filled with them. I think she's saving in case of a flood—I mean, we have more than enough to eat. Nobody goes hungry around here, and she certainly eats well. She's always putting food away as though she might not get another meal. I keep asking her, 'What are you doing that for?'"*
>
> —CAROL G.

a regular walk with her. If she can handle it, buy exercise videos that might keep her occupied for a while and use up some energy.

◆ Try to figure out what triggers the agitation—a particular activity, a certain room or place, or a time of day. Then be prepared next time you head into that zone, or avoid it all together.

◆ Be aware of any personal need or discomfort that might cause the agitation, such as hunger, a full bladder, fatigue, or thirst.

◆ Sometimes agitation is prompted by some unspoken concern. Your mother may be wringing her hands or nervously bouncing her leg up and down because she is worried about being late for an appointment or about getting home safely from a visit. If you can figure out what's worrying her, you may be able to calm her fears with reassurance.

◆ Reduce stimulating noise, bright glare, and commotion. Turn off the TV (you can buy headsets for the television so she doesn't have to listen to it). Move guests into a different room. Turn down the radio.

◆ See if there isn't something that might soothe her, like a cat or special pillow or sweater or photo album.

◆ Give her something to do, like shelling peas, stuffing envelopes, folding laundry, or polishing silver. Or make up a task. *Mom, I need all these pages folded in half. Could you help me?*

◆ Distract her. When she starts to pace, get her doing or thinking about something else—a song, a photo album, memory, a story she loves to tell.

◆ When it's time to stop, try relaxation techniques, such as massage or therapeutic touch, imagery, and soothing music.

WANDERING

A PERSON WITH DEMENTIA MAY START out on an errand and forget where she is going, and where she started from. Suddenly, she can't get home and doesn't know where she is. Or she might just amble aimlessly out the door and into the night.

If your parent simply needs to pace, give her ample space to pace

GRANDPA IS SCARING ME

A dearly beloved grandfather says bizarre things, or is mean or crass. He wets his pants or makes a mess of his food. It's hard enough for an adult to understand, but this disease can be frightening for children. It can also leave them with unhappy memories of someone who is dear to you.

Explain that Grandpa's brain is sick, and that he doesn't mean what he says and can't remember what's just happened. If possible, find some humor in any odd behaviors, excusing Grandpa for that loud belch or racy statement and giving him a supportive hug. If he is violent or turbulent, stay calm. Your reaction will help your kids stay calm as well, and it gives them the message that this is nothing to worry about.

Assure children that Grandpa still loves them, even though he may not be able to show it now. And encourage them to discuss their feelings about this with you. If you ache for your children to know your parent as he was, offer them a glimpse into the past with stories of your childhood and his life, and old photos.

Once they understand what is happening, children can be wonderful company for an older person with dementia, and a big help to you. They are often more forgiving than adults and may be able to play at the same level as your parent. A child might like to sing songs or play games that are manageable and calming for a grandparent.

For help explaining dementia to a young child, several books are available, including *The Sunsets of Miss Olivia Wiggins* by Lester Laminack, *The Memory Box* by Mary Bahr and David Cunningham, and *Grandpa Doesn't Know It's Me* by Donna Guthrie.

at home. Clear pathways. Make sure she has slippers, socks, or shoes that provide ample traction. Use nonskid strips, if necessary.

Even if your parent has never wandered before or shown signs of wandering, be sure she wears an identification bracelet or necklace. If wandering is a concern or becomes a regular problem, talk with your par-

ent's doctor because certain medications can make it worse. Follow some of the tips above for dealing with agitation, as the two are related. And don't forget, exercise and a ban on caffeine will help.

◆ Sign up with the Alzheimer's Association's Safe Return Program (888-572-8566 or www.alz.org). Your parent will receive identification cards and jewelry, and be entered into a national database, so that anyone who finds her knows whom to call. Local police departments also have immediate access to photos and information that will help them locate your parent.

◆ Along with an ID card, put a card in your father's pocket with instructions for him: "Dad, stay calm. Find a phone. Call this number." Be sure he always has some change, or give instructions for calling collect.

◆ Some caregivers find it helpful to put a sign on the door: "Jack, Do Not Leave," or simply, "STOP." But this may work only for a short time and only in the early stages.

◆ Disguise exits with posters, wallpaper, curtains, or other decorations.

◆ Alert neighbors and the local police to the situation. Have photographs of your parent on hand so that if he does get lost, you can hand them out. Ask neighbors to be aware if they see your parent strolling by.

◆ Lock doors with bolts placed high or low on the door, or use plastic childproof knobs. If this presents a fire hazard, install alarms on doors, or attach a bell to the door so it alerts you or others when the door is opened.

◆ Consider buying motion-sensitive and pressure-sensitive alarms (in medical supply stores) that alert you when your parent gets out of bed. You can also buy monitoring devices that sound an alarm when the person wearing the device leaves the house.

◆ While expensive, you can get tracking devices that help you find someone within a certain radius of your house. (These are available through several companies, which can be found online by searching under "tracking devices for the elderly").

◆ Install a sturdy fence around the property.

◆ If nothing else helps, consult your parent's doctor about the possibility of using medications to control wandering.

REPETITION

REPETITION IS THE CHINESE WATER torture of dementia. The first few drops land on the head with little impact, but as the minutes and hours pass, each drop, each repeated tale or movement, echoes more irritatingly and painfully than the last. Other people can't understand why you are getting so angry, and neither can you. But you are certain that if your parent says or does that particular thing one more time, you will scream.

Sometimes, like nudging the needle on a skipping record (for those of us who lived before tapes and CDs were around), you can nudge your parent out of whatever repetitious behavior is bothering you. Diversions help, or if your parent asks the same question over and over, either stop answering it or reply in a different way. (When she asks for the eightieth time, "When's

MY FATHER DOESN'T KNOW IT'S ME

As dementia weaves its way through your parent's brain, destroying his abilities and his memories, it will eventually get around to that cherished pocket that holds his memories of you. He may know who you are at one moment, but not at another. He may know your name, but forget that you are his daughter. This is the heartbreaking nature of dementia.

Suddenly, it seems that you no longer exist for your parent, and it may feel as if a part of you has died along with those memories. The magnetic forces that drew you to care for your parent, and kept you at it when things got rough, are weakened, or gone. Your father doesn't look at you with the same familiar gaze, full of knowledge and memories, but with the blank look of a stranger or the angry glare of a victim.

With all that you are losing, this is a debilitating blow. But remember, your parent needs you more than ever now. Not only does he need you to protect him because he can no longer fend for himself, but your warmth, your gaze, and your touch are powerfully reassuring for him, even if he can't say so, even if he doesn't know why. He has nothing left to give you now, and he needs everything from you. It is a lot to ask. Love him with whatever reserve you have left, for even though he doesn't remember your name or your past, you are his entire world now.

---

dinner?" instead of telling her one more time that it's at seven, you say, "We'll have dinner after Charlie comes home.") If the problem is a repeated motion, touch often works better than words. For example, if your parent is nervously stroking one elbow, rub her other arm or a leg for a moment.

When nothing works, focus your attention on something else. Take some deep breaths. Tune her out. Try to ignore her motions. Don't respond to her questions. In other words, when you can't divert her, be creative about diverting yourself.

ACCUSATIONS AND INSULTS

DEMENTIA DOESN'T SIMPLY OBLIT-erate people's personalities, it rearranges them. Certain traits become more pronounced, others fade away, and oddly enough, brand-new traits can appear. It's not uncommon for people with dementia to become mean and insulting. Your parent might complain that you never visit, that you don't feed him enough, that his wife is cheating on him, or that you've hidden things from him (which you may have, and for good reason). He might call people names, or he might be rude to strangers on the street, leaving you to apologize for him.

Given all that you are doing for him, such attacks can shatter the patience and control you are trying so hard to sustain. No matter how confused he may be, a parent's criticism hits a very sensitive nerve, and the insults may be virtually impossible to shrug off.

But shrug you must. Whenever your parent makes a biting remark, remember that he doesn't know what he is saying, or mean what he says. Try hard not to take such comments personally. Think of yourself as one of those blow-up clowns that you punch and they pop right back up—the blow was meaningless and did no harm.

Also, consider what might be behind your parent's comments, especially if the same criticism is made repeatedly. For example, people with dementia often accuse others of stealing things because that would explain why they can't find things. Your parent might claim that someone is keeping him prisoner because he is aware that he is losing his independence and can't understand why. He might accuse a spouse of infidelity because he feels inadequate as a mate. He might insist that you are mean because he feels frightened, alone, and insecure, or because he knows that he is increasingly dependent upon you and is angry about that. Not knowing where else to fire that anger, he fires it at you.

Next time your father accuses you of stealing his clock, rather than yelling back, simply accept the blame: "I probably did lose it. Let's see if we can't find it together." And rather than arguing, "I am not cruel to you!" console your parent and address his real fears: "I know the world feels cruel right now. I don't like this either. But we have each other and we will get through it together."

Remember, don't try to reason with your parent. Simply do what you can to reassure him that people love him and that he is safe.

Your father may not stop making the comments, but if you understand why he makes them, or accept that there is no reason or logic to his comments, you will be better equipped to put up with them.

Talk to others who care for him and explain all this to them. You may have to make up for your parent's anger and criticism by apologizing for him, and then being especially appreciative and complementary. If nothing else, perhaps you and these other workers can find some humor in it, seeing who bore the biggest brunt.

Special Issues

Certain behaviors and actions—incontinence, violence, inappropriate sexual behavior, hallucinations—can easily become too much for caregivers. If you encounter these problems, try some of the tips outlined below and throughout this chapter, and consult the local Alzheimer's Association and your parent's doctor.

If nothing helps and you simply can't handle it, know that you have a lot of company. It may well be time to find other housing and care for your parent.

AGGRESSION AND VIOLENCE

SOME OF YOUR PARENT'S ANGER AND aggression is understandable; life has taken a terrible turn, and each day is a series of failures, losses, and frightening experiences. But much of his behavior is due to damage to the part of the brain that regulates and reins in emotion. This can abolish inhibitions and disable the normal controls. As a result, your parent may not only behave badly, he may not realize that anything is wrong with what he is doing. Family members who no longer like this angry imposter, but who still have to care for him, face an agonizing conflict.

Derail his outbursts as best as you can. Look for cues that set off the rage, try to avoid them, and be ready to jump in and divert his attention. Remain as calm as you can because yelling back will only escalate the situation.

While it's unusual for a person with dementia to become physically violent, it happens. Remove or lock up potential weapons (knives, guns, baseball bats, umbrellas, scissors, etc.) and post emergency numbers by the telephones. Don't put yourself or others in danger under any circumstances. If your parent attacks you or someone else, do not try to disarm him or

> *My mother went through a violent stage, which was the scariest part of her dementia for me. She was a different person. It was horrible. She would yell, scream, and swear—at me, at the rest of the family, at the doctor. She would come right up to my face and threaten to hit me.*
>
> *When we were in public, she would get frustrated and there was no controlling her. I would take her to church and if somebody moved their head in front of her or talked, she would say, 'When is he going to shut up?' very loudly, you know.*
>
> *She would never have done that before, never be rude. It was horrible for all of us."*
>
> —LINDA K.

fight with him. Get away from him as quickly as possible. If necessary, call the police. When your parent can't be calmed down in any other way, aggression can be treated with medications, so talk with your parent's doctor about what to do.

If an outburst is physical but not dangerous—if your parent is storming around the room cursing violently, or banging his fists on the bed—let it happen. Provide a safe environment where he can explode, like in a room where there are no sharp edges, glass, or other dangerous items. Hopefully, he'll tire himself out quickly.

INAPPROPRIATE PUBLIC OR SEXUAL BEHAVIOR

INAPPROPRIATE PUBLIC BEHAVIOR IS very common with dementia; inappropriate sexual behavior is not. When either one occurs, decide first whether the behavior is worth making a fuss about. Sometimes what is construed as sexual behavior, such as sitting outdoors naked or rubbing one's crotch, may simply be an effort to get comfortable. It may be hot outdoors, and the crotch may itch.

If your parent's behavior is not hurting anyone—if your father is masturbating alone in the living room—try to ignore it, if you can. It's painful and bewildering for you, but you cannot force him to adhere to social norms that have disappeared from his mind. Ignoring him, whether it stops the behavior or not, will certainly save you a lot of aggravation.

When your parent's behavior has to be curbed, head it off before it starts. If he tends to play with his genitals in public, be sure that his hands are busy with something else. If he urinates in unusual places, buy him trousers without a fly (elastic-waisted pants or sweatpants) or with a belt—anything that is slightly difficult to open. Then as soon as you see him struggling with his belt or waistband, steer him toward the men's room.

Stay one step ahead of your parent. If you know that a long line or a wait at a restaurant will set your father off, for example, tell the waiter that you need to be served quickly. As soon as your mother starts berating a stranger or unbuttoning her dress on the street, suggest a diversion—one that she really enjoys, like having ice cream or visiting a grandchild.

Most important, don't make a fuss when your parent embarrasses you in public, as that will only draw more attention. Instead, gently convey the message that your parent is ill. Rather than lashing out at him, get him back on course, console him and calm him, apologize to anyone he offended, and exit quickly, if at all possible.

When your parent's sex drive is out of control, talk with the doctor. He may need medications to curb his desire.

DELUSIONS AND HALLUCINATIONS

YOUR MOTHER INSISTS THAT THE neighbor is trying to poison her. Your father tells you that he just spoke to Vanna White. As if you didn't have enough to worry about.

Delusions—believing things that are not true—are common in people with dementia largely because they tend to misinterpret what is happening around them. Your father may no longer understand the difference between a person on television and a person in real life. Your mother believes she is being starved because she can't remember her last meal.

Hallucinations—seeing things or hearing things that don't exist—are less common, but some people experience them. Your father says that there is a pig in the corner of his room, or

APPROPRIATE SEXUAL BEHAVIOR

In the early stages of dementia, in particular, relationships and flirting, romance, intimacy, and even sex may be quite appropriate. As long as your parent can still make somewhat reasonable decisions, is dealing with a person who is also relatively competent, and is not upsetting or abusing another person, love and intimacy are still normal and acceptable human needs.

If you are concerned, talk with someone from the nursing home or health-care agency, his doctor, or some other professional. Love and sex are wonderful if he can find them, and they are certainly within the bounds of acceptability.

It may be that your parent isn't having sex, but is forming liaisons. He may be flirting or just enjoying someone's company and attention. He may want a partner, someone to fill a void. That can be wonderful, too.

Unfortunately, your befuddled parent might call this companion by your mother's name (or call your mother by someone else's name). He might insist that some woman he just met is married to him, or that they are siblings, or that they have been together for years. As painful as this is, let it be if it makes him happy. He means no harm. His reality is skewed.

If your parent has a spouse, sexual problems may arise in their relationship. Your mother might not be interested because of the exhaustion and grief of caregiving, or because her spouse has changed so much. Or she might feel that her mate has become inappropriately sexual. Or perhaps she wants to have sex, but her spouse is no longer interested.

Sexuality issues become complicated when one spouse is ill, but these troubles are compounded when one is ill with dementia. Most people do not talk about these issues, but struggle silently with their feelings and desires, confusion and anger. Urge your "well" parent to talk with a professional counselor or doctor about sexuality issues. The local chapter of the Alzheimer's Association may be able to help.

tells you that elves speak to him. You can no more convince your parent that these things aren't true than someone could convince you that what you see is not there. Don't argue with your parent. In fact, in many cases, it's better to do just the opposite. If the hallucination is not frightening—and some are actually amusing or pleasant —let your parent tell you more about it and accept her word as true. If a delusion is not causing any trouble, go along with it or ignore it.

If the beliefs or visions are upsetting your parent, assure him that he is safe, that the goblins are friendly ones or that you will shoo the pig away. Take a bite of any "poisoned" food first or let your parent keep her own closet of food if she feels she is being starved.

As with other troubling behaviors, look for any possible underlying meaning—when she says that her bed is on fire, find out if the electric blanket is on too high. If she says that a home-care worker is trying to kill her, ask how the worker is going to do that. Maybe your parent feels that the aide is trying to suffocate her because she keeps all the windows closed and smokes all day.

Hallucinations sometimes go away if the person simply moves to another part of the room or house. Distractions can help. Increase lighting. Get rid of any noises that might be contributing to hallucinations. And cover mirrors or other props that might be prompting a vision or belief. If visions are coming from one part of the room, see if there isn't something in that corner

> " *My mother would wake up in the middle of the night screaming, 'Get them out of here! Get them out of here!' She would say she saw people, little children, at her bedside. I didn't know what was going on.*
>
> *At one point I had a minister come and talk to her. I didn't know what else to do. I thought maybe he could help get rid of any demons or spirits in her life, but it didn't help.*
>
> *Then one day it just stopped on its own. She stopped crying out. I asked her later about the little children, if she had seen them lately, and she didn't know what I was talking about. She told me I was nuts."*
>
> —MARY W.

that might be triggering the hallucination. Also, be sure your parent isn't watching upsetting or violent television shows. She might be having a hard time separating television from reality.

If all else fails and the delusions or hallucinations become a serious problem, talk with the doctor.

Chapter Twenty-Four

THE LAST
GOOD-BYE

Talking about Death • Caring for Your Parent Now
• Hospice • Treatment Choices • The Face of Death

....

A T SOME POINT, IT BECOMES CLEAR THAT YOUR PARENT
is neither invincible nor immortal, that despite your labor
and love, the best efforts of doctors and the prayers of
friends, she will not be around much longer. If you have been
giving ceaselessly and worrying constantly, or if your parent has
suffered miserably through illness and infirmity, this may not be
a completely unwelcome thought. At the same time, it is an agonizing
one. Inconceivable, in a way. How can this person who has been
with you from the start, cared for you, guided you, and fought you,
ever be gone? No matter how sick your parent is, no matter how
much or how little she can say or do now, she is still there and still
your parent. How could it ever be otherwise?

The approaching death of a parent may be deeply painful to
think about and even more difficult to talk about. In fact, you
might be tempted to deny it, to refuse to confront it. But as your
parent nears the end of her life, keep in mind the wise words of
Dr. Sherwin B. Nuland, author of *How We Die:* "Death belongs to
the dying and to those who love them." This death, your parent's

death, belongs not to hospitals, doctors, and nurses. It belongs to your parent, to you, and to other family members.

Your family has some control over this death—not perhaps over its cause or timing, but over how your parent dies and what sort of life she lives until that point. You can choose which medical treatments will be used and which refused, where your parent will be, how she will spend this time, who will be with her, what will be said, what comfort will be given, and, when it's over, what sort of memorial will honor her life.

Death is a process, a final passage of life, that demands both practical and emotional involvement from everyone. Do not turn away. You and other family members are facing a great loss, but you can still cherish these final days with your parent and help her find comfort and peace.

Death is not simply a grim and heartbreaking betrayal. No, when we are willing to face it, death is also a potent reminder that despite all of the aggravations in a day, life is precious—very, very precious. To whatever extent you are able, acknowledge this process, and, in doing so, celebrate life.

Beyond Denial

Although you may know on some level that your parent has only a limited time left to live, you might tiptoe around words like *terminal* and *hospice,* and certainly avoid a word like *dying.* You may find yourself saying, "Everything is going to be fine," when you know full well that it won't be. It's as if by saying the words we might make it happen, and by dodging them, we cling to hope.

But whether anyone says it openly or not, your parent knows what is happening. She understands that she is incurably ill or hopelessly frail and that her life is drawing to a close. In fact, she probably knows it better than anyone. But she may be doing exactly what you are doing—avoiding the subject for fear of upsetting those around her. She may be keeping quiet to protect you.

How sad to spend these last months, or weeks, or days, in silence, when there are practical matters to discuss, and when both of you might welcome the opportunity to share your fears and sorrow. This is a chance to express devotion, make apologies,

> *One afternoon I was wiping my father's face with a damp washcloth, to cool him. I was exhausted, and he was barely conscious. He was very thin and pale, but I could still see my father there, the young, strong man that I knew. I stroked his forehead, his cheekbones, the hollows and curves of his neck. His skin was always so soft.*
>
> *He was there, still there for me, but he wasn't going to be there much longer. I knew that. I could still love him and touch him and hug him, but just for now. For this moment. But maybe not again. And at that moment I loved him more than I have ever loved anyone in my life."*
>
> —MARJORIE C.

remember the wonderful things about your parent's life, and start saying good-bye.

PREPARATIONS

IF YOU TALK ABOUT NOTHING ELSE, discuss your parent's medical care. Hopefully he has signed advance directives. Perhaps you have promised him that you won't ever "let it be dragged out." You know what he wants. You know what to do. But do you?

If this is all you know and all you do, then the odds are high that he will still die in a hospital or nursing home, alone and in pain, receiving brutal treatments and suffering needlessly.

To avoid this nightmare and make your parent's death as gentle as it can be, it is essential that you do more.

◆ **Find those directives.** By now, your parent should have signed a living will outlining her wishes regarding medical care at the end of life, and a power of attorney for health care, authorizing someone to make medical decisions on her behalf. Find them. Be sure that you have a copy on hand, and that her doctor has one as well. If she hasn't signed them already, get them signed immediately. They are described in full on page 383.

◆ **Talk.** With any luck, you've already discussed your parent's wishes concerning medical care at some length. Now you need to talk some more, or, if you haven't started, you need to get started (pronto).

By this point, her doctor should be able to give you some idea of what the future holds and what sorts of decisions she and you may face. Given her current health and what is known about her future, would your parent want to be put on a respirator? Would she want artificial nutrition or hydration? Would she want to be resuscitated if her heart were to stop? Or would she like to be at home now, under the care of a hospice, with assurances that any discomfort and symptoms will be treated?

If you've talked before, bring this up as part of a continuing conversation. *Dad, do you remember when you said that you would never want to be on life support? Do you still feel that way?*

Otherwise, ask your parent what the doctor has told her, and what she thinks lies ahead, and see where she goes with that. Or let your parent know that you've spoken with her doctor and ask if she wants to hear about it.

If your parent can't understand the choices or communicate her wishes, you and other family members should discuss her situation immediately, at some length. Talk with her doctor and review possible scenarios, options, and likely outcomes.

> *My mother would say, 'I'm tired. I've had enough. If anything else happens, I don't want any more.' But I think she was thinking in terms of an operation. She was thinking of her brain surgery. I'm not sure. She didn't ever spell it out. She had had angina for years, but that wasn't what we considered to be her problem.*
>
> *When she had a heart attack, we just weren't ready for that. She went to the emergency room and was put on life support.*
>
> *We assumed we were pretty savvy. We felt that we knew what was going on. But we were stunned. I look back and wonder, 'What were we thinking? What happened?' But the whole thing just snowballed."*
>
> —JOANN C.

Think about who she is and what she would want. Then think about the actions you might take.

◆ **Spread the word.** Make sure that your parent's doctor and other family members are all aware of these discussions and plans, are clear about your parent's wishes, and are ready to abide by them. If even one sibling disagrees with a decision to withhold care, a doctor may insist on providing unwanted medical treatment. Yes, you can fight it, but life will be much easier for everyone if you all come to a consensus in advance.

If your parent is in a hospital or nursing home, be sure that his advance directives are on file there, and speak with nurses or aides involved in his care. Make sure they understand your parent's wishes or family's decision and that they will abide by them. Find out exactly what they will or will not do in specific situations. Be persistent in ensuring that his wishes will be honored.

◆ **Brace yourself.** Now for the big step. Talking is one thing, but you and others also need to be ready to act, one way or the other. You might be able to say that you'd never agree to aggressive and seemingly futile medical care, but could you really say no? You've promised that you'll "pull the plug," but do you understand what that means? Do you know what is involved? If a procedure offers some chance of lengthening her life, but will add to her pain, will you agree to it? If you are not going to put her on a respirator or allow resuscitation, what are you going to do? How will her pain be treated, her fear eased, and her soul calmed? How will you react to a crisis? Are you ready to let go? Are you and others around her ready, really ready, to say good-bye?

◆ **Don't wait for "there."** A common mistake people make is waiting. Waiting for some clear line between living and dying, between useful medical treatments and futile ones. When hospice is suggested, they say, "Oh, we're not there yet."

By waiting, however, people often find that "there" has come and gone. They are left standing in an ICU staring at a person full of tubes, wondering where "there" went and how they got "here." Or they call hospice, but not until the final hour, at which point hospice workers can only respond to the most urgent issues.

Unfortunately, there is often no clear-cut dividing line, some place where decisions are obvious. Instead, there are odds and possibilities and unknowns. It's up to you to learn all you can, weigh the possibilities, and make excruciating decisions. Don't wait. Start making them early.

◆ **Beware of hope.** When someone is facing the possibility of death, loved ones and doctors tend to tone down or hide the bad news, and inflate or invent the good. They do it in the name of hope, to give the patient hope, to keep up morale. *We can't tell her the prognosis, or call hospice because she might lose hope.*

> *I knew my father was extremely sick and that he probably wouldn't make it through the year. But we didn't talk about it. We talked about his illness and treatments, but not about his dying.*
>
> *About three weeks before he died, I noticed that he wasn't eating, and I mentioned his lack of appetite. He said, 'That's what happens in the terminal stage.' It was as if a window shattered. There was a silence that seemed to last several seconds. Finally I said, 'Are you afraid of dying?' And he said, 'No. I want to be sure that your mother is going to be all right. But I'm not afraid.' And that was it. We didn't say anything else. I just wrapped my arms around him and we held each other.*
>
> *That was the only time the word was said, but it was enough. It was as if a veil was removed. After that, every look, every touch was so intense and so close because we both knew, and we knew the other knew."*
>
> —MARJORIE C.

Hope is good. But lies and half-truths do not create hope; they create deception and often lead to unwanted medical treatments. Studies and anecdotal stories show that vast numbers of people get medical treatments they didn't want because doctors and families, in trying to maintain hope, have lied to them.

> " *I asked her about dying.*
> *I said, 'Do you think about*
> *dying much?' And she said, 'No, I*
> *really don't.' And that was it. That*
> *was the end of the conversation.*
>
> *I was blunter than I usually am,*
> *but I wanted to give her a chance to*
> *talk about it. I didn't get anything,*
> *but I know it didn't offend her*
> *either. We're just different. I enjoy*
> *introspection, thinking about life,*
> *and she doesn't. She's always been*
> *that way."*
>
> —BETTY H.

Certainly there is no reason to dump dreadful news on someone who is not ready to hear it or force someone to accept a fact that they simply can't. That's not the point.

Ask your parent what she thinks and what she wants to know. Let her determine what news she gets and how she wants to handle it. If she knows the facts and still wants to talk about cures and years of long life, let her. If she does not want to hear what the doctor has to say, she doesn't have to.

But do not tell her lies or hide the truth. The truth may hurt her, it may make her sad, but knowing allows her to prepare, to move forward, to accept what is happening, and to make decisions about her care. And as we've noted, she surely already knows more than you think she does.

Keep in mind, hope has many faces, and hoping for a cure or long life is only one of them. People can hope to live until a certain date, or hope to be free of pain, or hope that their life had value. They can hope for all sorts of things. Accepting that death is near, knowing the truth, does not mean the loss of hope.

OTHER CONVERSATIONS

MAYBE YOU'VE FOUND A WAY TO TALK with your parent about his medical care. Maybe you've been honest with him about his prognosis. But how do you talk about anything else? How do you stop commenting nervously on the weather and the hospital décor?

Standing at the bedside of someone who is terminally ill is agonizing. You may be able to grieve on some level, and even talk in muted tones about death with friends and family (or maybe not). But then, you get in that room with your parent, and a wall comes up. What do you say? You may want desperately to tell him you love him, that you'll miss him, that you'll never forget him. Or maybe you want to know what he's feeling, what's in his heart, or how you might help. But it's all too close, too stark, too massive.

It's fine to talk about the ugly blue vinyl chairs and the cool day outside, but if it all starts to feel a bit empty and false, go ahead, cross the border. You can jump in, or just dangle a toe in.

Conversations don't have to be long and heavy. At a time like this, a few words, a comment, a bit of reassurance, even a look, an embrace, or a touch can say a great deal. The important thing is that you allow communication. Don't lie or dodge your parent's efforts to talk. If possible, open the door for her.

Ask gentle, open questions that allow your parent to speak or not speak, to take the conversation wherever she needs it to be. Be open, honest, and ready to listen.

This is an important time for her to review her life and express her concerns. See page 529 for what she might be thinking and what you might discuss.

Quite often, important issues arise on their own, at unexpected times. Your parent might say out of the blue, "I'm going to miss you," or "I'm afraid." Or she might say something like, "I want you to know where my old tax returns are stored," or "I need to give you your birthday present early."

People in the late stages of illness sometimes broach the subject in more cryptic ways. Your parent may talk about a relative or a friend who is dead, or she might make references to traveling—getting tickets, packing bags, going on a boat, or leaving someone behind.

Be ready for these moments, because you can easily be caught off guard and shut your parent off by saying something like, "Oh Mom, don't talk like that." Be careful not to change the subject, disagree, discount her fears, or attempt to cheer her up. Instead, offer her a safe place to expose her feelings and concerns. More valuable than

PLEASE DON'T GO

You may find that you are not only having trouble talking openly about death, but that you are doing just the opposite. When the subject comes up, you state emphatically that she will get better. Or you plead desperately with her not to die, saying that she mustn't leave you.

In your own way, you are telling your parent that you love her and that you will be sad when she is gone. Your words are meant to be kind and affectionate, and your parent probably understands this. But be aware that such denial shuts your parent out. It leaves her no way to share her pain, love, or fears. Worse, it puts her in the role of protecting you; in addition to dealing with her own grief, she must now worry about you and your future.

If you want to tell your parent that you love her, that you wish things weren't this way, that you will miss her, do so. But if you find yourself pleading with her or denying the truth, think about how your words are affecting her and try to take a different approach next time.

> *I had promised him that I would never allow extraordinary medical procedures. No life support. He was a sick man. I knew that he would die of these problems. But I didn't know that, given his situation, life support was likely to be in his future. I was never told that for a person with breathing problems, in an emergency situation, a respirator would be indicated. I had this general idea that he didn't want to be on machines, but as far as specifics go, we hadn't discussed it.*
>
> *He was on a respirator and hooked to all sorts of tubes for twenty days. I watched him being tortured in front of me. I could hardly touch him because there were tubes everywhere.*
>
> *One day a doctor came in and saw me stroke his calves and said, 'Oh, he's getting a massage.' But I was touching him there because that was the only place where I could touch him. I couldn't even touch his face.*
>
> *Those are my memories. That's what I'm left with."*
>
> —KATHERINE D.

anything you say right now is what you allow your parent to say.

If you reflexively jump away from an opening, don't worry. You did what most people do. Simply bring the subject up yourself: "Do you remember when you told me that you would miss me?" Or listen carefully for another opening. But do not wait long, as time may be short now.

WHEN COMMUNICATION IS LIMITED

IF YOUR PARENT IS TOO SICK TO SPEAK much, or at all, don't just stand numbly by the door, or sit by her bed staring at her.

Look through family photo albums and describe the scenes and moments. Talk about your memories and fun and wonderful times you've had together. Hearing you and others reminisce and laugh will fill her heart.

Do this even if you think your parent can't understand or hear you. You can never be sure how much an ill person comprehends, and even if she doesn't understand your words, she will be soothed simply by your presence and your voice.

It is also okay to sit quietly at times. Read to yourself or aloud to her, work on your laptop computer, watch television quietly.

OPTING NOT TO TALK

DESPITE YOUR BEST INTENTIONS, IT may not be possible for you to discuss much of anything with your parent. Don't be hard on yourself. Sometimes the issues are too big. Certainly this is not the time to take on complex family dynamics. You might ask a question or offer simple forgiveness, but don't expect to resolve old problems now.

Sometimes talking openly about anything terribly important is out of the question. Candor comes naturally to some, but for others, it's too much. It may not be who your parent is, who you are, or what your relationship has been.

Talking about death requires that you accept that your parent is going to die. It means leaving the safe harbor of denial and exposing yourself to a whole set of razor-sharp emotions—shock, anger, despair, helplessness, and profound sadness.

Think carefully, because you may not have another chance. What is the worst thing that might happen if you spoke candidly? How will you feel later if you say nothing now? What might such an honest gesture mean to your parent? How might it help her? How might it help you? How might it hurt either of you? Whatever you decide is fine.

If it is your parent who doesn't want to talk—if you open this dialogue and he repeatedly changes the subject—then respect his decision. In this case, silence is a way of honoring your parent, of letting him deal with death in his own way.

> *The best therapy for us was the laughter. She and I loved to laugh together. Even toward the end, we were laughing. Those are the memories we share."*
>
> —KIM D.

Remember, you don't have to use words to let him know that you love him and that you will miss him. The look in your eyes, your embrace, your tears, and your tenderness will tell him what he most needs to know.

Your Parent's Perspective

To talk with your parent, and to care for him, you need to understand some of what he is going through. Of course, without facing death ourselves, it is almost impossible to imagine. But there are common themes.

◆ People are often more afraid of dying than of death. They are afraid of the process, of the unknown, and, more than almost anything else, of being alone. Your parent needs affection and assurance that you or others will be with her throughout this time.

◆ People are almost universally afraid of dying in pain. Straightforward information from a doctor or nurse about what is to come and how pain will be controlled, as well as promises from you that you will fight for ample pain control, should alleviate much of this fear. If she is not under the care of a hospice, ask the doctor for a consultation with a palliative care specialist, who will know all about controlling pain and symptoms.

◆ People are often afraid that they will be a burden to others as they grow sicker. Your parent needs to know that she is not a burden, that you or another loved one will gladly take care of her directly, or will continue to oversee her care in a hospital, hospice, or a nursing home.

◆ It's important now for people to review their lives—what life has meant, what its value has been, and how they will be remembered. They want to know that their lives have been worthwhile, that they have accomplished certain things, and that they were loved. Help your parent remember the good things in her life—friends, jobs, milestones, successes. If she's still alert, ask her about her life. How was it growing up on a farm? How did she choose her husband or her job? What is she most proud of? What are some of the most memorable moments of her life? (How far you go with all this depends on how far she wants to go.) Tape-record these conversations, for you will surely want to remember it all. Then let her know that her life was well lived and, in particular, that you respect, love, and admire her.

◆ Your parent will also want to know that she will be remembered, that she has left some legacy behind. Talk about the lessons she taught you and the memories that will be passed on to future generations. Then let her know that her grandchildren still talk about the time she took them to New York, or that they still repeat a story she used to tell. Or if she has gifts to pass on, legacies or treasures, help her accomplish that.

◆ Those who are dying also want to know that their loved ones will be okay, their affairs are in order, their dependents cared for, their battles reconciled. They want to know that nothing crucial will be left unsettled or unfinished. If you sense that your parent feels that she has left something undone, help her to bring it to a conclusion. Urge an estranged relative to speak to her, or help her dictate a note to someone she has distanced herself from.

Let your parent know that while you will miss her, you and others will be okay. As the end draws near, let her know that it is all right for her to go; give her permission to die peacefully.

FIVE STAGES

EACH PERSON RESPONDS TO ILLNESS and death in his or her own way; people react as differently to the end of life as they do to other major events. But there are several reactions that are more common. Knowing about them may help you respond to them. For the most part, you simply have to be understanding and allow them. Let your parent hide in denial and release his anger. Don't fight him or disagree with him. Don't tell him that his reactions are wrong. Acknowledge his rage and give him a place to vent it. If he talks about cures and a long life, don't disagree, but don't agree either. Just say, "That would be great. I hope so."

Keep in mind that the reactions noted here are by no means universal. People react to death as individually as they react to life. Also, while these responses are presented as sequential stages, many people bounce among them, moving, for example, through a period of denial, a few days of anger, and then back into denial. Some adopt several at one time, angry on one level and still denying on another.

◆ **Denial.** Sometimes the brain simply pulls down the shades and looks the other way, announcing to itself and the world, "This cannot be happening. It is not possible. There must be another explanation." This response is completely normal, developed through years of evolution to protect a person from news that is just too painful to bear.

Don't encourage your parent's denial, but allow it, especially early on. Urge him, gently, to face decisions that he must. But don't force information upon him needlessly. If he insists that he is going to get well when the doctor has told him otherwise, simply say, "That would be great, Dad. I certainly hope that's the case."

If your parent remains in denial, and it gets in the way of making medical decisions or taking proper care of him, you may have to push a little and/or make some plans and decisions for him. It's a lonely place to be, but one that you have to accept.

◆ **Anger.** Once your parent realizes that he is indeed dying, he may become angry—angry at himself for being ill, angry at others who are not ill, angry at God for letting this happen, angry at doctors who bear bad news, and angry at family and friends for any reason or no reason at all. Your parent may express his anger loudly, in fits of rage, or he may bottle it up. Again, allow him his reactions. You might even encourage his anger, giving him pillows to punch and a place to yell. When you become his target, don't escalate things by arguing with him.

◆ **Bargaining.** People who are terminally ill often go through a period of mental bargaining, usually with God or whatever higher power they believe in. *Let me get well, and I'll stop smoking, cheating, being unkind, etc.* Your parent might bargain for his health, or he might bargain for comfort, love, or time—perhaps he wants to be around for a specific event, such as an anniversary, a birthday, or a celebration. You may not know the specifics of the deal, but you may notice some change in his behavior. Perhaps he is suddenly taking an active role in his health care, doing everything he can to prolong his life.

Find out if there is a particular goal your parent has in mind. If he wants to see a loved one before he dies, help bring that about. If his bargaining involves lifestyle changes, such as eating well or exercising, encourage it, not as a way for him to cure his illness, but as a way for him to gain a sense of control over his life.

◆ **Worry and grief.** Realizing that there is no escaping death, no bartering with God, your parent may begin to mourn the loss of life and the loss of those around him whom he loves.

" My father had a wonderful death. That's a funny thing to say, but his whole countenance changed. He was a difficult and demanding man, and he made a lot of people angry during his life. But when he learned he had only a few months to live, he walked back through his life and reviewed it all. He became very sweet and tender. The minister came frequently to see him, and prayed with him. It made him very genuine and real, and you could say anything to him. We were very close during those weeks. I spent a lot of time up in his room, sitting at a card table trying to write. It was a lovely, sort of profound, relationship.

The minister told me much later that he'd never seen a person prepare himself for death as beautifully as my father had. I don't know where it came from, but I hope that I can do the same. It was a tremendous gift that he gave us all, at the end."

—BETTY H.

He may mourn things he failed to do in the past and dreams he will not be able to fulfill in the future. He may feel helpless, powerless, and deeply saddened. He may worry terribly about being a burden to you and other family members.

People sometimes feel anxious about specific issues (Will my grand-children be okay? Will I need life support? How will we pay for these medical bills?) and experience a loss of self-esteem due to illness. Some of these concerns may be eased with reassurance. But when people are grieving the loss of life, reassurance rarely alleviates the pain. A dying person cannot "cheer up," and he must be allowed to have this sorrow. He may want to share his sadness, but it's more likely he will be silent. You can share your parent's grief without words, perhaps by touching him tenderly or just sitting quietly by his side.

Sadness and grief are normal; true clinical depression, even at the end of life, is not. If your parent sinks deep into depression, feeling that all is hopeless and dark and the weight of life is too much to bear, talk with his doctor or a psychiatrist. Depression, even at this point, is treatable and definitely worth treating.

◆ **Resignation and acceptance.** At some point, many people become resigned, acknowledging what is happening and realizing that there is nothing they can do to change it. They may not necessarily accept it, but they are resigned to it.

For those fortunate enough to reach it, acceptance is a calm, almost peaceful time, when a person accepts that death is approaching. That is not to say that he welcomes death, but he is relieved that the struggle is over. He is no longer trying to extend his life or to get well. He is no longer depressed or angry. He may be preparing for his departure, seeking simply comfort and serenity.

If your parent has been sick for some time, he may have gone slowly and quietly through the other stages, or he may have skipped them completely. In either case, some people seem to go straight to acceptance.

Acceptance is best for your parent, and, if you are on the same page, it can be a wonderful time for your whole family. This is sad, but it can also be a time of intense love, humor, intimacy, and joyful memories. It can be almost "other-worldly," as if you have temporarily closed the door on day-to-day life and entered a place that only a privileged few get to share.

However, this time may be difficult for you if you have not reached a similar stage yourself. You may sense that your parent has given up when you think that he should still be fighting. You may feel his separation and long to bring him back.

But he is ready to go; he may already have begun to sever his earthly ties. As a result, he may want to see fewer and fewer people, not for any lack of feeling for them, but because he has said his good-byes already and is at peace with that. Saying good-bye again would require too much energy. He may also choose not to see certain people who have not accepted his dying; their denial may be too much for him to handle now.

If your parent refuses visitors, respect his wishes. If he chooses not to see you, try to understand his response and be happy for him that he has

---

> ## AROUND AND AROUND WE GO
>
> Keep a journal of what is happening and all you are feeling now. If you don't have time or don't want to write, buy a small tape recorder and keep it in the car, in the bathroom, or by your bed. Talk into it about whatever is on your mind. Record the painful emotions, the memorable comments, the tender looks, and the loving embraces. As unforgettable as this experience seems now, the details and the intensity will be lost if they are not recorded, and while they are painful, you may want to remember them in the future.

---

reached this stage of readiness. It is time to let him go. If you can, give him your blessing, whether aloud or in silence.

Caring for Your Parent Now

Whether your parent is in a hospital, a nursing home, or at home, there is much that you can do to care for her now:

◆ Be aware of her mental and spiritual health. In addition to talking with you, she should have the opportunity to talk to a counselor, social worker, psychiatrist, or clergyperson. (Even if she can't communicate, she might be consoled by their reassuring words.)

◆ Make the most of your parent's days. Think about what she might most appreciate. Does she want to be left in silence? Does she like to listen to music, the television, or the radio? Would she like someone to tell her stories about old times, read aloud to her or sing her favorite songs? Would she like to watch birds come to a feeder outside her window? If she can be moved, would she like to be driven along a waterfront, or would she like to lie on a lounge chair in the sun? Or would she simply like someone to sit quietly with her and stroke her? In tending to her physical care, don't lose sight of her daily needs and simple pleasures.

◆ Treat your parent with respect and dignity and ask others to do the same. Keep her informed about what is happening and give her as much control over decisions as possible. Respect her modesty, even if she seems

> *I don't know where she ends and I begin, our lives are so intertwined. Part of me is very much looking forward to losing her and being free. But frankly, I think that when she goes, I'll feel like, 'Oh, my God, I'm going to die now, too.'"*
>
> —Sasha L.

unaware of such matters. And ask people around her to call her by the name or title she is used to.

◆ Give your parent lots of affection. Touch is a powerful tonic—for both of you. Hold her hand, stroke her forehead, rest your head on her arm, kiss her cheek, or give her a gentle massage.

◆ Even if your parent can't express her thoughts, or if she seems oblivious to what is happening, assume that she hears and understands what is going on around her. Hearing is the last sense to go, so take private conversations out of the room and don't talk about your parent as if she were not there. Talk to her as you or others turn her, bathe her, and feed her. "I'm going to lift your right arm and put a pillow under it." That sort of thing.

◆ If your parent is bedridden, watch for bedsores. As she becomes frailer and spends more time in bed, her skin will become increasingly thin and fragile. The pressure and friction on bony spots—elbows, heels, buttocks, the back of the head—can cause sores that, if left untreated, are very painful. (See page 249 for more on bedsores.)

◆ Make sure her room smells fresh, and if she is at home, keep linens, commodes and other items clean.

◆ As your parent becomes sicker, take stock of your own emotional state, as well as hers. Death is a consuming process—for everyone involved. You and other family members need to get away from the preoccupation with illness and death and talk about other things. You need to eat well and get some sleep. And you should meet, even if it's only briefly, with a counselor, social worker, member of the clergy, hospice nurse, or another person trained in grief counseling and bereavement. If anyone involved becomes extremely anxious or depressed, he or she should see a psychiatrist or his or her personal doctor. These problems are nothing to be ashamed of and can be treated effectively with medication and counseling.

CARE AT HOME

IF YOUR PARENT AND FAMILY WANT to avoid the tubes, technology, and other invasions of hospital care, your parent may be able to move into a hospice, or she can stay in her home, with the help of a hospice or visiting nurses.

By making this choice, you give her the comfort of home and keep her free from unwanted medical treatments and the indignities of hospital life. She will be surrounded by the people she loves and have control over what she wants to do—sip a glass of sherry, watch television at three in the morning, have quiet time alone, or listen to Mozart.

At home, you create the opportunity for intimacy, for treasured moments of warmth and humor. You will be able to grieve, love, hurt, and care for your parent freely, privately, and completely. It will be, no doubt, a life-changing experience.

All this intimacy comes at a price, however. Such an undertaking often entails sleepless nights and challenging days of changing diapers, keeping track of medications, lifting and shifting your parent to prevent bedsores, and providing other demanding physical care. Even if health aides and nurses are enlisted to do the physical work, the constant proximity to death can be draining. These are long days and nights, spent watching your parent become sicker and weaker and closer to death.

Caring for a dying parent at home is hugely rich and rewarding, but it is not for everyone. When considering home care, think about whether you have the time and energy to give, and whether other family members and close friends might help. Think, too, about how you react to illness and whether you will be able to handle such immersion in the dying process.

If you are remotely interested in caring for your parent at home, call the local hospice. They can tell you what to expect, what help they can provide, and what your role will be. The sooner you call the more help they can offer.

Hospice

Hospice, the philosophy and practice of caring for people who are approaching death, is based on the belief that death is a natural and inevitable part of life and that at some point, rather than battling illness and fighting death at any cost, all efforts should be focused on enhancing whatever life remains.

With the help of a hospice, a person who is incurably ill and close to

> *When we brought my mother home from the hospital, there was all this equipment that had been delivered. We had a backup generator in case the electricity went out and tanks of oxygen. We had a commode and a special bed. I thought, 'What am I doing?'*
>
> *But we saw an improvement in her, almost right away. She perked up, being at home. She started her crocheting again. She could walk down the hall—she refused to use the walker—and sit in my room in the sun. She seemed so much happier. And I knew that what we were doing was right."*
>
> —NELLY O.

death is removed from the fast pace and machinery of a hospital and brought home (or to a homelike setting within a nursing home or a freestanding hospice center) to die more comfortably and peacefully.

Hospice nurses and doctors do not try to cure patients, and in general they discourage the use of aggressive medical treatments such as ventilators, feeding tubes, chemotherapy, radiation, and surgery. Instead, the focus of care is palliative, aimed at relieving pain and symptoms such as nausea, dizziness, and constipation. Most hospices will, however, arrange for invasive medical procedures (in conjunction with the patient's doctor) if those procedures

will ease pain or treat some secondary illness. Sometimes they will do it simply because a patient or family requests it.

Hospice nurses, who often work with a patient's primary physician or hospice doctor, are extraordinarily adept at managing pain without causing unnecessary grogginess. There is no getting around the fact that serious illness and the treatments aimed at combating it cause physical agony as well as mental anguish. But once under hospice care, patients generally do not suffer severe pain, except in rare circumstances.

As important as the physical care is the social, psychological, and spiritual support the hospice staff provides to both patients and their families. Nurses, aides, and social workers guide families through the daily regime and discuss the dying process, grief, and other emotional and practical issues with family members and the patient. They help resolve conflicts; offer financial guidance, pastoral support, and bereavement counseling; and in some instances even assist in planning funerals. Almost all hospice services, from companions to nurses to medical equipment, are covered by Medicare and other insurance.

There are more than two thousand hospice organizations across the country. Most offer home care and respite services. They typically have a medical director, nurses, home health aides, social workers, psychiatrists, nutritionists, speech and physical therapists, clergy, and volunteers, all of whom work with the family and patient, as well as the patient's own doctor. Whatever a family's specific needs, staff members are usually available twenty-four hours a day to answer questions or visit if there is an emergency.

Some hospices have residences where patients can stay either for the duration of their care or for a brief period when necessary. Others will make arrangements for short-term care, either by moving a patient temporarily into a nursing home or by arranging for nurses and aides to fill in at home while a family takes a break. Nearly half of all hospices have contracts with hospitals so that patients can be transferred if they need more extensive medical care.

The Myths of Hospice

Hospice care is not about giving up, or waiting for death, or overmedicating someone to the point of causing death. These are myths. Here are the facts:

◆ Hospice is state-of-the-art medical care. The only difference is that the goal of that care is to maximize comfort, mobility, and lucidity.

◆ People receiving hospice care do not necessarily die sooner than those receiving traditional hospital care. In fact, ironically, the evidence suggests that they actually live longer. Once people are free of pain and symptoms, surrounded by those they love, and relieved of their fear and anxiety, the desire to live is powerful.

◆ Giving people ample pain relief does not cause death. Certainly, a sudden megadose of morphine will stop a person's breathing. But when these drugs are given in gradually increasing doses, the body adjusts and can handle these doses.

◆ Hospice is about much more than giving morphine and waiting for death. It is about living whatever life is left to its fullest.

Hooking up with a Hospice

Before a patient is accepted for hospice care, Medicare and other insurance companies require that a doctor determine—as much as such a determination is possible—that the patient has less than six months to live.

If your family is interested, even if the timeline is still quite uncertain, contact the local hospice organization so you can learn the options, meet the staff, and, if desired, start making arrangements. As we've mentioned, the

> *Would we do it again?*
> *Yes, she was my mother.*
> *She was Michelle's grandmother. It's wearying, but it was a special time, during those months. There was an incredible closeness and tenderness among all of us. I was worried about Michelle because she's just a teenager, but she developed a bond with her grandmother."*
> —TERRY C.

mistake most people make is waiting too long.

To find a hospice, contact the National Hospice and Palliative Care Organization (800-658-8898 or www. nhpco.org). If there is a choice of hospices—many urban areas have more than one—ask about certification, staffing, credentials, and admission requirements. If the hospice does not have a residence, find out if it has a contract with a hospital or nursing home to offer inpatient care, if needed.

When There is No Hospice

If you are interested in caring for your parent at home, but there isn't an established hospice organization in the area or you don't like the one that is, don't despair. Hospice is not just an institution and a group of people, it is a philosophy of care. You can still take care of your parent at home; you will just need to do a little more legwork and organize your own support system.

Call a home-care agency and let them know that you are interested in hospice-type care. More and more home-care agencies are offering this sort of care to the dying, whether or not they are certified as hospices. Talk to your parent's doctor and contact a social worker, member of the clergy, or a psychotherapist who specializes in bereavement.

If your parent is in a hospital or a nursing home and you are not able to care for him at home, ask if the institution can offer hospice-type care,

AVOIDING 911

If you are caring for your parent at home, decide what you will do in an emergency. What will you do if his breathing stops? If he doesn't want to be resuscitated, then you shouldn't call an ambulance, because in most states paramedics must, by law, start resuscitation efforts. Admittedly, it's difficult to refrain from making such a call. In that frightening moment, people often find that they aren't quite ready to allow a parent to die, despite any previous plans, and they have an overwhelming desire to "save" him. It will help if you can prepare emotionally and practically for such an event. Think about what you would do and how you might say good-bye.

If you are worried that someone in the household might, in a state of panic, call 911, see if you can get a "nonhospital Do Not Resuscitate order," a legal document that releases paramedics from their obligation to resuscitate. (You can obtain a DNR order through your parent's doctor.) Post it in an obvious place where it will be spotted immediately.

or if hospice nurses can work with him within the institution. Sometimes hospitals or nursing homes have wings specifically for hospice care, or are willing to turn a room into a hospice-type facility, low on medical gear and high on hominess.

Preventing Burnout

Whether you realize it or not, you are living this death almost every minute of your day. Even during a break, sitting in another room, you may hear your parent's raspy breathing, feel the health aide's presence, or smell the soiled bedsheets. Your sleep may be interrupted, and you may have no time to eat, or little appetite for food.

Caring for someone at the end of life takes a tremendous toll on a person, but you may be so caught up in it that you aren't aware of how it is affecting you. If you want to keep caring for your parent, you have to take care of yourself, at least in some minimal way, even through this intensely demanding time.

Get help early. See if the hospice staff can arrange for a home health aide or companion. Most hospices provide aides directly, and, if not, they will arrange for one. They also have volunteers on hand who can help. You should also recruit other family members and close friends to take shifts, make meals, run errands, or do anything else that might be helpful to you now.

When others are caring for your parent, get away. Go for a walk, see a friend, run errands, sit on the beach, or go for a drive. If you don't pace

> *We felt we had to do it all ourselves, so we took shifts. I would stay with Mom until midnight, and then my daughter would sit with her. My sister would come during the day, and if she couldn't come, then one of my aunts would come. We were on this round-the-clock schedule, which was fine as long as everybody showed up for their time slot. It got to be, 'Okay, we've made it through today. Now let's hope everybody's in place again tomorrow.'*
>
> *In the end, that last week before she died, I found that I couldn't deal with it. I totally broke down. I hadn't had any sleep. I was exhausted. I started crying and couldn't stop. I called the hospice, and they sent someone over right away."*
>
> —Susan V.

yourself and remove yourself occasionally, at least for short periods, you will not last long at this undertaking. If you are concerned about leaving, consult the hospice nurses, who can often tell whether a dying person has weeks, days, or only hours to live. If it's hours, then stay, of course. If it's more, then go.

If your parent's care is onerous and continues for more than a couple of months, consider respite care. Nearly all hospices provide it or know how to get it. Your parent can be moved into a nursing home or a hospital temporarily, or you can hire round-the-clock aides to care for your parent at home. Take a few days and get away. Tend to your own needs and to other important relationships. Get your mind on something else. And get some sleep.

If you feel that you can't leave the house at all because your parent appears close to death, at least get out of earshot occasionally and get your mind on something else. Go have a cup of coffee, flip through a magazine, take a nap, soak in a hot bath. And be sure to have a good meal now and then. (Caregivers often forget to eat during this period, or they eat only junk food, which wears them down more quickly.)

Even during this grim time, don't be afraid to laugh. It may seem disrespectful, but it is not. Watch a comedy or read a funny book. Your emotional core needs strength, and laughing is a great recharger. Do it alone, with friends, or, yes, even with your parent. Laughter is welcome, even when death is near.

If you run out of stamina, if your parent continues to live for longer than you expected, if the emotional drain is too much, or if the care becomes too demanding, don't be ashamed to tell the hospice nurses how you feel and talk with them about possible solutions. Many terminally ill people who are cared for at home die in a hospital or nursing home because their care becomes too much for caregivers to bear. Give what you can, but recognize and respect your personal limits.

IN THE HOSPITAL

MOST PEOPLE TODAY DIE IN HOSPITALS. In the hospital, your parent will get intensive medical care and round-the-clock nursing care, which is usually covered by public or private insurance. The reality of death will be less stark, and the kind of hands-on care required of you is far less rigorous than if your parent were to die at home.

But hospitals have enormous drawbacks. For starters, it's hard to buck the system, and the system is founded on keeping people alive. Whatever the cost.

Also, they are impersonal and unfamiliar places that impose physical and emotional distance between patients and their loved ones. You won't be able to be there as often as you might like, or at the times you might like. When you are there, the medical machinery and staff intrusions get in the way of your having any private or intimate time together. You may be unable to hug your parent, hold her hand, or even find a body part that can be touched. Furthermore, you and your parent will have less control over her care and daily life.

But there are things you can do to regain some control, even in a hospital. (See Chapter Fourteen, on how to care for your parent in the hospital.)

◆ Be sure that your parent's living will and other directives are filed in her medical record and that the nurses and doctors overseeing her care are aware of them and prepared to follow them. You might write a large note

A NOTE ON PAIN

Pain is no simple matter, especially when death is near. It radiates from, and is compounded by, a number of sources: the disease; chemotherapy, surgery, and other medical interventions; emotional anguish and fear; exhaustion and fatigue; and the fear of pain itself. Dreading what may come, we tighten our muscles, clench our jaws, and, as a result, become physically and psychologically overwhelmed by the first twinge of pain.

Determine the roots of your parent's pain and address them. Be sure his questions about illness, dying, and pain medication are answered. Let him talk about troubled relationships or spiritual questions. Easing his emotional pain will, in turn, vastly ease his physical discomfort.

Whatever else you do, be adamant that your parent receives ample pain medication. Although doctors say that they believe in sparing patients from pain, they commonly limit narcotics because of all sorts of misguided beliefs.

Your parent should receive medication at regular intervals, before the pain begins (alleviating pain is more difficult than keeping it at bay in the first place), and extra doses of medication should be available at any indication of pain. Ask the doctor about a morphine pump that gives regular shots of pain relief while allowing the patient, if he is able, to push a button for additional doses when necessary. Studies show that patients who control their own pain medication actually use less medication and report less pain than those who do not have such control.

At this stage, no one should be concerned about addiction. Also, people become tolerant of these medications and can handle extremely high doses—doses that would, without such a gradual introduction, kill a person. Don't let anyone tell you that more medication will compromise her breathing or shorten her life. At this point, you need to be sure she is comfortable.

If your parent's pain is not adequately treated, ask for a consultation with a palliative care specialist. Most hospitals now have such doctors, as the specialty has become increasingly complex. Their mission is just this, to treat pain and symptoms.

> *I know they are short-staffed in hospitals, but my mother was not a demanding person. That was her big thing, not to bother anybody. But when she called for a bedpan or painkillers, the nurses responded very slowly. Then, one afternoon, I was there and she wanted to walk, and the nurse said she would have to wait until later. But 'later' never came.*
>
> *That did it. I said, 'I've had it. Let's get her home.'"*
>
> —JANE P.

and tape it over her bed, stating clearly what is not to be done and what is to be done in various circumstances. Include your phone (and cell phone) number.

◆ Be there as often as possible, and when you can't be there, find others who can be. You need to monitor her care closely, and, if she doesn't want certain procedures, you need to be sure they aren't performed.

◆ Unless you want all-out medical treatment for your parent, keep her out of the intensive care unit. The staff in these units will work to keep your parent alive under almost any circumstances, because that is what they are trained to do. These units are also not designed for comfort. The beeping monitors, bright lights, and bustle of personnel is unsettling, and it hinders the kind of communication and phys-

ical contact that is so desperately needed now. Many ICUs also have rigid rules about visiting, further impeding proximity and solace.

◆ While you need to be diligent in fending off certain treatments and tests, you need to be equally diligent in being sure your parent gets the care and attention she needs. Hospital staff are busy and often neglect the less urgent needs of patients.

Furthermore, studies show that dying patients (and their families) receive even less attention from hospital staff, and as the patient grows sicker, the attention dwindles further. Like the rest of us, and perhaps more than the rest of us, nurses and doctors are uncomfortable with death. They are also given little or no training in how to provide general comfort or to tend to the emotional needs of dying patients and their families. So they tend to distance themselves from dying patients, usually out of a sense of helplessness or failure. It falls on you to search out and then persist in getting your parent adequate care.

◆ Track down a hospital social worker or chaplain, or bring in one on your own. Either can help address the emotional and spiritual needs of your parent and family now.

◆ Encourage visitors, but keep visits short if they tire your parent. Remember, she may want someone to simply sit quietly with her.

◆ Make sure your parent is getting all the pain relief she needs. There is no reason to limit medication if it can make her more comfortable (see page 309).

◆ Ask the nurses if you or another family member can spend the night. Some hospitals have units where family members can sleep, while others may allow you to sleep in an extra bed or cot in your parent's room.

◆ If your parent is afraid of being left alone, or you don't like the thought of her being alone but can't always be with her, hire a companion or find a volunteer who will sit by her side.

Treatment Decisions

THE DOCTOR HAS LAID OUT THE choices. Your parent is too far gone to decide. So now, it's up to you. You thought you knew what to do, but standing at the bedside, with the clock ticking, your parent still warm to touch, and your heart breaking into a zillion pieces, it all looks completely different than expected.

"Extraordinary treatment," "futile," "no reasonable chance of recovery." These are the things you discussed. But now there are chances, albeit slim ones. Now it's not clear whether treatment is futile, or whether it might possibly, just possibly, help. What exactly is a "reasonable chance"? You need to know, because the other side of this— saying no, refusing life-sustaining treatment—feels very, very final.

Whether or not to jump-start the heart of an old and dying person with electric jolts when there is virtually no chance of survival is clear-cut. It's not only futile, but inhumane. But how does one know when a cancer treatment is no longer useful, when a dialysis machine should be turned off, or when using antibiotics to treat a case of pneumonia no longer makes sense?

If a treatment cannot improve the quality of your parent's life or extend a life that will be reasonably comfortable, if it only prolongs or exacerbates pain and suffering, then the treatment should be stopped or refused. But again, these are difficult phrases to define. For one person, being immobile and hospitalized without hope of recovery may make life unbearable. Another person might want to hang on, regardless of pain or indignity, to see an anniversary or the birth of a grandchild, or simply because the will to live has not yet been diminished by suffering or exhaustion.

There is no right answer. You're going to have to think about your parent's wishes and trust your own good judgment.

If you're uncertain and have the chance, take your time. If that means keeping your parent hooked to a machine for a few extra days, then go ahead and do so. You need time to make this decision and accept it.

Make sure you fully understand your parent's state, prognosis, and options. Get a second opinion. Talk with family members. And if it might

> " *The nurse called me at work and said that my mother was vomiting and had diarrhea. The nursing home needed my permission to start an IV line for fluid and nutrition. I was about to say yes when I stopped myself. Was this really what she would want? No. I knew my mother wouldn't want it. So I said, 'No. Give her whatever she will take on her own.'*
>
> *It was a very, very long day, and I didn't sleep at all that night. I live far away, and I'd been back and forth twice that week already, so all I could do was wait by the phone. She died the next day.*
>
> *Do I regret my decision? Not at all. Could I do it again? I hope so."*
>
> —CARL L.

help, get input from a trusted outsider, a professional with experience in these matters, such as a social worker or member of the clergy.

Then, when you have all the facts, think about who your parent is and what she values in life. Sit down beside her, put your hand on hers, and look into her face. Listen quietly for her voice. Hear her words, for you undoubtedly know them. You and your siblings, along with her spouse if he is around, know better than anyone else what she could tolerate and what she could not, what she would consider acceptable, how she felt about medical treatment, and how she felt about death. You know, if you listen hard enough, what she would want you to do.

If you turn this question away from your own needs, if you think not about what you want, but what she would want, you will make the right decision, whether that means ending treatment or continuing it.

Here are a few things to consider while you deliberate:

◆ By law, your parent has the right to refuse any and all medical treatment. If your parent is unable to speak for himself, his assigned health-care proxy is in charge. If there is no proxy, a doctor will usually turn to family members to make a decision.

Not only can you legally refuse treatment, you can also stop treatment that has been started. While it's more difficult to stop treatment than to reject it in the first place, it is possible, legal, and done routinely.

◆ This is your family's decision. It does not belong to the doctor who colored the choices with his or her own biases. It does not belong to the nurse who raised her eyebrows and made a slicing comment. It does not belong to a friend or acquaintance who believes they understand where you stand. It is private. It is yours. Do not be swayed.

◆ If you choose to withhold or stop a medical procedure or treatment, know that you are not in any way killing your parent; disease and old age are. That sounds simple, but you need to believe it in your heart.

We live in triumphant times, medically speaking, but all the scientific victories and discoveries and advances have left us in a horrible position. We, mere mortals, mere civilians, must make life-and-death decisions. They are made every day in every hospital in this country by people no better or wiser than you. The majority of deaths today occur after a decision has been made to end or refuse medical treatment. And that is a power none of us wants.

As you sit, pondering what to do, some little voice inside may keep insisting that by forgoing some treatment, you are cutting short her life. But your parent is going to die soon no matter what you do. You are simply deciding how far to push the envelope and trying to find the gentlest and least painful route possible. Your decision, thought out and bravely held, is your gift to her.

◆ Consider the goal of any treatment decision. Define what you want to accomplish. Are you aiming to prolong life, to preserve independence, to instill comfort? Once you know your goal, decisions about specific treatments should be clearer.

WHEN THERE'S DISAGREEMENT

IF YOUR FAMILY CAN'T DECIDE WHAT to do about your parent's medical care, or if your wishes regarding treatment clash with those of the doctor and you have no power of attorney giving you the authority to make decisions about her health care, contact the hospital ombudsman, the social worker, or the hospital's medical ethics committee.

You can also contact Last Acts Partnership (800-989-9455 or www.last actspartnership.org) for counseling, legal advice, and support. Last Acts Partnership works to protect patients' rights concerning end-of-life care, whatever the patient's wishes may be. You can also contact the National Right to Life Committee (202-626-8800 or www.nrlc.org), which opposes euthanasia and will help you keep your parent on life support or secure aggressive medical treatment.

Understanding Some Options

What does it mean to "pull the plug"? What is a DNR? What is "life support"? Learn all this, if you can, before you face a crisis.

◆ **Life support.** The phrase commonly refers to a ventilator, also known as a respirator, which is a large machine, about the size of a mini-refrigerator, that forces oxygen in the lungs through a tube that is inserted into the nose or mouth, or directly into the windpipe (trachea). While people are often put on life support temporarily and then successfully weaned, a very sick elderly person is not likely to get off the machine and resume breathing independently.

The tubes are irritating, and the compression of air is uncomfortable. Also, patients on ventilators usually

A NOTE ON SUICIDE

If your parent is interested not only in ending treatment, but wants to speed up his dying by committing suicide, be certain that he is not suffering from any sort of dementia, depression, or other mental disorder. His own doctor or, better yet, a psychiatrist can determine whether he is fit to make such a decision. (Doctors often fail to diagnose depression, especially in patients who are terminally ill.)

Be sure that your parent fully understands the course of his disease and the scope of pain relief and comfort care available. Most people who choose suicide do so to avoid pain, humiliation, and disability. But often their visions of the future are inaccurate. Pain can almost always be conquered, and feelings of humiliation can often be spared when loved ones speak openly to one another. Have your parent talk at some length to a hospice nurse or other medical professional who is well versed in issues of death about what his future holds and what care is available.

Be sure, too, that he is not doing this simply to protect you and others from the burden of his care. While this work certainly is challenging, most people are glad to have the chance to give in this way.

If you conclude that his desire to commit suicide is based on reasoned thinking and full information, then you are left with little recourse but to support him as best as you can. His doing this may trouble and anger you. You may feel painfully helpless. But even if you do not agree with his decision, stay with him. Don't abandon him. Your parent needs you now, and you will surely regret it if you fail to support him.

Although physician-assisted suicide is generally illegal, some doctors will help a patient commit suicide if the patient is terminally and incurably ill, and is deemed to be mentally competent to make such a decision. Some will supply ample doses of narcotics without comment, while others will provide directions for and even personal help in using them.

---

need catheters in their bladders, tubes for hydration and nutrition, and an array of links to various monitors. Mucus must be sucked up regularly and their lungs monitored for infection.

◆ **Pulling the plug.** When life support is withdrawn, people are not actually pulling a plug. "Pulling the plug" is a coarse way of saying that treatment will be stopped, and machines turned off, with the understanding that death will follow. It seems drastic, but this death does not have to be painful. In fact, is it likely to be less painful than if the treatment were continued.

A patient is given sedatives and painkillers. Then, once the drugs have taken effect, the air is turned down and the ventilator is stopped. Once the tube is removed, the patient might be given oxygen to keep him comfortable.

Family members can stay with him, talk with him, hold him, lie with him. Sometimes people die immediately; sometimes they continue to breathe on their own for hours or even days.

◆ **DNR.** When a person becomes severely and irreversibly ill, the family and doctor (or the patient) may draft a Do Not Resuscitate, or DNR, order. This means that if the person's breathing or heartbeat should stop, there will be no attempt to revive her. DNR orders are usually made when the family, patient, and doctor believe that resuscitation would only delay the inevitable and leave the person severely and permanently incapacitated.

A DNR is not the same as a living will. A living will outlines a person's wishes. A DNR is a medical order issued by a physician regarding specific treatments that are not to be used.

◆ **CPR.** Cardiopulmonary resuscitation is performed when a person's heart or lungs stop working. On the street, this means pushing on a person's chest and performing mouth-to-mouth resuscitation. Within a hospital or nursing home, it is a loud, frantic,

and violent procedure. Air is forced into the lungs through something called an Ambu-Bag, and a lifeless heart is jolted with electric paddles. If the patient survives this, and most elderly people don't, he is hooked up to life support machinery.

The chance of an acutely ill, elderly person surviving resuscitation is about 15 percent, and the chance of that person ever leaving the hospital is between 0 and 5 percent.

◆ **Artificial hydration and nutrition.** Most people can't help but think of food and water as basic comfort care. For many, removing or refusing such treatment is more difficult than cutting off a ventilator.

The fact is, artificial nutrition and hydration—pumping liquids and nutrients into a body—is an aggressive and invasive medical treatment. It does not, in any way, resemble a sip of water or home-cooked meal. It is painful and involves complications and risk. And for your parent, at this stage of life, it is dangerous.

The human body, once it has finished its initial struggle to live, is remarkably adept at dying. People who are close to death lose their appetites and don't want more than a small sip of water to wet their mouths and lips. The organs are shutting down. The body no longer needs food and water. And indeed, it does not want them.

Forcing nutrients and fluids into a body that can no longer digest, circulate, or dispose of them can lead to all sorts of complications, including

> *My mother was in a coma for ten days in the hospital. I knew we were finally saying good-bye because I saw her dying before me, little by little, and I just wanted her to go. I wanted it to be over. After all those years of watching her be strangled by this disease, I knew she was finally going to be set free."*
>
> —SALLY T.

shortness of breath, a backlog of water into the lungs, severe constipation or diarrhea, bloating, and infections.

In the end, the effort makes the person less comfortable, not more.

Stopping these treatments once they have been started is not thought to be painful or distressing. Dying patients who grimace because of a wound do not show signs of hunger or thirst. In fact, when such intake is reduced, the body releases endorphins, natural pain-relievers. Dehydration, which causes the patient to lapse into a coma and die peacefully, is called "nature's anesthetic."

◆ **Comas and persistent vegetative states.** The neat border between life and death becomes blurred when most of the brain, but not quite all of it, is damaged or destroyed, and a patient falls into the twilight zone of a coma or a persistent vegetative state. It may be easier to cope with the emotional turmoil if you understand the biology of what has happened.

In older patients, these states usually are caused by strokes, heart attacks, or Alzheimer's disease. When a person is in a coma, most of the brain no longer functions. The comatose person behaves much like someone under heavy anesthesia. She does not respond consciously to stimuli, such as shouting or poking, although she may be able to breathe on her own.

Once in a deep coma for more than a month or two, patients usually enter what is referred to as a persistent vegetative state. Few recover from this, and none fully. In the case of an older person, the chance of recovery is virtually nil. At this point the brain stem, the most rudimentary portion of the brain, which controls basic bodily functions, is all that remains alive. The lungs take in oxygen, the heart beats, and the body eliminates waste, but the person has no consciousness, no self-awareness, no thought process. Studies using sophisticated scanners that measure brain activity show that patients in persistent vegetative states do not feel pain, though they may jerk reflexively when pinched.

The situation is sheer hell for family and other loved ones. The person is there, soft and warm to touch and hold, and, in some sense, alive. She may even have normal sleep-wake patterns, and her muscles may react involuntarily. Her eyes may open and blink. She may cough or yawn. Her lips may even curl into a smile. It's almost impossible for families to believe that this person can't think, feel, or communicate. It's a horrifying trick played out by medicine and human biology.

The last stage of this continuum between life and death occurs when the brain completely stops working, a state that doctors sometimes refer to as "brain dead." Although the term seems to leave room for doubt or hope, there is no difference between this and death. The term "brain dead" is often used when a person remains hooked to a respirator, heart machine, and other gadgets that keep blood oxygenated and pumping, usually so his organs can be used for transplantation. The brain, however, is no longer functioning and the person is, in fact, dead.

What Death Looks Like

What does death look like? How do you know when the end is near? What can you expect to see? What will your parent experience?

In wonderful old movies, a dying person is propped up on clean, downy pillows, her hair is in place, her face is tired but still attractive, and she gazes lovingly at someone before gracefully lowering her lashes and heaving a last sigh. In the real world, death is less picturesque. A lot less.

The scenario is different for each person. Some people die slowly, some go unexpectedly in their sleep, some lapse into a coma, and others are alert right up to the end. More often than not, death is not a dramatic moment, but a slow process, a gradual departure.

> " During the last week, Dad couldn't talk or respond. The hospice nurses told us that he had only hours to live, but five days passed like this. The tension of thinking every moment, 'This is it,' for such a long time got to be too much.
>
> A hospice worker told us that we had been spending so much gratifying time with Dad—talking about what he meant to us, about experiences we'd shared and how much we loved him, and reading his favorite Robert Frost poems—that he was fighting to stay alive. She said, 'He's going to hang on as long as this stuff keeps coming. He's loving it. There is so much energy here. You have to leave him; only then will he be free to leave.'
>
> She suggested that each of us go in and say good-bye. And rather than clutching him close to us, that we stroke him very lightly, moving from his head, down his arms and out beyond his body into the space of the room. This was a very physical way of letting go. Each of us did this and we went to bed around midnight, more calm ourselves. Around 2 A.M. he died very peacefully."
>
> —RUTH S.

As a person becomes sicker, he gets weaker. He becomes less mobile and usually becomes incontinent. Many dying people have trouble swallowing and eventually refuse nearly all food and drink. As the person eats less and less, he becomes thinner and thinner, until his face is quite sunken and sallow. (Remember, this disinterest in food and water is natural and helpful.)

Make sure your parent's mouth is always fresh and moist. Give her ice chips or small amounts of water and wipe her teeth, gums, and tongue with a damp cloth, or use disposable mouth swabs.

Several other symptoms, such as breathing difficulty, nausea and vomiting, constipation, confusion, and infections, are common as death nears, but most can be treated so they do not cause severe discomfort, distress, or pain. If you are aware of such symptoms, alert the doctor or nurse. Your parent may also become achy and stiff from being in bed, so it is important to move him regularly—over on his side, to a chair, sitting up, lying flat, with legs elevated, and so on.

Your parent will become less aware of what is happening—because of both the illness and pain medication—and he may drift in and out of consciousness. Sleep patterns are often disrupted, so he may stay awake at odd hours of the night and sleep soundly in the middle of the day. Communication may be limited. At times your parent may stare off as though he is thinking about something, his eyes may look glassy, and you may not be able to draw his attention.

Some dying people appear to have what has come to be called a near-death experience. They see and chat with people who have died, or talk about

> " *At about 1 A.M. my sister woke me and said, 'She's choking. Something is happening.' I ran in and found my mother dying. I held her for a moment and then she died. And that was it. She was gone.*
>
> *Bonnie and I just looked at each other and looked at Mom. We didn't cry right away. We just stood there. It had been a long haul. And now it was over. She was dead. It seemed very matter-of-fact, almost anticlimactic.*
>
> *We pulled a blanket up, tucked her in, and then we made some tea and sat in the living room. It hit us both at the same time and we just started to cry. The exhaustion, the reality of this death, looking around that familiar room. After all we had done, our mother was gone.*"
>
> —SUSAN V.

being in some distant place. This may startle you, but usually these experiences are quite pleasant, or at least not unpleasant. Your parent may also twitch or jerk occasionally, but this is nothing to worry about. It is usually not a sign of pain, just a restless muscle.

In the last days or hours, your parent's fingers, toes, elbows, nose, lips, and other extremities may feel cold and turn a bluish gray. At the same time, his temperature may rise, and he may have bouts of sweating (be sure to sponge your parent off and keep the sheets clean and dry).

His breathing may be labored and, as secretions gather in his throat and the throat muscles relax, he may make a gurgling sound when he breathes, something known as a death rattle. It sounds a little like someone sucking up the last bits of a drink into a straw. This noise does not mean that your parent is having any discomfort, but it may be frightening for you. Drugs can dry the secretions, but this is only for your comfort, not his.

Eventually there may be gaps in his breathing—he will stop breathing for a few seconds (and so will you), then gasp for another breath and continue breathing normally for a while. Near the end, these pauses will become longer until the breathing stops altogether.

The final moment is often quiet and uneventful, though a few biological reactions can take place that will be less upsetting if you are prepared for them. Sometimes the bowels and bladder release. The eyes and jaw may remain open. Sometimes people let out a howl or yell, not a cry of pain or despair, but simply a last muscular spasm of the voice box.

Sometimes people appear to make a last, energetic effort just before they die—sitting up, trying to stand, gasping for another breath—which may upset those who are watching, but you should know that such activity is largely reflexive, and not a conscious effort on the part of the dying person.

If you are aware that your parent is dying, it's hard to know what to do during these last hours, minutes, and seconds. You may feel paralyzed, awkward, and intensely helpless. You may feel shock. Focus your energies on making your parent feel loved and safe. By now he will have little, if any, ability to communicate, but it is likely that he can still sense your voice and your embrace. Give him a peaceful exit. Speak gently to him and let him know that you are there, that he has nothing to fear, that he is safe, that you love him, that he has had a good life, and that he is free to go. Hold him or touch him, and give him all the love in your heart.

The Moment after Death

Your parent has taken his last breath and you are standing beside him. Whether you are weeping or numb with shock, you face the question of what to do next.

Actually, you don't have to do anything. If you are in the hospital, you don't need to call for a nurse. If you are at home, you don't have to contact anyone right away. There is no need to whisk the body away.

You can sit with your deceased parent, hold him in your arms, touch his hands and face, say good-bye, and weep. You may want to wait for other family members to arrive so they, too, have this moment to say good-bye. You may want to pray, take part in another religious ritual, or tend to your parent's body in some way. You can pick out clothing for his burial (which

" *Death, being part of that passage, was a turning point for me. It gave me strength. Facing it, what it brings.*

I know a lot of people saw my mother—a skeleton—saw her discomfort, and left the room and didn't know anything else. Their only thought was, 'Oh, my God, I'm going to deteriorate and be in such discomfort.' But when you're there, through the whole process, you see that that is just a minor part. The rest of it is coming to terms and having your good-byes.

At one point, just before she died, I was lying next to her, and with the last bit of energy, she kind of turned on her side and gave me a huge hug. She hadn't moved in over a day. It was amazing how she got those long arms wrapped around me. I don't know how she did it. But that was my good-bye.

She died that night. She looked absolutely beautiful. She was in her own bed. She had this peaceful expression. She was beautiful."

—Kim D.

most funeral homes require) or, if you choose, dress him, or even bathe and groom him. Some people find that such a task is actually a healing and tender final gift. Do whatever feels right for you. This time and these acts belong solely to you and your family.

When you are ready, call the nurse or your parent's doctor. You may want to call a member of the clergy. Don't worry if it's the middle of the night. Most clergy would rather come when they are needed than on the following morning when the crisis is over. Also, call a funeral home. Once your parent has been declared dead by a doctor, nurse, or coroner, the funeral home can pick up his body and begin the process of filing a death certificate and preparing the body for burial or cremation. (If it's late at night, they may not come until morning.)

As soon as you are able, call members of your parent's immediate family. Do not hesitate to "bother" someone who is on vacation or at work. Most people want to be told as soon as possible, and feel cheated or deprived if they are not notified of the death until days after it has happened. If the family is a large one, make a list of people to be called and ask other family members to share the task. Most people will want to know whether a funeral or a memorial service has been scheduled and will understand when you keep the conversation brief.

WHEN YOU ARE NOT THERE

IF YOU HAD HOPED TO BE WITH YOUR parent when she died, and weren't— whether you were far away or just made a quick trip to the store—you may feel cheated out of something, or guilty that you didn't extend your last visit.

Don't berate yourself. People often die after loved ones, who have sat with them for hour after long hour, leave for a moment. Perhaps they don't want their loved ones to watch. Perhaps they can't ease into death with the stimulation of a loved one about.

Your parent may have chosen, in some way, to die when you weren't present. This is something you will never know. But you did nothing wrong. You gave your parent love and care long before that final moment, and that is what matters.

It may ease your mind to hear an account of the last days or moments of her life, so ask the doctor, nurses, or whoever was in the room at the time, to tell you about every detail while the memory is still fresh in their minds.

Chapter Twenty-Five

THE AFTERMATH

Finding a Funeral Director • The Obituary
• Cemeteries • Services • Taking Care of Business

A FTER A PARENT HAS DIED, IN THE MIDST OF YOUR GRIEF or before you have had a chance to even realize what's happened, there is work to be done—people to be called, services to be planned, obituaries to be written. While these tasks may seem overwhelming, they can also be therapeutic.

Funeral and memorial services are valuable rituals, allowing your family to deal with the reality of your parent's death, to share your tears and memories, and to see, in the midst of your emotional disarray, that life still has some order. Picking out music, choosing readings, and even making arrangements for the body all give you a chance to think about your parent and to honor her life. A service also allows people who may not be part of the inner circle, or who may not have seen your parent for some time, to mourn his death, remember his life, and pay their respects.

You don't have to take the traditional route; you can be creative and come up with a plan that suits your parent and your family. Do what feels right to you, but do take an active part in planning this last farewell.

Finding a Funeral Director

For most people, the first step in planning a funeral is to talk to a funeral director, who will guide you through the process. (However, in most states, you do not need a funeral director; you can plan this on your own.) Find a funeral director who has a good reputation. While some are trustworthy and reliable, many are scoundrels who inflate prices, charge for services that were never provided, and urge survivors to spend more than is necessary. A mourning family is easy prey.

Ask friends or family for recommendations. The Funeral Consumers Alliance (see page 667) may know of trusted funeral homes in the area. If you want to go yet another step, the local regulatory board will know which funeral homes have complaints filed against them.

Look for a locally owned and operated funeral home, which is apt to give you more personal service. Large national corporations have bought up enormous numbers of small, local funeral homes in recent years, and some still seem local, even though they are not.

Once you have a few names, get a price list from each because prices can vary dramatically. Funeral homes have to, by law, give you prices, even over the phone. They will usually e-mail or fax the list to you as well. For more details on funerals and costs, see Appendix J, page 666.

If you are planning a funeral from a distance, and the Funeral Consumers Alliance is not familiar with the area, the National Funeral Directors Association (800-228-6332 or www.nfda.org) has a list of funeral homes. You might also ask reputable funeral directors in your area for a recommendation, as they often know funeral directors in other places.

In general, it's best to meet with a funeral director at his or her offices. Too often, funeral directors come to a family's home, size up their worth, and price accordingly.

At this point, if you are planning to have services, you should contact any member of the clergy or person who will officiate, and begin planning the program. If the minister, priest, rabbi, or other official did not know your parent well, describe who he was in some detail so the service feels personal. If you do not have anyone in mind, the funeral director should be able to make recommendations.

The Obituary

Write the obituary in any way you wish, but know that many newspapers will rewrite it. Some will send or e-mail you a form to fill out. Otherwise, the funeral director can help you.

An obituary should include the full name of your parent, his date of birth, schooling, career (where he worked, in

ACCEPT ALL HELP

If, during this time, people ask if they can do anything to help—and many people will—by all means say yes. Ask them to babysit, run errands, prepare a meal, call people about the time and place of the service, or pick up and put up out-of-town guests.

If they are close friends of your parent's or yours, ask them to write down their memories of him, especially if they start reminiscing over the phone to you. You may be too raw and preoccupied to absorb such stories, but you will want to hear them later. Save all notes and recorded memories for yourself and other members of the family.

what positions, and during what years), memberships in organizations, military service, awards received, hobbies, the full names of his siblings, children, spouse, and other survivors, and the date and cause of death. You should include the time and place of a funeral or memorial service, and note the fund or charity where people can send donations in lieu of flowers. You may want to send a photo as well. (Some newspapers charge a fee to print death notices, which include information about the services, and a few charge to print full obituaries.)

Local newspapers and school alumni magazines may print longer and more personal obituaries, in which case you should provide more detailed information about your parent's past, personality, gifts, and traits. You might include anecdotal stories, especially ones that occurred in that town or at that school.

Handling the Body

If your parent had specific wishes about how his body is to be handled, they should be honored. If not, what would make you and others in the family most comfortable?

If your parent's wishes and yours conflict, think about the strength of your parent's convictions—was he simply trying to be organized and helpful, or did he have personal or religious feelings about this? While you should respect his choices, the funeral and other final rituals are truly meant for those left behind. Some of the options you should know about:

◆ **Autopsy.** An autopsy is an examination of the body performed by a coroner, medical examiner, or physician, usually when a death is regarded as suspicious or unnatural. However, a doctor might suggest an autopsy if such an examination would be useful for medical research or teaching purposes. You must give your permission before such an exam is performed.

Ask the doctor what the procedure entails in your parent's case. Will the body remain largely intact? Will you still be able to have a viewing?

The decision depends solely on your own beliefs and feelings. If you think your parent would want to give this one last contribution to medicine, or if you want to and you don't mind any disfigurement that might occur, then this is a noble gesture. But if the idea makes you squeamish, don't feel pressured into it.

◆ **Organ donation.** Even elderly people can become donors. Hearts, kidneys, pancreases, lungs, livers, skin, eyes, and bone marrow are all needed. Medical schools and research institutes also like to have bodies for research and education. (If your parent dies at home, with hospice, you may have to make arrangements for donations in advance.)

For more information, contact the Coalition on Donation (804-782-4920 or www.shareyourlife.org).

◆ **Interment.** Interment is the traditional form of burial. The body is placed in a casket and buried in the ground, usually in a cemetery.

◆ **Entombment.** The casket is put in a mausoleum, a structure usually made of marble, stone, or concrete, with rows of crypts or, in some cases, individual rooms for caskets.

◆ **Cremation.** The body is placed in a box and then put in a special crematory furnace where, over several hours, intense heat reduces it to a few

> *It felt so distant looking at these things in the funeral parlor. There was no connection to my father. It was like going to Caldors. So we decided to build one ourselves.*
>
> *We bought beautiful pine boards and built the interior frame like a boat because my father was a boater. It had crown moldings, wood panels, and hinges of hand-forged brass, and nice handles that I bought in India twenty years ago. I always loved them. And rope handles for carrying it. We lined the interior with this thick soft blanket, sort of like a bedspread, that had been given to my father years ago.*
>
> *All my brothers and sisters and the grandchildren helped. We worked straight through the night, sawing, sanding, polishing, and varnishing.*
>
> *It was a wonderful experience. I can't really explain it. We laughed and cried. We talked about Dad and things we'd done. It gave the funeral a whole different feeling, having a focus like that. It gave the family a connection to the process because everyone had a part in it."*
>
> —PETER W.

pounds of bone fragments and ashes. The ashes, or "cremains," are then returned to the family in a box of cardboard, metal, or plastic, or placed in an urn or other container (known as an inurnment).

✔ A FUNERAL CHECKLIST

☐ Make a list of people who should be notified. Split it up and have others do some of the calling.

☐ Choose a funeral director.

☐ Decide the date of the service or services. Pick a day when all immediate family members can be present, leaving time to make the necessary preparations.

☐ Write an obituary and send it to local newspapers and other appropriate publications (alumni or company magazines, and newspapers in other places he has lived).

☐ Decide whether the body will be cremated, buried immediately, or embalmed for viewing.

☐ If the body or ashes are to be buried, find out if your parent owns a plot or if there is a family plot. If not, visit local cemeteries. Find out the rules of the cemetery. (For example, do you need a grave liner? Can you hold a service on the weekend or evening?)

☐ Decide whether you want a viewing, graveside service, funeral, and/or memorial service.

☐ Pick out a casket or urn.

☐ Choose the place for services— a church, synagogue, or other religious building; the funeral home; a private home; or a rented hall or club—and make sure it is available.

☐ Decide whom you would like to officiate and then meet with them to plan what will be included in the services—prayers, songs, readings, and speakers.

☐ Select music. Will there be instruments, an organ, a choir, a soloist? Do you need to pass out songbooks, hymnals, or sheet music? Talk to the music director or organist at the church and to relatives who might know your parent's favorite hymns.

☐ Decide what kind of flowers, candles, guest books, or other extras you would like and where

The ashes are buried in the earth, put in a niche at a cemetery or church columbarium, kept by family or friends, or scattered in some meaningful place. (It is illegal to sprinkle ashes in some places, so check with local health officials first.)

Cremation simply speeds up the natural process of decay (all bodies, even those that are buried in expen-

you will buy them. (Do you want photos, letters, or other reminders of your parent's life on display at the service?)

☐ Ask people to serve as pallbearers and/or ushers at the service, if necessary.

☐ If your parent was a veteran, you may want to notify the local American Legion for a military component at the funeral.

☐ If there is to be a graveside service, decide whether the casket or urn will be lowered into the grave or placed in the columbarium while people are present and, if so, who will do this task—family members or people from the cemetery or funeral home.

☐ Ask a neighbor who will not be attending the services, or the police, to keep an eye on your parent's home (and perhaps yours) during the services. Thieves often learn about funerals to find out which houses will be empty.

☐ Decide whether there will be a gathering after the service. (If so, where and when? Will everyone be invited or just a select few? Will a meal be served or just coffee? Do you need a caterer or bartender?)

☐ If you want a program for the funeral, write it and get it printed. (Sometimes funeral directors keep sample programs on hand. They should also be able to recommend printers.) Be sure to order a few extra copies for friends and family who will be unable to attend the service.

☐ Think about where visitors will stay and how they will get from the airport or train station to the services. You are not responsible for this, but it's helpful, if you can, to make recommendations. If necessary, write up directions and e-mail them to everyone.

☐ If you have chosen an earth burial, then at some point you need to select a grave marker or headstone. (This can be done later, however.)

sive caskets, decay), and it is less expensive than an earth burial. You can still have all the rites of a funeral if you so choose—a viewing before the cremation, a memorial service, and burial in a cemetery with a gravestone. Most religions now allow cremation, although the Greek Orthodox and Jewish conservative and orthodox faiths oppose it.

If you choose to have a visitation and funeral prior to cremation, you can rent a casket with a removable liner from the funeral home, usually for about a third of the retail price. If you do not want a viewing, you can buy a simple casket of wood, pressboard, cardboard, or canvas. (You can buy a cardboard casket over the Internet for about $20. Fill it with a soft, lovely blanket and it will be just right.) Don't let a funeral director convince you that you need a casket for cremation because you don't, in any state.

Stick to your guns if anyone tries to convince you that your parent should not be cremated. There are people, as well as unsavory funeral home directors, who try to dissuade this practice.

◆ **Embalming.** People began embalming bodies in this country during the Civil War, when the bodies of soldiers had to be shipped long distances. The custom has continued, but is not necessary in most cases. Embalming is sometimes required when a body is going to be transported a long distance, when there is to be a viewing, or when the dead person carried certain communicable diseases. It does not prevent the body from decaying; it only delays the process.

During an embalming, the body is washed and disinfected. Blood and other body fluids are drained out and chemicals—perfumed formaldehyde, glycerin, alcohol, and water—are injected into the arteries to make the

BENEFITS FOR VETERANS

Military veterans are entitled to a free burial (including opening and closing of the grave, care of the grounds, headstone, and grave marker) in a national cemetery. These benefits extend to spouses and children of veterans as well. Some states have also established state veterans cemeteries.

If your parent is buried elsewhere, the Department of Veterans Affairs will reimburse families of qualified veterans several hundred dollars for funeral and burial expenses, for a plot or inurnment. In some cases, a small amount may be reimbursed for the cost of transporting the body from a VA nursing home or hospital. The VA will also provide a grave marker, cover some of the cost of a gravestone, and send a large American flag to drape over the casket. A funeral director or the regional VA office should be able to help you apply for these benefits. To reach the regional office, contact the VA at 800-827-1000 or www.cem.va.gov

(Be leery of any private cemeteries offering free burials to veterans. They often charge other fees that cancel out any savings.)

tissue gel and to prevent the growth of bacteria. The undertaker then prepares the body for the viewing by dressing it and applying makeup. If you want, he or she can repair any damaged areas, plump sunken skin, and replace missing hair. Find out what is to be done, otherwise your parent may be unrecognizable. *Mom never wore red lipstick a day in her life! And is that a wig she's wearing?*

The Cemetery

Most communities have a municipal cemetery as well as several cemeteries owned by religious or private organizations. Veterans have the added option of being buried at a national cemetery.

Your parent may have made plans for his burial (if he has not told you, look through his important papers and safe-deposit box to see if he has already reserved a cemetery plot). If not, choose a cemetery that appeals to you. Though, if price is a determining factor, compare prices as well; be sure that the price includes any hidden extras.

Within a cemetery, you can buy a single grave plot or a family plot. Some cemeteries also sell space in a mausoleum, an above-ground building that has crypts for caskets, or a columbarium, which has stacks of niches for urns of ashes. Find out if the cemetery requires some sort of grave liner or vault, and if it has any restrictions on markers, monuments, or plantings.

A PRIVATE REMEMBRANCE

If you can't go to the funeral, hold your own service where you live. Invite a few close friends to come over and share in a memorial. Put out photos, flowers, and candles. Ask a member of the clergy to come. Have a reception. Or have your own private memorial so you can say your good-byes.

Some cemeteries, for example, are set up like gardens and allow only flat markers and no headstones.

A growing number of cemeteries now offer a full range of services, with a funeral home on the premises and, in some cases, a crematorium, flower shop, and gravestone supplier.

Services

The service should be whatever, whenever, and wherever you want it to be. People usually schedule the service within a week or two of the death because they need it then, emotionally, and why wait? But you can put it off several weeks or even months if you want to. Or, you can have a cremation or burial service soon after the death, and then hold a memorial service months later when you have the energy to make arrangements, and

CHILDREN AND FUNERALS

While children are often excluded from funerals, wakes, and memorial services, they often want to be included in the ritual, and they stand to learn from it. Describe what the event will be like and let them decide for themselves if they want to attend. Most children, even as young as four or five, can make such decisions for themselves. If the service is going to be quite long—too long for a child to sit still or remain quiet—bring a supply of toys and snacks, or include the child for only part of the service and arrange for a sitter to be nearby.

In the weeks after the funeral, give your child a chance to talk about your parent. You might give her a photo or help her make a scrapbook about her grandmother's life (as soon as you can handle such a project). Don't be surprised if your child has nightmares. They are normal and they will end. But they are apt to occur whether he does or doesn't attend the services. (For more on children and grief, see page 576.)

when friends and family can all be present.

Once you know when you want to hold the service, you have to decide what it will be. A funeral or memorial usually follows the tradition of your parent's religion. But you can personalize even a formal service by giving it whatever touch you feel is appropriate. You can hold communion; have speakers; read poems, prayers, or letters; or play music that has special meaning. You might hold a memorial walk or have an open, unstructured service that allows people in the congregation to stand and share memories and thoughts about your parent. You can tell jokes or funny stories. You might have people each carry a certain flower or humor-ous bauble if that's more fitting, and place them on the gravesite. At some services, the body is placed in a white casket (made of cardboard) and guests arrive with markers, crayons, paints, and pens and write notes, draw pictures, and otherwise decorate it. At others, each person takes a turn digging out a scoop of dirt in the earth where the coffin will be laid.

This service can and should be whatever you want it to be. It is, after all, for you and others who are mourning this death and honoring this life.

As you decide what the mood and the message will be, think about what you want out of this service. Do you want a joyous gathering that celebrates and remembers your parent's life or a solemn, religious service that attempts to help people come to terms with death? Or both?

A service can last for ten minutes or half a day. In the Jewish tradition of shivah, the family stays at home for seven days after the funeral service to receive guests. Funeral ceremonies and receptions are often held at a funeral home, a private home, a hall, a church, or a synagogue, but they can be held at any favorite spot—on the beach, in a park, near a summer cottage.

Viewing. The casket is usually present at a funeral—opened or closed —and not present at a memorial service. Either type of service may be preceded by a viewing or wake.

An open casket, which allows people to see and touch the body, gives people an opportunity to accept the reality of death, to see, quite literally, that this person is gone, and to say good-bye. It may be helpful for family and close friends who were not present at the time of death and who feel that they missed something important, but it is certainly not for everyone.

Taking Care of Business

If you weren't taking care of your parent's business before he died, you can only hope that he was well organized, because there is a lot of paperwork to be done now. Most of it doesn't have to be done immediately. Take time to grieve, and then attend to these tasks when your head and heart are a little more stable.

◆ **Contact relevant parties,** such as your parent's lawyer, financial planner, or accountant. If your parent didn't have a lawyer, you may need to hire one now.

◆ **Locate the will** by checking her safe-deposit box, files, and desk drawers, or by calling your parent's lawyer. If there is no will and no lawyer, then

FILING COMPLAINTS

Funeral directors are regulated by state licensing boards and by the Funeral Rule of the Federal Trade Commission. If you have questions, have trouble with a funeral home, or feel that you have been misled or cheated in any way, you should contact the funeral home directly first. If that doesn't solve the problem, contact the Funeral Consumer's Alliance (800-765-0107 or www.funerals.org).

You can also file a complaint with the state consumer protection agency, state funeral examining or licensing board, and/or the FTC. To file a complaint with the FTC or to get more information, call 877-382-4357 (FTC-HELP), or go online to www.ftc.gov.

the estate will be doled out according to state laws.

◆ **Check with the probate clerk's office** in your parent's town to get a list of deadlines. If your parent has property in more than one state, be sure to check with the probate clerk's office in each state.

◆ **Contact your parent's bank** to close accounts and to find out if there is a safe-deposit box. These boxes are closed at the time of death in some states, but you may be able to check the box for a will and list the contents for tax purposes.

◆ **Get five to ten copies of the death certificate** from the funeral director or health department. You will need these when reporting your parent's death to insurance companies, the Social Security office, the IRS, veterans affairs, etc.

◆ **Find your parent's marriage certificate** if your parent's spouse is alive and will be applying for benefits. The town clerk in the town where your parents were married should be able to provide copies if you can't find them in your parent's files. You may also need birth certificates for any dependent children, which are available from the town clerk's office in the town where the children were born.

◆ **Notify insurance companies** (life, health, mortgage, accident, auto, credit card, employer policies). File all claims, switch any policies over to a spouse's name, and/or change the names of beneficiaries. Do this early so beneficiaries can receive their money as soon as possible. (Some health insurance policies provided by an employer can be continued in a spouse's or in children's names.)

◆ **Contact the Social Security and Veterans Affairs offices.** You may receive a death benefit to cover funeral costs and other benefits to help a surviving spouse. Contact the Social Security Administration (800-772-1213 or www.ssa.gov) for information, and if your parent served in the military, contact the local Veterans Affairs office (800-827-1000 or www.va.gov).

◆ **Contact former employers.** Your parent may be owed pension benefits, salary, or pay for unused vacation or sick leave.

◆ **Make a list of all assets.** You will need to gather titles and deeds to any property, automobiles, boats; ownerships or partnerships in businesses; stocks, bonds, savings accounts, and checking accounts; profit-sharing plans, pension plans, and retirement accounts. You'll need to change the name on any titles and deeds if property is transferred to a surviving parent or child.

◆ **List all debts** from mortgages, unpaid bills, charge accounts, etc. Cancel all credit cards and pay the balance out of the estate.

◆ **Find a copy of your parent's most recent income tax return.** If your parent was required to file a tax return, you will have to file one for the year in which he died. You can get an extension, if necessary. Call the local IRS office for information. Federal taxes are also due on larger estates. There are usually state estate and inheritance taxes as well.

◆ **Revise the will of a surviving spouse.** The will of a surviving spouse may have to be changed if it lists your deceased parent as a beneficiary. Likewise with any insurance policies. She will also need to adjust anything held under joint names, such as bank accounts, property, credit cards, etc.

Dividing the Estate

Most wills note only that property be "divided equally" among the children. Money divides easily, but it's up to siblings to find an equitable way to split up possessions. If not done with great care, this can severely damage family relationships, especially if a will is poorly written or siblings are not on good terms. The division of valuable items, as well as worthless sentimental ones, can lead to bitter disagreements and hurt feelings that don't fade easily. Your father's high school sweater or your mother's old diary may suddenly become an invaluable icon. Or you may find yourselves reverting to childhood roles and feeling things are "unfair." Even those who thought that their parents' assets weren't particularly valuable, that the family's relationships were

> " The hard part was cleaning out the house. We came across all these little reminders, bits and pieces of our childhoods and memories of Dad. That was upsetting. My sister and I took care of it at our own slow pace. We met at the house three or four times over the course of a month or more, taking one room at a time. Then we would always go out for a beer when we were done. There was a lot of crying and a lot of laughing that went on. Dividing things up didn't divide us. If anything, it made us closer."
>
> —ALICIA B.

strong, or that their own hearts were generous, can be drawn into battle.

When you divide your parent's belongings, do it ever so carefully. Spend some time beforehand remembering what is truly important (the ratty old sweater or your relationship with your brother), what your parent would have wanted, and how you can enter this field with your fists unclenched.

And before you start, get your siblings to agree upon some ground rules. (You might also want to go out for dinner together and have a couple of stiff drinks and a few good laughs before you dig in.) Some suggestions:

◆ If possible, wait a few weeks until the grief has subsided. Emotions won't be so volatile and perceptions so askew. Immediately after a parent's death, yellowed letters, war medals, and moth-eaten scarves may seem unbelievably precious.

◆ Assign some value to each item so everyone knows its relative worth and walks away with items of roughly the same cash value. Hire an appraiser, if necessary. (You will probably have to hire an appraiser anyway, as part of probate proceedings.)

◆ If the appraiser assigns zero value to sentimental items, as he or she probably will, pull them out to divide separately.

◆ Before heading to the house or apartment, have each person write down three to five items that she or he most wants, in the order of preference. It may be that what is most important to one person may not be particularly important to another. If so, the crucial items can be divided before you even get there, without contest.

◆ Ask an outsider—a friend or professional—to monitor the division of the estate. Find someone whom everyone trusts and who is a good mediator.

◆ Decide together who will be present when items in the house are distributed. Are spouses invited? Children? Friends? You may or may not want in-laws putting in their two cents' worth.

◆ For those who cannot be present, you might photograph or video-tape items in advance and let the absentees make a list of their preferences. They might have a relative or friend stand in their place.

◆ Once you've sorted through the most desirable items, go through the house picking through the rest. You might draw straws to determine who goes first in a given room, and then take turns choosing items. You can rotate the order so each person has at least one chance to choose first in a room.

◆ Plan several breaks if the house is large or if there is a potential for disagreements.

◆ If beneficiaries are unable to agree, the executor usually divides assets in "approximately equal shares." If there are irreconcilable differences, then the property is sold and the heirs receive cash.

Chapter Twenty-Six

GOOD GRIEF

Stages of Grief • Growing from Grief • Reviewing Your Relationship with Your Parent • The Surviving Parent • Children and Grief

YOUR PARENT IS GONE. HE WAS OLD AND SICK, AND IT WAS probably time. Yet the loss is jarring. Your world has changed. A big piece is missing.

Grief rolls in like a series of waves, washing you in sorrow, confusion, anger, relief, and regret. It may pulse through you evenly or crash down on you when you least expect it. You may feel as though your very core has been shattered and that life will never be the same again. In fact, it won't be. With time, the hole will grow smaller and less painful, but a bit of it will always remain.

You can't control your grief, shake it off, or speed it up, and you shouldn't try. Grief is a necessary and valuable process that allows you to accept this loss, say good-bye to your parent, and move on with your life and other relationships. It is not something to race through or escape from. Allow yourself to feel it in your own way and at your own pace.

Stages of Grief

While each person's grief is unique, psychologists have mapped out a number of common reactions. You may experience only a few of them and do so in no particular sequence, bobbing from one emotion to another and then returning to old feelings you thought had long disappeared. But these descriptions should assure you that your reactions are normal, and they should also give you some insight into the feelings of others who may be mourning your parent's death.

◆ **The immediate impact.** Numbness, forgetfulness, inattentiveness, agitation, denial, disbelief, and shock are often the first reactions. There is a sense that this didn't happen or couldn't have happened. The truth that your parent is dead seems real only at certain moments.

In the immediate days after a death, some people feel intense pain, while others respond with cool detachment. Some become disoriented and have trouble making decisions, while others become adept organizers. Some are unable to do much, while others are hyperactive, scrubbing kitchen counters, cleaning out closets, playing basketball, and losing themselves in other physical tasks. Your reaction is not a measure of how much you loved your parent. Each person will respond in his or her own way, at his or her own pace.

As you digest the reality of your parent's death, you may feel angry at him for leaving you or overcome by guilt for things you said or did or failed to say or do. And you may feel resentment or jealousy toward others who still have their parents.

Acute grief causes physical repercussions as well, weakening the immune system, tipping hormones out of balance, upsetting one's appetite, and disrupting sleep. Some people become physically sick in the early stages of mourning, and suffer from chronic headaches, the flu, or other illnesses.

In the days and weeks after your parent's death, take time off from work and other responsibilities, if you can, to care for yourself. Spend time with family and good friends. The more support you have, the better you will cope. Be willing to ask for a shoulder to cry on when you need it. Most people want to help and feel complimented that you trust them enough to ask.

Resist the temptation to be stoic about your loss. No matter what your relationship with your parent was like, you have suffered a great blow. At the same time, don't force it. People may tell you to "get it out" to cry and feel

> **"** *My mother died nine years ago and I still wonder, 'Where is she? Where did she go?' I can't seem to let go of this feeling that she is still there, somewhere."*
>
> —BARBARA K.

the hurt, but dragging painful emotions to the surface before you are ready may not be helpful. Your heart and soul need time in order to digest this. Experience only as much as you want to, and at your own pace. Some people like to immerse themselves in memories of the deceased parent so they can grieve more intensely, while others prefer to avoid such hurtful reminders.

> *After my father died, we went into the living room and collapsed on the couch and, to be perfectly honest, we started laughing. That sounds horrible, I know, but we were completely exhausted. We had worried so much and cried so hard that I don't think we had any other emotions left."*
>
> —TINA R.

◆ **The aftershocks.** In the weeks after the funeral, family members return to their homes, friends no longer offer words of condolence, and employers run out of sympathy. Everyone may think it's time for you to be your old self again, but you may still be grieving and unable to carry on with business as usual. Give it time. Some people experience grief only after the formalities and commotion subside. For others, the initial pain gives way to despair,

NO REGRETS

When a parent dies and there is no longer a chance to do more or do differently, people sometimes feel guilt. Perhaps you got angry at a father who was confused, or fed up with a mother who needed a lot of care. Perhaps you didn't visit as often as you think you should have, or maybe you wished for your parent's death.

Be realistic. Put in the same situation again, it is likely that you would think the same thoughts and behave in the same way. And honestly, would a slightly different approach or a few more visits have made a genuine difference in your relationship or your parent's care? Certainly any thoughts you had about your parent's death did not hasten or affect his dying and probably had little real impact on your relationship.

Remember all you did for your parent, how much you gave, and what you shared. Think about the days of worry, the calls, the care, the unending love and support. Now that this time is over, you have only to be proud.

> **❝** *I have kept myself so busy since she died, perhaps because there has been so much to do, perhaps because I want to be distracted. But now I find myself crying sometimes when I'm driving home from work.*
>
> *During that quiet time alone the reality sets in that she's not here anymore."*
>
> —Nelly O.

hopelessness, and depression. Some become irritable, and others become anxious and restless.

Unless you welcome them, say no to invitations, extra assignments, and social obligations. Continue to make yourself a priority.

You may find yourself yearning and searching for your parent, visiting his grave or his favorite spots, trying in some way to stay close to him. Some people adopt the habits and mannerisms of the dead person and, in a few cases, even the symptoms of the person's final illness. (Such an obsession, along with its symptoms, will pass.)

For months after the death, you may think that you see your parent out of the corner of your eye, or sense for a moment that you hear her come into the house. You may forget she is gone and pick up the phone to call her. It's not uncommon to have dreams about the deceased person, which are usually upsetting but may also be reassuring.

Your parent's death may cause you to reexperience other losses in your life, of loved ones who died, friends who moved away, close relationships that were severed. This compounds the pain and adds to the confusion. And yet, if those losses weren't fully mourned when they happened, this may be an opportunity to grieve and let them go, too.

After a loved one dies, people often speculate about the phenomenon of death, the meaning of life, and their own spiritual or religious beliefs. It may help to talk with a member of the clergy even if you have no connection with a particular religious institution.

Having said all this, it is quite possible that you are not grieving at all now, that instead you feel relief. Don't feel guilty about any lack of sorrow. If your parent was sick for a long time, in great pain, or lost to dementia, you may have finished your grieving process some time ago.

◆ **Letting go.** After some time, sleeping or eating problems, crying bouts, despair, or depression may persist, but to a far lesser degree. This tends to be a time of reflection and growth. With the acute pain gone, people often review their relationship with the parent they have lost and reminisce about time spent together. Friends and mates may try to get you to focus on the present or the future now, but this review is an essential part of saying good-bye.

Recognizing your parent for who she truly was and reconciling, or at least accepting, your differences will help you detach. It may also help you sort through your own personality traits—in what ways you are like or unlike your parent and how you might change.

Logic suggests that the more you loved your parent, the more deeply you will grieve her death, and conversely, that a troubled relationship means you will grieve less and perhaps even welcome this departure. But often just the opposite is true. If the relationship was full of conflict, you may be left with unresolved anger and dueling emotions of love and resentment. But now there is no one to confront. You will have to reconcile the relationship on your own. If the turmoil persists, a support group or psychotherapy can be invaluable in resolving such a struggle. Mental health centers, hospices, and community centers sometimes offer bereavement groups and counseling.

◆ **Moving on.** Now life begins to return to normal. If you have allowed yourself to grieve, accepted the loss, and adjusted to the changes in your life, you should be able to face each day with more energy and spirit. You won't think of your parent as often. In fact, you may go through many days without thinking of him at all. Sorrow may come only at rare moments now—at a wedding, a celebration of a new job, the birth of a child, and other important events your parent cannot witness. And your memories of your parent should be

> " *In the beginning, I welcomed the pain I felt when I thought about my mother. I wanted to remember her, to think about her, and I thought that as long as I felt the pain, she was still with me, still alive in some way. I was afraid that when I stopped hurting, she would be gone. It seemed like a betrayal to stop mourning.*
>
> *Now I realize that it's okay not to grieve. The memories have faded, but they never go away. She'll always be with me, a part of me.*"
>
> —BARBARA K.

more pleasant now—memories of her as a younger, more vital woman, instead of those visions of how she was at the end of her life.

Growing from Grief

The death of a parent can arouse far more complicated emotions than the death of a friend. It is not simply a matter of feeling sorrow and then getting back into the old groove. Life will never be the same. Whatever sort of relationship you had with your parent, your life is different now. In some ways it may be worse, and in other ways you may find that it is better.

DRUGGING GRIEF

Think twice before using drugs or alcohol to dull your emotional pain. Grieving is a necessary and natural response to a loss, and dulling the pain may only prolong or postpone it. Sleeping pills in particular can cause dependency and severe reactions. If you are suffering from clinical depression or from sheer exhaustion because you can't sleep, medication may be necessary for a short time, but be sure to use it in low doses and only under the supervision of a doctor.

◆ **Newfound independence.** Whether you are seventeen or seventy-five, when your only surviving parent dies, you become an orphan. That may leave you feeling, at least for a time, afloat, rootless, and profoundly alone. You may have lost a safety net, a confidant, or a link to your childhood. The awareness that you are truly on your own, that you are no longer someone's child, can be a crushing and unexpected aspect of grief, but with time it can also be an impetus for new growth and bolder independence. If your father guided you financially or your mother fed your ego, you will have to learn to do these things for yourself now. And if you had a stressful relationship with your parent—if your mother was domineering or your father always made you feel inadequate—the loss can actually be liberating.

◆ **A clearer view of one's self.** A parent's death brings you face-to-face with your own mortality. You don't have a buffer against the future anymore.

You are now the older generation, and therefore the next in line to go.

You may have already studied your own wrinkles and white hairs. You may have settled into retirement and your "golden years." You may have even contemplated your own death. Will I be like she was? Will my children care for me? Without children, who will care for me? With the death of your parent, these ruminations and questions become a little more stark.

This confrontation with mortality can depress you, but it can also serve as a clarion call to recognize how precious life is and to make the most of it—and perhaps to do better in old age than your parent did.

◆ **Redirected energy.** The job of caregiver, although draining, may have given you a sense of purpose as it consumed your days. The loss of that role can require a great deal of adjustment. If you have been at it for some time, you may have distanced yourself from friends or cut back on your hours at work, and become accustomed to a superhuman pace. Now there is a void.

Slowing down, finding new meaning in your life, and reestablishing broken ties will take time. It requires patience and awareness. Find worthwhile tasks for yourself, and be careful not to fill the vacuum by trying to take over the care of yet another person, such as a surviving parent who is managing all right on her own.

◆ **Changes in family structure.** Certain family patterns and rituals may disappear with your parent. You no longer know what your sister is up to because your mother isn't there to spread the news. Holiday plans are now open because Thanksgiving was always spent at your father's house. While the change is disorienting, getting together as a family is now a choice, and perhaps a chance to create your own traditions.

With time, old roles may disappear and family alliances shift. A sister who was closer to Dad may create a new, stronger relationship with Mom, which in turn may threaten a brother's intimate relationship with her. Or siblings who fought about a parent's care may develop new bonds now that the parent is gone.

This is a time of testing and sampling. Let it happen and participate in it. While it may be uncomfortable at first, your family needs to establish new rituals and relationships.

◆ **Review of other relationships.** In the midst of all this sorting-through, your relationship with your

> *" I had a very difficult relationship with my mother. I struggled in those last years to get close to her, to build some sort of loving mother-daughter relationship, and nothing ever worked. We were never close.*
>
> *Given how little we had together, I was amazed at how much I missed her. After she died there was a big hole, this big, empty hole in my life that I couldn't seem to fill or escape. I am still trying to figure out what that is about. Do I miss her, or do I miss the relationship I never had with her?"*
>
> —JANE M.

mate may come under review, and problems in the relationship may loom large. Remember that your spouse cannot fill the void that your parent's death has left, or know what you are feeling unless you tell him. As you detach from your parent, you will be better able to see your mate for all he is and all he cannot be.

Your relationship with your own children may also come under scrutiny. You may worry about what kind of a parent you are or have been. Are you repeating your parent's mistakes? Are you a good role model? Are you able to offer your children the positive things your parent gave you? Think about these questions and work on your own shortcomings. You do not

REVIEWING YOUR RELATIONSHIP WITH YOUR PARENT

After your grief has subsided, you may find it helpful to explore your parent's life and to consider any unresolved issues between the two of you. Approach these projects only when you are ready and only if doing so feels right for you.

◆ **Write.** Set aside time when you won't be interrupted to keep a journal or write letters to your deceased parent. Tell him whatever is on your mind. Say all the things you never had the nerve to say. Tell him how he angered you or what you appreciated about him. And when you are ready, tell him good-bye.

◆ **Interview.** Talk with your parent's relatives and friends about his life, his childhood, his professional life, his relationships. Pursue whatever interests you and delve into areas that you may have avoided when your parent was alive.

◆ **Commemorate.** Create rituals to honor and remember your parent. Visit her grave, frame photos, return to a favorite spot, plant a memorial tree or garden, or have a family gathering on the anniversary of her death.

◆ **Join.** Get involved with a support group or attend seminars on grief (hospice organizations sometimes hold or know about such meetings). It will give you a chance to talk about issues with people who understand them.

◆ **Explore.** Review your relationship with your parent, and perhaps with others in the family. Write down memories of your parent, focusing on both the good and bad. Describe your relationship and how it changed, or failed to change, through the years. What did you do together? How did you make decisions? Make a list of your parent's traits and the things you agreed and disagreed about. Think about what values or traits of your parent live on in you. Go back and review what you wrote several days later, and add any new thoughts.

have to repeat your parent's mistakes. You can emulate only her best qualities. Make this a time for growth and enrichment, not despair.

The Surviving Parent

Some widows or widowers become extremely depressed and isolated in the months, and even years, following the death of a spouse, especially after the funeral is over and friends and family have resumed their own lives. They may have trouble sleeping and eating normally and may become physically ill. And they often face overwhelming practical hurdles—how to manage finances, cook for one, do household repairs that a mate always took care of, or relate to friends who are still couples. While you need time for your own grief, you also need to support your surviving parent and figure out your new role in her life.

◆ **Stay in touch.** Call regularly and visit as often as possible. Share your grief and allow her to share hers. As you do this, remember that her relationship with her spouse as well as her role as caregiver was very different than yours—probably far more intense and exhausting. Let her deal with her grief and express her feelings in her own way, without comparison or reproach.

◆ **Get her out.** While your parent may not have the energy or the will to go out, social contact is very impor-

> *In the spring after my mother's death, I was planting a tree when I realized that it was my mother's birthday. So I called it Mary's Tree. And I tended to it, and fed it and watered it with care and love.*
>
> *When I'm in the backyard, I look up at this tree, which is quite tall now, and I say, 'Hi, Mary.' And it helps."*
>
> —RITA W.

tant now. Encourage her to see friends and include her in family gatherings.

◆ **Foster independence.** Control your impulse to supply more protection than your parent needs. You may have a lot of caregiving energy on your hands, or you may assume that your mother can't survive on her own. Be careful. She has to adjust, learn about her new life as a single person, and regain her confidence and independence. If you take over her affairs or deluge her with advice, it may offend her or cripple her. Love and support her, but let her learn to live her own life.

◆ **Limit decisions.** In general, a surviving parent should not make any major decisions, such as moving, changing jobs, or selling a home, immediately after a spouse's death. It's better to get through most of the grieving process (which can take a year or more), let things settle, and sort out finances first. In the confusion of mourning, people sometimes make decisions they later regret.

◆ **Stay healthy.** Encourage your parent to see her doctor regularly and to take care of her physical health. Poor health will make her more susceptible to depression and illness. If she is using antidepressants or sleeping pills, be sure that she understands their side effects and potential dangers.

◆ **Keep an eye on the holidays.** The holidays, especially around Christmas and Hanukkah, can be particularly difficult. Stay in close contact. Call and visit often. Let her talk and listen quietly.

Mark your calendar with your parent's wedding anniversary, his birthday, the anniversary of your other parent's death, and other special dates, and try to be in touch on these days as well. They are often painful and lonely times for a surviving spouse.

◆ **Support groups and counseling.** While she may be feeling too vulnerable to attend a support group at first, your parent may benefit from some one-on-one support. Most hospice programs offer or know of grief and bereavement counseling and support groups. To find a hospice nearby, contact the National Hospice and Palliative Care Organization (800-658-8898 or www.nhpco.org). AARP also has a Grief and Loss Program (888-687-2277 or www.aarp.org), which connects people with volunteers who have suffered similar losses and can offer emotional support as well as practical

information. It also has online support groups. When she is ready, a bereavement or support group for widows can provide guidance, emotional support, and friendships. Senior centers, family counseling centers, hospice centers, and churches and synagogues often run or know of such groups.

◆ **Get her involved.** As she starts to heal emotionally, urge your mother to take classes, work, travel, and get involved in whatever activities interest her. With time and encouragement, she will find in herself the will to enjoy living again.

◆ **Allow for change and growth.** You may find that your parent undergoes a surprising personality change now that her spouse is gone. A mother who played second fiddle may prove to be quite capable and even assertive. One who was introverted may become extroverted. Living with your deceased parent may have repressed some of her personality traits and encouraged others. Any perceivable change is likely to be troubling for you—you may prefer the "old Mom"—but let your parent find out who she is as a single person, and then let that person thrive.

Children and Grief

No matter how we may try to shield them, children, even very young children, are profoundly affected by dying and death. They are affected

BOOKS THAT HELP

A number of books can help a child come to grips with old age, illness, and death. (They should be read in addition to, not instead of, open dialogue at home.) Some good ones are:

For preschool children:

The Dead Bird by Margaret Wise Brown, illustrated by Remy Charlip (Young Scott Books)

The Tenth Good Thing about Barney by Judith Viorst, illustrated by Erik Blegvad (Atheneum)

For children five to eight:

Annie and the Old One by Miska Miles, illustrated by Peter Parnall (Little, Brown and Company)

Nana Upstairs and Nana Downstairs by Tomie dePaola (Putnam)

My Grandpa Died Today by Joan Fassler (Human Sciences Press)

Something to Remember Me By by Susan V. Bosak, illustrated by Laurie McGaw (Communications Project)

Love You Forever by Robert N. Munsch, illustrated by Sheila McGraw (Firefly Books)

For children eight and up:

A Taste of Blackberries by Doris Buchanan Smith (Thomas Y. Crowell Co.)

Charlotte's Web by E. B. White, illustrated by Garth Williams (Harper & Row)

The Birds' Christmas Carol by Kate Douglas Wiggin (Houghton-Mifflin)

Little Women by Louisa May Alcott (Grosset & Dunlap)

---

indirectly by your distress, and directly by their own loss. There are no magic words, there is no right way to address this issue. Give your children room to express and explore their feelings, and then respond to their questions as honestly as you can. (See page 184 for more on dealing with children when a grandparent is ill.)

◆ **Start the conversation.** Sometimes children don't ask questions because they don't know what questions to ask. They simply know that the household is astir and they are scared by it. Explain briefly (very briefly if a child is quite young) what is happening—why Mommy is upset, why the child has been sent repeatedly to a friend's house—and ask if he has questions. Then listen, really listen to those questions, and answer them as honestly and simply as you can.

◆ **Leave the conversation** open for further discussion. A few days later you might ask the child if he has any more questions or if there is anything more he wants to talk about. Be aware that children may ask the same questions over and over. Answer them over and over. Sometimes it takes a few repetitions for the information to sink in.

◆ **Be honest.** Avoid saying things like "God took him away," "She is asleep and won't ever wake up," or "He went on a long trip and will never come back." Children take things literally. (You may end up with an atheist, insomniac, or homebody.) Or, if you tell a child that a grandparent is up in the clouds watching over the family, he may worry about practical matters, like where Grandpa is on clear days or whether an all-knowing Grandpa sees every private thing he does.

Explain that Grandpa was old, his body was very sick and it stopped working, so he no longer eats, breathes, or talks. Use examples from the child's own experience, like the death of a pet. You might add that the deceased person lives on in everyone's memories, or find an explanation that reflects your religious beliefs.

Be sure to explain that Grandpa is in no pain, that, in fact, he is out of pain; that death is not a punishment, but a natural thing that happens to everyone eventually; that death is not contagious; and that the child is in no way responsible for the grandparent's death. These are all frequent concerns of children.

◆ **Let them be children.** Although it may be hard for you, allow your children to play and laugh at this time. They are not being disrespectful; they are only being children.

Let them find their own way to grieve. Young children sometimes use play to work through their feelings and questions. They may have a doll or stuffed animal that "dies," which they then bury. Or they may lie still, pretending they are dead, as they try to figure out what it means to be dead. They may also express their grief by misbehaving or withdrawing. Everyone deals with hurt and confusion in his or her own way, and children need the leeway to grieve in whatever way they can.

Early in adolescence, children learn to be cool, and believe that it is uncool to reveal one's fear or pain. If your child reacts in this way, don't corner or push him into admitting something he doesn't want to admit. Instead, talk about what you are feeling. Hearing about your emotions may help him deal with, and perhaps even talk about, his.

Chapter Twenty-Seven

You're Next

Can You Afford to Grow Old?
• Taking Care of Your Body
• Keeping Your Mind Sharp • Living Fully

THROUGH IT ALL, ONE QUESTION LOOMS. IT TRAILS SILENTLY behind you, wakes you at 3 A.M., and whispers to you as you stare at the hunched, sagging shadow that is now your parent. How will you deal with your own old age?

How will you make sure that you get the care you need? How will you avoid your parent's mistakes? How will you create a different, perhaps gentler and, who knows, maybe even joyful final chapter of life? And perhaps most important of all, how will you protect your children from some of what you've been through? Or, heavens, if you don't have children, then what?

Whether you are thirty or seventy, there is work to be done. (Certainly if you are seventy! For Pete's sake, get going!) There are documents to sign, papers to find, issues to discuss, insurance to evaluate, money to save, and moves to consider. Have you updated your will (or even written one)? Do you need long-term care insurance? Have you signed a power of attorney?

If you want to make your late years the best they can be, and if you want to protect your family from the trials of caregiving, then you have to face, head-on, some extremely difficult subjects. You have to think about growing old, and growing frail, and even dying.

Don't roll your eyes in defeat, or put this off for another day. Do some real planning. It's the only way to protect yourself and your loved ones. Learn the options. Make decisions. And give clear instructions. Don't delay.

Of course, you also need to start taking better care of yourself, both physically and mentally. This is critical stuff that directly affects how you age and, well, whether you even get the chance to age.

But that's not all. No, no. There's much more. In fact, if you walk away from this experience gleaning nothing more than retirement basics, the stuff put out by accountants and estate lawyers, you will have missed the point. For beyond the legal forms and retirement accounts, beyond the megavitamins and yoga classes, there is a life to be lived.

How we age, how we live our last years, what burdens or gifts we bestow on others, and, finally, how we die, is not dependent upon the size of a pension, the complexity of a will, or how many miles we jog. It is determined largely by how we live. In the end, what really matters—for us and for those who eventually care for us— is what sort of people we have become, what we have done with our time on this earth, and, most important of all, whether we have loved our family and friends fully.

The Business Stuff

It's all fine and good that people are living longer than ever before, and that scientists expect this trend to continue. In fact, scientists say that in the foreseeable future they will have drugs that actually slow the aging process. As a result of these and other advances, more and more people will be seeing one hundred. Perhaps even you.

That's great, but how are you going to pay for all those years? The average life expectancy for a person who is sixty-four is another eighteen years. Within a short time, that figure could easily be twenty-five, or even thirty years. The point is, if you retire sometime in your sixties, you will need enough money to pay for twenty or thirty, maybe even forty, years of life. You don't want your children to foot that bill (even if they could), and you don't want to live on the streets. So what are you going to do?

SAVE!

IF THERE'S ONE THING THAT WILL make life easier later, it's saving money now. It is an absolute must. It should be one of your highest financial priorities. You can't count on Medicare and Social Security. They don't even begin to cover an elderly person's bills, and plans are in the works to cut them back further. You need your own nest egg, and a hefty one at that.

Most people do not save nearly enough for retirement. Many boomers who are living well today are going to end up spending their old age in poverty (and being a tremendous burden to their kids) because they simply refused to save. You do not want to be one of them. It's a miserable life. Start putting money away right now. Today.

Retirement pros will tell you that you need about 80 percent of your current annual budget (adjusted for inflation) when you retire. But retirees will tell you this is hogwash. Maybe you won't have a mortgage or college tuitions to pay, but you will have time on your hands. You'll want to travel, eat out, and visit your grandkids. And don't forget about the heart pills, dentures, walkers, health aids, and, yes, that nursing home, which may cost close to $300,000 a year by the time you need it.

Eighty percent of your current budget just won't cut it. No, you'll need the whole enchilada.

> " *I've seen firsthand what an incredible responsibility it is to take this on, as a caregiver, and that is not anything I'd want for my daughter. Absolutely. I would not want her to care for me. Never.*
>
> *What I want to do is create a facility for my friends and me to buy into, where we'd have all the services we'd need. I want to figure that out and put it together.*
>
> *I've saved quite a bit, but I have to put this together because I will never put my daughter through what I've been through.*"
>
> —SYD S.

So how much is enough? Let's say you and your spouse are fifty, and together you make $80,000 a year, and you want to retire in fifteen years, when you are sixty-five. You each expect to live, say, until seventy-five. Assuming you get Social Security, you should have about $800,000 in various accounts and pension plans to cover your retirement expenses.

If this makes you feel a bit sick to your stomach, that's good, because it's time to wake up. You need to look at your savings, pensions, and assets, figure out what you have, what you need, and then take action.

On a cheerier note, it isn't too late. Money you save can add up faster than you imagine. Stop pinning your hopes on lottery tickets and do some serious saving instead. You can do it in fairly painless ways, one small step at a time. Forget $4 cups of coffee. Turn down your thermostat. Skip the masseuse. Don't eat out. Quit smoking (double benefit). Shop around for gas, clothes, and groceries. Use coupons. Weatherize your house. Forgo the designer bottled water (fill a water bottle at home). Avoid "dry clean only" clothes. Rent movies and make your own popcorn. It's amaz-ing what these little cutbacks will do for your budget.

Let's say you buy lunch from a deli on most workdays, spending $6 a day, or $120 a month. If you switch to making a bag lunch that costs only $2 (and may be healthier), you'll save $80 a month. Over five years, at 6 percent interest, that's over $5,500 saved. And that's just a little lunch money. It's hardly noticeable. But it adds up. Imagine if you saved in other ways as well.

RETHINKING RETIREMENT

While the government pushes back the age of retirement (from sixty-five to sixty-seven), some people are making plans to retire even younger. But if you retire at sixty-five or, heaven forbid, earlier, what are you going to do with all that time? With the average life expectancy expanding, and people staying healthy and independent until eighty, ninety, and even one hundred, you could spend an awfully long time in retirement. Forgetting for a moment how you'll pay for those years, what will you do with them? Play golf? Knit? Travel? Watch the telly? For twenty or thirty years? Is this really a good plan? Have you thought this out?

Examine your plans. When do you want to retire? Why do you want to retire then? What will you do? What happens if you keep working? Might you launch a second career or continue working part time? Or, if you already saved plenty, maybe you could devote a decade or two to community service? Perhaps you could go back to school. Who will you be with during these years? Who will you live near? How will you spend the day?

It's a new world out there. The idea that you can work until sixty-five, then kick back and enjoy life for ten years, at which point you suddenly drop dead, just isn't realistic. We have to start looking at sixty-five as not an ending but a new beginning, perhaps simply a change of venue.

If you want to age well, and stay off your children's backs, make plans. Stay active. And rethink sixty-five.

Since saving money is a bit like dieting—a good idea for a week or two, but it grows old quickly—take the decision out of your hands. Have a certain amount deducted automatically from your paycheck and deposited directly into a retirement or other savings account. Certainly put the maximum allowed into any company 401(k) or other matching pension plan. While you're at it, chuck your credit cards. Then, you don't have the option of spending more than you should. The money and the cards are simply not there.

Numerous Web sites have retirement calculators that will show you how much you need to save each year to meet your future needs. Don't get depressed and figure it's not worth trying. Everything you can save and put away and invest will be of enormous help. Do whatever you can. Keep in mind, these calculators and worksheets provide only rough estimates that will change each year, depending upon inflation, interest rates, and the market. So stay on top of it.

REVIEW YOUR ASSETS

WHETHER YOUR FINANCES ARE IN good shape or nonexistent, sit down with an accountant or other financial adviser, and review the situation. Look at where you are and where you need to be. Examine your company benefits—pensions, Social Security, 401(k)s, insurance, etc. Consider various retirement accounts and how they might affect your savings plan and your taxes.

And talk about credit counseling, if need be.

Also, rethink any investments. As you near retirement, your portfolio should become increasingly conservative. You might want to consider some sort of annuity. (An annuity pays an annual benefit each year, every year, until you die, rather than a simple savings or "contribution" plan.) These may not make you rich, and they certainly aren't right for everyone, but when interest rates are reasonably high, they are worth considering.

SIGN THOSE DOCUMENTS

SEE CHAPTER SEVENTEEN ON SIGNING a will, durable power of attorney, living will, and power of attorney for health care. You should absolutely, without a doubt, have these, regardless of your assets, age, or plans.

◆ A will. About 70 percent of adults don't have a will, which means that a court and the laws of the state determine what happens to their property when they die, and, if they have young children, who will be responsible for them. Be sure you have a will, and update it regularly. Name an executor, name guardians for children, and spell out clearly how any money, property, and belongings are to be divided.

You can draw up a simple will with a generic form or will-writing software. Or, a safer bet, you can hire a lawyer to do it for somewhere between $500 and $3,000, depending upon the complexity of your estate.

> " *My mother talked all the time about how she didn't want to be a burden to us kids and how she would NEVER move in with any of us. She would see other people depending on their kids and be very critical of them.*
>
> *But that's all she did. Talk. She never made a plan or took any action. Her emphysema got worse, and her diabetes got worse, and she just kept talking about how she didn't want us to have to care for her. But she never dealt with it in any practical way.*
>
> *So of course, we all had to take care of her, and it was a ton of work.*
>
> *My husband and I are very proactive about this. I'm a bit neurotic about it, to be honest. We have long-term care insurance and an account that we put money into every month for our old age. We have been clear with the girls that we want to be in an assisted-living home or nursing home; as we get a bit older, we'll probably pick one out and start making arrangements. Whatever it takes, we do not, ever, want them taking care of us like that.*
>
> —Betsy M.

◆ **Durable power of attorney.** Every adult should have a durable power of attorney, absolutely. If you should get hit by a hockey puck or if a flowerpot should fall on your head, this document gives someone the power to write checks, access accounts, and otherwise carry on with your affairs. You can adjust the document so that it pertains only to specific accounts or powers, if you want.

Without a durable power of attorney, your family may find that you need care and they can't pay for it. They will have to go to court to have you declared legally incompetent, which is expensive and time-consuming, not to mention emotionally harrowing.

◆ **Advance directives.** As for those dreaded advance directives (living will and power of attorney for health care, which outline your wishes for care at the end of life and give someone the power to make medical decisions on your behalf), it's time to get going. You've got to have them.

Don't just blindly put pen to paper. Think long and hard about this. It's easy to say, "I don't want any extraordinary care when I'm at the end of the road," but it's often difficult to tell whether a person is at the end of the road. And how close to the end do you need to be? Perhaps an operation or ventilator or other procedure has a chance of extending life, some. What's a "reasonable" chance, in your mind, and what sort of life would be worth extending? These are intensely difficult issues that require a good deal of thought.

You can get copies of advance directives for your state through Last Acts Partnership (800-989-9455 or www.lastactspartnership.org). See page

383 for more on signing, and talking about, advance directives.

◆ **Letters of instruction.** In addition to signing these legal documents, write letters of instruction to your loved ones. Attach one to your will that explains why you divided things the way you did, your thoughts on how you want them to handle things, or extra information they might need about clearing out your house or dealing with a business, an art collection, or pets. Attach a note to your living will as well, explaining what you want loved ones to consider when making decisions about your medical care at the end of life, relieving them of uncertainty and guilt at a horrible time.

Store all these documents where family members or other loved ones can find them when they need them. Generally a safe-deposit box is *not* a good idea, as your children won't be able to get into it and many states seal safe-deposit boxes when someone dies. A firebox or office file may be better. Be sure a relative and/or your attorney knows where it is. (Your attorney should have the originals, or at least copies, of all these documents.)

MEET WITH AN ATTORNEY

AN ATTORNEY CAN GET THE AFORE-mentioned documents for you and draft a will. While generic forms and will-writing software are fine in some cases, in most situations it makes sense to spend a little money and have it done right.

> " *My daughters came over after their father died and said, 'Think about what should go to whom because everybody's been fighting over Dad's stuff.' They had me write it all out and sign it. And then they said, 'Think about what casket and what music you want.'*
>
> *It was hard. I thought, 'Here I am, planning my demise.' You have no idea the feeling I had doing that. I wasn't prepared for it. It pulls you up short and makes you think, 'I'm going to die one day.'"*
>
> —MAE H.

If you have substantial assets, consider ways to protect them from taxes. Although there are plans to repeal the federal estate tax, and it is slipping away each year, you can't be sure what lies ahead. You can minimize estate taxes by giving money to your heirs now, establishing various trusts, shifting assets into your children's names, or buying life insurance. Be sure that you are in a good position to pay for your retirement and any care you might need, however, before giving anything away.

There are also ways to avoid probate, which can make life easier for your children and other survivors, especially if you live in a state with onerous probate laws, or if you have properties in more than one state.

If your assets are moderate to meager and you are getting on in

ALL IN ONE PLACE

If you really want to be kind to your children, get your finances in order, your documents signed, and your plans laid out, then put all necessary paperwork and information neatly in one file or binder notebook. It will be the greatest gift you give them. You don't need to give it to them now, of course, especially as you will be updating it regularly. But let them know where it is so they can find it when they need it. Or, if they are young, let a sibling, close friend, or trusted attorney know where to find it.

Your binder should include your will or instructions for finding your will if it is elsewhere; original copies of your advance directives and power of attorney; a list of all assets and debts; names and numbers of attorneys, investors, accountants, etc.; information about accounts and credit cards; burial instructions; personal instructions about your home, pets, belongings, or other property; old tax forms or information on where they are located; insurance policies; company benefits; information about a business; military/veteran papers; deeds and titles; etc. (See page 12 for a complete list of important papers that caregivers or survivors might need.)

years, you should speak with an elder law attorney about making plans to go on Medicaid and finding other ways to pay for old age.

WHERE WILL YOU GROW OLD?

IF YOU ARE UNDER SIXTY, YOU CAN probably skip this section. If you are over sixty, it's time to start thinking about where you will live in your retirement, and beyond. Do you hope to stay in your current home until the day you die? Is it suited for, or could it be renovated for, say, a wheelchair? Is it near family? Are there ample services in the community for elderly people?

If not your home, then where? If you don't want to burden your children, think this through and make at least some preliminary plans now. You've been through some of this with your parent. You know the lingo. Now put yourself in his shoes. Where would you want to be at that age? Is your plan feasible? How would it affect your children or other potential caregivers?

If you want to stay in your community, but your own home isn't the best choice for some reason, check into other housing possibilities. Look at group, assisted-living, and nursing homes. Talk to friends about what they might do, or if they want to set up some new, creative arrangement for a group. You don't need to sign up for anything, but know what's out there and what your options are.

If you're thinking of moving or building a new house sometime soon, and this is where you think you'll stay, consider whether it will be suitable for you in your gray and golden years. Don't build a house that you'll have to abandon just when you've made it feel like home. Be sure there is a bedroom on the first floor, wide hallways, a large bathroom, low cabinets, lever handles, etc.

HOW WILL YOU PAY FOR LONG-TERM CARE?

As you know by now, Medicare and other health insurance do not pay for most long-term care, nursing-home, assisted-living, and home care. And yet, most people do, at some point, need this sort of help. (Nearly 70 percent of people over sixty-five end up needing some help getting through the day.) Such care can cost from $30,000 to more than $100,000 a year, and rates are expected to triple over the next twenty years. So by the time you need it, such care might cost $300,000 a year!

Long-term care insurance will pay for some, but certainly not all, care. However, many people shouldn't bother with it, particularly those who may qualify for Medicaid by the time they need care, or those who have plenty of money to pay for such care themselves.

Remember, this is insurance. Number crunchers have figured out the odds. You could pay tens of thousands of dollars for it and never use it. If, for example, you buy a policy at sixty and pay $3,000 a year in premiums, but don't enter a nursing home until eighty-two (the average age of admission), then you've shelled out $66,000 that could have been earning interest for coverage that you might not even need. On the other hand, you could pay one premium and suddenly need three years in a nursing home. What you are paying for, largely, is peace of mind.

An extensive investigation by *Consumer Reports* found that the policies were too expensive and risky for most people. It recommended that someone not even consider such insurance much before age sixty (unless you are at high risk of heart disease, diabetes, or some other disease, or you are a smoker). If you buy while you're still relatively young, you may end up paying premiums for thirty years or more. (Of course, the premiums are lower the earlier you buy.) Furthermore, policies bought twenty or thirty years before they are needed could become obsolete, given all the unknowns in this fledgling field. If you wait too long, until you're quite old, however, you may not be eligible or the rates may be prohibitive. Somewhere between sixty and sixty-five is generally a good time to buy because it's not too late, and it's not too early. You'll still qualify, and the rates are reasonable. At sixty-five you should expect to pay about $3,000 to $4,000 a year for such insurance. (See page 368 for

> " I know I shouldn't say this, but I don't think it's so horrible for kids to have some responsibility for their parents. I took care of my mother and it wasn't easy, but I wouldn't have it any other way. She's my mother. I wanted to care for her. So should my kids have to take care of me? I can say no, of course not, but some little voice in me thinks, why not? Isn't this what family is all about?"
>
> —SUSAN R.

a full description of long-term care insurance.)

Keep in mind that retirement saving, health insurance and, for those with dependents, life insurance and disability insurance should take precedence.

While pondering long-term care insurance, consider the possibility of a life-care, or continuing-care, community, or perhaps some more creative option. Life-care communities are large complexes that offer the full spectrum of retirement services and care. It's an alternative to long-term care insurance that is, at this point, primarily for the wealthy.

EVEN BURIAL PLANS

YES, YES, YES, YOU HAVE TO FACE IT all. It will be a help to your family if you can give them even a few general instructions on what to do when you are gone. Typically, Dad is lying in bed, his jaw hanging open, and his pulse gone; the nurse takes a closer look and announces that, yes, he is, indeed, dead; the family is directed to call a funeral home so they drag out the Yellow Pages and find the name of a local funeral home; and then, after a few hours of shock, they turn to each other and say blankly, "Do you have any idea what he wanted us to do?"

You don't want to tie their hands. Funeral and burial rituals are meant to soothe survivors. Don't plan the entire affair, down to the last detail, or draft a plan that will trouble them. While you might like to be sprinkled over a landfill, your children might not think that is such a great idea. You might dream of cremation, but your spouse thinks it's disgusting.

Talk about it. If you have thoughts on, say, cremation versus interment, or if you would love a particular hymn sung, tell them. Perhaps you truly couldn't care less. Well, then, tell them that. But some instructions, one way or the other, some conversation about it, will be helpful.

Think about organ donation or donating your body to research. Would an autopsy be permissible if, for some reason, the doctor wants to do one? Do you want to be cremated, interred (buried whole, in a casket), or entombed (put in a mausoleum or some such structure)? Where do you want to be buried? If cremated, what should your family do with the ashes?

Do you care if your survivors hold a viewing, funeral service, graveside

PREPAYING FOR FUNERALS

Don't do it. Funeral homes advertise this option with vigor, and it seems at first blush like a sensible approach. But it's generally a bad idea, and not necessary. The problems with prepaying are many. States have different laws about such arrangements, and some have no laws at all, leaving this turf unregulated.

Where does the money go? Into an escrow account or into the funeral director's pocket? (Sometimes the funeral home gets the interest on any account, but your estate pays the taxes on these gains.) How can you be sure that what is promised will actually be covered? What if you move? What if the funeral home goes out of business or is bought? All it spells is trouble.

Generally, the executor of an estate (as named in a will) has access to the deceased's assets and can use them, first and foremost, to pay for burial expenses. Prepaying isn't necessary.

If, for some reason, you feel it is imperative to set aside money specifically for this purpose, put money in a "payable on death," or POD, account. This is simply a bank account (checking, savings, CD, money market) under the name "Fred Smith POD Fred Smith, Jr." Junior has no access to it during his father's life, but has access to it immediately after death. It doesn't go through probate (but is subject to the usual taxes).

How much money do you need to put into it? Well, that depends upon what sort of funeral you want to have, or what sort of a shindig your family might want to have. For a simple cremation and nothing else, $1,000 is plenty. For flowers, food, services, and a casket, somewhere between $6,000 and $10,000 should be fine. Of course, if you want a top-of-the-line casket and a sit-down dinner for two hundred, you're in another league altogether. For more on funerals, burials, and the like, see pages 554 and 669.

service, or memorial service? Should anyone in particular officiate at the service? Are there any readings, music, etc. that you want to part of this service?

What about a cemetery plot (which you can buy in advance)? A grave monument? Anything special you want written on your headstone? (Come on now, you can do this. Have a stiff drink and contemplate it.)

Finally, is there anything you would like outside of a traditional service and proceedings? Maybe you'd like each guest to bring a yellow rose, your favorite, and place it in your grave; or they could each jot down some favorite memory of you that that could go in a book for your grandchildren.

Once you've thought it out and talked about it, write it down, especially if there might be any squabbling or confusion among family members. Some state laws recognize written wishes, sort of like a living will, and those wishes must be honored. Some states allow you to legally name someone who, like a health-care proxy, has the authority to make funeral decisions for you. A state funeral consumer group or funeral regulatory agency may know if there are actual forms for doing this.

Again, do not store these papers with your will or in a safe-deposit box. A will is typically not read until after a funeral, and a safe-deposit box may be sealed after your death. Leave them with family members and your attorney, and keep a copy in your own files. (Put it in that binder mentioned previously.)

TALK, DISCUSS, EXPLAIN!

SAVING MONEY GETS THE FIRST exclamation point, and talking with your family gets the second. Talk with your spouse or closest ally at length, and repeatedly over time, about all of this. As your kids get into their twenties, start talking with them as well.

You don't have to lay out the details of your finances or a list of exact plans for your old-old age, but let them know that you have saved for certain things, what that money is for, how you expect it to be used, what you want in your final years, and how your family should proceed if, at some point, they need to handle your affairs. Talk with them about all that's outlined in this chapter: Where you have stored important documents, your wishes concerning end-of-life care, your thoughts on where you might live late in life, any burial directions, etc.

Be very clear and matter-of-fact. Call a formal family meeting, if necessary, and invite any professional advisers who might help clear things up. Make sure you have compiled the aforementioned binder and let them know where it is.

Open communication—now and then repeatedly over the years—will help your children, and you, more than just about anything else you do.

The Body Stuff

A good part of why one person lives to be ninety-eight with their own teeth intact, and another is bedridden at seventy-two, is genetics. And this is something you can't do a whole lot about.

But you still have power and control over much of the aging process. A study by the MacArthur Foundation found that genetics play a much smaller role than people had thought. According to the study, up to 70 percent of physical aging is the result of lifestyle. People who age well, who suffer the fewest ailments and infirmities, who remain active and have the best time in their old-old age, are those who exercise, eat well, and stay active and involved. It's that simple. Most ailments that hinder people in old age, including arthritis, Alzheimer's, osteoporosis, diabetes, cancer, stroke, heart disease, insomnia, and depression are associated in large part to diet and exercise.

So, take care of yourself. You know how. Eat plenty of vegetables and fruits, get lots of fiber and fluids. Stick to foods that are low in fat and salt. Take some extra calcium.

And exercise. Stretch, flex, and lift. Take long walks. Try yoga, weight lifting, or basketball. Get outdoors. Get fresh air. Stretch your lungs and your muscles. This makes a tremendous, *tremendous* difference.

ANTIAGING MIRACLES

Yes, you can suck down bottles of glutathione, picolinate, manganese, d-alpha tocopherol succinate, coenzyme Q10, HGH, DHEA, and whatever else you can find, and hope it all blends together to create the fountain of youth.

Or, if you're really opposed to mortality, you can freeze your corpse in the hope that one day the cure to what killed you will be discovered, along with a safe way to defrost you. Some people sock away a set of their DNA in the hope of becoming rebuilt or cloned at a later date. And others believe that through "cybernetic immortality," they can download all their thoughts, memories, desires, impulses, biases, and everything else that makes them who they are onto a computer. Then, when their bodies are kaput, the cyber-them can go on, teaching their children, writing their books, and calling their friends.

Most antiaging approaches are less far-flung. But the majority of them are, nevertheless, a huge waste of time, energy, and money (money that could be tucked into a retirement account instead). Many are downright dangerous. We live in a death-defying, age-fearing time, and businesses have spotted prey. The promises are hard to resist, but be a smart, skeptical, and realistic consumer.

Stay healthy and active. Eat your broccoli. Work your muscles. Use your mind. Skip the chocolate. Take a daily multivitamin. But don't be fooled. Don't waste these years buying into scams. And don't let dreams of immortality distract you from what really needs to be done—living your life, taking care of yourself, and planning for the inevitable.

Oh yes, and lose weight. Obesity is quickly becoming the number one cause of death in America, and if it doesn't kill you, it will make your golden years dreadful, between the diabetes and heart disease and arthritis.

While you're at it, buckle your seat belt. Limit the booze. And definitely, toss the cigarettes.

You've heard it all, but you won't believe what a difference it makes until you really set yourself to the task. Not only will it make for better golden years, because you'll live longer, have fewer ailments, be more independent, and have fewer memory problems, it will also make you feel younger, more energetic, less stressed, a bit sharper, and more optimistic right now, today. It will make old-old better, but also help make your middle years pretty darn good.

Lack of exercise and poor diet are more detrimental to your body than the passing years themselves. Yes, bodies age. But they age a whole lot faster when they are stagnant and surviving on donuts. And as you may have noticed by now, older bodies simply can't get away with the nonsense that younger bodies can. A few more calories each day and you'll feel them (and see them) immediately. No exercise? You'll find that you get winded climbing the stairs, that you can't touch your shins (much less your toes), and that everything feels a little stiff. You won't sleep as well, and you'll be perfectly suited for a good bout of depression.

While you're tending to your body, be sure to get good medical care.

Don't put off that pelvic exam or prostate test. Find a good doctor, have regular checkups, and be alert to signs of trouble. (And don't forget the dentist!) This, too, has been shown to have an enormous impact on how we age (or don't get to age).

The Mind Stuff

Once again, use it or lose it. Brains are not all that different from the rest of the body; they need exercise. Plus, using your mind is fun and makes you a more interesting person. Oh sure, you use your mind while working, reading, talking with friends, doing the crossword puzzle, and traveling, and this is great. But use it for new things, as well.

Doing the same old thing every day—whether it's crunching numbers, editing manuscripts, or writing business reports—exercises only one part of your mind, a part that is already well defined. Stretch some neglected synapses. Learn Spanish, take an oil painting course, pick up chess, join a fencing club, make Thai meals, study Mayan culture, go to a lecture on eastern philosophy.

Not only is it critical to keep your mind active, but it's important to remain productive, to feel that you contribute to society in some way. Volunteer in a school overseas, with an environmental group, at a hospital. Teach children, disabled people, or other adults. Get involved in politics, or social causes.

Tapping into your creative juices is also beneficial, even if you've never done anything creative in the past. Take up sculpting or writing or dance.

All of this will keep you young and fend off forgetfulness and confusion. Get involved. With people, with life, with learning.

As for Alzheimer's, everyone's biggest fear, well, age itself is the biggest risk factor. Genes are certainly involved, meaning that you're at higher risk if others in your immediate family have it.

But there are other risk factors that you can control. Mounting evidence shows that various facets of lifestyle, diet, and exercise all play a role in dementia. Head injury increases the risk, so wear a helmet when you bike or ski; that's an easy one. High cholesterol has been linked to Alzheimer's, which means you should avoid saturated fats, stick to lean meats and fish, and, again, enjoy your fruits and vegetables. Some studies suggest that eating one serving of fish once a week lowers the risk of Alzheimer's, and others show that the antioxidants (such as vitamins C and E) found in many fruits and vegetables (berries, broccoli, carrots, citrus fruits) lower the risk. Exercise has also been shown to keep Alzheimer's at bay, as have stress-relieving activities (meditation, deep breathing, imagery). These are the same things that will help fend off other ailments common in old age and make your life better all-around.

The Living Stuff

Now that you've signed off with the lawyer, stocked your fridge with spinach and carrots, finished your yoga class, and studied Nietzsche, it's time to get down to the really critical stuff. It's time to live life. Pick yourself up by your shabby old bootstraps, let go of your gripes and regrets, and get out there. Seize the day.

Planning for your walker days, editing wills, and talking about, well, death, isn't a rollicking fun time. But doing it—acknowledging the future and even recognizing your mortality— teaches you, more than anything else, about life. To age well, and die well, and not be a big drag on your family, you need to live well.

LAUGH

A LOT. HARD. AND OFTEN. It's incredible medicine for body, mind, heart, and soul.

LOVE AND FORGIVENESS

AT THE END OF THE DAY ONLY ONE thing matters, and that is your friends and family. Your sister might make you angry. Your kids might drive you crazy. And you might not have time, not right now, anyway, for your friends. Well, change your bloody ways. Because there is nothing, nothing at all, more important.

These relationships will make your life richer now, but in your old age they will make your life worth living. If you don't have time, make it. Call an old friend. Visit your brother. Take time out for your kids. And never be stingy with words like "I'm sorry," "You're forgiven," and "I love you."

Foster your relationships. Nourish them. Water them and feed them. Work at them and enjoy them. Because when you're sitting in your wheelchair with little hair and no teeth and only a faint memory, the fact that you were promoted at work, or won a race, or made money, or revamped your house, or cleaned out your basement won't mean a damn thing. But having loved ones, having true friends, will.

FIND YOUR SOUL

YOU DON'T HAVE TIME FOR STRUCtured religion, or maybe you attend religious services, but you're just going through the motions. Or maybe the whole thing seems like a silly waste of time. Whatever your views, whatever your background, whatever your practice, spend a little time each week with your soul.

It's not easy. We live in a fast world and are blasted constantly by distractions, time frames, deadlines, noise, and pressure. It's there, wherever we go. The cell phone. The pager. The e-mail. The video player. The fax. The Internet. The CDs and DVDs. Whether we're sitting in our cars, or waiting at a station, or walking down the street, or eating in a restaurant, or standing in our kitchens, the noise—the interference—is there.

Take a moment away from it. Sit quietly. Very quietly. And listen. Do you hear it? Is it still there? What is it saying? As the minutes pass, if you can clear your head of the commotion, you will begin to hear it, the voice of your soul. And, if you give it a chance, it will ease your stress and remind you of what's important, of why you live, of what you need to do, and of what you believe.

We all get our strength from different places and believe in different things. But whatever we believe in, whether it's God or Buddha or nature or just the human spirit, that strength leaks out of us, and the inner voice becomes silent when we ignore it.

What does this have to do with growing old? Everything. It is this voice that guides us to where we need to be, and gets us through times of turbulence, pain, and loneliness. It will help now, and it will certainly help when your knees hurt and your eyes don't work, and the Grim Reaper is whispering your name. It is this voice, your soul, your beliefs, and your spirituality that will give you strength and solace.

LAUGH

EVERYTHING ELSE—THE FRIENDS, THE forgiveness, the personality improvement, and maybe even a certain form of spirituality—will happen on its own if you find the humor in life, and have at least one good laugh every day.

CHECK YOUR PERSONALITY

CANTANKEROUS. CURMUDGEON. Cranky. Surly. Grouchy. Grumpy. Crabby. What do these words bring to mind? It's the seven dwarfs at ninety. If some of these adjectives already apply to you, imagine what words they'll be using when you arrive with your cane on the steps of Twin Oaks Memorial Home.

It's not just about being a nice person so your kids don't call Jack Kevorkian too soon. It's about being the person you want to be. It's about being tolerant and kind, or creative and wild, or ambitious and bold. It's about knowing that people can change, even at your age. It's about making choices about who you are and feeling good about yourself.

Think about what kind of person you want to be, why you want to be that way, and how you might achieve that. When you're lying on your deathbed, what will you regret about your actions? And, yes, how would you like to be remembered?

You can't change yourself completely, and there are traits that you simply have to live with. But, the point is, you aren't powerless over yourself. And the other point is, you do not have to become your mother. Or your father. You really don't.

BE ADAPTABLE

IF YOU SPEND TIME WITH GERIATRIcians, nursing-home administrators, and hospital nurses, they will tell you that the people who age best are adaptable. They adapt easily to sickness, to infirmity, and to changes in their housing or lifestyle. These adaptors are also less of a burden to their families.

With age, most people become entrenched in their ways, more stubborn and unbending with each passing year. But just as we can stretch our bodies and become more flexible, we can stretch our personalities and become more adaptable.

Work at letting go of things, and going with the flow from time to time. Try it in small ways. Let go of the reins occasionally. Let others make plans, don't make a fuss when plans are suddenly changed, and rearrange your own rigid routines and habits from time to time. With time, you may find that you are more resilient, more agreeable, and better prepared to face the changes that certainly lie ahead.

LOVE THYSELF

GIVE YOURSELF A BREAK. WE ARE ALL so darn hard on ourselves. Forgive yourself. Like yourself. Give yourself credit. Know what is wonderful about you. If you need to, write yourself a letter about what you like about yourself. Go ahead, love yourself.

Do it now, and do it when you are ninety-eight. Sure, you should know your shortfalls, and maybe even work to improve them. But know your plusses too. Know all that is great about you, at forty and fifty, or eighty and ninety. Know that you are good, and that you have value. Give yourself a hug.

CROSS THE GENERATION GAP

MAKE FRIENDS WITH PEOPLE OF DIF-ferent ages. Spend time with children (volunteer at a preschool, be a Big Brother, substitute teach at the high school), invite an older colleague to lunch, socialize with someone ten years younger than yourself.

Being with younger people keeps you young (because you start behaving like them!) and, in some cases, allows you to teach and pass on some of what you've learned over the years. Being with people who are older might just teach you a thing or two as they pass on their wisdom, and it should remind you that your own wrinkles and aches aren't really so bad (stop complaining).

LAUGH

DON'T FORGET.

CHANGE YOUR ATTITUDE ABOUT OLD AGE

ALL THOSE NASTY REMARKS YOU make about old people are going to come back and haunt you one day.

Yes, it seems that negative stereotypes about old age are actually bad for you. That's right. And you know you're guilty. You've made cracks about old drivers who can't see over the dash, and senile old men who fall asleep at the dinner table, and little old ladies who can't sort their change much less find their canes. You know you have.

And you've spent a bundle dyeing your hair and buying wrinkle creams and stocking up on gingko so you don't have to be one of them.

Well, studies suggest that people who view aging in a positive light live years longer than those who view it negatively. (And unfortunately, most of us fit into the latter category.)

The time has come to change your views.

We live in a culture that has gone from respecting our elders to despising them. We hide them away in nursing homes and watch, with horror and disgust, as they hobble across the road. And we do everything in our power to pretend it won't happen to us. Fighting age is a multibillion dollar industry, and it is growing by leaps and bounds. The more it grows, the more we all fight and deny old age, the more we distance ourselves from those who are already there.

People who don't dread old age, who accept it as just another stage of life, who view themselves as wiser and richer as they age, and who still see themselves as valuable members of society when they are old, live longer. A lot longer, or so it seems. In one study (by researchers at the Yale School of Medicine), this positive attitude about old age added 7.5 years to a person's life. It was shown to have a greater impact on longevity than blood pressure, cholesterol, weight loss, smoking, and exercise.

So rethink your views. Do it because it might extend your life. But more important, do it because these views are wrong and small-minded. We make an enormous mistake, on so many levels, by eschewing the elderly, ridiculing them, and viewing old age in a harsh and negative light.

For all that is rotten about old age, elderly people have special insights and joys, and much to teach us. Age breeds wisdom, moving poorly breeds thoughtfulness, loss breeds strength. No matter how poorly they might drive, elderly people have much to contribute to our lives and to our communities.

By changing our views, by respecting the elderly and caring for them adequately, by recognizing our own aging process and seeing our gains as well as our losses, we will all be richer.

Be kind to your parent, be polite to the old lady digging for change, respect the elderly gentleman at the head of the table, and don't make a wide arc when passing the nursing home.

Be nice because, whether you like it or not, you're next.

THE YELLOW PAGES OF HELP

Appendices A–J

APPENDIX A
Useful Organizations

ACCESSIBILITY

AARP
601 E St. NW
Washington, D.C. 20049
888-687-2277
www.aarp.org
AARP has information on "universal design" on its Web site, explaining ways to make a home safer and more accessible for an elderly person, and a checklist to be sure that a home meets a person's current needs.

ABLEDATA
8630 Fenton St., Suite 930
Silver Spring, MD 20910
800-227-0216
www.abledata.com
This federally funded program has an enormous database of assistive technology and rehabilitation equipment, as well as information about the price and manufacturer or distributor. ABLEDATA's Web site also offers a useful resource center and "reading room," and has some consumer reviews of products.

DisabilityInfo.gov
www.disabilityinfo.gov
This Web site of the federal government informs people living with disabilities about their rights and options.

National Rehabilitation Information Center
4220 Forbes Blvd., Suite 202
Lanham, MD 20706
800-346-2742
www.naric.com
This federally funded resource provides information about accessibility and rehabilitation, facilities, funding, organizations, and other issues.

National Resource Center on Supportive Housing and Home Modification
213-740-1364
www.homemods.org
Based in California, this center has information about home modification and accessibility products, as well as a database of programs and contractors who specialize in such work and will do renovations and maintenance work for seniors at a discount.

Paralyzed Veterans of America
801 18th St. NW
Washington, D.C. 20006
800-424-8200, or Health Care Hotline: 800-232-1782
www.pva.org
This private, nonprofit advocacy group provides information on getting benefits, living with a disability, modifying a home, and other topics. It also makes referrals to local services.

ADULT DAY SERVICES

**National Adult Day Services
Association**
22 Grant St., Suite L
Herndon, VA 20170
800-558-5301
www.nadsa.org
The association can refer you to
adult day service (also known as
adult day care) in your parent's area.

AFRICAN AMERICAN
SERVICES

**National Caucus and Center
on Black Aged**
1220 L St. NW, Suite 800
Washington, D.C. 20005
202-637-8400
www.ncba-aged.org
The center works to improve the
quality of life for African American
seniors and other low-income or
minority seniors. While it provides
no services directly to the public, it
has programs in job opportunities
and training, health care, housing
options, and long-term care.

ALCOHOL AND DRUG
ABUSE

Al-Anon Family Groups
1600 Corporate Landing Pkwy.
Virginia Beach, VA 23454
888-425-2666
www.al-anon.org
These groups help family members
and friends of alcoholics to cope. The
organization makes referrals to local
chapters and sends out brochures

about the effects of alcoholism on
families. The newsletter *Al-Anon
Speaks Out* is available without
charge online at Al-Anon's Web site.

Alcoholics Anonymous
P.O. Box 459
Grand Central Station
New York, NY 10163
212-870-3400
www.alcoholics-anonymous.org
The national office can direct you
to a local AA chapter. AA assists
alcoholics in becoming and remaining sober through self-help groups.

**National Clearinghouse for
Alcohol and Drug Information**
P.O. Box 2345
Rockville, MD 20847
800-729-6686
www.ncadi.samhsa.gov
This federal clearinghouse has publications on alcoholism and drug use.
The main focus of the information
is prevention, but there are some
materials on treatment as well.

**National Council on Alcoholism
and Drug Dependence**
20 Exchange Pl., Suite 2902
New York, NY 10005
800-622-2255
www.ncadd.org
The council works to fight the
stigma of alcoholism. They offer
information on the disease, support
to family members of alcoholics, and
referrals to local services.

**National Institute on Alcohol Abuse
and Alcoholism**
5635 Fishers La., MSC 9304
Bethesda, MD 20892
301-443-3860
www.niaaa.nih.gov

Run by the National Institute of Health, this organization offers information on alcoholism's harmful effects. Among other things, its Web site offers free publications, links to related sites, and a thesaurus of alcohol and drug terms.

ALZHEIMER'S DISEASE

Alzheimer's Association
225 N. Michigan Ave., Suite 1700
Chicago, IL 60601
800-272-3900
www.alz.org
Also known as the Alzheimer's Disease and Related Disorders Association, this organization provides information and referrals to local chapters, which in turn refer people to local services and support groups. The information and services are helpful to families dealing with other forms of dementia as well.

**Alzheimer's Disease Education and Referral Center
(ADEAR Center)**
P.O. Box 8250
Silver Spring, MD 20907
800-438-4380
www.alzheimers.org
Directed by the National Institute on Aging, this center has information on all aspects of Alzheimer's Disease.

Alzheimer's Resource Room
www.aoa.gov/alz
This Web site, run by the U.S. Administration on Aging, provides information about Alzheimer's, tips for caregivers, and links to other sites.

National Institute of Neurological Disorders and Stroke
P.O. Box 5801
Bethesda, MD 20824
800-352-9424
www.ninds.nih.gov
Part of the National Institutes of Health, this office has information about stroke and other brain disorders, such as Parkinson's, Alzheimer's, and epilepsy and makes referrals to local clinical research centers.

ARTHRITIS AND OSTEOPOROSIS

Arthritis Foundation
P.O. Box 7669
Atlanta, GA 30357
800-283-7800
www.arthritis.org
The foundation provides information and makes referrals to local chapters that sponsor support groups, events, and classes.

National Institute of Arthritis and Musculoskeletal and Skin Diseases Information Clearinghouse
1 AMS Circle
Bethesda, MD 20892
877-226-4267
www.niams.nih.gov
This federal clearinghouse is part of the National Institutes of Health and has publications covering a host of disorders and diseases that affect bones, joints, and skin.

National Osteoporosis Foundation
1232 22nd St. NW
Washington, D.C. 20037
800-223-9994
www.nof.org

This organization has information on the causes, prevention, detection, and treatment of osteoporosis.

NIH Osteoporosis and Related Bone Diseases—National Resource Center
1232 22nd St. NW
Washington, D.C. 20037
800-624-2663
www.ostco.org
Part of the National Institutes of Health, this center has information on osteoporosis, as well as other bone diseases.

ASIAN SERVICES

National Asian Pacific Center on Aging
1511 Third Ave., Suite 914
Seattle, WA 98101
206-624-1221
www.napca.org
This national advocacy organization offers several employment programs.

ASSISTED LIVING

(see Nursing Homes and Assisted Living)

CANCER

American Cancer Society
1599 Clifton Rd. NE
Atlanta, GA 30329
800-227-2345
www.cancer.org
Staff members can answer questions on a broad range of subjects, such as cancer detection, treatment, and the latest research. The Web site has

information about diagnoses, treatments, trials, as well as emotional support and local chapters, which can refer you to local services.

National Cancer Institute
Suite 3036A
6116 Executive Blvd., MSC 8322
Bethesda, MD 20892-8322
800-422-6237
www.nci.nih.gov
The NCI helpline and Web site provide information on the detection and treatment of cancer, finances, and home care. It gives referrals to local organizations, cancer centers, and support groups.

National Coalition for Cancer Survivorship
1010 Wayne Ave., Suite 770
Silver Spring, MD 20910
877-622-7937
www.canceradvocacy.org
This private, nonprofit group is a survivor-led advocacy organization. It offers information on cancer treatments, costs, and insurance coverage, and refers people diagnosed with cancer to support groups.

CAREGIVER SERVICES

AARP
601 E St. NW
Washington, D.C. 20049
888-687-2277
www.aarp.org
AARP provides all sorts of information on caregiving, financial and legal matters, and a variety of other issues facing the elderly and their families. Most of their pamphlets are free and much of the information is available on their Web site.

Children of Aging Parents
1609 Woodbourne Rd., Suite 302A
Levittown, PA 19057
800-227-7294
www.caps4caregivers.org
CAPS provides information on caregiving and referrals to support groups, geriatric care managers, and other resources. There is a small charge for brochures and copies of articles from the group's newsletter, which is published six times a year. (An individual membership costs $25 a year.)

Eldercare Locator
800-677-1116
www.eldercare.gov
Run by the U.S. Administration on Aging, this is a good place to start looking for local services. Its helpline and Web site will tell you how to reach the area agency on aging that oversees services to the elderly in your parent's hometown.

Family Caregiver Alliance
690 Market St., Suite 600
San Francisco, CA 94104
800-445-8106
www.caregiver.org
Started in California, the alliance runs a National Center on Caregiving and provides information on a wide variety of topics useful to anyone caring for an elderly person.

National Alliance for Caregiving
4720 Montgomery, 5th Floor
Bethesda, MD 20814
www.caregiving.org
The alliance is involved in research and public education. Its Web site offers information and support to caregivers, and rates books and other resources.

National Association of Professional Geriatric Care Managers
1604 N. Country Club Rd.
Tucson, AZ 85716
520-881-8008
www.caremanager.org
Primarily a trade association for care managers, this group provides referrals to geriatric care managers.

National Association of Social Workers
750 1st St. NE, Suite 700
Washington, D.C. 20002
www.socialworkers.org
This is a trade association for social workers, but on its Web site it provides referrals to local social workers who specialize in geriatrics.

National Family Caregiver Support Program
www.aoa.gov/prof/aoaprog/
caregiver/caregiver.asp
The Administration on Aging, in an attempt to centralize information, runs this Web site, which primarily provides links to a vast array of other helpful Web sites.

National Family Caregivers Association
10400 Connecticut Ave., #500
Kensington, MD 20895-3944
800-896-3650
www.nfcacares.org
Caregivers get free membership to the NFCA, which entitles them to a newsletter and a pamphlet on caregiving. Other materials are available for a fee. The association also works to affect public policy.

Well Spouse Foundation
63 W. Main St., Suite H
Freehold, NJ 07728
800-838-0879
www.wellspouse.org
The foundation offers support to
people caring for a sick spouse who
need a little emotional care themselves.
Members are directed to support
groups, can be assigned pen pals if
desired, and receive a newsletter.

DEATH AND DYING

Aging with Dignity
P.O. Box 1661
Tallahassee, FL 32302
888-594-7437
www.agingwithdignity.org
This organization, established in
1996, created the "Five Wishes"
document designed to help people
express how they'd like to be treated
if they ever fell seriously ill and were
unable to speak for themselves.

End-of-Life Choices
P.O. Box 101810
Denver, CO 80250
800-247-7421
www.endoflifechoices.org
Originally the Hemlock Society,
End-of-Life Choices promotes the
right to physician-assisted suicide
and other ways of hastening death.
It has information and publications
as well as telephone counseling and
referrals to local chapters and other
local organizations.

Last Acts Partnership
1620 Eye St. NW, Suite 202
Washington, D.C. 20006
800-989-9455
www.lastactspartnership.org

Last Acts Partnership, formerly
Partnership for Caring, provides
information about end-of-life care
and advance directives (legal forms
that include a living will and durable
power of attorney for health care)
that are up-to-date and specific to
each state. Staff lawyers, nurses, and
social workers are available to counsel
families.

National Right to Life Committee
512 10th St. NW
Washington, D.C. 20004
202-626-8800
www.nrlc.org
The committee, a grassroots organization that opposes abortion and
euthanasia, has drafted a "Will to
Live" form for each state. The form
states a person's wishes to be kept
on life support regardless of the
medical prognosis. The committee
also provides help for people seeking
treatment that a doctor or hospital
refuses to provide.

DEMENTIA

(see Alzheimer's Disease)

DENTISTRY

American Dental Association
211 E. Chicago Ave.
Chicago, IL 60611
312-440-2500
www.ada.org
The ADA's Web site allows you to
find a local dentist and provides
a glossary of oral health. There's
information available on dentures
and oral changes caused by aging.

**National Institute of Dental and
Craniofacial Research**
45 Center Dr., MSC 6400
Bethesda, MD 20892
301-496-4261
www.nidcr.nih.gov
Part of the National Institutes
of Health, this institute offers
general information to the public
on dentistry and periodontal care.

DIABETES

**American Association of Diabetes
Educators**
100 W. Monroe, Suite 400
Chicago, IL 60603
800-338-3633
www.aadenet.org
This is a professional association for
diabetes educators—health workers
trained and certified to teach diabetics
how to manage the disease. The
association provides referrals to local
diabetes educators.

American Diabetes Association
1701 N. Beauregard St.
Alexandria, VA 22311
800-342-2383
www.diabetes.org
The association provides information
on diabetes, from medical treatment
to financial concerns, and can direct
you to state chapters for referrals to
local doctors and support groups.

**National Diabetes Information
Clearinghouse**
1 Information Way
Bethesda, MD 20892
301-654-3327
www.diabetes.niddk.nih.gov

Sponsored by the National Institute
of Diabetes and Digestive and Kidney
Diseases, the clearinghouse has information on all aspects of diabetes.

DIGESTIVE DISEASES

**National Digestive Diseases
Information Clearinghouse**
2 Information Way
Bethesda, MD 20892
800-891-5389
www.digestive.niddk.nih.gov
This information service of the
National Institute of Diabetes and
Digestive and Kidney Diseases
offers brochures, scientific articles,
and other information on digestive
diseases, from indigestion and gas
to ulcers and gallstones.

DRIVING

AAA Foundation for Traffic Safety
607 14th St. NW, Suite 201
Washington, D.C. 20005
800-305-7233
www.aaafoundation.org
The foundation has information,
pamphlets, and videos on driving
and safety. One of the items aimed
at older drivers is a booklet containing
a self-exam to test driving knowledge
and skills, and information about a
flexibility training program. They have
a Web site, www.seniordrivers.org,
directed toward senior citizens.

National Safety Council
1121 Spring Lake Dr.
Itasca, IL 60143
800-621-7619
www.nsc.org

The council offers a course for elderly drivers called "Coaching the Mature Driver." Call or visit the Web site to find out where it is offered locally.

EXERCISE

American Alliance for Health, Physical Education, Recreation, and Dance
1900 Association Dr.
Reston, VA 20191
800-213-7193
www.aahperd.org
The alliance publishes books on exercise and other physical activity, including books for the elderly and the disabled.

American Physical Therapy Association
1111 N. Fairfax St.
Alexandria, VA 22314
800-999-2782
www.apta.org
A professional association, the APTA makes referrals to local certified physical therapists.

Arthritis Foundation
P.O. Box 7669
Atlanta, GA 30357
800-283-7800
www.arthritis.org
The foundation has information on exercise and rehabilitation, and makes referrals to local chapters, which often offer exercise classes.

National Senior Games Association
P.O. Box 82054
Baton Rouge, LA 70884
225-766-6800
www.nsga.com

The NSGA is a not-for-profit organization dedicated to promoting healthy lifestyles for active adults 50 and over through education, fitness, and sport. They organize the Senior Olympic Programs nationwide.

President's Council on Physical Fitness and Sports
Department W
200 Independent Ave. SW
Room 738-H
Washington, D.C. 20201
202-690-9000
www.fitness.gov
The council provides information on physical fitness and exercise programs.

FINANCES

BenefitsCheckUp
www.benefitscheckup.org
This Web site screens for federal, state, and local private and public benefits and entitlement programs for people fifty-five and over. The online questionnaire matches people with programs for which they are eligible. It also provides information about prescription drug programs that can help save money.

Centers for Medicare & Medicaid Services
7500 Security Blvd.
Baltimore, MD 21244
877-267-2323
www.cms.hhs.gov
Contact this center or search its Web site for up-to-date information on both Medicare and Medicaid.

**Certified Financial Planner
Board of Standards
1670 Broadway, Suite 600
Denver, CO 80202
888-237-6275
www.cfp.net**
This regulatory board oversees the
licensing of certified financial planners.
It has information about financial
planning, provides referrals to CFPs,
and lets you check on a CFP's current
standing or file a complaint.

**Financial Planning Association
1615 L St. NW, Suite 650
Washington, D.C. 20036
800-282-7526
www.fpanet.org**
This trade association offers information for the general public on
selecting a financial planner, retirement planning, financial security
in old age, and more. It also gives
referrals from its list of members.

**GovBenefits
www.govbenefits.gov**
This Web site provides private, online
screening to determine eligibility for
government benefits. If you qualify
for a program, the Web site provides
necessary contact information.

**Internal Revenue Service
800-829-1040
www.irs.gov**
Tax information and forms are
available online. Or you can call
the IRS at 800-829-1040 for tax
information, or 800-829-3676 to
order publications and tax forms.

**Medicare Hotline
800-633-4227
www.medicare.gov**

The Web site and hotline has all
sorts of information about Medicare,
Medigap, Medicaid, and nursing
homes.

**National Association of Personal
Financial Advisors
3250 N. Arlington Heights Rd.,
Suite 109
Arlington Heights, IL 60004
www.napfa.org**
NAPFA provides referrals to local
financial advisors, who charge a fee
for drawing up a plan.

**National Association of
Securities Dealers
800-289-9999
www.nasd.com**
This association can inform you
of any complaints filed against a
brokerage firm or individual broker.

**National Foundation for
Consumer Credit
801 Roeder Rd., Suite 900
Silver Spring, MD 20910
800-388-2227
www.nfcc.org**
The foundation makes referrals to
local Consumer Credit Counseling
Service offices, which provide free
or low-cost counseling on budgeting
and debt management.

**Pension Rights Center
1140 19th St. NW, Suite 602
Washington, D.C. 20036
202-296-3776
www.pensionrights.org**
The center provides workers,
retirees, and their families with
information and legal guidance
regarding pensions.

**Securities and Exchange
Commission**
450 5th St. NW
Washington, D.C. 20549
202-942-7040
www.sec.gov
Anyone giving advice on stocks
must be registered with the SEC.
The Web site provides information
on researching brokers, filing
complaints, and other issues..

Social Security Administration
Office of Public Inquiries
Windsor Park Bldg.
6401 Security Blvd.
Baltimore, MD 21235
800-772-1213
www.ssa.gov
Call to arrange for direct deposit
of Social Security checks, to notify
the agency of a change of address,
to check benefits, or for general
information on Social Security,
SSI, or disability benefits.

Society of Financial Service
Professionals
270 S. Bryn Mawr Ave.
Bryn Mawr, PA 19010
800-392-6900
www.financialpro.org
The society provides names of
members—insurance or financial
advisers—in your area. It also has
a list of questions to ask when
selecting a financial adviser.

FOOT CARE

American Podiatric Medical
Association
9312 Old Georgetown Rd.
Bethesda, MD 20814
800-366-8227
www.apma.org

For information on foot care and
disease, referrals to podiatrists.

FUNERALS

Funeral Consumers Alliance
33 Patchen Rd.
South Burlington, VT 05403
800-765-0107
www.funerals.org
This group offers guidance on
planning inexpensive and dignified
funeral and memorial services. It can
also direct you to a local consumer's
funeral society in your area.

National Funeral Directors
Association
13625 Bishop's Dr.
Brookfield, WI 53005
800-228-6332
www.nfda.org
This association offers guidance in
locating a funeral director and planning memorial services and burials.

GAY AND LESBIAN
SERVICES

SAGE (Senior Action in
a Gay Environment)
305 7th Ave., 16th Fl.
New York, NY 10001
212-741-2247
www.sageusa.org
This is the nation's oldest and
largest social service and advocacy
organization for lesbian, gay, bisexual,
and transgender seniors. Based in
New York City, SAGE's SageNet helps
people locate similar programs
nationwide.

GENERAL

AARP
601 E St. NW
Washington, D.C. 20049
888-687-2277
www.aarp.org
AARP is one of the largest and most powerful lobbying and educational organizations in the country. It has information on a wide range of topics such as housing options, home care, caregiver stress, and financial plights. There are money-saving programs for members, such as a travel service and a mail-order pharmacy, and volunteer programs and services. Call or visit the Web site to find out about local chapters, membership benefits, and publications.

Administration on Aging
www.aoa.gov/eldfam/eldfam.asp
Through the "Elders and Families" portion of its Web site, the AOA provides links to other programs and Web sites, covering topics from Alzheimer's to volunteering.

FirstGov for Seniors
www.firstgov.gov/topics/seniors
FirstGov is the door to an enormous government information network, providing links to millions of Web pages on a vast array of topics. FirstGov for Seniors focuses on senior issues ranging from legal and financial issues to health and travel.

National Consumers League
1701 K St. NW, Suite 1200
Washington, D.C. 20006
202-835-3323
www.nclnet.org
This nonprofit organization educates the public about a variety of issues, from food and drug safety to financial services to consumer fraud, as well as Medicare, Medicaid, and other insurance issues.

National Council on the Aging
300 D St. SW, Suite 801
Washington, D.C. 20024
202-479-1200
www.ncoa.org
This private, nonprofit organization initiates programs, trains professionals, and advocates on behalf of the elderly. The NCOA has "institutes" for professionals and volunteers, including the National Institute of Senior Centers, the National Institute of Senior Housing, and the National Institute on Financial Issues and Services for Elders. While largely administrative, the NCOA makes referrals to local services and has information on caregiving and related topics (living arrangements, support groups, social services, legal and financial support, nutrition, and health).

HEALTH AND MEDICINE

Center for Food Safety
and Applied Nutrition
5100 Paint Branch Pkwy.
College Park, MD 20740
888-723-3366
www.cfsan.fda.gov
Maintained by the U.S. Food and Drug Administration, this center offers information about food products and general nutrition. There is information available specifically for seniors.

HealthFinder
P.O. Box 1133
Washington, D.C. 20013
www.healthfinder.gov
This Web site, created by the
Department of Health and Human
Services, provides all sorts of general
health information.

Merck & Co.
www.merck.com
This pharmaceutical company prints
the *Merck Manual of Geriatrics*.
Updated regularly, the book is available on the Web. While intended for
doctors, the information is useful for
any consumer. Also on this site, you
can find the *Merck Manual of Medical
Information*, which is a more general
medical book for consumers.

**National Center for Complementary
and Alternative Medicine**
P.O. Box 7923
Gaithersburg, MD 20898
888-644-6226
www.nccam.nih.gov
This branch of the National
Institutes of Health offers scientific
information on alternative and complementary medicine, as well as
alerts and advisories.

National Health Information Center
P.O. Box 1133
Washington, D.C. 20013
800-336-4797
www.health.gov/nhic
The center, sponsored by the
Department of Health and Human
Services, is a referral service that
links people with questions about
illness, health, or health insurance to
the appropriate organizations.

National Institute on Aging
Bldg. 31, Room 5C27
31 Center Dr., MSC 2292
Bethesda, MD 20892
800-222-2225
www.nia.nih.gov
The NIA, a division of the National
Institutes of Health, supports research
on aging and health. It produces several free publications, including
dozens of "Age Pages" (also available
online) with information on various
geriatric health issues.

National Library of Medicine/Medline
8600 Rockville Pike
Bethesda, MD 20894
888-346-3656
www.nlm.nih.gov
www.medlineplus.gov
(for consumer information)
The National Library of Medicine's
entire database, referred to as Medline,
is available online at this Web site. It
can also take you to "Medline Plus,"
which has less technical health information for consumers.

**National Organization for
Rare Disorders, Inc. (NORD)**
55 Kenosia Ave.
P.O. Box 1968
Danbury, CT 06813
800-999-6673
www.rarediseases.org
This nonprofit clearinghouse makes
referrals to national organizations for
rare disorders and provides information about them. The first request is
free, but there is a minimal charge
for subsequent requests.

NIH Senior Health
www.nihseniorhealth.gov
Developed by the National Institute
on Aging and National Library of

Medicine, this Web site has health information for older adults.

People's Medical Society
P.O. Box 868
Allentown, PA 18105
610-770-1670
www.peoplesmed.org
The society protects the rights of patients and their families by monitoring the practices of doctors, nurses, hospital administrators, and others in the medical field. Call for information on patients' rights and how to file a complaint.

WebMD
www.webmd.com
This Web site is a credible source of medical information, with access to over 100 medical journals. For more detailed technical information, WebMD's sister site, Medscape (www.medscape.com), is directed toward health-care providers.

HEALTHY AGING

Go60.com
335 Old Quarry Rd. N.
Larkspur, CA 94939
415-464-0511
www.go60.com
This Web site offers insight, advice, tips, and information with the aim of helping older people age well, stay active, and keep on learning. It features senior news and health information that is updated regularly, as well as links to other related Web sites.

SPRY (Setting Priorities for Retirement Years) Foundation
10 G St. NW, Suite #600
Washington, D.C. 20002
202-216-0401
www.spry.org
The SPRY Foundation is an independent, nonprofit research and educational organization that helps people prepare for successful aging. They focus on physical wellness, mental health, financial security, and life engagement.

HEARING AND SPEECH

American Academy of Audiology
800-222-2336
www.audiology.org
The academy's Web site allows you to locate an audiologist in your area.

American Academy of
Otolaryngology—
Head and Neck Surgery
1 Prince St.
Alexandria, VA 22314
703-836-4444
www.entnet.org
The academy, a professional association for otolaryngologists, makes referrals to local doctors and provides general information about head and neck surgery.

American Hearing Research
Foundation
8 S. Michigan Ave., Suite 814
Chicago, IL 60603
312-726-9670
www.american-hearing.org
The foundation provides information on specific hearing disorders and makes referrals to local otolaryngologists.

American Speech-Language-
Hearing Association
10801 Rockville Pike
Rockville, MD 20852
800-638-8255
www.asha.org
A membership organization for audiologists and speech pathologists, the
association provides general information on speech and language disorders
and makes referrals to audiologists
and speech pathologists.

American Tinnitus Association
P.O. Box 5
Portland, OR 97207
800-634-8978
www.ata.org
The association makes referrals to
local hearing specialists and self-help
groups and has staff and volunteers
who can answer individual questions.
The Web site also has general information about tinnitus.

Association of Late-Deafened Adults
1131 Lake St. #204
Oak Park, IL 60301
877-907-1738 or
TTY: 708-358-0135
www.alda.org
This membership organization
publishes a newsletter, has an
online "chat room," and sponsors
an annual convention.

Better Hearing Institute
515 King St., Suite 420
Alexandria, VA 22314
800-327-9355
www.betterhearing.org
This nonprofit organization publishes educational brochures and
pamphlets on various aspects of
hearing loss.

Captioned Media Program
1447 E. Main St.
Spartanburg, SC 29307
800-237-6213 or
TTY: 800-237-6819
www.cfv.org
The U.S. Department of Education
sponsors this program, which loans
videos with captioning free of charge
to people who have hearing loss.

Healthy Hearing
www.healthyhearing.com
This Web site has vast information
on hearing loss, hearing aids,
implants, and other hearing issues.

HEAR NOW
9745 E. Hampden Ave., Suite 300
Denver, CO 80231
800-648-4327
www.sotheworldmayhear.org
This private, nonprofit group supplies
hearing aids and cochlear implants,
without charge, to low-income people.

Hearing Aid Helpline
16880 Middlebelt Rd., Suite 4
Livonia, MI 48154
800-521-5247
www.ihsinfo.org/consumerresources
The helpline is run by the International
Hearing Society, a professional association for "hearing instrument specialists" (people who fit hearing aids). The
society has information on hearing loss
and treatments, and provides referrals
to specialists who are members of the
society.

League for the Hard of Hearing
50 Broadway, 6th Floor
New York, NY 10004
917-305-7700 or
(TTY) 917-305-7999
www.lhh.org

This organization offers information about assistive technology, advocacy, communication therapy, and early identification of hearing loss.

National Aphasia Association
29 John St., Suite 1103
New York, NY 10038
800-922-4622
www.aphasia.org
The association promotes public awareness of aphasia, a disorder that interferes with a person's ability to use or comprehend words. It makes referrals to local support groups and to representatives who can link you to local services.

National Association of the Deaf
814 Thayer Ave.
Silver Spring, MD 20910
301-587-1788 or
TTY: 301-587-1789
www.nad.org
The NAD is a membership organization that advocates for deaf and hard-of-hearing people and their families through its scholarships, teacher certification, youth and volunteer programs, legal services, and other projects.

National Institute on Deafness and
Other Communication Disorders
Information Clearinghouse
31 Center Dr., MSC 2320
Bethesda, MD 20892
800-241-1044 or
TTY: 800-241-1055
www.nidcd.nih.gov
Part of the National Institutes of Health, this clearinghouse provides information on disorders related to hearing, balance, smell, taste, speech, and language.

Self Help for Hard of Hearing People
7910 Woodmont Ave., Suite 1200
Bethesda, MD 20814
301-657-2248 or
TTY: 301-657-2249
www.hearingloss.org
The group distributes information on hearing loss, including tips on coping and help for family members. Its bimonthly journal keeps people abreast of news from regional chapters and support groups.

HEART DISEASE

American Heart Association
7272 Greenville Ave.
Dallas, TX 75231
800-242-8721
www.americanheart.org
The association provides referrals to local CPR courses and offers information on blood pressure, cholesterol, stroke, heart disease, diet, nutrition, exercise, and other topics.

National Heart, Lung, and Blood
Institute Information Center
P.O. Box 30105
Bethesda, MD 20824
301-592-8573
www.nhlbi.nih.gov
Part of the National Institutes of Health, this center provides information on ailments of the heart, lungs, and blood.

HISPANIC SERVICES

National Association for
Hispanic Elderly
234 E. Colorado Blvd., Suite 300
Pasadena, CA 91101
626-564-1988
www.anppm.org

The association advocates for the Hispanic elderly, especially those living on low incomes. It has brochures and other information in Spanish and may be able to give referrals.

National Hispanic Council on Aging
2713 Ontario Rd. NW
Washington, D.C. 20009
202-265-1288
www.nhcoa.org
This organization educates and advocates for the aging Hispanic community.

HIV

National Association on
HIV Over Fifty (NAHOF)
23 Miner St.
Boston, MA 02215
617-233-7107
www.hivoverfifty.org
This association offers support and medical information for people over 50 who are HIV positive.

HOME CARE

National Association for
Home Care and Hospice
228 7th St. SE
Washington, D.C. 20003
202-547-7424
www.nahc.org
This professional organization represents a wide range of home-care organizations. It gives referrals and offers tips on choosing a home-care agency.

National PACE Association
801 N. Fairfax St., Suite 309
Alexandria, VA 22314
703-535-1566
www.natlpaceassn.org
Programs of All-inclusive Care for the Elderly (PACE) provide a broad menu of programs and services, from transportation to adult day services to home care, so that elderly people who are eligible for nursing-home care can stay in their own homes instead. Only a few areas have PACE programs; they are listed on the Web site.

National Private Duty Association
8604 Allisonville Rd., Suite 260
Indianapolis, IN 46250
317-844-7105
www.privatedutyhomecare.org
The association represents home-care companies that are not certified by Medicare and generally do not offer skilled nursing care. Such private duty companies are listed on this Web site.

Visiting Nurse Associations
of America
99 Summer St., Suite 1700
Boston, MA 02110
800-426-2547
www.vnaa.org
The VNAA represents nearly 500 visiting nurse associations across the country that offer skilled nursing care, therapy, hospice care, counseling, home health aides and homemakers, nutrition counseling, and chore services.

HOME MODIFICATION

(See Accessibility)

HOSPICE

Hospice Association of America
228 7th St. SE
Washington, D.C. 20003
202-546-4759
www.hospice-america.org
Part of the National Association for
Home Care and Hospice, this trade
association has brochures, videos,
and books on hospice care, as well
as information online.

Hospice Foundation of America
2001 S St. NW, #300
Washington, D.C. 20009
800-854-3402
www.hospicefoundation.org
The foundation works to improve
public policy concerning hospice
care. It provides information on
hospice, how to choose a hospice
agency, and referrals to local
hospice services.

**National Hospice and Palliative
Care Organization**
1700 Diagonal Rd., Suite 625
Arlington, VA 22314
800-658-8898
www.nhpco.org
This organization represents hospices
across the country. Through its
Helpline and Web site, it provides
information about hospice care and
makes referrals to local hospices.

HOUSING

**(see also Nursing Homes and
Assisted Living)**

**American Association of Homes
and Services for the Aging**
2519 Connecticut Ave. NW
Washington, D.C. 20008
202-783-2242
www.aahsa.org
The association has some consumer
information on housing options, caregiver issues, and community services.

**Continuing Care Accreditation
Commission**
1730 Rhode Island Ave. NW,
Suite 209
Washington, D.C. 20036
866-888-1122
www.ccaconline.org
This commission has a list of CCRCs,
of full-life centers, that are accredited.

**National Shared Housing
Resource Center**
www.nationalsharedhousing.org
The center provides information
about shared housing and makes
referrals to local organizations that
help bring together roommates. Use
the Web site to locate the address
and phone number of your state's
regional coordinator.

HUNTINGTON'S DISEASE

**Huntington's Disease Society of
America (HDSA)**
158 W. 29th St., 7th Floor
New York, NY 10001
800-345-4372
www.hdsa.org
This society publishes information
about all aspects of Huntington's
disease and offers medical referrals
to genetic counseling clinics, nursing
homes, neurologists, and local chapters that can link individuals to local
support groups and services.

INCONTINENCE

**American Foundation for
Urologic Disease, Inc.**
1000 Corporate Blvd., Suite 410
Linthicum, MD 21090
800-828-7866
www.afud.org
The foundation educates patients by
providing information on urinary
tract infections, incontinence, diseases
and disorders of the prostate and
bladder, and other urinary tract and
rectal disorders.

**International Foundation for
Functional Gastrointestinal
Disorders**
P.O. Box 170864
Milwaukee, WI 53217
888-964-2001
www.iffgd.org
The foundation has brochures, articles, and other information (some of
which are on their Web site) on irritable bowel syndrome, constipation,
diarrhea, fecal incontinence, and
other disorders of the bowels.

National Association for Continence
P.O. Box 1019
Charleston, SC 29402
800-252-3337
www.nafc.org
This nonprofit organization has
brochures, books, videos, and tapes
giving detailed information about
incontinence. It also has a catalog of
special products and a national listing of doctors who specialize in
incontinence. Much of this information is available on the association's
Web site.

**National Kidney and Urologic
Diseases Information
Clearinghouse**
3 Information Way
Bethesda, MD 20892
800-891-5390
www.kidney.niddk.nih.gov
Sponsored by the National Institute
of Diabetes and Digestive and
Kidney Diseases, the clearinghouse
provides up-to-date information on
incontinence, as well as other disorders and diseases of the kidneys,
prostate, and urinary tract.

Simon Foundation for Continence
P.O. Box 835-F
Wilmette, IL 60091
800-237-4666
www.simonfoundation.org
A consumer education organization,
the foundation puts out books,
videos, tapes, newsletters, and
reprints of articles on urinary
incontinence.

INSURANCE

AARP
601 E St. NW
Washington, D.C. 20049
888-687-2277
www.aarp.org
AARP has a lot of up-to-date
information on its Web site about
Medicare, Medigap, and managed
care.

Center for Medicare Advocacy
P.O. Box 350
Willimantic, CT 06226
860-456-7790
www.medicareadvocacy.org
This center offers free legal help
primarily to Connecticut residents

struggling with the Medicare bureaucracy. But it provides general advice to people from other states, makes referrals to similar organizations in other states, and has quite a bit of information on its Web site.

Federal Long Term Care Insurance Program (FLTCIP)
Long Term Care Partners
100 Arboretum Dr.
Portsmouth, NH 03801-7833
800-582-3337
www.ltcfeds.com
This Web site offers free informational kits about the Federal Long Term Care Insurance Program (for Federal and U.S. Postal Service employees, active and retired members of the uniformed services, and qualified relatives), downloadable applications, and a calculator that determines how much insurance will cost based on your age and the benefits you choose.

Health Care Coach.com
www.healthcarecoach.org
A project of the National Health Law Program, this Web site has information on getting health insurance, filing claims, and patients' rights.

Insurance Information Institute
110 William St.
New York, NY 10038
800-331-9146
www.iii.org
This industry-sponsored hotline answers questions concerning home and life insurance, as well as government insurance programs.

Medicare Hotline
800-633-4227
www.medicare.gov

The hotline and Web site answers questions about Medicare, Medigap, and state insurance departments. It also reports on Medicare fraud and other illegal practices.

Medicare Rights Center
1460 Broadway, 17th Floor
New York, NY 10036
212-869-3850
www.medicarerights.org
This independent organization offers information and free counseling services to people with questions, concerns, and problems regarding Medicare.

LEGAL ISSUES

American Bar Association
541 N. Fairbank Ct.
Chicago, IL 60611
800-285-2221
www.abanet.org/public.html
The ABA primarily serves lawyers, but it provides information to the public through its Web site and a number of brochures. It makes referrals to local bar associations that have more specific information and often make referrals. Its Commission on Law and Aging (202-662-8690 or www.abanet.org/aging) has brochures and technical books available to the public and makes referrals to local agencies and legal aid societies.

National Academy of
Elder Law Attorneys
1604 N. Country Club Rd.
Tucson, AZ 85716
520-881-4005
www.naela.com
This organization will refer you to elder law attorneys (who specialize in issues facing the elderly) in your area.

LUNG DISEASE

American Lung Association
61 Broadway, 6th Floor
New York, NY 10006
800-586-4872
www.lungusa.org
The association provides information about lung diseases such as asthma, emphysema, tuberculosis, and cancer. It makes referrals for medical care, support groups, smoking cessation programs, and other local services. The above number will lead you to a local office and local services. To speak with a lung health professional, call 800-548-8252.

National Heart, Lung, and Blood Institute Information Center
P.O. Box 30105
Bethesda, MD 20824
301-592-8573
www.nhlbi.nih.gov
As part of the National Institutes of Health, this center provides information about ailments of the heart, lungs, and blood.

MEDICAID AND MEDICARE

(See Insurance)

MENTAL HEALTH AND SUPPORT GROUPS

American Association for Geriatric Psychiatry
7910 Woodmont Ave., Suite 1050
Bethesda, MD 20814
301-654-7850
www.aagponline.org

This association makes referrals and, on its Web site, has information about depression, dementia, and other mental health issues.

American Association for Marriage and Family Therapy (AAMFT)
112 S. Alfred St.
Alexandria, VA 22314
703-838-9808
www.aamft.org
AAMFT makes referrals to local therapists who specialize in problems facing families of the elderly.

American Psychiatric Association
1000 Wilson Blvd., Suite 1825
Arlington, VA 22209
703-907-7300
www.psych.org/public_info
The association has brochures on numerous issues (which can be downloaded online).

American Psychological Association
750 1st St. NE
Washington, D.C.. 20002
800-964-2000
www.helping.apa.org
APA's Help Center provides information about psychology, relationships, stress, and coping, and makes referrals to state associations, which can provide names of local clinical psychologists.

Depression and Bipolar Support Alliance
730 N. Franklin St., Suite 501
Chicago, IL 60610
800-826-3632
www.dbsalliance.org
This organization offers information on mood disorders, and referrals to support groups and local chapters.

National Alliance for the Mentally Ill
Colonial Place Three
2107 Wilson Blvd., Suite 300
Arlington, VA 22201
800-950-6264
www.nami.org
NAMI provides information on
mental illness and referrals to local
support groups and services.

National Association of
Social Workers
750 1st St. NE, Suite 700
Washington, D.C. 20002
202-408-8600
www.naswdc.org
The association makes referrals to
local care managers, therapists, and
other social workers.

National Institute of Mental Health
6001 Executive Blvd., Room 8184,
MSC 9663
Bethesda, MD 20892
866-615-6464
www.nimh.nih.gov
NIMH is a research institute that provides information to the general public
on a wide variety of issues through its
Web site and information line.

National Mental Health Association
2001 N. Beauregard St., 12th Floor
Alexandria, VA 22311
800-969-6642
www.nmha.org
The association provides information
on mental health issues and makes
referrals to local organizations.

National Self-Help Clearinghouse
365 5th Ave., Suite 3300
New York, NY 10016
212-817-1822
www.selfhelpweb.org

This clearinghouse directs people to
national or regional organizations
that can connect you to a local support group. If no local groups exist,
the National Clearinghouse can help
you start a group.

NATIVE AMERICAN SERVICES

Eldercare Locator
800-677-1116
www.eldercare.gov
In addition to the hundreds of area
agencies on aging across the country,
there are more than 240 Native
American agencies on aging, known
as "Title VI," that serve elderly members of federally recognized tribes.
They can be found through the
Eldercare Locator.

National Indian Council on Aging
10501 Montgomery Blvd. NE,
Suite 210
Albuquerque, NM 87111
505-292-2001
www.nicoa.org
Formed by tribal chairmen in 1976,
the NICOA is a nonprofit advocacy
group for American Indian and
Alaska Native elders. The council
offers employment training and job
opportunities.

NURSING HOMES AND ASSISTED LIVING

American Health Care Association
National Center for Assisted Living
www.longtermcareliving.com
These two organizations, which represent long-term care providers, created

this Web site to help consumers plan for, cope with, and pay for long-term care.

Assisted Living Federation of America
11200 Waples Mill Rd., Suite 150
Fairfax, VA 22030
703-691-8100
www.alfa.org
ALFA represents about 5,000 assisted living facilities. It provides consumers with general information and referrals to its members.

Medicare's Nursing Home Compare
800-633-4227
www.medicare.gov/NHCompare
This resource is run by Medicare and allows users to search for nursing homes across the nation and view quality measures, inspection results, and staff information about them.

National Citizens' Coalition for Nursing Home Reform
1424 16th St. NW, Suite 202
Washington, D.C. 20036
202-332-2276
www.nccnhr.org
This coalition of advocacy organizations, ombudsman programs, and individuals works to improve nursing-home care. Its Web site offers guidance in selecting nursing homes and filing complaints, explains laws regulating nursing homes, and provides referrals to local ombudsman programs.

National Long Term Care Ombudsman Resource Center
1424 16th St. NW, Suite 202
Washington, D.C. 20036
202-332-2275
www.ltcombudsman.org
This resource center educates both the consumers and providers of nursing-

home care. They provide consultation, information, and referrals.

NUTRITION AND MEAL SERVICES

American Dietetic Association's Nutritional Hotline
120 S. Riverside Plaza, Suite 2000
Chicago, IL 60606
800-366-1655
www.eatright.org
Call the hotline for up-to-date information on nutrition, to speak with a registered dietitian, or for a referral to a local dietitian.

Food and Nutrition Information Center
National Agricultural Library
Room 105
10301 Baltimore Ave.
Beltsville, MD 20705
301-504-5719
www.nal.usda.gov/fnic
Part of the National Agricultural Library, this center is run by professional nutritionists and aims to distribute the most current information on food and nutrition. The Web site offers educational materials, government reports, and research papers in printable format.

National Meals on Wheels Association of America
1414 Prince St., Suite 302
Alexandria, VA 22314
703-548-5558
www.mowaa.org
The association makes referrals to local meal-delivery programs and congregate or group dining programs. Consumers can also order frozen meals.

NutritionGov
www.nutrition.gov
This Web site provides access to the U.S. Department of Agriculture's online National Nutrient Database. There, nutritional information is offered specifically to senior citizens.

OCCUPATIONAL THERAPY

American Occupational Therapy Association
P.O. Box 31220
4720 Montgomery Dr.
Bethesda, MD 20824
301-652-2682
www.aota.org
This professional association has consumer information on topics such as making a home safe, recovery, Alzheimer's disease, and living with disabilities.

OSTEOPOROSIS

(See Arthritis and Osteoporosis)

PARKINSON'S DISEASE

American Parkinson Disease Association
1250 Hylan Blvd., Suite 4B
Staten Island, NY 10305
800-223-2732
www.apdaparkinson.org
The association provides information on Parkinson's disease and links people to local APDA chapters.

National Institute of Neurological Disorders and Stroke
P.O. Box 5801
Bethesda, MD 20824
800-352-9424
www.ninds.nih.gov
Part of the National Institutes of Health, this office provides information about stroke and other brain disorders, such as Parkinson's, Alzheimer's, and epilepsy. It reports on the latest scientific research and makes referrals to local clinical research centers.

National Parkinson Foundation
1501 9th Ave. NW
Bob Hope Rd.
Miami, FL 33136
800-327-4545
www.parkinson.org
This foundation reports on all aspects of Parkinson's disease and makes referrals to local services and medical experts specializing in the disease.

Parkinson's Disease Foundation
710 W. 168th St.
New York, NY 10032
800-457-6676
www.pdf.org
This organization sponsors research and professional education, educates the public about Parkinson's disease, and makes referrals to specialists.

SKIN

American Academy of Dermatology
P.O. Box 4014
Schaumburg, IL 60168
888-462-3376
www.aad.org

The academy has information on specific skin diseases and refers people to dermatologists.

National Arthritis and Musculoskeletal and Skin Diseases
1 AMS Circle
Bethesda, MD 20892
877-226-4267
www.niams.nih.gov
Part of the National Institutes of Health, this organization provides information on many disorders and diseases affecting the skin.

SLEEP

National Sleep Foundation
1522 K St. NW, Suite 500
Washington, D.C. 20005
202-347-3471
www.sleepfoundation.org
This foundation has information on sleep disorders and makes referrals to local sleep clinics. (They ask that you write, rather than call, for information if you don't use the Internet.)

STROKE

American Physical Therapy Association
1111 N. Fairfax St.
Alexandria, VA 22314
800-999-2782
www.apta.org
APTA has a bibliography on strokes and makes referrals to rehabilitation centers.

American Speech-Language-Hearing Association
10801 Rockville Pike
Rockville, MD 20852
800-638-8255
www.asha.org
The association has information and makes referrals to pathologists and organizations.

American Stroke Association
7272 Greenville Ave.
Dallas, TX 75231
888-478-7653
www.strokeassociation.org
Call for referrals to local chapters, which have information on stroke and support groups.

National Aphasia Association
29 John St., Suite 1103
New York, NY 10038
800-922-4622
www.aphasia.org
The association has information on aphasia and makes referrals to support groups and other associations.

National Institute of Neurological Disorders and Stroke
P.O. Box 5801
Bethesda, MD 20824
800-352-9424
www.ninds.nih.gov
The institute provides information on stroke and other brain disorders, such as Parkinson's, Alzheimer's, and epilepsy, and makes referrals to local clinical research centers.

National Stroke Association
9707 E. Easter La.
Englewood, CO 80112
800-787-6537
www.stroke.org

The association offers information on strokes and makes referrals to medical experts, support groups, rehabilitation centers, and other services.

VETERANS

Department of Veterans Affairs
800-827-1000
www.va.gov
Veterans can call this office for general information about benefits and eligibility and for referrals to regional offices and VA medical centers.

VISION

American Academy of
Ophthalmology
P.O. Box 7424
San Francisco, CA 94120
800-222-3937
www.aao.org
The academy provides information on eye diseases and makes referrals to ophthalmologists, some of whom offer low-cost eye care to people over sixty-five.

American Council of the Blind
1155 15th St. NW, Suite 1004
Washington, D.C. 20005
800-424-8666
www.acb.org
This council advocates for the blind and makes referrals to state affiliates and other organizations that provide information, services, and equipment to the blind.

American Foundation for the Blind
11 Penn Plaza, Suite 300
New York, NY 10001
800-232-5463
www.afb.org
The foundation provides referrals to rehabilitation centers, state agencies, low-vision clinics, and other services, and has information on the emotional and practical aspects of coping with vision impairment and loss.

American Macular Degeneration
Foundation
P.O. Box 515
Northhampton, MA 01061
888-622-8527
www.macular.org
This foundation works for the prevention, treatment, and cure for macular degeneration, and offers information about the disease.

Association for Macular Diseases
210 E. 64th St., 8th Floor
New York, NY 10021
212-605-3719
www.macula.org
The association is run by volunteers who provide emotional support, information, and referrals.

Blinded Veterans Association
477 H St. NW
Washington, D.C. 20001
800-669-7079
www.bva.org
The association helps veterans get VA benefits, rehabilitation, and other services.

Glaucoma Foundation
116 John St., Suite 1605
New York, NY 10038
212-285-0080
www.glaucomafoundation.org

This foundation offers information about glaucoma and connects sufferers to support groups. Its newsletter, *Eye to Eye,* is available at their Web site free of charge.

Glaucoma Research Foundation
490 Post St., Suite 1427
San Francisco, CA 94102
800-826-6693
www.glaucoma.org
The foundation provides information and referrals to local glaucoma specialists. Through its Glaucoma Support Network, it provides online chat groups and support.

Lighthouse International Center for Vision and Aging
111 E. 59th St.
New York, NY 10022
800-829-0500
www.lighthouse.org
Contact the Lighthouse for information on every aspect of vision loss and eye disease, as well as for referrals to state agencies, local services, support groups, and low-vision centers.

Macular Degeneration Foundation
P.O. Box 531313
Henderson, NV 89053
888-633-3937
www.eyesight.org
This foundation's Web site offers the latest news and clinical trials on macular degeneration.

National Association for the Visually Handicapped
22 W. 21st St., 6th Floor
New York, NY 10010
800-677-9965
www.navh.org

This association provides information on vision, eye diseases, low-vision aids, and the emotional aspects of vision loss. It offers referrals to low-vision specialists and clinics, and it has a lending library of large-print books and a catalog of visual aids that can be ordered by mail.

National Eye Institute
31 Center Dr., MSC 2510
Building 31, Room 6A32
Bethesda, MD 20892
301-496-5248
www.nei.nih.gov
The Institute, which supports research projects, has information on eye disease and the latest research and treatments.

National Federation of the Blind
1800 Johnson St.
Baltimore, MD 21230
410-659-9314
www.nfb.org
The federation runs a number of programs for the blind, provides information on blindness (including medical, social, emotional, legal, and financial issues), and makes referrals to services and support groups.

National Library Service for the Blind and Physically Handicapped
Library of Congress
800-424-8567
www.loc.gov/nls
The library lends out books on tape, on disk, and in Braille (as well as equipment for playing tapes and disks) to people with vision loss. All of this is free. (They prefer not to be contacted by mail.)

Prevent Blindness America
500 E. Remington Rd.
Schaumburg, IL 60173
800-331-2020
www.preventblindness.org
Through its toll-free line and Web site, this organization provides information on eye diseases and referrals to local support groups.

Vision Council of America
1700 Diagonal Rd., Suite 500
Alexandria, VA 22314
800-424-8422
www.visionsite.org
This nonprofit group works to increase public awareness about vision care. It has some information on eye disease and aging.

VOLUNTEERING, WORKING, AND LEARNING

AARP
601 E St. NW
Washington, D.C. 20049
888-687-2277
www.aarp.org/scsep
AARP is one of ten national sponsors of the Senior Community Service Employment Program, a project funded by the U.S. Department of Labor to provide job training and placement services to low-income seniors (defined as 55 and up). Its Web site includes a list of the other nine sponsors.

Elderhostel
11 Avenue de Lafayette
Boston, MA 02111
877-426-8056
www.elderhostel.org

Elderhostel, a nonprofit organization, offers a huge array of educational and travel packages to people fifty-five and older, including those with disabilities.

ExperienceWorks
2200 Clarendon Blvd., Suite 1000
Arlington, VA 22201
866-397-9757
www.experienceworks.org
This organization, one of the largest sponsors of the Senior Community Service Employment Program, offers training and employment programs to senior citizens, and also runs www.geezer.com, a Web site that allows seniors to market their crafts and handmade products over the Internet.

Points of Light Foundation and
Volunteer Center National Network
1400 I St. NW, Suite 800
Washington, D.C. 20005
202-729-8000
www.pointsoflight.org
The foundation can refer you to volunteer centers in your parent's area.

Senior Corps
Corporation for National
and Community Service
1201 New York Ave. NW
Washington, DC 20525
800-424-8867
www.seniorcorps.org
This service runs federal volunteer programs, including the Foster Grandparent Program, the Senior Companion Program, and the Retired Senior Volunteer Program (RSVP).

Senior Job Bank
www.seniorjobbank.org

This nonprofit referral system helps coordinate seniors wishing to work with possible employers or those searching for volunteers.

SeniorNet
www.seniornet.org
Senior Net educates adults over fifty about computers and the Internet through online courses and tutorials or their learning centers.

Senior Service America
8403 Colesville Rd.
Suite 1200
Silver Spring, MD 20910
301-578-8900
www.seniorserviceamerica.org
Senior Service America is a nonprofit organization that provides job training and placement services to seniors across the country. It has programs to place low-income seniors in community services jobs, and other older workers in jobs with the U.S. Environmental Protection Agency.

Service Corps of Retired Executives (SCORE)
409 3rd St. SW
6th Floor
Washington, D.C. 20024
800-634-0245
www.score.org
Through SCORE, retired and working volunteers provide free counseling to small business owners.

Volunteers of America
1660 Duke St.
Alexandria, VA 22314
800-899-0089
www.volunteersofamerica.org
The national office can link you to one of its local volunteer programs.

WOMEN'S SERVICES

National Women's Health Information Center
8550 Arlington Blvd.,
Suite 300
Fairfax, VA 22031
800-994-9662
www.4women.gov
This organization is dedicated to women's health. It offers information for aging women and makes referrals to specialists.

Older Women's League
1750 New York Ave. NW,
Suite 350
Washington, D.C. 20006
800-825-3695
www.owl-national.org
OWL is a grassroots organization advocating for economic and social equality of midlife and elderly women. It offers information on issues such as women's health and caregiving, and provides some referrals.

APPENDIX B
State Units on Aging
and Long-Term Care Ombudsmen

The state unit on aging can tell you about programs and services for the elderly in your parent's state and direct you to the area agency on aging that serves her community. These local agencies, which actually go by a variety of names, will refer you to local services and provide general information. They might put you in touch with a case manager who can help with the particulars of your parent's situation, determining her needs and hooking her up with services (transportation, meals, homemakers, adult day services, etc.). They can also tell you about caregiver support, legal assistance, and elder abuse prevention programs.

Long-term care ombudsmen help people who are searching for long-term care residences and respond to specific complaints about nursing homes, assisted-living homes, and other long-term care facilities. The state ombudsman should either be able to help you directly or put you in touch with a local ombudsman.

For more information, contact the Eldercare Locator (800-677-1116 or www.eldercare.gov).

ALABAMA

Department of Senior Services
770 Washington Ave.
RSA Plaza, Suite 470
Montgomery, AL 36130
334-242-5743
www.adss.state.al.us

LTC Ombudsman
Same Address/Phone

ALASKA

Commission on Aging
P.O. Box 110209
Juneau, AK 99811-0209
907-465-4879
www.alaskaaging.org

LTC Ombudsman
550 W. 7th Ave.
Suite 1830
Anchorage, AK 99501
907-334-4480

ARIZONA

Aging and Adult Administration
1789 W. Jefferson St.
Phoenix, AZ 85007
602-542-4446
www.de.state.az.us

LTC Ombudsman
Same Address
602-542-6454

ARKANSAS

**Division of Aging
and Adult Services
Arkansas Dept of
Human Services**
P.O. Box 1437
Slot S-530
1417 Donaghey Plaza S.
Little Rock, AR
72203-1437
501-682-2441
www.state.ar.us/dhs/
aging

LTC Ombudsman
P.O. Box 1437
Slot 1412
Little Rock, AR 72203
501-682-8952

CALIFORNIA

Department of Aging
1600 K St.
Sacramento, CA 95814
916-322-5290
800-510-2020 (in state)
www.aging.state.ca.us

LTC Ombudsman
Same Address
916-323-6681

COLORADO

**Aging and
Adult Services
Department of
Human Services**
1575 Sherman St.
Ground Floor
Denver, CO 80203-1714
303-866-2636
www.cdhs.state.co.us

LTC Ombudsman
The Legal Center
455 Sherman St.
Suite 130
Denver, CO 80203
800-288-1376

CONNECTICUT

**Division of Elderly,
Community, and
Social Work Services**
25 Sigourney St.
10th Floor
Hartford, CT
06106-5033
860-424-5277
www.dss.state.ct.us/
divs/eldsvc.htm

LTC Ombudsman
Same Address
860-424-5200

DELAWARE

**Dept of Health &
Social Services
Division of Services
for Aging and Adults
with Physical
Disabilities**
1901 N. DuPont Hwy.
New Castle, DE 19720
302-577-4791
www.dsaapd.com

LTC Ombudsman
Same Address
302-255-9390

DISTRICT OF COLUMBIA

Office on Aging
One Judiciary Square
9th Floor
441 4th St. NW
Washington, DC 20001
202-724-5622
www.dcoa.dc.gov

LTC Ombudsman
601 E St. NW, A4-540
Washington, DC 20049
202-434-2140

FLORIDA

**Department of
Elder Affairs**
Building B, Suite 152
4040 Esplanade Way
Tallahassee, FL
32399-7000
850-414-2000
http://elderaffairs.state.
fl.us

LTC Ombudsman
Same Address
888-831-0404

GEORGIA

**Division of
Aging Services
Department of
Human Resources**
2 Peachtree St. NE
9th Floor
Atlanta, GA 30303-3142
404-657-5258
www2.state.ga.us/
Departments/DHR/
aging.html

LTC Ombudsman
Same Address
888-454-5826

HAWAII

**Executive Office
on Aging**
No. 1 Capitol District
250 S. Hotel St.
Suite 109
Honolulu, HI
96813-2831
808-586-0100
www2.state.hi.us/eoa

LTC Ombudsman
250 S. Hotel St.
Suite 406
Honolulu, HI
96813-2831
Same Phone

IDAHO

Commission on Aging
P.O. Box 83720
Boise, ID 83720-0007
208-334-3833
www.idahoaging.com

LTC Ombudsman
Same Address/Phone

ILLINOIS

Department on Aging
421 E. Capitol Ave.
Springfield, IL 62701
217-785-2870
www.state.il.us/aging

LTC Ombudsman
Same Address
217-785-3143

INDIANA

**Bureau of Aging and
In-Home Services**
402 W. Washington St.
P.O. Box 7083
Indianapolis, IN
46207-7083
317-232-7020
www.in.gov/fssa/
elderly/aaa

LTC Ombudsman
Same Address
800-545-7763

IOWA

**Department of
Elder Affairs**
Clemens Bldg.
3rd Floor
200 10th St.
Des Moines, IA
50309-3609
515-242-3333
www.state.ia.us/
elderaffairs

LTC Ombudsman
Same Address
515-242-3327

KANSAS

Department on Aging
New England Bldg.
503 S. Kansas
Topeka, KS 66603-3404
785-296-4986
800-432-3535
www.agingkansas.org/
kdoa

LTC Ombudsman
900 SW Jackson St.
Suite 1041
Topeka, KS 66612
785-296-3017

KENTUCKY

**Division of Aging
Services**
275 E. Main St. 5C-D
Frankfort, KY 40621
502-564-6930
www.chs.state.ky.us/
aging

LTC Ombudsman
Same Address/Phone

LOUISIANA

**Governor's Office of
Elderly Affairs**
P.O. Box 80374
Baton Rouge, LA
70898-0374
225-342-7100
www.louisiana.gov/
elderlyaffairs/

LTC Ombudsman
Same Address
225-342-6872

MAINE

**Department of Human
Services**
35 Anthony Ave.
State House, Station #11
Augusta, ME 04333
207-624-5335
www.state.me.us/dhs/
elder.htm

LTC Ombudsman
1 Weston Ct.
P.O. Box 128
Augusta, ME 04332
207-621-1079

MARYLAND

Department of Aging
State Office Bldg.
Room 1007
301 W. Preston St.
Baltimore, MD
21201-2374
410-767-1100
800-243-3425 (in state)
www.mdoa.state.md.us

LTC Ombudsman
Same Address/Phone

MASSACHUSETTS

**Executive Office of
Elder Affairs**
1 Ashburton Pl.
5th Floor
Boston, MA 02108
617-222-7451
800-243-4636
www.800ageinfo.com

LTC Ombudsman
Same Address
617-727-7750

MICHIGAN

**Office of Services
to the Aging**
P.O. Box 30676
7109 W. Saginaw
Lansing, MI
48909-8176
517-373-8230
www.miseniors.net

LTC Ombudsman
Same Address
517-335-0148

MINNESOTA

Board on Aging
444 Lafayette Rd.
St. Paul, MN 55155-
3843
651-296-2770
www.mnaging.org

LTC Ombudsman
121 E. 7th Pl., Suite 410
St. Paul, MN 55101
651-296-0382

MISSISSIPPI

**Aging and Adult
Services**
750 N. State St.
Jackson, MS 39202
601-359-4925
800-948-3090
www.mdhs.state.ms.us/
aas.html

LTC Ombudsman
Same Address
601-359-4927

MISSOURI

**Department of Health
& Senior Services**
P.O. Box 570
615 Howerton Ct.
Jefferson City, MO
65102-0570
573-751-6400
www.health.state.mo.us

LTC Ombudsman
Same Address
800-309-3282

MONTANA

**Senior and Long Term
Care Division**
Department of Public
Health & Human
Services
P.O. Box 4210
111 Sanders, Room 211
Helena, MT 59620
406-444-4077
www.dphhs.state.mt.
us/sltc

LTC Ombudsman
Same Address
800-551-3191

NEBRASKA

**Division of Aging
Services**
**Dept of Health &
Human Services**
P.O. Box 95044
301 Centennial Mall S.
Lincoln, NE 68509
402-471-4623
800-942-7830
(Nebraska only)
www.hhs.state.ne.us/
ags/agsindex.htm

LTC Ombudsman
Same Address/Phone

NEVADA

**Division of
Aging Services
Department of
Human Resources**
3416 Goni Rd., Bldg.
D-132
Carson City, NV 89706
775-687-4210
www.aging.state.nv.us

LTC Ombudsman
445 Apple St. #104
Reno, NV 89502
775-688-2964

NEW HAMPSHIRE

**Division of Elderly and
Adult Services**
State Office Park S.
129 Pleasant St.
Brown Bldg. #1
Concord, NH 03301
800-351-1888
603-271-4680
www.dhhs.state.nh.
us/DHHS/DEAS/
default.htm

LTC Ombudsman
Same Address
603-271-4704

NEW JERSEY

**Division of
Senior Affairs
Department of Health
& Senior Services**
P.O. Box 807
Trenton, NJ 08625-0807
877-222-3737
www.state.nj.us/health/
senior

LTC Ombudsman
Same Address
609-943-4026

NEW MEXICO

State Agency on Aging
La Villa Rivera Bldg.
228 E. Palace Ave.
Ground Floor
Santa Fe, NM 87501
505-476-4799
800-432-2080
(in-state only)
www.nmaging.state.
nm.us

LTC Ombudsman
1410 San Pedro NE
Albuquerque, NM 87110
505-225-0971

NEW YORK

Office for the Aging
2 Empire State Plaza
Albany, NY 12223-1251
518-474-7012
www.aging.state.ny.us

LTC Ombudsman
Same Address
518-474-0108

NORTH CAROLINA

**Department of Health
and Human Services
Division of Aging**
2101 Mail Service Center
Raleigh, NC 27699-2101
919-733-3983
www.dhhs.state.nc.us/
aging

LTC Ombudsman
Same Address
919-733-8395

NORTH DAKOTA

**Department of Human
Services
Aging Services Division**
600 E. Boulevard Ave.
Dept. 325
Bismarck, ND
58505-0250
701-328-2310
800-472-2622
www.state.nd.us/
humanservices/
services/adultsaging

LTC Ombudsman
Same Address
800-451-8693

OHIO

Department of Aging
50 W. Broad St.
9th Floor
Columbus, OH
43215-5928
614-466-5500
www.goldenbuckeye.com

LTC Ombudsman
Same Address
614-466-1221

OKLAHOMA

**Aging Services Division
Department of Human
Services**
P.O. Box 25352
312 NE 28th St.
Oklahoma City, OK
73125
405-521-2327
www.okdhs.org/aging

LTC Ombudsman
312 NE 28th St.
Oklahoma City, OK
73105
405-521-6734

OREGON

Senior & Disabled Services
500 Summer St. NE, E02
Salem, OR 97301-1073
503-945-5811
800-282-8096
www.dhs.state.or.us/
seniors

LTC Ombudsman
3855 Wolverine NE
Suite 6
Salem, OR 97305
503-378-6533

PENNSYLVANIA

Department of Aging
555 Walnut St.
5th Floor
Harrisburg, PA
17101-1919
717-783-1550
www.aging.state.pa.us

LTC Ombudsman
Same Address
717-783-7247

PUERTO RICO

Governor's Office of Elderly Affairs
P.O. Box 50063
Old San Juan Station
San Juan, PR 00902
787-721-5710

LTC Ombudsman
Same Address
787-725-1515

RHODE ISLAND

Department of Elderly Affairs
John O. Pastore Center
Benjamin Rush Bldg.
#55, 2nd Floor
35 Howard Ave.
Cranston, RI 02920
401-462-0500
www.dea.state.ri.us

LTC Ombudsman
422 Post Rd., Suite 204
Warwick, RI 02888
401 785 3340

SOUTH CAROLINA

Department of Health & Human Services
P.O. Box 8206
1801 Main St.
Columbia, SC
29202-8206
803-898-2500
www.dhhs.state.sc.us

LTC Ombudsman
Same Address
803-898-2850

SOUTH DAKOTA

Office of Adult Services and Aging
Richard F. Kneip Bldg.
700 Governors Dr.
Pierre, SD 57501-2291
605-773-3656
www.state.sd.us/
social/asa

LTC Ombudsman
Same Address/Phone

TENNESSEE

Commission on Aging and Disability
Andrew Jackson Bldg.
Suite 825
500 Deaderick St.
Nashville, TN 37243-0860
615-741-2056
www.state.tn.us/
comaging

LTC Ombudsman
Same Address/Phone

TEXAS

Department on Aging
P.O. Box 12786
Austin, TX 78711
512-438-3200
www.tdoa.state.tx.us

LTC Ombudsman
Same Address
512-438-4356

UTAH

Division of Aging & Adult Services
P.O. Box 45500
120 N. 200 West St.
Salt Lake City, UT
84145-0500
801-538-3910
www.hsdaas.state.ut.us

LTC Ombudsman
Same Address/Phone

VERMONT

**Department of Aging
and Disabilities**
Waterbury Complex
103 S. Main St.
Waterbury, VT
05671-2301
802-241-2400
www.dad.state.vt.us

LTC Ombudsman
264 N. Winuski Ave.
P.O. Box 1367
Burlington, VT 05402
802-863-5620

VIRGINIA

**Department for
the Aging**
1600 Forest Ave.
Suite 102
Richmond, VA 23229
804-662-9333
www.aging.state.va.us

LTC Ombudsman
530 E. Main St.
Suite 800
Richmond, VA 23219
804-644-2923

WASHINGTON

**Aging and Adult
Services Administration
Department of Social
& Health Services**
P.O. Box 45600
Olympia, WA
98504-5050
360-725-2310
800-422-3263 (in-state)
www.aasa.dshs.wa.gov

LTC Ombudsman
1200 S. 336th St.
P.O. Box 23699
Federal Way, WA 98093
800-562-6028

WEST VIRGINIA

**Bureau of Senior
Services**
1900 Kanawha Blvd. E.
Holly Grove, Bldg. 10
Charleston, WV 25305
304-558-3317
www.state.wv.us/senior
services

LTC Ombudsman
Same Address/Phone

WISCONSIN

**Bureau of Aging and
Long Term Care
Resources
Department of Health
and Family Services**
1 W. Wilson St.
Room 450
Madison, WI
53707-7851
608-266-2536
www.dhfs.state.wi.us/
aging

LTC Ombudsman
1402 Pankratz St.
Suite 111
Madison, WI 53704
800-815-0015

WYOMING

**Division on Aging
Department of Health**
6101 Yellowstone Rd.
Room 259B
Cheyenne, WY 82002
307-777-7986 or
800-442-2766
http://wdhfs.state.wy.
us/aging

LTC Ombudsman
756 Gilchrist
P.O. Box 94
Wheatland, WY 82201
307-322-5553

APPENDIX C

State Health Insurance Counseling and Assistance Programs (SHIPs)

SHIP programs, which go by different names in each state, offer information to residents about the various Medicare plans, Medigap policies, Medicare billing and appeals, and understanding your rights under Medicare

If you have trouble contacting the SHIP program in your parent's state, contact the area agency on aging (see Appendix B) or Medicare (at 800-MEDICARE or at www. medicare.gov).

ALABAMA

Alabama Department of Senior Services
800-243-5463
www.ageline.net

ALASKA

Medicare SeniorCare
800-478-6065 (in-state only) or 907-269-3680
www.hss.state.ak.us/dsds/seniorcaresio.htm

ARIZONA

State Health Insurance Assistance Program
800-432-4040 or 602-542-6595
www.de.state.az.us/aaa/programs/ship

ARKANSAS

Seniors Health Insurance Program
800-224-6330 or 501-371-2782
www.state.ar.us/insurance/srinsnetwork/seniorshlth_p1.html

CALIFORNIA

Senior Advocacy Services
800-303-4477 (in-state only) or 707-526-4108
www.cahealthadvocates.org

COLORADO

Colorado State Health Insurance Assistance Program
888-696-7213 or 303-899-5151
www.coloradomedicare.com

CONNECTICUT

CHOICES
800-994-9422 (in-state only) or 860-424-5245
www.ctelderlyservices.state.ct.us/ProgramsFrm.htm

DELAWARE

ELDERinfo
800-336-9500 (in-state only) or 302-739-6266
www.state.de.us/inscom/eldindex.htm

DISTRICT OF COLUMBIA

Health Insurance Counseling Project
202-739-0668

FLORIDA

Serving the Health Insurance Needs of Elders (SHINE)
800-963-5337 or
850-414-2000
www.elderaffairs.state.
fl.us/doea/english/
shine.html

GEORGIA

Georgia Cares
800-669-8387
www.state.ga.us/
departments/dhr/
agingcares.html

HAWAII

SagePLUS
888-875-9229 or
808-586-7299
www2.state.hi.us/eoa/
programs/sage_plus/
index.html

IDAHO

Senior Health Insurance Benefits Advisors (SHIBA)
800-247-4422 (in-state only) or 208-334-4350
www.doi.state.id.us/
shiba/shibahealth.aspx

ILLINOIS

Senior Health Insurance Program
800-548-9034 (in-state only) or 217-785-9021
www.ins.state.il.us/Ship/
ship_help.htm

INDIANA

Senior Health Insurance Information Program
800-452-4800 (in-state only) or 317-232-5299
www.in.gov/idoi/shiip

IOWA

Senior Health Insurance Information Program
800-351-4664
www.shiip.state.ia.us

KANSAS

Senior Health Insurance Counseling of Kansas
800-860-5260 or
316-337-7386
www.agingkansas.org/
shick

KENTUCKY

Kentucky State Health Insurance Assistance Program
877-293-7447
www.chs.ky.gov/Aging/
programs

LOUISIANA

Senior Health Insurance Information Program
800-259-5301 (in-state only) or 225-342-5301
www.ldi.state.la.us

MAINE

Maine State Health Insurance Assistance Program
800-262-2232
www.state.me.us/dhs/
beas/hiap/welcome.htm

MARYLAND

Senior Health Insurance Assistance Program
800-243-3425 (in-state only) or 410-767-1100
www.mdoa.state.md.us/
Services/ship.html

MASSACHUSETTS

Serving the Health Information Needs of Elders (SHINE)
800-243-4636
www.800ageinfo.com
(then click on "shine")

MICHIGAN

Medicare/Medicaid Assistance Program
800-803-7174
www.mymmap.org

MINNESOTA

State Health Insurance Assistance Program
800-333-2433 or
651-296-2770
www.mnaging.org/
seniors/healthinsurance/
SHIP.html

MISSISSIPPI

Mississippi Insurance Counseling Assistance Program (MICAP)
800 948 3090

MISSOURI

State Health Insurance Assistance Program
800-390-3330
www.mpcrf.org/
beneficiaries/medicare_
help.asp

MONTANA

State Health Insurance Program
800-551-3191 (in-state only) or 800-332-2272

NEBRASKA

Nebraska Senior Health Insurance Information Program (SHIIP)
800-234-7119
www.nol.org/home/
NDOI

NEVADA

State Health Insurance Assistance Program
800-307-4444
www.nvaging.net/ship/
ship_main.htm

NEW HAMPSHIRE

Health Insurance Counseling, Education and Assistance Services
800-852-3388 (in-state only) or 603-225-9000
www.nhhelplinc.org/
hiceas

NEW JERSEY

State Health Insurance Program
800-792-8820 (in-state only) or 877-222-3737
www. state.nj.us/health/
senior/ship.shtml

NEW MEXICO

Aging & Long-Term Services Department
800-432-2080 (in-state only) or 505-827-7640
www.nmaging.state.nm.
us/benes.html

NEW YORK

Health Insurance Information, Counseling & Assistance Program (HIICAP)
800-333-4114
www.hiicap.state.ny.us

NORTH CAROLINA

Seniors' Health Insurance Information Program
800-443-9354 (in-state only) or 919-715-0319
www.ncshiip.com

NORTH DAKOTA

Senior Health Insurance Counseling Program (SHIC)
800-247-0560
(ask for SHIC)
www state nd us/ndins/
consumer/details.asp?
ID=58

OHIO

OHIO Senior Health Insurance Information Program (OSHIIP)
800-686-1578 or
614-644-3458
www.ohioinsurance.gov

OKLAHOMA

Senior Help Insurance Counseling Program (SHICP)
800-763-2828 (in-state only) or 405-521-6628
www.oid.state.ok.us/
consumer/index.html

OREGON

Senior Health Insurance Benefits Assistance (SHIBA)

800-722-4134 (in-state only) or 503-947-7979
www.oregonshiba.org

PENNSYLVANIA

APPRISE Health Insurance Counseling Program
800-783-7067
www.aging.state.pa.us/aging/cwp/view.asp?a=3&q=175451

RHODE ISLAND

Senior Health Insurance Program
401-462-0508

SOUTH CAROLINA

Bureau of Senior Services
800-868-9095 or 803-898-2850
www.dhhs.state.sc.us

SOUTH DAKOTA

Senior Health Information and Insurance Education
800-536-8197
www.state.sd.us/social/ASA/SHIINE

TENNESSEE

State Health Insurance Assistance Program
877-801-0044 or 615-741-2156
www.state.tn.us/comaging

TEXAS

Health Information, Counseling, and Advocacy Program
800-252-9240 or 512-438-3200
www.tdoa.state.tx.us/BenefitsBasics/BenefitsBasicHICAP.htm

UTAH

Health Insurance Information Program
800-541-7735 (in-state only) or 801-538-3910
www.hsdaas.utah.gov/health_ins_info.htm

VERMONT

Northeastern Vermont AAA
1161 Portland St.
St. Johnsbury, VT 05819
802-748-5182

State Health Insurance Assistance Program
800-642-5119 (in-state only) or 802-751-0428
www.medicarehelpvt.net

VIRGINIA

Virginia Insurance Counseling and Assistance Program (VICAP)
800-552-3402
www.vda.virginia.gov

WASHINGTON

Statewide Health Insurance Benefits Advisors Helpline (SHIBA)
800-397-4422
www.insurance.wa.gov/consumers/shiba

WEST VIRGINIA

Senior Health Insurance Network (SHINE)
877-987-4463 or 304-558-3317
www.state.wv.us/seniorservices/Shine

WISCONSIN

Medigap Helpline
800-242-1060
www.dhfs.state.wi.us/aging/BOALTC/MEDIGAP.HTM

WYOMING

Wyoming State Health Insurance Information Program (WSHIIP)
800-856-4398 or 307-856-6880
www.wyomingseniors.com/WSHIIP.htm

APPENDIX D
State Medicaid Offices

Medicaid, government health insurance for the poor, is administered by each state. While the federal government sets some guidelines, the specific rules for eligibility, what is covered, and special services or programs varies from state to state.

For more information about Medicaid, contact the state Medicaid office listed here, the local department of social services, or the Centers for Medicare & Medicaid Services (877-267-2323 or www.cms.hhs.gov).

ALABAMA

**Medicaid Agency
of Alabama**
800-362-1504
www.medicaid.state.al.us

ALASKA

**First Health Recipient
Services**
800-780-9972
www.hss.state.ak.us/dpa/
programs/medicaid

ARIZONA

**Arizona Health Care
Cost Containment
System (AHCCCS)**
800-654-8713
(in-state only)
800-523-0231
(out-of-state)
www.ahcccs.state.az.us

ARKANSAS

Arkansas Medicaid
800-482-5431
www.medicaid.state.ar.us

CALIFORNIA
Medi Cal
916-552-9797
(about benefits)
916-552-9200
(about eligibility)
www.dhs.ca.gov/mcs/
medi-calhome

COLORADO

**Medicaid Customer
Service**
800-221-3943
www.chcpf.state.co.us

CONNECTICUT

**Department of Social
Services**
860 424 5250
www.dss.state.ct.us

DELAWARE

**Division of Social
Services**
800-372-2022 (in-state
only) or 302-255-9500
www.state.de.us/dhss/
dss/medicaid.html

DISTRICT OF COLUMBIA

**Income Maintenance
Administration**
202-724-5506

FLORIDA

**Agency for Health Care
Administration
Consumer Hotline**
888-419-3456
or
**Department of
Children and Families**
800-342-0825
www.fdhc.state.fl.us/
Medicaid/index2.shtml

GEORGIA

**Division of Medical
Assistance**
800-211-0950
www.ghp.georgia.gov
(click on "member
information")

HAWAII

Med-QUEST
808-586-5390

IDAHO

211 Idaho CareLine
800-926-2588
www2.state.id.us/dhw/
medicaid

ILLINOIS

**Health Benefits
Hotline**
800-226-0768
www.dpaillinois.com/
medical/medicaid.html

INDIANA

**Hoosier Healthwise
Helpline**
800-889-9949
www.healthcarefor
hoosiers.com

IOWA

**Department of Human
Services**
800-972-2017
www.dhs.state.ia.us/
FinancialHealthand
WorkSupports/health
care.asp

KANSAS

**Kansas Medical
Assistance**
800-766-9012
www.srskansas.org/
services/HCP_index.htm

KENTUCKY

**Medicaid Member
Services**
800-635-2570
www.chs.ky.gov/dms/
or
www.cfc.ky.gov/help/
medicaid.asp

LOUISIANA

State Medicaid Office
888-342-6207
(in-state only)
225-342-3891
(out of state)
www.dhh.state.la.us/
offices/?ID=92

MAINE

MaineCare
800-977-6740 (in-state)
207-623-2300
(out-of-state)
www.state.me.us/dhs/
bfi/MaineCare.htm

MARYLAND

**Medical Assistance
Beneficiary Services**
800-492-5231
www.dhr.state.md.us/
fia/medicaid.htm

MASSACHUSETTS

MassHealth
800-841-2900
www.state.ma.us/dma/

MICHIGAN

Michigan Medicaid
800-642-3195
(in-state only)
517-335-5477
(out of state)
www.michigan.gov/mdch
(look for "Medicaid"
under the "site map")

MINNESOTA

**Medical Assistance
Information Line**
800-657-3659
www.dhs.state.mn.us/
HealthCare/asstprog/
mmap.htm

MISSISSIPPI

Division of Medicaid
800-421-2408 (in-state
only) or 601-359-6050
www.dom.state.ms.us

MISSOURI

Recipient Services
800-392-2161
www.dss.mo.gov/dms/
pages/description.htm

MONTANA

Medicaid Helpline
800-362-8312
www.dphhs.state.mt.
us/hpsd/medicaid/
index.htm

NEBRASKA

**Medicaid Eligibility
System**
800-642-6092 or
402-471-9147
www.hhs.state.ne.us/
med/medindex.htm

NEVADA

Welfare Division
702-486-5000
dhcfp.state.nv.us

NEW HAMPSHIRE

Medicaid Program
603-271-5254
www.dhhs.state.nh.us/
dhhs/medicaidprogram/
default.htm

NEW JERSEY

**Medical Assistance
Hotline**
800-356-1561
www.state.nj.us/
humanservices/dmahs/
index.html

NEW MEXICO

**Medicaid Client
Services**
888-997-2583 or
505-827-3100
www.state.nm.us/hsd/
mad/Index.html

NEW YORK

Medicaid Helpline
800-541-2831 or
518-747-8887
www.health.state.ny.us/
nysdoh/medicaid/
medicaid.htm

NORTH CAROLINA

CARE-LINE
800-662-7030 (in-state
only) or 919-733-4261
www.dhhs.state.nc.us/
dma

NORTH DAKOTA

Medical Services
800-755-2604
(in-state only)
701-328-2321

OHIO

**Medicaid Consumer
Hotline**
800-324-8680
www.jfs.ohio.gov/ohp/
index.stm

OKLAHOMA

Health Care Authority
800-522-0114
www.ohca.state.ok.us/
Consumer/Medicaid/
Overview/consmed_
view.htm

OREGON

**Oregon Medical
Assistance Health
Services**
800-527-5772 (in-state
only) or 503-945-5772
www.dhs.state.or.us/
healthplan

PENNSYLVANIA

Pennsylvania Helpline
800-692-7462
www.dpw.state.pa.us/
omap/dpwomap.asp

RHODE ISLAND

**Department of Human
Services Information
Line**
401-462-5300
www.dhs.ri.us/dhs/
elderly/dmaelder.htm

SOUTH CAROLINA

**Health and
Human Services**
888-549-0820
www.dhhs.state.sc.us

SOUTH DAKOTA

Medicaid
605-773-3495
www.state.sd.us/social/
index.htm

TENNESSEE

**TENNCare
Information Line**
800-669-1851
www.state.tn.us/human
serv/medi.htm

TEXAS

Medicaid Hotline
800-252-8263
www.hhsc.state.tx.us/
medicaid/index.html

UTAH

**Medicaid Information
Line**
800-662-9651
http://health.utah.gov/
medicaid/

VERMONT

**Health Access Member
Services**
800-250-8427
www.path.state.vt.us/
Programs_Pages/Health
care/medicaid.htm

VIRGINIA

**Medical Assistance
Unit**
804-726-7380
www.dss.state.va.us/
benefit/medicaid_
coverage.html

WASHINGTON

**Medical Assistance
Customer Service**
800-562-3022
wws2.wa.gov/dshs/online
cso/abdmedical.asp

WEST VIRGINIA

Client Services
800-642-8589 (in-state
only) or 304-558-2400
www.wvdhhr.org/bcf/
family_assistance/
medicaid.asp

WISCONSIN

**Medicaid Recipients'
Services Hotline**
800-362-3002
www.dhfs.state.wi.us/
medicaid/index.htm

WYOMING

**EqualityCare Client
Helpline**
800-251-1269
or
Office of Medicaid
307-777-7531

APPENDIX E
A Hospital Patient's Bill of Rights*

1 The patient has the right to considerate and respectful care.

2 The patient has the right to and is encouraged to obtain from physicians and other direct caregivers relevant, current, and understandable information concerning diagnosis, treatment, and prognosis.

Except in emergencies when the patient lacks decision-making capacity and the need for treatment is urgent, the patient is entitled to the opportunity to discuss and request information related to the specific procedures and/or treatments, the risks involved, the possible length of recuperation, and the medically reasonable alternatives and their accompanying risks and benefits.

Patients have the right to know the identity of physicians, nurses, and others involved in their care, as well as when those involved are students, residents, or other trainees. The patient also has the right to know the immediate and long-term financial implications of treatment choices, insofar as they are known.

3 The patient has the right to make decisions about the plan of care prior to and during the course of treatment and to refuse a recommended treatment or plan of care to the extent permitted by law and hospital policy and to be informed of the medical consequences of this action. In case of such refusal, the patient is entitled to other appropriate care and services that the hospital provides or transfer to another hospital. The hospital should notify patients of any policy that might affect patient choice within the institution.

4 The patient has the right to have an advance directive (such as a living will, health care proxy, or durable power of attorney for health care) concerning treatment or designating a surrogate decision maker with the expectation that the hospital will honor the intent of that directive to the extent permitted by law and hospital policy.

Health care institutions must advise patients of their rights under state law and hospital policy to make informed medical choices, ask if the patient has an advance directive, and include that information in patient records. The patient has the right to timely information about hospital policy that may limit its ability to

*These rights can be exercised on the patient's behalf by a designated surrogate or proxy decision maker if the patient lacks decision-making capacity, is legally incompetent, or is a minor.

implement fully a legally valid advance directive.

5 The patient has the right to every consideration of privacy. Case discussion, consultation, examination, and treatment should be conducted so as to protect each patient's privacy.

6 The patient has the right to expect that all communications and records pertaining to his/her care will be treated as confidential by the hospital, except in cases such as suspected abuse and public health hazards when reporting is permitted or required by law. The patient has the right to expect that the hospital will emphasize the confidentiality of this information when it releases it to any other parties entitled to review information in these records.

7 The patient has the right to review the records pertaining to his/her medical care and to have the information explained or interpreted as necessary, except when restricted by law.

8 The patient has the right to expect that, within its capacity and policies, a hospital will make reasonable response to the request of a patient for appropriate and medically indicated care and services. The hospital must provide evaluation, service, and/or referral as indicated by the urgency of the case. When medically appropriate and legally permissible, or when a patient has so requested, a patient may be transferred to another facility. The institution to which the patient is to be transferred must first have accepted the patient for transfer. The patient must also have the benefit of complete information and explanation concerning the need for, risks, benefits, and alternatives to such a transfer.

9 The patient has the right to ask and be informed of the existence of business relationships among the hospital, educational institutions, other health care providers, or payers that may influence the patient's treatment and care.

10 The patient has the right to consent to or decline to participate in proposed research studies or human experimentation affecting care and treatment or requiring direct patient involvement, and to have those studies fully explained prior to consent. A patient who declines to participate in research or experimentation is entitled to the most effective care that the hospital can otherwise provide.

11 The patient has the right to expect reasonable continuity of care when appropriate and to be informed by physicians and other caregivers of available and realistic patient care options when hospital care is no longer appropriate.

12 The patient has the right to be informed of hospital policies and practices that relate to patient care, treatment, and responsibilities.

The patient has the right to be informed of available resources for resolving disputes, grievances, and conflicts, such as ethics committees, patient representatives, or other mechanisms available in the institution. The patient has the right to be informed of the hospital's charges for services and available payment methods.

APPENDIX F
Touring a Nursing Home, Assisted-Living Facility, or other Residence

When touring nursing homes, assisted-living homes, or other homes for the elderly, be sure that any residence you consider is near family and friends. Visitors are critical. Look for a place where your parent will be safe and comfortable, keeping in mind her particular needs and preferences (especially if she cannot join you on the hunt). What is really important to her? Gardens? Books and lectures? Good friends who might be in the same facility? Religious affiliations? Proximity to her doctor and the ability to continue on in his or her care? You might want to take along a list of things to look for and questions to ask. No facility will meet all your requirements, so decide what is most important. Also, see page 432 for more on finding the right nursing home.

Here are some of the questions and issues you should consider:

At First Glance

◆ Is the residence conveniently located for anyone who might visit your parent regularly? If your parent is still able to get around, is it near shops or restaurants? Is it near public transportation?

◆ Are the buildings, grounds, and interiors clean, well kept, and well maintained? Do the premises smell fresh, airy, and odor-free? Or do they smell of chemicals meant to conceal odors? (At least a few rooms will smell of urine because some patients are incontinent, but the odor should be minimal and limited only to a few rooms.)

◆ Is the residence well lit, attractive, and cheery? Does it feel comfortable and homey?

◆ Is the building safe? Are there clearly marked fire exits, smoke alarms, fire doors, and fire alarms? Are evacuation plans clearly displayed? Is there ample security?

◆ Is it set up to prevent accidents, and manageable for those with canes, walkers, or wheelchairs? Are there grab bars by the toilets and beds and handrails along the hallways? Are pathways kept clear of clutter? Are there ramps, wide hallways, and elevators? Are toilets wheelchair accessible? Are residents required to climb stairs? Are furnishings sturdy?

◆ Is the building, and particularly the residents' rooms, kept at a comfortable temperature?

◆ How is the noise level? Is a television

constantly blaring in the only public room? Are disruptive or noisy residents allowed to dominate public spaces?

◆ What are the grounds like? Is there a garden or nearby park? Are there benches and paths? Is there a solarium? Do residents have ready access to these areas?

◆ Do residents use the common areas, or do they all stay in their own rooms? If they don't use common areas, why don't they?

◆ Be sure to venture beyond the first wing of rooms, which are often the nicest, most recently renovated ones. Ask to see the entire home, including any dementia unit and Medicaid wing.

The Residents

◆ How are residents dressed? Are their clothes clean and appropriate for the weather or temperature? Are they wearing scanty clothing in public places, or left in soiled or wet clothing?

◆ What is the level of functioning—physical and mental—of the residents? Will your parent find people at his general level of functioning?

◆ Do residents and their families say they are happy here? What do they like best about this residence, and what troubles them? Do they like the staff? Do they have warm relationships with the staff?

◆ Is there a sense of community? Do residents interact with each other and seem to have friends?

◆ Are the residents busy, involved in activities and using common rooms?

◆ Do residents in need of help receive it quickly?

◆ Are residents encouraged to be independent, to care for themselves and make decisions for themselves as much as possible?

◆ Is there a written plan of care for each resident? How is the plan determined, how often is it reassessed, and how closely is it followed?

◆ Are schedules flexible? For instance, can your parent stay up and watch television until 1 a.m. and have a snack at midnight, if that is his habit?

◆ Do residents and families have a voice in how the home is managed? Is there a resident and/or family council? When was the last time it recommended a change that was adopted? Can you attend a meeting? (If so, do.)

The Staff

◆ Is there enough staff? Does the staff seem harried and overworked? Are patients neglected and chores left undone, or does the staff-to-patient ratio seem okay? An ideal ratio in a nursing home is one staff to five patients during the day, one to ten in the evening, and one to fifteen at night—higher on dementia wards. There should be at least one registered nurse available on every shift. Most nursing homes don't meet these standards, but they should not be far off. Be sure the listed staff are actually providing direct care to residents; administrators, custodial workers, and other staff do not count. "Staff" should be registered nurses, licensed practical nurses, and certified nursing assistants.

◆ Does the staff treat the residents with respect, kindness, and affection? Is the same care and courtesy given to all alike?

◆ Is the staff friendly, accommodating, and courteous when you visit? Are they open and direct in answering your questions?

◆ Do staff and administrators appear to enjoy their work?

◆ Do members of the staff and administration know residents by name and interact easily with them?

◆ Is there a full-time social worker on staff?

◆ Do staff members seem content, and do they receive support from colleagues and supervisors? (The morale of the workers will make a big difference in the quality of care your parent receives.)

◆ What is rate of turnover?

◆ Does the staff have experience in dealing with people who have the same disabilities as your parent? How do they handle incontinence, insomnia, confusion, blindness, etc.?

◆ Are staff assigned to residents and do they develop relationships with them, or will your parent be dealing with different people daily?

◆ How are family members regarded by the staff—with respect or as a nuisance? Ask other family members who are visiting or talk with a member of the family council, if there is one.

◆ Does the staff encourage phone calls, so you can routinely inquire about your parent's well-being?

Medical Care

◆ What are the arrangements for medical care, dentistry, psychiatric services, foot care, eye care, preventative care, and other health-related needs? Do residents receive regular checkups by a doctor or nurse? Can they continue to use their personal doctors, if they so choose? (By law, they can.)

◆ Is a physician on call at all times for emergencies?

◆ Is there a hospital within a reasonable distance?

◆ What percentage of patients are restrained—physically with straps or chemically with sedative drugs—at any given time? (See page 000 for more on use of restraints.)

◆ What percentage of the residents are incontinent, and how is incontinence handled? Are patients put on a regime to improve continence? (If a large number of patients are incontinent— half or more—it may be because the staff uses diapers and catheters in place of good toileting habits.)

◆ Do you notice any patients with sores, wounds, or other problems that may not have received medical attention?

◆ Are residents allowed to self-administer medications?

Rooms

◆ Are bedrooms private or shared? Are bathrooms private or shared?

◆ How are rooms assigned and roommates matched? Do residents have any choice? If roommates don't get along, can they change?

◆ Are the rooms pleasant? Is there enough space? Are there windows and views?

◆ Are the rooms furnished nicely? Is there a comfortable bed, a bureau and closet for personal belongings, a lamp, and a sitting chair? Are personal furniture and furnishings allowed?

◆ Do the rooms reflect their individual inhabitants? Are residents encouraged to decorate their rooms with their own touches and fill them with personal mementos? Or do they look sterile and institutional?

◆ Is there privacy? Are there curtains around the beds in shared rooms?

◆ Is there a locked place to store valuables?

◆ Are there emergency call buttons that can be easily reached from both the bed and toilet?

◆ In general, are visits encouraged and visitors made to feel welcome? What are the rules regarding visiting hours and visitors? Can visitors come for meals? Are young children allowed? Can residents have private time in their rooms with mates or spouses? Are there private places where you can be alone with your parent?

◆ What are the rules regarding smoking?

◆ Are pets allowed?

◆ What accommodations are there for televisions and telephones?

◆ If someone goes on Medicaid, can he be evicted? Would he be moved to another section of the nursing home? (If so, tour this section as well.)

Meals

◆ Are meals nutritious and well balanced? Is the food fresh and relatively appetizing? Is it served at an appropriate temperature? Is there variety and choice in the daily menus? Is the menu that is posted adhered to?

◆ Is there a registered dietitian on staff, or one who consults with the cook regularly?

◆ Can the kitchen accommodate special diets (kosher, low-salt, fat-free, soft foods)?

◆ Is the kitchen clean?

◆ Are the hours for meals flexible? Is food available between meals?

◆ Can residents keep food of their own? Where?

◆ Will the staff help residents who have trouble eating on their own?

◆ Do patients confined to beds have help or company at meals?

♦ Is the dining room attractive, neat, and intimate? How is seating decided? Can residents choose their own dining companions?

Activities

♦ What are residents doing when you visit? Are they bored, staring at a television set? Or are they engaged in projects and activities?

♦ Is there a monthly activity calendar and does it offer a wide range of choices? Are there frequent movies, lectures, classes, outings, games, and meetings that your parent might enjoy, given her interests and abilities? If there is an activity during your visit, how many people are involved, and why aren't more taking part in it?

♦ Is the activities director willing to offer new classes or organize new events based on a resident's interests?

♦ Are there exercise classes, physical trainers, or physical therapists?

♦ Is there a library? Lounge? Card room? Exercise room?

♦ Is the nursing home involved with the community? For example, are there school groups that visit on holidays? Cultural activities from the community? An adopt-a-grandparent program? Are volunteer visitors encouraged?

♦ What are the rules on leaving the grounds? Are residents encouraged to spend time outdoors? Are there planned outings? How are residents monitored if they leave the building?

♦ What sort of transportation is available to residents?

♦ What provisions are there for religious worship? Are there services in-house? Can residents go to churches or synagogues in the community? Is transportation provided? Do clergy visit frequently?

♦ Can residents do paid or volunteer work?

♦ Do residents who are confined to their rooms because of illness or disability receive any kind of physical and social stimulation? Does someone help get them to activities?

Dementia

♦ Are there special units or services for people with dementia?

♦ Are these simply regular units that are locked so people can't wander off, or are they special units that truly offer an array of services and special arrangements suited to people with dementia?

♦ Are they kept separate from other residents?

♦ Is the area set up to allow for pacing and wandering?

♦ Are doors, hallways, bathrooms, kitchens, and hazards all clearly marked?

♦ Is the staff specially trained to deal with people with dementia? What does that training consist of?

♦ What is the staff-to-patient ratio? (It should be higher than in the rest of the nursing home, certainly.) What is that ratio at night?

How does the staff handle agitation? Incontinence? Inappropriate public behavior? Outbursts? Anxiety? Repetition? Does the staff sound well versed in these issues?

Are there activities, exercise classes, and outings planned regularly? Would any of these activities or classes interest your parent?

Are residents encouraged to remain independent? Are there opportunities for them to cook, fold laundry, clean their own rooms, set tables, and otherwise stay involved and feel useful? Likewise, are they encouraged and assisted in taking care of themselves—bathing, grooming, dressing, toileting—so they retain a sense of independence?

Do residents get outside for fresh air as often as they like?

Can they have pets?

If your parent moves into one of these units, how much extra will it cost? (Get this in writing.)

Costs

Is this nursing home fully certified to participate in Medicare and Medicaid? If only a wing or a certain number of beds are certified, what will happen if your parent goes on Medicaid while he is living in the facility? Is he guaranteed a bed, or might he be discharged?

What are the entry fees, monthly fees, and additional costs? Find out exactly what is included and what is extra, such as laundry, haircuts, special meals, outings, physical therapy, dental visits, lab work, medical equipment, and prescription drugs.

How long will your parent's bed be reserved in the event that she needs to be hospitalized or is temporarily absent for some other reason? What happens if she exceeds that limit? (This is particularly important if your parent is on Medicaid, as the facility's time limit may be quite short or it may not hold a bed at all. If your parent loses her place, the residence must give her the first Medicaid bed available, but you need to be persistent to make sure that she gets it.)

What has the increase in monthly fees been over the past three years? What sort of increases are expected in the coming years?

Can contracts be terminated? Under what conditions? What is the refund policy?

If a resident is discharged, how many days notice is given? Who receives such notice?

How stable is this residence financially? (Ask to see the most recent annual report and/or financial records. You may also want to ask the state's long-term care ombudsman about the financial stability of a particular nursing home.) What happens to your parent if the home becomes part of another facility or goes out of business?

Do residents maintain control over their personal finances?

APPENDIX G
A Nursing-Home Resident's Bill of Rights

To participate in Medicare or Medicaid, nursing homes must meet standards outlined in the Nursing Home Reform Law (the Omnibus Budget Reconciliation Act, 1987). Among the law's provisions:

Residents Have a Right to:

◆ be treated with dignity and respect

◆ exercise their rights, file complaints, or voice grievances without fear of discrimination, restraint, interference, coercion, or reprisal, and to expect prompt efforts for the resolution of grievances

◆ equal access to care and services without discrimination

◆ privacy concerning their personal and medical care, telephone calls, visits, letters, and meetings with family and resident groups

◆ inspect and purchase photocopies of their records

◆ confidentiality regarding their medical and personal records

◆ full information about their health, and the right to participate in decisions regarding their care and treatment

◆ refuse treatment and refuse to participate in experimental research

◆ information concerning Medicare and Medicaid benefits and how to apply

◆ information regarding all facility services and charges

◆ information regarding advocacy groups and ombudsman programs

◆ manage their own financial affairs; they are not required to deposit personal funds with the facility

◆ choose a personal physician

◆ self-administer drugs unless determined unsafe by an interdisciplinary team

◆ perform or refuse to perform services for the facility; payment for any work done must be at or above prevailing rates

◆ advance notice of any change in room or roommate

◆ share a room with a resident spouse

◆ choose their own activities, schedules, and health care and any other aspect affecting their lives within the facility

◆ organize or participate in resident councils or other groups

◆ be free from verbal, sexual, physical, or mental abuse, corporal punishment, and involuntary seclusion.

The Nursing Home Must:

◆ not require a third-party guarantee of payment or accept any gifts as a condition of admission or continued stay

◆ not require residents to waive their right to receive or apply for Medicare or Medicaid benefits

◆ provide a copy of the latest inspection report and any written plans to correct violations

◆ provide residents with individualized financial reports quarterly and upon request

◆ protect resident funds with a security bond

◆ notify residents when their balance comes within $200 of the Medicaid eligibility limit

◆ not charge Medicaid residents for items or services covered by Medicaid, including routine personal hygiene items and services

◆ not use physical restraints or psychoactive drugs for discipline or convenience; restraints must not be used without a doctor's written orders to treat medical symptoms or to ensure the safety of the resident and others

◆ provide access to any relevant agency of the state or any entity providing health, social, legal, or other services

◆ use identical policies regarding transfer, discharge, and services for all residents

◆ not discharge or transfer a resident unless his needs cannot be met, safety is endangered, services are no longer required, or payment has not been made

◆ notify a resident of reason(s) for transfer or discharge and provide sufficient preparation to ensure a safe transfer or discharge

◆ provide written notice of state and facility bed-hold policies before and at the time of a transfer

◆ follow a written policy for readmittance if the bed-hold period is exceeded

◆ thoroughly investigate all alleged violations and report the results

◆ provide a private space for residents' group meetings, and then listen to and act upon requests of the group

◆ provide social services to maintain each resident's highest level of well-being

◆ provide a safe, clean, comfortable, homelike environment

◆ allow residents to use personal belongings to the extent possible

◆ provide housekeeping and maintenance services; clean bath and bed linens; private closet space; adequate and comfortable lighting and sound levels; comfortable and safe temperature levels.

APPENDIX H
State Citizen Advocacy Groups for Nursing-Home Reform

Citizen advocacy groups deal primarily with policy issues, although most will help you find a good nursing home and advocate for your parent.

This list is reprinted with permission from the National Citizens' Coalition for Nursing Home Reform in Washington, D.C. For more information, the coalition can be reached at 202-332-2276 or www.nccnhr.org. (Not all states have citizens' coalitions. If you are interested in starting one, contact NCCNHR.)

ALASKA

CARING
2420 Chinook Ave.
Anchorage, AK 99516
907-345-0515

ARKANSAS

Arkansas Advocates for Nursing Home Residents
9901 Satterfield Dr.
Little Rock, AR 72205
501-225-4082

Arkansas Advocates for Nursing Home Residents
135 Hillview Dr.
Fairfield Bay, AR 72088
501-884-6728
www.aanhr.org

CALIFORNIA

Foundation Aiding the Elderly
P.O. Box 254849
Sacramento, CA 95865
916-481-8558

California Advocates for Nursing Home Reform
1610 Bush St.
San Francisco, CA 94109
415-474-5171
www.canhr.org

CONNECTICUT

Connecticut Citizens Coalition for Nursing Home Reform
80 Jefferson St.
Hartford, CT 06106
860-278-5688

Advocates for Loved Ones in Nursing Homes
224 Ledyard St.
New London, CT 06320
860-739-5859

DISTRICT OF COLUMBIA

Washingtonians for Improvement of Nursing Homes
4425 Nannie Helen Burrough Ave. NE
Washington, DC 20019
202-397-1120

FLORIDA

Fighting Elder Abuse Together (FEAT)
591 Jupiter Blvd. NW
Palm Bay, FL 32907
321-984-8883

Coalition to Protect America's Elders
8094 Buck Lake Rd.
Tallahassee, FL 32317
850-216-2727
www.protectelders.org

Advocates Committed to Improving Our Nursing Homes
4714 Euclid Ave.
Tampa, FL 33629
813-837-1714

Quality Care Advocates, Inc.
P.O. Box 494224
Port Charlotte, FL 33949
941-743-0987

GEORGIA

Georgia Council on Aging
2 Peachtree St. NW
Atlanta, GA 30303
404-657-5348
www.gcoa.org

ILLINOIS

Tender Loving Care in Long-Term Care
620 N. Walnut St.
Springfield, IL 62702
217-523-8488
www.tlcinltc.org

Nursing Home Monitors
6111 Vollmer Ln.
Godfrey, IL 62035
618-466-3410
www.nursinghome
monitors.org

Illinois Citizens for Better Care
220 S. State St. #800
Chicago, IL 60604
312-663-5120

INDIANA

United Senior Action
324 W. Morris St.
Suite 114
Indianapolis, IN 46225
317-634-0872

IOWA

Advocacy Network for Aging Iowans
4554 NW 114th St.
Urbandale, IA 50322
515-727-0667
www.agingiowans.org

Iowans for Nursing Home Reform
3707 SE 24th Ct.
Des Moines, IA 50320
515-288-9403

KANSAS

Kansas Advocates for Better Care
913 Tennessee St. #2
Lawrence, KS 66044
800-525-1782
www.kabc.org

LOUISIANA

Citizens Care
P.O. Box 56041
New Orleans, LA 70156
504-894-9607

MARYLAND

Voices for Quality Care (LTC)
P.O. Box 6555,
Waldorf, MD 20603
888-600-2375

MASSACHUSETTS

Massachusetts Advocates for Nursing Home Reform
P.O. Box 42
Hingham, MA 02043
781-598-1969
www.manhr.org

Cape United Elderly
P.O. Box 954
Hyannis, MA 02601
508-771-1727

MICHIGAN

Citizens for Better Care
4750 Woodward Ave.
Suite 410
Detroit, MI 48201
313-832-6387
http://cbcmi.org

Michigan Campaign for Quality Care
5886 Highgate Ave.
East Lansing, MI 48823
517-333-0221

ACTION! Coalition for Improvement of Nursing
P.O. Box 51463
Livonia, MI 48185
734-522-5424

MINNESOTA

Advocacy Center for Long-Term Care
2626 E. 82nd St.
Bloomington, MN 55425
952-854-7304
www.advocacycenter.net

MISSOURI

Missouri Coalition for Quality Care
P.O. Box 7165
Jefferson City, MO 65102
888-262-5644
www.mcqc.com

NEBRASKA

Nebraska Advocacy Services, Inc.
134 S. 13
Lincoln, NE 68508
402-474-3183

Nebraska Advocates for Nursing Home Residents
10050 Regency Circle
Omaha, NE 68114
402-397-3801

NEW MEXICO

New Mexicans for Quality Long Term Care
P.O. Box 1712
Belen, NM 87002
505-864-7534

NEW YORK

Coalition of Institutionalized Aged and Disabled
425 E. 25th St.
New York, NY 10010
212-481-7572
www.ciadny.org

FRIA
18 John St.
New York, NY 10038
212-732-4455
www.fria.org

Long Term Care Community Coalition
242 W. 30th St.
New York, NY 10001
212-385-0355
www.nhccnys.org

NORTH CAROLINA

Friends of Residents in Long Term Care
883-C Washington St.
Raleigh, NC 27605
919-782-1530
www.forltc.org

OHIO

Families for Improved Care, Inc.
3440 Olentangy River Rd.
Columbus, OH 43202
614-267-0777
www.familiesfor
improvedcare.org

OKLAHOMA

Oklahomans for Improvement of Nursing Care Homes
1423 Oakwood Dr.
Norman, OK 73070
405-364-5004
www.nhadvocates.org

PENNSYLVANIA

CARIE
100 N. 17th St.
Philadelphia, PA 19103
215-545-5728
www.carie.org

RHODE ISLAND

Alliance for Better Long Term Care
422 Post Rd.
Warwick, RI 02888
401-785-3340
www.bulletinboards.
com/view (use the
password: abltc)

TENNESSEE

East Tennessee Coalition on Advocacy, Inc.
9111 Cross Park Dr.
Knoxville, TN 37923
865-691-2551

East Tennessee Coalition on Advocacy, Inc.
701 Chateaugay Rd.
Knoxville, TN 37923
865-531-4638

TEXAS

United People for Better Nursing Home Care
P.O. Box 13124
Arlington, TX 76094
817-265-1234

Texas Advocates for Nursing Home Residents

P.O. Box 3653
Wichita Falls, TX 76301
940-723-7431
www.tanhr.org

**Texas Advocates
for Nursing Home
Residents**
1015 Wavecrest Dr.
Houston, TX 77062
281-488-5291
www.tanhr.org

**United Senior
Advocates**
9406 Cathedral
Houston, TX 77051
713-734-4594

**Texans for
The Improvement
of Long Term Care**
4545 Cook Rd. #303
Houston, TX 77072
281-933-4533

**Texas Advocates
for Nursing Home
Residents**
500 E. Anderson Ln.
Austin, TX 78752
512-719-4757
www.tanhr.org

**Texas Advocates
for Nursing Home
Residents**
P.O. Box 68
DeSoto, TX 75123
972-572-6330
www.tanhr.org

**Advocates for Nursing
Home Reform**
16908 S. Ridge Ln.
Austin, TX 78734
512-266-0056

**Garland/Richardson
Association of
Family Co.**
3705 Oakridge Circle
Garland, TX 75040
972-495-9022

**Texas Advocates
for Nursing Home
Residents**
9727 Ballin David Dr.
Spring, TX 77379
281-701-2904

VIRGINIA

**Citizens Committee
to Protect the Elderly**
407 Oakmears Crescent
Virginia Beach, VA
23462
757-518-8500
www.citizenscommittee.
org

**Virginia Friends &
Relatives of NH
Residents**
1426 Claremont Ave.
Richmond, VA 23227
804-644-2804

TLC for Long Term Care
P.O. Box 523323
Springfield, VA 22152
703-569-1746
www.tlc4ltc.org

**Citizens' Committee
to Protect the Elderly**
P.O. Box 3
Virginia Beach, VA 23458
757-518-8500

**Friends & Relatives
of Nursing Home
Residents**

110 Sun Beau Ct.
New Market, VA 22844
540-740-4121

WASHINGTON

**Family Advocates for
NH Improvement**
10955 W. Villa Monte Dr.
Mukilteo, WA 98275
888-647-3367

**Citizens for the
Improvement of
Nursing Homes**
4649 Sunnyside N.
Seattle, WA 98103 6900
206-545-7053

**Resident Councils
of Washington**
220 E. Canyon View Rd.
Belfair, WA 98528
360 275 8000
www.residentcouncil.org

WISCONSIN

**Citizen Advocates for
Nursing Home
Residents**
P.O. Box 188
Slinger, WI 53086-0188
414-783-7161

WYOMING

**Concerned Citizens
for Quality Nursing
Home Care**
240 S. Wolcott St.
Casper, WY 82601
307-266-6659

APPENDIX I
Dietary Details for the Elderly

Here are the nuts and bolts—or nuts and grains, if you will—of a good diet. For more information on nutrition and diet, see page 73.

Dietary Components

PROTEIN

WHILE MOST PEOPLE GET PLENTY OF protein, the elderly often have lower levels of protein in their bodies than their more youthful counterparts because they don't make as much of it as they used to.

Proteins are lengthy molecular strings of tiny amino acids. They make up many hormones, form cell walls, and serve as the major structural basis of many body tissues—skin, hair, muscles, and tendons. To repair or grow new cell walls, the body needs ample protein.

Most of the twenty amino acids that the body needs to make proteins are manufactured internally, but at least nine of them—the "essential amino acids"—must come from outside sources. The most complete sources of protein are meat, chicken, fish, dairy, and eggs. But rice, peanuts, kidney beans, peas, and tofu are all rich in protein too.

FIBER

ANYONE WHO'S HEARD OF CONSTI-pation has heard of fiber, and most older people know constipation all too intimately. Fiber keeps things moving, through the body and out. It is helpful in preventing and treating constipation, diverticular disease, and irritable bowel syndrome. It helps lower blood cholesterol and stabilizes blood sugar levels. And it seems to lower the risk of certain cancer and cardiovascular disease. A miracle food.

Fiber is the indigestible part of plants. It is found in roughage—fruits, vegetables, and grains. Bran, which is the outer coating of whole wheat, corn, and oats, is high in fiber, with wheat bran having the highest fiber content. In the intestines, fiber acts like a sponge, soaking up liquids (but your parent has to drink those fluids so there is something to soak up) and making the bowel contents softer and, thus, easier to move. Most adults should eat about 20 to 35 grams of fiber each day, so get out the prunes!

Take it slow. Your parent should not suddenly start pouring bran on his food to reach his daily requirement or to treat a case of constipation. A sudden and **unusually** large dose will tie his stomach in knots and give him gas. Instead, he should start slowly, adding a little more to his diet each day and drinking plenty of water to help the fiber do its job. Your parent should also try several sources of fiber, such as vegetables, fruits, whole-grain bread, cereal, and pasta, rather than gulping down a bowl of high-fiber cereal every morning and calling it quits. High-fiber cereals are helpful, but if overused they can interfere with the absorption of important trace minerals. Also, it is best to get fiber from foods, rather than from pills.

Look at the label on various foods to find out exactly how much fiber they contain. (Convenience foods, which are popular among the elderly, are almost always fiberless.)

FLUIDS

DRINKING WATER SEEMS ALMOST like a waste of time—no calories, no vitamins, no nutrients. But the human body is about 70 percent water, and it's important to keep it that way. Fluids keep the volume of blood high, keep the digestive track running smoothly, and help the kidneys work effectively. A lack of fluids can lead to dehydration, constipation, confusion, and dry skin, mouth, and eyes.

Drinking adequate fluids can be a challenge at any age, but for the elderly it is more of one because with age, people lose their sense of thirst. They don't feel thirsty, so they don't drink. Furthermore, some medications increase the need for fluids.

Food	Amount	Grams of Fiber
Dried apricots	100 grams	24
All-Bran or 100% Bran cereal	1 cup	23
Prunes	100 grams	16
Green peas, cooked	½ cup	7.7
Grape-Nuts cereal	⅓ cup	5
Corn	⅔ cup	4.2
Lentils (cooked)	½ cup	4
Carrots (raw)	1 medium	3.7
Potatoes, cooked	⅔ cup	3.1
Apple	1 small	3.1
Grapefruit	½	2.6
Strawberries	½ cup	2.1
Broccoli, cooked	¾ cup	1.6
Grapes	16	0.4
Rice, white, cooked	1 cup	0.4

Many elderly people also forgo fluids because going to the bathroom can be a tiresome trip. If your parent is incontinent, he may become obsessed with avoiding liquids. But drying the body out is not the way to treat incontinence and usually just makes it worse.

Your parent shouldn't wait until she feels thirsty to drink; she should make an effort to drink at regular intervals or simply sip at something throughout the day. She'll know if she's getting enough fluids because her urine will be pale yellow, rather than dark yellow.

Water is so cheap, so available, and, with a few ice cubes and a squeeze of lemon, so good. A bit of juice mixed with seltzer makes a wonderful treat. Your parent should always have a glass of something close at hand. If she sucks on hard candies all day because her mouth is dry or has a bad taste, or if she worries about bad breath, get her to sip on a glass of minty water instead. (If you're worried about the purity of tap water, call the EPA's Safe Drinking Water Hotline, 800-426-4791.)

Limit caffeine, which acts as a diuretic (expelling liquids from the body) and also buzzes the central nervous system, speeding up the heart rate and making a person jittery. Sorry, but alcohol does *not* count as a serving of fluids. Also, be cautious about herbal teas, especially odd, uncommon brews. Most are fine, but some are medicinal and may not mix well with the drugs your parent takes.

CARBOHYDRATES

CARBOHYDRATES ARE THE SUGARS and starches that fuel the body, not just for running around the track but for processing and operating even when you are just lying on the couch. Carbohydrates come from cereals, fruits, potatoes, rice, pasta, bread, corn, and dried beans and peas. Sugar and white flour also have lots of carbohydrates, but cakes and cookies should be limited for the most part, as they are full of fat and lack any real nutritional value.

CALCIUM

IF YOU ARE FEMALE AND DOING A little aging yourself, you might join your parent in some high-calcium meal planning. Calcium makes bones strong, which is important for all elderly people, but particularly for women, whose bones tend to atrophy after menopause. Weakened bones, known as osteoporosis, often leads to fractured bones, which in an elderly person is extremely serious. (See page 255 for more on osteoporosis.)

The recommended dose of calcium for an elderly person is 1,200 milligrams

Food	Serving Size	Milligrams of Calcium
Plain yogurt	1 cup	400
Sardines (with bones)	3 ounces	370
Collards	1 cup	360
Milk	1 cup	300
Hard cheese	1 ounce	150–200
Cottage cheese	1 cup	140
Broccoli, raw	1 cup	130

a day, and yet most get less than 600 milligrams of calcium a day in their diet. Your parent should consider taking calcium supplements. Calcium citrate seems to cause fewer side effects.

Be sure your parent also gets ample vitamin D—at least 600 I.U. (international units) a day. Vitamin D, which enables the body to absorb calcium, is made by the body in response to direct sunlight and is found in certain foods. (Too much vitamin D—more than 2,000 I.U. a day—can harm the liver and might even lower bone mass.)

The best source of calcium is low-fat or nonfat dairy products, but the mineral is also in dark green, leafy vegetables, such as broccoli, collard greens, mustard greens, and kale. It is also in tofu, salmon, and sardines (with the bones), oysters, dried beans and peas, and citrus fruits. Some brands of orange juice and bread are now fortified with calcium.

VITAMINS

VITAMINS HELP ALL THE SYSTEMS OF the body run efficiently, but all bodies do not need vitamins equally. Elderly people have different dietary needs than their younger counterparts, in part because of changes in weight, activity, and the body's ability to absorb vitamins. While the research is still scant, scientists now know that older people are often lacking in a number of essential vitamins, particularly folate and vitamins B-6, B-12, D, and E.

Vitamins come in two types, fat-soluble and water-soluble. Fat-soluble ones (A, D, E, and K) are stored in fat, where they can be retrieved for use at a later time, so people don't need them daily; they can eat them on Monday and use them up on Wednesday. Water-soluble ones (C and the B vitamins) can't be stored in the body and should be consumed daily.

SODIUM

SODIUM HELPS TO REGULATE THE body's water level and keeps the heart in rhythm and the nerves conducting. While some people have low sodium levels, the vast majority get far more than they need in the form of simple table salt.

Even if your parent doesn't sprinkle it on vigorously at home, there are inordinate amounts of sodium in most prepared and processed foods, frozen dinners, deli cheese, cured meats, and snack foods. Many sauces and broths are also high in salt, as are soy sauce, ketchup, mustard, olives, and pickles.

Too much sodium leads to high blood pressure, heart disease, stroke, kidney damage, and fluid retention. Plus, lowering one's sodium intake might slow the loss of calcium from the bones.

So lead your parent away from processed foods and hide the salt shaker. To liven up food, add herbs, spices, or lemon. If he must have prepared foods, check the labels. Frozen entrees usually have less sodium, and some of the others are labeled "low-sodium."

Vitamin	Daily RDA* (for adults over 50)	Foods That Provide It
Vitamin A/Beta carotene Foods that are rich in beta carotene, an antioxidant the body converts into vitamin A, are thought to lower the risk of cancer and heart disease. However, too much vitamin A appears to increase the risk of fractures, so check with the doctor before taking a supplement with vitamin A.	5 to 6 milligrams of beta carotene (800 to 1,000 retinol equivalents of vitamin A)	Cantaloupe, apricots, carrots, squash, sweet potatoes, tomatoes, broccoli, spinach and dark green vegetables, liver, cheese, egg yolks, fortified milk
Vitamin B-6 B-6 strengthens the immune system.	1.6 to 2 milligrams	Whole-grain breads and cereals, beans, nuts, chicken, avocado, liver, legumes, potatoes, bananas, spinach, fish
Vitamin B-12 Older people often have atrophic gastritis, which hinders absorption of B-12 and, as a result, can cause confusion. Vitamin B-12 is need to keep blood and nerves healthy.	2.4 micrograms	Liver, kidney, beef, eggs, cheese, milk, and shellfish (Because older people often have trouble absorbing B-12 from animal sources, they should try fortified breakfast cereals or take supplements of the vitamin.)
Folate, or folic acid A deficiency causes depression and fatigue, and may increase the risk of stroke, heart disease, and some cancers.	180 to 200 micrograms	Dried peas and beans, oranges, whole grains, liver, kidneys, nuts, wheat germ, and dark green, leafy vegetables
Vitamin C Vitamin C may lower the risk of heart disease and cancer, but too much can block absorption of B-12.	60 milligrams	Citrus fruits, strawberries, tomatoes, cantaloupe, potatoes, broccoli, brussel sprouts, cabbage, spinach, and other dark green vegetables
Vitamin D Vitamin D helps the body to absorb calcium, which strengthens bones. It is made in the skin after exposure to sunlight. Older people, particular those who are homebound or live in nursing homes, do not produce as much vitamin D.	600 I.U. (international units)	Fortified milk, egg yolks, liver, and oily fish (such as salmon, sardines, herring, and tuna) Twenty minutes of direct sunlight, without sun lotion
Vitamin E Vitamin E may lower the risk of cataracts, help prevent heart disease, and slow progression of Alzheimer's disease. Deficiency can lead to anemia.	8 to 10 I.U.	Vegetable oils, dark green, leafy vegetables, wheat germ, and nuts

Recommended Dietary Allowances from the National Academy of Sciences

IRON

TOO LITTLE IRON SHOULDN'T BE A problem unless your parent has an ulcer, hemorrhoid, or some other condition that causes bleeding, or is taking large doses of antacids, which hinder the body's absorption of iron. Your parent may also be iron deficient if she is what dietitians refer to as a "tea-and-toaster"—an elderly lady who sits around sipping tea and nibbling on toast. The bread may be fortified with iron, but ingredients in the tea combine with the iron to form another substance that is excreted by the body, and in the process iron is lost.

Too much iron can contribute to heart attacks in some cases, so your parent shouldn't take extra doses of iron without her doctor's orders.

FAT AND CHOLESTEROL

FAT, THAT ALMOST FOUR-LETTER word, is actually a necessary part of every diet. It is used by the body to supply energy and maintain cell structure, and it helps the body absorb certain vitamins. It also makes food more appealing and helps it slide down the throat more easily, which is particularly important for elderly people who have trouble swallowing.

Unfortunately, because it tastes so good, most people get more than enough fat without trying, and could stand to eat a whole lot less of the stuff. Too much fat increases the risk of heart disease, diabetes, and some cancers. While the risk is greatest for younger people, elderly people, especially those suffering from high cholesterol levels or obesity, should be concerned as well. Because they tend to be sedentary, elderly people do not burn off fat easily.

Fat, which is made primarily of something known as fatty acids, is saturated or unsaturated depending upon the number of hydrogen atoms attached to the fat molecules. Saturated fat raises blood cholesterol levels, and should be kept to a bare minimum. It comes primarily from animals. That is, saturated fat is found in meat, especially fatty meat and poultry skin, and high-fat dairy products (cheese, whole milk, cream, butter). It is also found in the oils of tropical plants, such as coconuts and palms.

Unsaturated fats, which include monounsaturated and polyunsaturated fats, do not raise cholesterol levels. In limited amounts, they are part of a good diet. These fats come from peanut, olive, canola, sunflower, and corn oils, as well as olives and many kinds of nuts. Some fish, such as salmon, tuna, and mackerel, contain something known as omega-3 fatty acids, which appear to be good for the heart.

The easiest rule, which applies in most cases, is that if something is solid at room temperature (butter, lard, animal fat, and milk products) it should be avoided or consumed sparingly.

That infamous fatty substance, cholesterol, should be kept to a minimum, especially if your parent has heart disease. It can clog arteries and cause heart disease or stroke.

Cholesterol is made in the liver from saturated fats, or absorbed directly from foods such as liver and other organ meats, egg yolks, and high-fat dairy products. Cholesterol roams the body wrapped in a package called a lipoprotein. High-density lipoproteins (HDLs) are "good" in that they actually transport cholesterol out of the body and reduce the risk of heart disease. Low-density lipoproteins (LDLs), or very low-density lipoproteins (VLDLs), are "bad" because they tend to be slovenly and sit around on cell walls, narrowing the passageways. (Warning: A product can have "no cholesterol," but still be loaded with saturated fats and, therefore, raise cholesterol levels in the body.)

While it's always good to have a low-fat, low-cholesterol diet, there is evidence that people over seventy who have no signs of heart disease probably either have low cholesterol or are genetically protected in some way from the effects of high cholesterol. If your parent has been working at keeping his cholesterol down with diet, exercise, and medication, he should keep up his efforts, as they may be keeping him alive. But if he has no symptoms of heart disease, he might not need to start aggressive efforts to lower it now. In fact, for some elderly people, the benefit of protein from eggs, cheese, and other high-cholesterol foods might outweigh any adverse effects of high cholesterol. Have your parent talk to his doctor.

(Another warning: Foods are often advertised as "low-fat," but know that this does not mean low-calorie or not fattening. There might not be as much fat in a low-fat muffin as a regular one, but there is still fat in it, and there might be extra sugar added, making it heavily caloric.)

What to Eat

Eating at your parent's age basically means eating the same good foods we should all be eating, but smaller amounts of them, and further restricted amounts of fat. This does not have to be boring; healthy food can be delicious. Honestly. Here is a list of what a good day's diet includes, adjusted from the usual food pyramid to meet the needs of elderly people.

NOTE: A "serving" is not whatever amount you dump on a plate; in fact, it is a pretty small portion of food. Check labels to see how much of a food makes up a serving. Sometimes packages sold as single servings are actually two or more servings (but it will say this on the nutrition label).

Also, be careful not to confuse cooked and uncooked serving sizes, as the amounts are different. Four ounces of raw meat, for example, is only about three ounces once it is cooked. People who are less active should eat the smallest number of servings suggested for each food group, and those who are active can eat additional servings. Most elderly people should be staying to the lower number.

THE SIX FOOD GROUPS

Food Group	Sample Servings	Notes
Fluids (8 servings a day)	8 ounces (1 glass) of water, juice, milk, broth	Fluids are so important, especially for the elderly, who often lose their sense of thirst.
Bread, pasta, rice, grains (6-9 servings a day)	1 slice bread or a roll ½ cup cooked pasta or rice 1 ounce dry cereal ½ cup cooked cereal, like oatmeal	Choose whole-grain foods—whole-grain bread, brown rice, oatmeal, popcorn, whole-wheat crackers, whole-wheat pasta, whole barley, tabouli salad. Skip doughnuts, croissants, sugary cereal, muffins, and other desserts masquerading as breakfasts. Try something new, like couscous, polenta, bulgur, and other grains.
Vegetables (3 or more servings a day)	½ cup carrots, sweet potato, squash or cooked spinach 1 cup lettuce	Fresh is best. Frozen is fine. But limit canned foods, which are often high in sodium and sugar. Do not overcook or soak vegetables. Dark green, red, orange, or yellow vegetables (spinach, green-leaf lettuce, sweet potatoes, squash) have the most nutrients.
Fruit (2 or more servings a day)	½ grapefruit or melon 1 orange or banana ¼ cup dried apricots, prunes, or raisins ¾ cup orange juice	Again, choose fresh over frozen, and limit canned in syrup. Whole fruits are better than juices, which contain little or no fiber. Fruits with deep colors (strawberries, mangoes, peaches) have the most nutrients.
Dairy (3 or more servings a day)	8 ounces (1 cup) milk 2 cups cottage cheese 1½ ounce hard cheese (about a one-inch cube) 1 cup plain yogurt	Use nonfat or low-fat products. Ice cream and cheesecake are not substitutes for the dairy category. A number of substitutes are available for people who are lactose intolerant.
Meat and beans (2 or more servings a day)	1½ cups cooked dried beans, peas, or lentils 2 to 3 ounces of fish, poultry, or lean meat ⅔ cup nuts 2 eggs	Choose beans, peas, and lean meats. Limit bacon, salami, bologna, and other fatty meats, as well as organ meats, such as liver and kidneys. Use tuna canned in water, not oil. Remove skin from poultry. Skip yolks, if possible.

APPENDIX J
Funeral Choices and Costs

Money may seem like a crass subject at a time like this, but you should consider the bottom line. You can spend an exorbitant amount of money now, given your frame of mind and with so little time to think.

While a simple cremation should not cost more than $1,000, more elaborate funerals typically run around $6,000 and up. Once flowers, limousines, meals, booze, and other extras are added on, it can easily exceed $10,000. Indeed, the casket alone can run well over $10,000. Add a service and a reception that includes a full meal and you can spend over $30,000.

The main problem is not the caterer or the flowers, which might be important to you; the main problem is that funeral directors often take advantage of mourning families by overcharging, adding on unnecessary services, and convincing them to pay for services that they really don't need or want.

Compare prices and negotiate. There is absolutely nothing wrong with getting the best price possible. In fact, if your parent was at all frugal, he would want you to shop around. Do it in his spirit. Bring someone with you who can be impartial and is less emotionally invested; he or she can do the negotiating.

Funeral homes are required, under the Funeral Rule of the Federal Trade Commission, to give you prices and even to quote them over the phone. Or you can have them sent to you. Cemeteries are not bound by the same rules, but most will quote prices.

The Funeral Rule also requires full disclosure of all prices and gives consumers the right to buy individual goods and services, rather than "packages" that might include services you don't want.

The funeral home must also give you an itemized list of the total cost of the funeral, although the director may have to provide a "good faith estimate" for any services not directly provided (reception, clergy, flowers, etc.).

The following list will give you some idea of the services and goods that you might need. Prices range depending upon where you live, what you opt for, and who's running the show.

◆ **Funeral director's services.** This fixed charge is not optional if you use a funeral director. It covers overhead and the funeral director's time. It can run from a few hundred dollars (which is what it should be) to several thousand dollars.

◆ **Care of the body.** A funeral home must seek permission before embalming a body and, unless it is required for some reason, you do not have to pay for the service if you did not authorize it.

Dressing the body and putting it in the casket is usually, but not always, included in the price of embalming, but find out what is covered. You may be charged extra for having hair and makeup done and restoring a body that is damaged by autopsy or disease.

Embalming usually costs between $200 and $500, while other work on the body can cost $50 on up.

♦ **Transportation.** The transportation price quoted may cover only the price of getting the body to the funeral home; most funeral homes charge an additional fee for transporting the body to the church, gravesite, or crematorium, and for other transportation, such as picking up the death certificate or burial permit. You will also have to pay extra for services such as a hearse, a limousine for the family, a flower car, or a motorcycle escort for the funeral procession.

Simply having a local funeral home pick up a body from the house shouldn't cost more than about $100. A hearse might cost closer to $200, and a limousine, about $150 or $200.

♦ **Services.** You can hold services in a private home, church, synagogue, or rented hall, or you may be able to hold them at the funeral home or in a public, outdoor space. Be sure that any price quoted includes everything, because funeral homes may suddenly charge additional fees for the use of

FUNERAL CONSUMER GROUPS

Nonprofit funeral and memorial societies exist in nearly every state. They are run by volunteers. Many have contracts with funeral homes that offer low-cost funerals or discounts to society members. All offer reassuring guidance and information, and most have price lists from local funeral homes and examples of package deals. They can also tell you how to plan a funeral on your own, how to arrange a low-cost funeral using a funeral director, what state laws require, and what to do when there's trouble. To find a local group, contact the Funeral Consumers Alliance (800-765-0107 or www.funerals.org).

lounges, parking lots, offices, dressing rooms, and chairs.

Again, prices vary widely, but a viewing, funeral service, memorial, or graveside service shouldn't cost much more than $500.

♦ **Miscellaneous items.** The funeral director will usually require a cash advance to pay for anything he has to buy from a third party on your behalf, such as organists, pallbearers, death notices, obituaries, and copies of the death certificate. You can also order acknowledgment cards through the funeral home.

◆ **Receptions, flowers, food.** You can spend as much or as little as you want to on flowers, guest books, music, food and alcohol. Once you rent a hall and offer full meals and open bar, it'll cost over $50 per guest.

◆ **Caskets.** Walking through rows of caskets is unsettling and impersonal, to say the least. If you decide what you want and how much you want to spend in advance, it will expedite the process. If it's too unpleasant a task, do it over the phone, over the Internet, or ask a friend or relative to do it for you.

Caskets come in wood, metal, fiberglass, or plastic. The wooden ones may be hardwood (mahogany, walnut, cherry, oak), softwood (pine), or plywood; they may be solid wood or veneer. The metals include stainless or rolled steel, or copper bronzes of varying thicknesses (the lower the "gauge," the thicker the steel). They may be lined with cloth: twill, crepe, velour, or velvet (although you can use your favorite cloth, quilt, or comforter). Some have mattresses in them, and you can opt for a spring contraption that raises and lowers the body for viewing.

You will also have to decide if you want the casket to be sealed, which is usually done with a rubber gasket, to prevent water from leaking in and rust from forming. As with embalming, sealing a casket—no matter how tight

or with what materials—does not prevent the body from decaying. Some unscrupulous funeral directors will talk about preserving the body in order to sell more expensive caskets, but their claims simply are not true.

Prices vary widely. At the lower end, a cardboard casket sells for under $20, and a pine box might be $200 (a do-it-yourself pine box kit is under $20).

Funeral directors have learned that most consumers buy one of the first three models they see, usually the middle-priced model of the three. And so, ingenious salesmen that they are, they usually show people three higher priced models right away. Lower priced models may not even be on display at all. Or they are hidden in a corner, covered with dust.

Before showing you any actual caskets, funeral directors must, by law, show you a list of caskets with descriptions and prices. Look at this carefully. Ask if there are lower priced models not on the list (which there often are). And then select three or four to look at, rather than marching dutifully behind and letting the funeral director lead the way.

It's up to you. Buy only what you want. Your love for your parent is not measured by the amount of mahogany, silver, satin, or velvet you sink into the ground. If you want a simple, inexpensive casket, ask for it.

Don't be afraid or embarrassed to negotiate over the price of caskets. Most funeral homes jack up their prices substantially, but faced with the prospect of losing a customer, they will usually come down. Negotiating may be more than you can handle now, but if you want to or want someone else to do it for you, you should know that people do it all the time and that it is perfectly acceptable, even in a time of mourning.

You can buy a casket elsewhere, which is usually much cheaper than buying it from the funeral director. Funeral directors are not allowed to charge any "nondeclinable fees" beyond the director's fee, which means they cannot charge for "casket handling" if you buy a casket elsewhere.

Numerous companies now sell caskets over the Internet. Scanning through Web sites in the privacy of your own home may be much easier than walking through a funeral home's showroom. You can buy one and have it shipped directly to the funeral home, and you won't be charged a fee. Or, you can scan Web sites just to get an idea of options and prices before heading to the funeral home's showroom.

Finally, more and more people are discovering that they can make their own caskets, or have a simple one made by a local carpenter and then decorate it as they please, to make it more personal.

◆ **Vaults and liners.** Some cemeteries require that you buy a grave liner or vault to prevent the ground from sinking as the casket deteriorates. You can buy these from the funeral director, the cemetery, or a third party.

A liner is a simple concrete box that costs several hundred dollars.

Sealing or lining the concrete with asphalt adds several hundred dollars to the price. A vault of ungalvanized steel costs almost twice as much as concrete, and a vault of galvanized steel triples the price.

The funeral director may advise you to choose a steel vault in order to preserve the body. Again, nothing prevents a body from decomposing; this is simply a way of jacking up the price. Also, if the funeral director tells you that the cemetery requires the heavier vault, check for yourself.

◆ **Cremation.** A cremation should be relatively inexpensive. You do not need a casket or embalming, unless you have a viewing. Funeral homes may charge you $100 to $200 for a simple box (although, as we've noted, you can buy one elsewhere for less than $20). If you are being charged too much and you have the energy, call the crematorium directly and ask about prices.

The ashes ("cremains") will be returned to you in a cardboard box unless you select an urn, which can cost anywhere from $100 to $1,000. You can get quite carried away here, if you want to. As people began opting for cremation, funeral directors had to find a way to keep making money. And so, you can buy solid bronze urns or custom-designed urns shaped like cowboy boots, golf club bags, hunting trophies, you name it. You can buy clusters of urns so that each family member can have their own handful of ashes, or cremation jewelry, in case you want to carry a

DO-IT-YOURSELF FUNERAL

You can do as much or as little of this as you want. Some people find it therapeutic and meaningful, not to mention a lot less expensive, to plan the funeral, build the casket, and bury the body themselves. This home style of dealing with death is an age-old tradition, and it is just as natural, difficult, and rewarding as allowing someone to die at home.

Most states allow you to arrange the funeral and burial or cremation without a funeral director, as long as you comply with public health codes.

Home burials are described in the book *Caring for Your Own Dead* by Lisa Carlson or you can get information from the Funeral Consumers Alliance.

sprinkle around in a locket. You can even pay to put the ashes in a mausoleum vault built especially for urns.

◆ **Immediate burial and direct cremation.** Many funeral homes offer package deals that are usually simple and inexpensive. The body is buried in the ground or cremated immediately after death, and there is no viewing or embalming. You can then hold a memorial service, with all the fixings you choose, at a later date.

Prices include the funeral director's fees, transportation of the body, care of the body, and a simple container or casket. They usually do not include the cost of any cash advance items, such as medical examiner's fees or death certificates. Funeral homes offer wide variations on these themes, so be sure you understand exactly what is included in the plan you select. Neither of these options should cost much more than $1,000.

◆ **Cemeteries.** The price of cemetery plots and services depends largely upon the cost of land and labor in the area. Visit several and be sure that you will get the plot or crypt shown to you. (And don't be talked into a larger family plot, a common selling tactic, if you don't want one.)

In addition to the cost of a plot or space in a mausoleum, you may have to buy a vault or liner. You might also be charged a few hundred dollars for "perpetual care." This money is usually put in a permanent trust to pay for the upkeep of the grounds. Some cemeteries charge for opening and closing the grave (several hundred dollars) and for installing the gravestone or marker (again, several hundred dollars).

You will have to pay for any gravestone, bench, or marker you choose. You can also pay extra to have the grave decorated on holidays, or to have a slot for a vase installed by the grave. You may also be charged extra for burials on weekends or during the evening.

INDEX

B

D

N

O

P

NOTES

NOTES

WE WELCOME YOUR VIEWS

HOW TO CARE FOR AGING PARENTS tries to address the wide range of concerns and questions that caregivers face, in as much detail as possible. But there is always room for improvement. Please let us know your thoughts on the book—advice that was helpful, questions that weren't addressed, facts we might have missed—so that we can make adjustments and include your views in any future editions. We look forward to hearing from you.

Write to:

> *How to Care for Aging Parents*
> c/o Workman Publishing Company
> 708 Broadway
> New York, New York 10003-9555

To contact the author, order books, or find helpful Internet addresses, visit our Web site: http://www.careforagingparents.com